# The Essential Physics of Medical Imaging Study Guide

**JERROLD T. BUSHBERG, PhD**

*Clinical Professor of Radiology and Radiation Oncology*
*University of California, Davis*
*Sacramento, California*

**J. ANTHONY SEIBERT, PhD**

*Professor of Radiology*
*University of California, Davis*
*Sacramento, California*

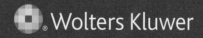
Wolters Kluwer

Philadelphia • Baltimore • New York • London
Buenos Aires • Hong Kong • Sydney • Tokyo

*Acquisitions Editor:* Nicole Dernoski
*Product Development Editor:* Eric McDermott
*Editorial Coordinator:* Varshaanaa SM
*Production Project Manager:* Barton Dudlick
*Senior Manufacturing Manager:* Beth Welsh
*Marketing Manager:* Kirsten Watrud
*Manager, Graphic Art and Design:* Stephen Druding
*Prepress Vendor:* Straive

9 8 7 6 5 4 3 2 1

Printed in Mexico

**Cataloging in Publication data available on request from publisher**

**ISBN: 978-1-9751-0326-2**

shop.lww.com

We are dedicating the first edition of the *The Essential Physics of Medical Imaging Study Guide* to the faculty and residents (past, present, and future) of the Department of Radiology at the University of California, School of Medicine, and UC Davis Health. Their contributions to our profession and encouragement over the years to continue to develop teaching material in medical physics, radiation protection, and radiation biology are deeply appreciated.

**J.T.B.** AND **J.A.S.**

# Authors

## Jerrold T. Bushberg, PhD

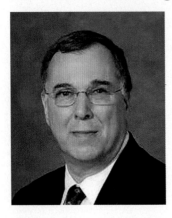

Jerrold T. Bushberg is a clinical professor of Radiology and Radiation Oncology at the University of California (UC), Davis, School of Medicine. He served as associate chair of Radiology (Radiation Biology & Medical Health Physics) until 2018 and was awarded Emeritus status by the UC Davis Chancellor as Director of Medical/Health Programs at that time. Dr. Bushberg is chair of the Board of Directors and senior vice president of the United States National Council on Radiation Protection and Measurements. He is an expert on the biological effects, safety, and interactions of ionizing and nonionizing radiation and holds multiple radiation detection technology patents. With over 35 years of experience, he has served as a subject matter expert and an adviser to government agencies and institutions throughout the nation and around the world including the U.S. Department of Homeland Security; the U.S. EPA's Radiation Protection Division; the National Academy of Sciences; the FDA's Center for Devices and Radiological Health; the World Health Organization's Radiation Program, Geneva; and the International Atomic Energy Agency, Austria, in the areas of ionizing and nonionizing radiation protection, risk communication, medical physics, and radiological emergency medical management. A former Commander in the U.S. Naval Reserve, among other assignments, CDR Bushberg served as Executive Officer of CBNR120 Pacific, a highly skilled multidisciplinary military emergency response and advisory team. Dr. Bushberg is an elected fellow of the American Association of Physicists in Medicine and the Health Physics Society. He has published numerous journal articles, book chapters, as well as other enduring academic material outside the domain of medical physics covering such diverse topics as emergency medical response to radiological terrorism and electromagnetic interference of wireless telecommunications systems with cardiac pacemakers. Dr. Bushberg is certified by several national professional boards with specific subspecialty certification in radiation protection and medical physics and currently serves as a director of the American Board of Medical Physics and served as its vice-chair from 2015 to 2018. Dr. Bushberg has received numerous honors and awards including NCRP's Warren K. Sinclair Medal for Excellence in Radiation Science in 2014 and the Christiansen Distinguished Alumnus award from the School of Health Sciences at Purdue University in 2016. Before joining the faculty at UC Davis as technical director of Nuclear Medicine, Dr. Bushberg was on the faculty of Yale University School of Medicine in the Department of Radiology where his research was focused on radiopharmaceutical development. Dr. Bushberg has responsibility for medical postgraduate education in medical physics as well as ionizing and nonionizing radiation biology and radiation protection.

## J. Anthony Seibert, PhD

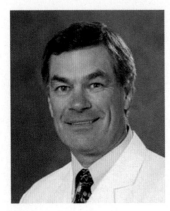

J. Anthony Seibert is a professor of diagnostic imaging physics at the University of California (UC) Davis Health in Sacramento, California. Dr. Seibert leads initiatives in x-ray fluorography, CT, digital mammography, projection imaging, interventional radiology, imaging informatics, and the tracking/assessment of radiation dose through automated registries.

Dr. Seibert received his PhD in radiological sciences from UC Irvine in 1983, with a focus on quantitative digital fluoroscopic imaging. He has served on the faculty of UC Davis since January 1983, conducting research in digital imaging and directing education in medical physics for graduate students and radiology residents.

Dr. Seibert is a voice for medical physicists, advancing opportunities for collaboration and quality improvement among specialties. An experienced leader Dr. Seibert has served as chair of the Society for Imaging Informatics in Medicine

(SIIM) (2004–2006), third vice president of the Radiological Society of North America (RSNA) (2009), president and chair of the American Association of Physicists in Medicine (AAPM) (2010–2012), and chair of the board of trustees of the American Board of Imaging Informatics (2012–2013). He has been active with the American Board of Radiology (ABR) since 1995, volunteering on several Diagnostic Medical Physics Committees and as chair for the Part I and Part 2 exam committees. Dr. Seibert was elected to the ABR as a Trustee for Medical Physics in 2013, and in 2017, he moved to the ABR Board of Governors.

Dr. Seibert leads educational symposiums for the AAPM, the International Atomic Energy Agency, and the National Council on Radiation Protection and Measurements, where he also serves as a council member. He is a fellow of the AAPM, American College of Radiology, SIIM, and the International Organization for Medical Physics. The author of more than 120 peer-reviewed articles and 200 published abstracts, Dr. Seibert has served as a reviewer for Medical Physics, as well as editorial board member and reviewer for Radiology and RadioGraphics. In 2019, Dr. Seibert received the Gold Medal award from the RSNA.

# Contributors

**Craig K. Abbey, PhD**
Researcher
University of California, Santa Barbara
Santa Barbara, California
(*Chapter 4 Image Quality; Appendix G Convolution and Fourier Transforms*)

**Stephen Balter, PhD**
Professor of Clinical Radiology, Physics in Medicine
Columbia University
New York, New York
(*Chapter 9 Fluoroscopy*)

**Wesley E. Bolch, PhD**
Distinguished Professor of Biomedical Engineering
J. Crayton Pruitt Family Department of Biomedical Engineering
University of Florida
Gainesville, Florida
(*Chapter 16 Radionuclide Production, Radiopharmaceuticals, and Internal Dosimetry; Chapter 17 Radiation Detection and Measurements; Appendix F Radiopharmaceutical Characteristics and Dosimetry*)

**Lawrence T. Dauer, PhD**
Associate Attending Physicist
Memorial Sloan Kettering Cancer Center

New York, New York
(*Chapter 21 Radiation Protection; Appendix I Radionuclide Therapy Home Care Guidelines*)

**William D. Erwin, MS**
Senior Medical Physicist
University of Texas MD Anderson Cancer Center
Houston, Texas
(*Chapter 18 Nuclear Imaging— The Gamma Camera*)

**Kathryn D. Held, PhD**
President
National Council on Radiation Protection and Measurements
Bethesda, Maryland
Associate Radiation Biologist/Associate Professor
Massachusetts General Hospital/ Harvard Medical School
Boston, Massachusetts
(*Chapter 20 Radiation Biology*)

**Nivene Hojeij, BS**
California State University
Sacramento, California
(*Chapter 2 Radiation and the Atom*)

**Youngkyoo Jung, PhD**
Associate Professor of Radiology

University of California, Davis
Sacramento, California
(*Chapter 12 Magnetic Resonance Basics: Magnetic Fields, Nuclear Magnetic Characteristics, Tissue Contrast, Image Acquisition*)

**Osama Mawlawi, PhD**
Professor of Imaging Physics and Chief of Nuclear medicine Physics
University of Texas MD Anderson Cancer Center
Houston, Texas
(*Chapter 19 Nuclear Tomographic Imaging—Single Photon and Positron Emission Tomography [SPECT and PET]*)

**Gianna Porro, BS**
College of Health Sciences
Purdue University
West Lafayette, Indiana
(*Chapter 3 Interaction of Radiation with Matter*)

**Charles E. Willis, PhD**
Retired Associate Professor
University of Texas MD Anderson Cancer Center
Houston, Texas
(*Chapter 7 Radiography*)

# Acknowledgments

We are grateful to our publisher Wolters Kluwer, Lippincott Williams & Wilkins, and (in particular) Sharon R. Zinner, who encouraged us to develop the fourth edition and the study guide, and Nicole Dernoski, who took over as our acquisitions editor. We would also like to thank our editorial coordinator team, led by Emily Buccieri, and our development editor, Eric McDermott, for their tireless efforts to bring the fourth edition and study guide to fruition. We would also like to take this opportunity to note the passing of Jonathan Pine who served as our senior executive editor during the development of the third edition. His endless capacity to provide encouragement and assistance was truly inspirational and greatly appreciated. He is missed by many.

During the development of the fourth and previous editions of the textbook, *The Essential Physics of Medical Imaging*, many experts generously gave their time and expertise. Without their help, the fourth edition of the textbook would not have been possible, and their efforts were essential for the creation of the study guide. The authors would like to express their gratitude for the invaluable contributions of the following individuals:

**Shadi Aminololama-Shakeri, MD**
University of California, Davis

**Erin Angel, PhD**
Canon Medical Systems

**Ramsey Badawi, PhD**
University of California, Davis

**John D. Boice Jr, ScD**
Vanderbilt-Ingram Cancer Center

**John M. Boone, PhD**
University of California, Davis

**Kevin S. Buckley, MSc**
Prospect Charter Care LLC
George Burkett, MEng
University of California, Davis

**Simon R. Cherry, PhD**
University of California, Davis

**Michael Corwin, MD**
University of California, Davis

**Michael Cronan, RDMS**
University of California, Davis

**Brian Dahlin, MD**
University of California, Davis

**Robert Dixon, PhD**
Wake Forest University

**Thomas Ferbel, PhD**
University of Rochester

**Brian Goldner, MD**
University of California, Davis

**R. Edward Hendrick, PhD**
University of Colorado

**Andrew Hernandez, PhD**
University of California, Davis

**Corey J. Hiti, MD**
University of California, Davis

**Jiang Hsieh, PhD**
General Electric Medical Systems

**John Hunter, MD**
University of California, Davis

**Sachin Jambawalikar, PhD**
Columbia University Irving Medical Center

**Kalpana Kanal, PhD**
University of Washington, Seattle

**Richard L. Kennedy, MSc**
The Permanente Medical Group

**Frederick W. Kremkau, PhD**
Wake Forest University School of Medicine

**Linda Kroger, MS**
University of California Davis Health System

**Steven M. LaFontaine, MS**
Therapy Physics, Inc.

**Ramit Lamba, MD**
University of California, Davis

**Edwin M. Leidholdt Jr, PhD**
University of California, Davis

**Karen Lindfors, MD**
University of California, Davis

**Mahadevappa Mahesh, PhD**
Johns Hopkins University

**Cynthia McCollough, PhD**
Mayo Clinic, Rochester

**John McGahan, MD**
University of California, Davis

**Michael McNitt-Gray, PhD**
University of California, Los Angeles

**Fred A. Mettler Jr, MD, MPH**
University of New Mexico School of Medicine

**Stuart Mirell, PhD**
University of California, Los Angeles

**Norbert Pelc, ScD**
Stanford University

**Nancy Pham, MD**
University of California, Davis

**Paul Schwoebel, PhD**
University of New Mexico

**D. K. Shelton, MD**
University of California, Davis

**Jeffrey Siewerdsen, PhD**
Johns Hopkins University

**Mani Tripathi, PhD**
University of California, Davis

**Jay Vaishnav, PhD**
Canon Medical Systems

**Steve Wilkendorf, RDMS**
University of California, Davis

**Sandra Wootton-Gorges, MD**
University of California, Davis

**Kai Yang, PhD**
Harvard University

# Contents

# Basic Concepts

# Introduction to the Study Guide

## 1.0 INTRODUCTION

As Dr. Mettler mentioned in the Foreword to the fourth edition of the textbook *The Essential Physics of Medical Imaging* (EPMI), the textbook's title was never completely accurate as both "Essentials" and "Physics" are a bit misleading. The fourth edition of the textbook is over 1,100 pages including over 1,000 figures (plus multipart figures), with more than 150 tables and 275 equations. The text also includes a thorough review of the radiation sciences related to medical imaging as well as comprehensive treatments of radiation protection and radiation biology. We also realized that over the years, the target audience has broadened from our original focus on radiologists in training to include biomedical engineers, medical physicists, and other imaging scientists. Hence, the breadth of discussion has grown to fully embrace this broader readership. To address the original goal of providing a concise compendium of information that focuses more on the didactic needs of radiologists, other physicians, and clinical medical physicists who will be preparing for their professional board examinations, we have developed the EPMI Study Guide. Each chapter of the Study Guide covers the same topic as its companion chapter in the main textbook, organized into three sections. Section I contains a summary of the textbook chapter's key points with illustrations and tables to convey the concepts. Section II contains sample questions and explanatory answers for that chapter's material, which are keyed (hyperlinked in the e-edition) to the textbook for more in-depth information. Section III has a list of key equations, symbols, quantities, and units that are introduced in the chapter. We hope that the EPMI Study Guide will serve the original intent of the "Essentials" and that the fourth edition of the EPMI textbook will complement the Study Guide for those who desire to understand the material at a deeper level.

## 1.1 SECTION I: CHAPTER SUMMARY

1. Organization
   a. Introduction
      (i) Most chapter introduction sections are relatively short, simply describing the major topic that will be covered. For example, in Chapter 13, Magnetic Resonance Imaging: Advanced Image Acquisition Methods, Artifacts, Spectroscopy, Quality Control, Siting, Bioeffects, and Safety the introduction reads:

> ### 13.0 INTRODUCTION
>
> Advanced pulse sequences and fast image acquisition methods; methods for perfusion, diffusion, and angiography imaging; spectroscopy; image quality metrics; common artifacts; MR siting; and MR safety issues are described and discussed with respect to the underlying physics.

**(ii)** In some chapters, a more descriptive overview is presented to properly orient the reader to the topics that will follow. For example, for Chapter 8—Breast Imaging: Mammography:

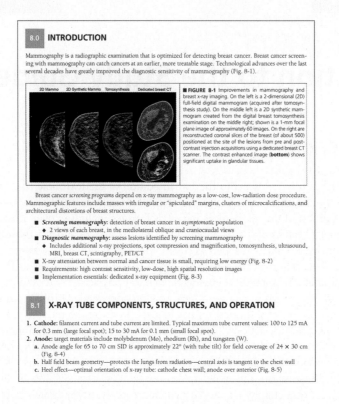

**2. Symbols**

**a.** While the chapter numbers and titles are identical to the fourth edition textbook, not all figures, tables, and equations are used in the Study Guide. When a figure, table, or equation number in the Study Guide is different from that in the fourth edition textbook, its original textbook reference number is displayed alongside the Study Guide number with the following symbol as shown in the examples:

**(i)** Figure 5-6 in the Study Guide is Figure 5-15 in the Textbook.

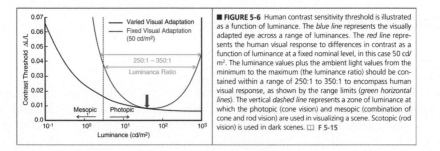

**(ii)** Table 8-2 in the Study Guide is Table 8-5 in the Textbook.

**TABLE 8-2 DIGITAL BREAST TOMOSYNTHESIS IMAGE STORAGE REQUIREMENTS—60 cm COMPRESSED BREAST THICKNESS, 24 × 30 cm FIELD SIZE—THREE MANUFACTURER IMPLEMENTATIONS** ▯ T. 8-5

| DBT | INDIRECT DETECTOR, 0.100 mm | | | DIRECT DETECTOR, 0.085 mm | | | DIRECT DETECTOR, 0.070 mm | | |
|---|---|---|---|---|---|---|---|---|---|
| *Acquisition* | *Matrix* | *# Images* | *Size (MB)* | *Matrix* | *# Images* | *Size (MB)* | *Matrix* | *# Images* | *Size (MB)* |
| Projections | 2,394 × 2,850 | 9 | 120 | 2,816 × 3,584 | 26 | 507 | 2,560 × 4,096 | 15 | 315 |
| Planes | 2,394 × 2,850 | 145 | 1,900 | 2,816 × 3,584 | 61 | 821 | 2,560 × 3,328 | 66 | 1,120 |

*Note*: Detector element binning (2 × 2) is used by some manufacturers in the acquisition of the planar images, with reconstruction of the tomosynthesis planes at a smaller pixel pitch (*e.g.*, 140 to 100 μm).
Data from Tirada N, Li G, Dreizin D, et al. Digital breast tomosynthesis: physics, artifacts, and quality control considerations. *Radiographics*. 2019;39:413–426. doi: 10.1148/rg.2019180046.

**(iii)** Equation 15-3 in the Study Guide is Equation 15-4 in the Textbook.

$$A = \lambda N$$

[15-3]   📖 E. 15-4

## 1.2   SECTION II: QUESTIONS AND EXPLANATORY ANSWERS

**Examples:** An example of the Questions and Answers sections are shown below. Note that the location of additional material related to the explanations given in the Study Guide is indicated after each of the explanatory answers.

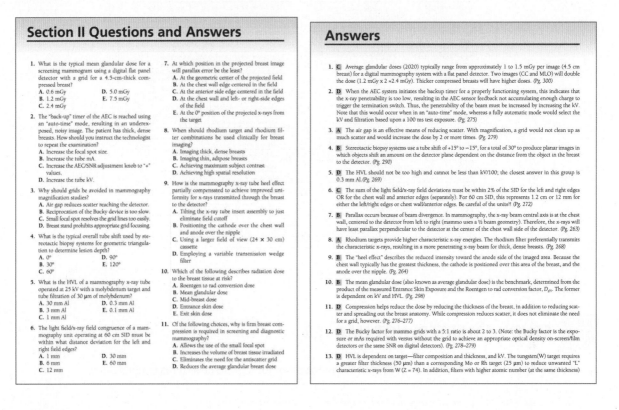

## 1.3   SECTION III: KEY EQUATIONS, SYMBOLS, QUANTITIES, AND UNITS

**1.** Section III has a list of key quantities and equations along with additional comments to assist in comprehension and their location in the fourth edition textbook for further reference. A table of symbols, quantities, and units is also provided for quick reference. An example of Section III for Chapter 8
—Breast Imaging: Mammography is shown below. Due to the extensive number and common use of acronyms in Chapter 5—Medical Imaging Informatics (some are actually initialisms rather than acronyms, a distinction we do not make in the Study Guide), a table of acronyms and their meaning are provided for that chapter.

## Section III Key Equations and Symbols

| QUANTITY | EQUATION | EQ NO./PAGE/COMMENTS |
|---|---|---|
| Focal spot effective length (line focus principle) | Effective length = actual length × sin θ is the "effective" anode angle | Eq. 6-2/Pg. 196/Focal spot length varies in the cathode-anode direction and is smaller on the anode side (Fig. 6-16) |
| Breast entrance surface dose: $Z$ (mGy) | $\approx X$ mGy(per 100 mAs) $\times \dfrac{Y \text{ mAs}}{100}\left(\dfrac{50 \text{ cm}}{D \text{ cm}}\right)^2$ | Eq. 8-1/Pg. 270/X-ray tube output, $X$, is measured at a standard distance (e.g., 50 cm) per 100 mAs. Inverse-square law correction applied for distance $D$ (source to breast surface). |
| Contrast degradation factor (CDF) | $\text{CDF} = \dfrac{C_s}{C_0} = \dfrac{1}{1 + \text{SPR}}$ | Eq. 8-2/Pg. 278/The amount of contrast achieved in the presence of scatter relative to contrast with no scatter. SPR = Scatter to Primary ratio (see Fig. 8-18) |
| Magnification, M | $M = \dfrac{\text{Image size}}{\text{object size}} = \dfrac{\text{source to image dist.}}{\text{source to object dist.}}$ | Eq. 7-2/Pg. 225/Fig. 8-20, Pg. 281. typical values run from 1.5× to 2.0× |
| Stereotactic lesion depth, Z | $Z = \dfrac{X}{2\tan 15^\circ}$ | Fig. 8-29 caption/Pg. 291/X is lesion shift distance in stereo pair images acquired at +15° and −15° |
| Mean Glandular Dose (MGD) | $D_g = X_{ESAK} \times D_{gN}$ | Eq. 8-3/Pg. 298/$D_g$ = MGD; $X_{ESAK}$ = Entrance Surface Air Kerma; $D_{gN}$ = conversion factor, derived from Monte Carlo transport algorithm. $D_{gN}$ tables dependent on kV, HVL, target/filter, thickness, tissue composition (Table 8-6, Pg. 299.) |
| Mean Glandular Dose (MGD) | $MGD = Kgcs$ | Eq. 8-4/Pg. 299/K = Entrance Surface Air Kerma; $g$ = fraction $K$ absorbed by glandular tissue; $c$ = correction for % glandularity; $s$ = factor to account for target/filter |

| SYMBOL | QUANTITY | UNITS |
|---|---|---|
| kV | Voltage applied to x-ray tube | volt, kilovolt |
| mAs | Tube current—time product | ampere-seconds |
| $s$ | Exposure time | second |
| θ | Anode angle | degree |
| HVL | Half Value Layer | mm Aluminum |
| SPR | Scatter to Primary Ratio | unitless |
| $M$ | Magnification | unitless |
| SID | Source-Image Distance | cm |
| SOD | Source-Object Distance | cm |
| OID | Object-Image Distance | cm |

## 1.4　STUDY SMARTER, NOT HARDER

Abraham Lincoln captured the concept of effective preparation for a given task in his famous quote,

*"Give me six hours to chop down a tree and I will spend the first four sharpening the axe."*

Like any new subject, there are effective and ineffective ways of studying. The ultimate goal is to integrate the information in a way that is not only useful in answering test questions but more importantly provides a deeper understanding of the core principles that will allow you to explore the many subtleties, exceptions, and applications of these topics in greater detail. Much research has been done and many books have been written on effective studying and integration of new technical information. The information below is a short synopsis of the most common recommendations from these sources.

1. **Employ Active Studying Techniques**
   Active studying is any activity that gets you more engaged with the subject matter.
   a. Rather than simply underlining or rereading what you think are the important points of a chapter, put them together in the form of questions, pictures, maps, or diagrams related to the material to provide another layer of association between related concepts. For example, when thinking about the core principles of radiation protection, you might put together your own PowerPoint slide to look something like Figure 1-1.
   b. Form study groups of 4 to 5 individuals with similar study goals and habits. Take turns within the group to present the material to each other and work on problems together.

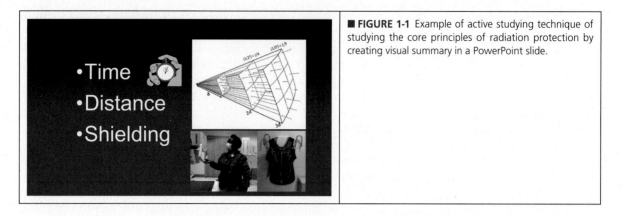

■ **FIGURE 1-1** Example of active studying technique of studying the core principles of radiation protection by creating visual summary in a PowerPoint slide.

   **c.** Watch YouTube videos on some of the concepts that may be difficult to visualize. For example, in MRI, the differences between image space and K-space can be a challenging subject for some students. This YouTube video, https://www.youtube.com/watch?v=IBUS0am7h5I, is one of many that provide a more in-depth look at the subject with clinical examples of how changing various acquisition parameters affects image quality.

   **d.** Go to free educational sites like the Board Review Section of AuntMinnie.com and work questions with your study group.

   **e.** Have fun while playing cards and learning medical imaging physics with a Medical Physics Imaging poker deck of cards available from medicalphysicsfiqures.com (Fig. 1-2).

   **f.** Do practice examinations (*e.g.*, medicalphysics.org).

   **g.** Access the wealth of information available from RSNA Radiographics, which is provided at the RadioGraph-

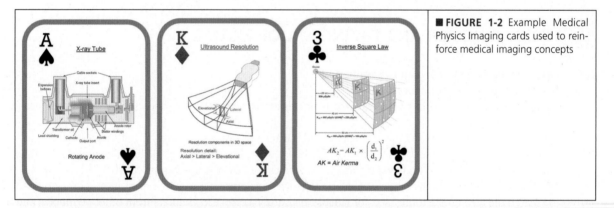

■ **FIGURE 1-2** Example Medical Physics Imaging cards used to reinforce medical imaging concepts

ics American Association of Physicists in Medicine Diagnostic Radiology Residents Physics Curriculum Article Index https://pubs.rsna.org/page/radiographics/aapm-physics.

   **h.** Listen to and discuss podcasts such as the Radiology Core Exam Review available at https://anchor.fm/mohammad-halaibeh.

**2. Create the proper environment for the type of study you are doing.**

   **a.** Individual study

     **(i)** Location, location, location: a quiet, relaxing space with good lighting where you can focus and where there will be minimal interruptions and distractions.

     **(ii)** A small public library and your home are examples of good and bad choices, respectively, for all the reasons mentioned above.

     **(iii)** If background noise is your thing to drown out the world around you, bring along some earbuds.

     **(iv)** Set reasonable time objectives. For most people, concentrated studying beyond 90 to 120 min without a break begins to show a rapid drop in return on investment of the time beyond that period. Even a break of 15 min of light physical activity (walking is great, or a power nap), will make you much more productive and improve content retention and integration.

   **b.** Group Study

(i) Active studying is done in this environment, and once the group is formed, there should be a leader to keep it organized. This responsibility can be shared but everyone must know who it is.

(ii) It should be convenient to all and have some of the same characteristics as individual study locations (*e.g.*, relaxing space, good lighting, minimal interruptions and distractions). Some of your activities may be loud, so pick a place where you are not likely to not disturb others.

(iii) Group size of 4 to 5 is ideal, but other sizes can work as well depending on how the groups are organized.

(iv) Select the most positive (not necessarily the "smartest") people for your group. Enthusiasm and the willingness to help others without judgment or ask what others may think of as "dumb" question is invaluable. In our experience, what you or some advanced student might think of as a "dumb" question is one that most of the class has without the nerve to ask it.

(v) Periodically, set some time aside to talk among yourselves about how the group study activities are going and what works, and what could be improved upon. Share your ideas with other groups both inside and outside your discipline.

3. **Study Aides**

   a. Tag your notes, so that later you can find them easily with a quick keyword search. Here are some of suggested tags and their meanings:

   (i) ?! = I've never heard of it! Should I believe it?

   (ii) $$ = high yield info

   (iii) ?? = do not understand, come back to again!

   (iv) ~F = formula to remember

   b. Use memory enhancing tools

   c. Flash cards (digital, paper, or whatever works for you). The key is to be open to and constantly look for new learning method.

## 1.5  PREPARING FOR AND TAKING MAJOR EXAMS

1. **Two to three weeks before a major examination**

   a. Identify strengths and weaknesses

   (i) Do practice exams to identify areas requiring additional understanding (see Section II and medical-physics.org).

   (ii) Make sure you understand the concept behind the answer, not just the answer to the question. A question about a concept can be asked in many different ways. Understanding the fundamentals behind the questions is the key to knowing the answer regardless of how the question is constructed.

   (iii) If there are concepts that are still out of reach, look for other sources of explanation. Use Google to search the web on the topic; look for videos on youtube.com; read chapters from other textbooks; and read articles in the medical physics educational series for radiology residents that are published periodically in radiographics and other resources from RSNA (see 1.4.1.g).

2. **The day before the examination**

   a. Carefully review all the rules and the examination instructions.

   (i) Understand the question types (*e.g.*, single best answer multiple choice; point and click; fill-in-the-blank; multiple select multiple choice).

   (ii) Understand the rules for navigating the examination, as there might be "blocked" questions where the ability to go back to a previous question is not allowed.

   (iii) Remote exams might require the completion of groups of questions that must be answered completely, prior to continuing the examination in order to provide breaks.

   (iv) Be aware of any other rules that have changed due to the unique aspects of remote exams in terms of security (*e.g.*, must have a camera on at all times showing the candidate and display and must allow third-party software to control the computer during the examination).

   b. Sleep

   (i) In the last two decades, a tremendous amount of research and information has been obtained that has confirmed the hypothesis that getting adequate about of "quality" sleep is an essential component of maintaining overall good health. The research has furthered our understanding that maintaining regular quality sleep is not only a requisite for optimal cognitive performance but its absence has deleterious effects on many of systems in the body. Sleep is a restorative and preparatory activity. While you sleep, your brain is cataloging information and healing your body. It decides; deciding what's important to hold onto and what can be let go. Your brain creates new pathways that help you navigate the day ahead and healing your body. Sleeping is also an essential part of healing of body systems like blood vessels and optimizing and maintaining functional metabolism and immunity. That being said, it is also known that making up for the lack of sleep is not a 1:1 proposition. You can't simply go to bed an hour earlier the next day to make up for a 1 hour debt. According to a fairly recent study (Kitamura et al., 2016), it takes 4 days to fully recover from 1 hour of lost sleep.

**(ii)** Some of the other most often mentioned preparation tips include setting your alarm; wearing comfortable clothes; and ensuring all preparations are confirmed regarding requirements for taking the test and relaxation techniques such as listening to your favorite music, repeating positive affirmations, and meditation along with focused breathing.

3. **During the exam**ination
   a. Time allocation
   **(i)** Dividing the number of questions by the time allotted provides a rough estimate of how much time you should spend answering each question. You should periodically check the time to see that you are not falling behind and if you have skipped some of the more difficult questions, make sure that all questions have been answered by the end of the examination period.
   b. Changing your first answer
   **(i)** The common adage that you should always trust your initial instinct with multiple choice questions is not supported by the research. The data across 33 separate studies indicate that there is absolutely nothing wrong with changing your initial answer (Benjamin et al., 1984).
   **(ii)** This is especially true if other questions in the examination bring additional information to mind.
   c. Unit analysis
   **(i)** When uncertain about the relationship of variables in an equation, organize them in the numerator and denominator so that when you cancel units, the answer is in the correct units for the quantity the answer should be in.

## REFERENCES

Benjamin LT, Cavell TA, Shallenberger WR. Staying with initial answers on objective tests: is it a myth? *Teach Psychol*. 1984;11:133–141. 10.1177/009862838401100303.

Kitamura S, Katayose Y, Nakazaki K, Motomura Y, Oba K, Katsunuma R, Terasawa Y, Enomoto M, Moriguchi Y, Hida A, Mishima K. Estimating individual optimal sleep duration and potential sleep debt. *Sci Rep*. 2016;6:35812. doi: 10.1038/srep35812.

# Radiation and the Atom

## 2.0 INTRODUCTION

- Radiation refers to energy that propagates through space or matter. Two important categories of radiation in medical imaging are electromagnetic radiation (EMR) and subatomic particulate radiation.
- Diagnostic imaging began with the discovery of x-rays by German mechanical engineer and physicist Wilhelm C. Rontgen approximately 115 years ago. While the immense scope and enormous impact of this discovery could not have been imagined at the turn of the 19th century, the word of its discovery and early applications spread rapidly across the world, and Rontgen received the first Nobel Prize in Physics in 1901.
- While other imaging modalities will be discussed, the x-ray, in its many embodiments (*e.g.*, radiography, CT, fluoroscopy, mammography), is still the most common form of energy used in radiology.
- With x-ray imaging, only a small fraction of the initial number of x-rays generated by the x-ray tube are transmitted toward the body, and only a small fraction of those (approximately 1%) exit and are recorded on an image receptor.
- Even fewer photons are detected and localized to create images in diagnostic nuclear medicine. In contrast to x-ray imaging where the recorded signal has been transmitted *through the body*, photons used in nuclear medicine (mainly in the form of high-energy EMR, *e.g.*, gamma [γ]-rays) are emitted from radiopharmaceuticals (pharmaceuticals, chemicals, or other substances labeled with radioactive materials) *inside the body* that were administered by inhalation, orally, or intravenously prior to imaging. The images created reveal the radiopharmaceutical's biodistribution, thus providing diagnostic information to the radiologist.
- Magnetic resonance imaging (MRI) utilizes strong magnetic fields and pulsed radiofrequency (RF) EMR to excite protons and to localize return signals, producing images which represent and are highly sensitive to the local variations in biochemical detail arising from differences the proton density and magnetic field properties of the different types of tissues that comprise internal organs (*e.g.*, fat, water, muscle, gray matter).

## 2.1 CLASSICAL ELECTROMAGNETISM

1. **Classical electrostatics**: Branch of physics that studies the interactions between stationary electric charges using an extension of the classical Newtonian model.
2. **Maxwell's equations:** Four widely used mathematical equations that describe how electric and magnetic fields propagate and interact, and how they are influenced by objects they encounter.
   a. Established the foundation for fields such as *special relativity* and *quantum mechanics*.
3. **Electron energy levels:** One of the revelations to come out of quantum mechanics was the concept that a particle that is bound (confined spatially, like orbital electrons of an atom) can only have particular discrete values of energy.
   a. Orbital electron binding energies describe the energy required to overcome the attractive force of the protons' positive electric field and eject electrons from specific orbitals in atoms. The lowest energy level an electron can have in this bound state is $-13.6$ eV, meaning that at least 13.6 eV of energy would need to be transferred to the electron to liberate it from the atom. In general, energy levels can also refer to the state of the atomic nucleus or vibrational or rotational energy levels in molecules.
   b. **Energy units**—In medical imaging, this energy is typically measured in multiples of electron volts (eV); 1 keV = 1,000 eV; 1 MeV = 1,000,000 eV
      (i) The formal definition is 1 eV equals the kinetic energy acquired by an electron as it accelerates across an electrical potential difference (voltage) of one volt in a vacuum.

(ii) One eV is an incredibly small amount of energy. When you apply a force ($F$) to lift the 4th edition of our textbook (2.7 kg) by one foot ($F = ma$, where $m$ is mass in kg and $a$ is the acceleration due to gravity approximately 10 ms$^{-2}$), you do work ($W = Fd$) of approximately: 2.7 kg × 10 ms$^{-2}$ × 0.3 m = 8.1 J, which is about $5.1 \times 10^{19}$ eV. However, as discussed in Chapter 3, if that same amount of energy were transferred to the book in the form of ionizing radiation, the dose of radiation the book would have received in Gray (Gy where 1 Gy = 1 J/kg) would be (8.1 J/2.7 kg) = 3 Gy. While not a lot of energy, it is a very large dose of radiation from a viewpoint of its potential for biological damage. As discussed in Chapter 20, if this dose were to be applied to the whole body at one time, the chance of survival would be approximately 50% in 30 days.

## 2.2  ELECTROMAGNETIC RADIATION

1. **Electromagnetic radiation (EMR)** is a traveling sinusoidal wave consisting of inseparable, self-sustaining oscillating electric and magnetic field components that propagate together at the speed of light ($c$) approximately $3.8 \times 10^{8}$ ms$^{-1}$ in a vacuum (Fig. 2-1)

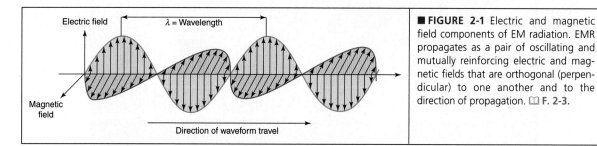

**■ FIGURE 2-1** Electric and magnetic field components of EM radiation. EMR propagates as a pair of oscillating and mutually reinforcing electric and magnetic fields that are orthogonal (perpendicular) to one another and to the direction of propagation. ▢ F. 2-3.

2. **Wave characteristics of electromagnetic radiation** (Fig. 2-2)
   a. **Wavelength ($\lambda$):** distance between any two identical points on adjacent cycles (typically in $nm$)
   b. **Amplitude (A):** maximal height or magnitude
   c. **Intensity (I):** power/area, which is proportional to the square of the amplitude
   d. **Period (T):** the time to complete one cycle of a wave (time for wave of $\lambda$ to pass a fixed point)
   e. **Frequency($\nu$):** number of periods that occur per second, inversely equal to the period: $\nu = 1/T$. Measured in multiples of hertz (Hz); MHz—$10^{6}$, GHz—$10^{9}$, THz—$10^{12}$
   f. **Energy (E):** $E = h\nu$, where $h$ is Planck's constant (see Section 2.3.1)
   g. **Phase:** temporal shift of one wave relative to another
   h. **Speed ($c$) of EMR:** is constant in a given medium
      (i) Frequency and wavelength are inversely proportional

$$c = \lambda\nu \tag{2-1}$$

(ii) Velocity ($v$) of EMR in a medium with a refractive index ($n$)

$$v = c/n \tag{2-2}$$

$n$ for selected media: vacuum, $n = 1.0$; water @ 20°C, $n = 1.33$; olive oil, $n = 1.46$; diamond, $n = 2.42$

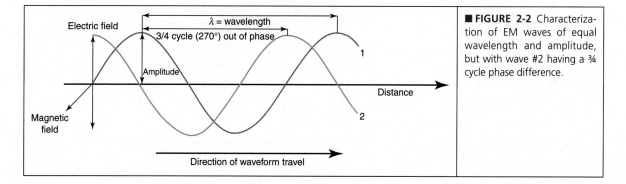

**■ FIGURE 2-2** Characterization of EM waves of equal wavelength and amplitude, but with wave #2 having a ¾ cycle phase difference.

3. **The electromagnetic radiation spectrum**

   **a.** EMR is commonly used at different frequencies for a wide variety of applications. Examples in order of increasing energy and frequency include radio waves, infrared waves, visible light, ultraviolet rays, x-rays, and gamma rays (Fig. 2-3).

   **(i)** EMR can propagate through matter but does not require matter for its propagation.

   **(ii)** EMR is emitted every time a charged particle accelerates.

   **(iii)** EMR obeys the laws of optics at all frequencies, which include refraction, reflection, dispersion, interference, and diffraction.

4. **Penetration of electromagnetic radiation in tissue**

   **a.** The energy of the EMR must be able to penetrate and interact with the organ and tissue of interest to interrogate the physical or chemical structure of organs and tissues within the body through imaging with EMR (Fig. 2-4).

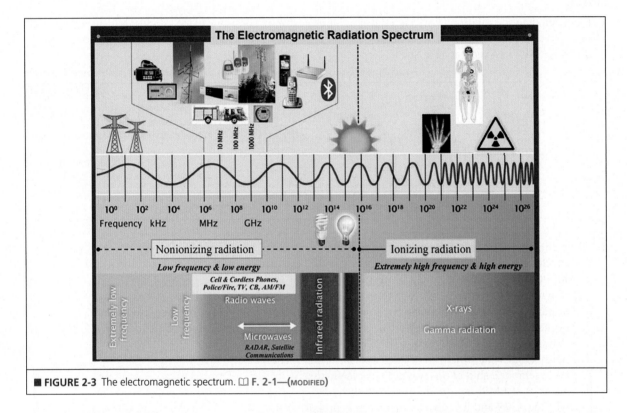

■ **FIGURE 2-3** The electromagnetic spectrum. 📖 F. 2-1—(MODIFIED)

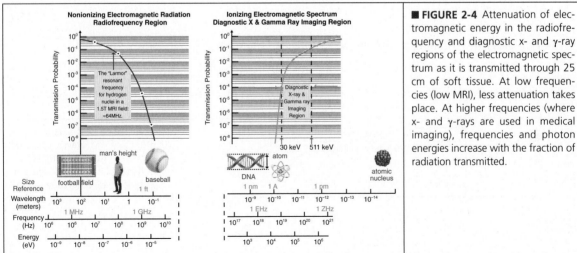

■ **FIGURE 2-4** Attenuation of electromagnetic energy in the radiofrequency and diagnostic x- and γ-ray regions of the electromagnetic spectrum as it is transmitted through 25 cm of soft tissue. At low frequencies (low MRI), less attenuation takes place. At higher frequencies (where x- and γ-rays are used in medical imaging), frequencies and photon energies increase with the fraction of radiation transmitted.

## 2.3 BEHAVIOR OF ENERGY AT THE ATOMIC SCALE: ONE OF THE MOST IMPORTANT DISCOVERIES IN THE HISTORY OF SCIENCE

1. **Energy quanta and the photon:** Max Planck ushered in the dawn of quantum mechanics with his suggestion that energy could only be emitted or absorbed in multiples of some minimal finite discrete packets of energy he called *quanta* (called the term *photon* in 1926), the smallest quantity of EMR.
   a. Energy of a photon is given by

   $$E = h\nu = \frac{hc}{\lambda}$$

   [2-3]

   where Planck's constant, $h$, = $6.626 \times 10^{-34}$ J-s = $4.136 \times 10^{-18}$ keV–s
   b. When $E$ is expressed in keV and $\lambda$ in nanometers (*nm*)

   $$E(\text{keV}) = \frac{1.24}{\lambda(\text{nm})}$$

   [2-4]

2. **Particle characteristics of electromagnetic radiation:** In 1905, Albert Einstein postulated that Planck's quanta were acting like physical particles—namely photons. This elucidation is now known as the ***photoelectric effect.*** Einstein was awarded the Nobel Prize in Physics in 1921 for this discovery.
3. **Wave-particle duality** (proposed in 1924 by future Nobel Laureate Louis de Broglie)
   a. All particles exhibit wave-like properties, and all waves exhibit particle-like properties.
   b. Wave characteristics are more apparent when EMR interacts with objects having dimension similar to the photon's wavelength (Fig. 2-5A).
   c. Particle characteristics of EMR, on the other hand, are more evident when an object's dimensions (*e.g.*, an electron of $10^{-18}$ m) are much smaller than the photon's wavelength (Fig. 2-5B).

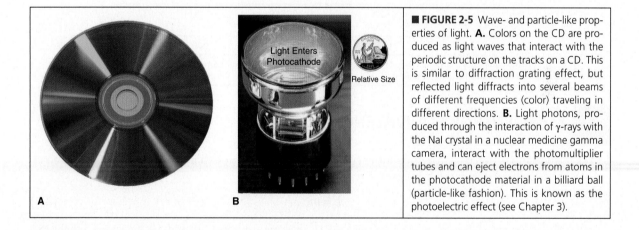

■ **FIGURE 2-5** Wave- and particle-like properties of light. **A.** Colors on the CD are produced as light waves that interact with the periodic structure on the tracks on a CD. This is similar to diffraction grating effect, but reflected light diffracts into several beams of different frequencies (color) traveling in different directions. **B.** Light photons, produced through the interaction of γ-rays with the NaI crystal in a nuclear medicine gamma camera, interact with the photomultiplier tubes and can eject electrons from atoms in the photocathode material in a billiard ball (particle-like fashion). This is known as the photoelectric effect (see Chapter 3).

## 2.4 IONIZING AND NONIONIZING RADIATION

1. *Ion:* an atom or molecule that has lost or gained one or more electrons and has a net electrical charge.
2. *Ionizing radiation*: photons of higher frequencies in far UV region of spectrum (shorter than 200 nm) with sufficient energy per photon to eject electrons from their atomic shells (*e.g.*, x- and γ-rays).
3. *Nonionizing radiation:* EMR with photon energies in and below the UV region (*e.g.*, visible, infrared (IR), terahertz (THz), microwave (MW), and radio frequency (RF) waves). Energy transfer occurs as electron excitation and photochemical reactions (IR, optical and UV) and heating due to increased molecular vibration and induced currents (THz, MW and RF).
4. *Ionization energy:* minimum energy to remove the outermost atomic electron in its ground state (approximately 13.6 eV).
5. *Average energy expended per ion pair (***W***)* is larger than the minimum ionization energy due to nonionizing energy losses from excitation and small kinetic energy transfers (approximately 33.7 eV).

## PARTICULATE RADIATION

Particulate radiations import to radiology and nuclear medicine are shown in Table 2-1.

1. *Proton:* found in nuclei of all atoms, positive electric charge identical to nucleus of H atom
2. *Electron:* in atomic orbit, charge equal in magnitude but opposite (negative), approximately 1/1,800 mass of proton
3. *Beta particles:* electrons emitted by the nuclei of radioactive atoms; beta-minus particles ($\beta^-$) indistinguishable from orbital electrons except for their origin
4. *Beta-plus particles* ($\beta^+$) or *positrons*: positively charged electrons; a form of "antimatter" that ultimately combines with electrons in a unique transformation in which their rest mass ($m$) is converted through annihilation to an equivalent amount of energy in the form of two oppositely directed 511 keV photons
5. *Neutron:* uncharged nuclear particle, mass slightly greater than proton; released in nuclear fission and can be used to irradiate stable nuclides in order to produce radioactive nuclides "radionuclides"
6. *Alpha particle*: a He nucleus with 2 protons and 2 neutrons giving a +2 charge; typically, harmless when external to the body, although can cause extensive cellular damage within the body if the dose is sufficient

**TABLE 2-1  PROPERTIES OF PARTICULATE RADIATION**

| PARTICLE | SYMBOL | ELEMENTARY CHARGE | REST MASS (amu) | ENERGY EQUIVALENT (MeV) |
|---|---|---|---|---|
| Alpha | $\alpha$, $^4\text{He}^{2+}$ | +2 | 4.00154 | 3,727 |
| Proton | p, $^1\text{H}^+$ | +1 | 1.007276 | 938 |
| Electron | $e^-$ | −1 | 0.000549 | 0.511 |
| Negatron (beta minus) | $\beta^-$ | −1 | 0.000549 | 0.511 |
| Positron (beta plus) | $\beta^+$ | +1 | 0.000549 | 0.511 |
| Neutron | $n^0$ | 0 | 1.008665 | 940 |

An elementary charge is a unit of electric charge where 1 is equal in magnitude to the charge of an electron. The amu, atomic mass unit, defined as 1/12th the mass of a carbon-12 atom.

## MASS-ENERGY EQUIVALENCE

1. The relationship between the mass and the energy in any system is expressed in one of the most famous equations in science based on Einstein's ground-breaking work:

$$E = mc^2 \qquad [2\text{-}5]$$

   where $E$ = energy in joules (J) (where 1 kg m$^2$s$^{-2}$ = 1 J), $m$ = mass at rest (kg), and $c$ = the speed of light in a vacuum (approximately $2.998 \times 10^8$ m/s). The implication is for any mass at rest of $m$ (kg), there is an equivalent of energy $E$ (J) equal to its mass (kg) times the speed of light squared (m$^2$s$^{-2}$).
2. A notable equivalence of mass and energy: the electron, with $m = 9.109 \times 10^{-31}$ kg, $E = 0.511$ MeV = 511 keV
3. Atomic mass unit (amu), 1 amu = 1/12 the mass of $^{12}$C atom = 931.5 MeV

## STRUCTURE OF THE ATOM

1. **The nature of atomic constituents**
   a. The atom is composed of an extremely dense positively charged nucleus, containing protons and neutrons, and an extranuclear cloud of light, negatively charged electrons
   b. Number of protons = number of electrons, so atom is electrically neutral in its normal "typical" state
   c. The atom is comprised of largely unoccupied space, in which the volume of the nucleus is only $10^{-12}$ (a millionth of a millionth) the volume of the atom
   d. Number of electrons in the valence shell of the atom determines its reactivity, or the tendency to form chemical bonds with other atoms

## 2. Electron orbits

**a. *The Bohr model*:** Early model of the electron orbitals

**(i)** Each electron occupies a discrete energy state in a given electron shell, assigned the letters K, L, M, N, …, with K denoting the innermost shell, in which the electrons have the lowest (*i.e.*, most negative) energy states and the highest binding energy (Fig. 2-6).

**(ii)** Electrons do not actually revolve in orbits but exist as 3-dimensional waves around the nucleus as a "cloud" of probabilities until something interacts with the cloud and collapses the wavefunction, causing the electron's position to suddenly appear.

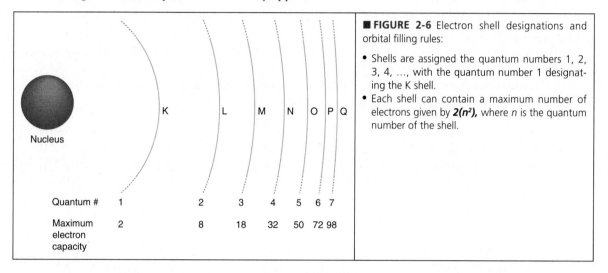

■ **FIGURE 2-6** Electron shell designations and orbital filling rules:

- Shells are assigned the quantum numbers 1, 2, 3, 4, …, with the quantum number 1 designating the K shell.
- Each shell can contain a maximum number of electrons given by **$2(n^2)$**, where *n* is the quantum number of the shell.

**b. *Quantum mechanical model*:** a 3D wave associated with all matter, including electrons in an atom

**(i)** The Schrödinger wave equation provides the atomic structure where the location of an orbital electron is described in terms of the probability it will occupy a given location within the atom.

**(ii)** At any given moment, there is even a probability, albeit extremely low, that an electron can be within the atom's nucleus; however, the highest probabilities are associated with Bohr's original atomic radii.

**(iii)** An electron can have only certain discrete energies inside an atom that agree with the experimental observation of the line spectra in which atoms exhibit and account for the characteristic red and yellow light that neon and sodium bulbs produce.

## 3. Electron binding energy

**a.** Orbital energy: energy required to eject (remove) an orbital electron completely from the atom.

**(i)** For radiation to be ionizing, energy transferred to the electron must equal or exceed its binding energy.

**b.** Binding energy of inner most shell (K) is greater than outer shells; binding energy also increases with the number of protons in the nucleus (atomic number) (Fig. 2-7).

**c.** Energy required to move an electron from the innermost electron orbit (*K* shell) to the next orbit (*L* shell) is the difference between the binding energies of the two orbits (*i.e.*, $E_{bK} - E_{bL}$ equals the transition energy).

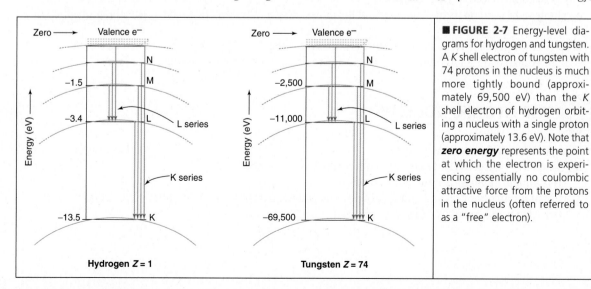

■ **FIGURE 2-7** Energy-level diagrams for hydrogen and tungsten. A *K* shell electron of tungsten with 74 protons in the nucleus is much more tightly bound (approximately 69,500 eV) than the *K* shell electron of hydrogen orbiting a nucleus with a single proton (approximately 13.6 eV). Note that ***zero energy*** represents the point at which the electron is experiencing essentially no coulombic attractive force from the protons in the nucleus (often referred to as a "free" electron).

## 2.8    RADIATION FROM ELECTRON TRANSITIONS

*Electron cascade:* describes the movement of electrons from their normal shell (energy state) to a different shell following the transfer of energy in the form of an x- or γ-ray photon or interaction with a charged particle. The vacancy created is usually filled by an electron transitioning from an outer, more distal shell. Energy of each transition is equal to the difference in binding energy between the original and final shells of the transitioning electron. This energy can be released by the atom as EMR in the form of *characteristic x-rays* or by transferring the energy to an even more weakly bound electron in the same atom and ejecting it (*Auger electron*).

1. **Characteristic X-rays**
   a. Electron transitions between atomic shells can result in the emission of EMR in both the ionizing and non-ionizing portions of the EM spectrum.
      (i) Electron binding energies depend on atom's atomic number and the orbital shell it occupies.
   b. *Characteristic* or *fluorescent x-ray* naming convention
      (i) According to orbital in which the vacancy occurred (*e.g.*, K, L, M) and the originating shell of the electron that filled the vacancy (*e.g.*, adjacent shell subscript is α; nonadjacent shell subscript is β (*e.g.*, $L \rightarrow K$ transition = $K\alpha$, $M \rightarrow L$ transition = $L\alpha$, $M \rightarrow K$ transition = $K\beta$) (Fig. 2-8A)
      (ii) Energy of the characteristic x-ray ($E_{x\text{-}ray}$) is the difference between the electron binding energies ($E_b$) of the respective shells, as shown in **Eq. 2-6**

$$E_{\text{characteristic x-ray}} = E_{b\,\text{vacant shell}} - E_{b\,\text{transition shell}}$$

[2-6]

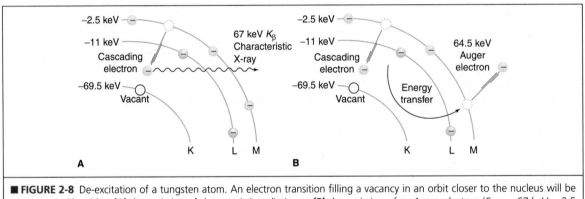

■ **FIGURE 2-8** De-excitation of a tungsten atom. An electron transition filling a vacancy in an orbit closer to the nucleus will be accompanied by either **(A)** the emission of characteristic radiation or **(B)** the emission of an Auger electron ($E_{\text{auger}}$ = 67 keV − 2.5 keV = 64.5 keV).

2. **Auger electrons and fluorescent yield:** Auger electron emission predominates in low Z elements
   a. Characteristic energy released is transferred to an orbital electron, typically occurring in the same shell as the cascading electron (Fig. 2-8B).
   b. Fluorescent yield, ω, is the probability of the emission of a characteristic x-ray; 1−ω is the probability of an Auger electron emission.
   c. ω probability: less than 1% for elements with Z less than 10; approximately 15% for calcium (Z = 20); approximately 65% for iodine (Z = 53) and approaching 80% for Z greater than 60.

## 2.9    THE ATOMIC NUCLEUS

1. **Composition of the nucleus**
   a. Composed of protons and neutrons, collectively known as *nucleons*
      (i) *Atomic number (Z):* number of protons
      (ii) *Mass number (A):* total number of protons and neutrons (note—**N**: number of neutrons)
      (iii) *Chemical symbol (X)* gives the construct:

$$^{A}_{Z}X_{N}$$

b. *Isotopes:* atoms of the same element with the same proton number but a different number of neutrons.

c. *Atomic mass:* based on the atomic mass unit (amu) =1/12 the weight of $^{12}C$. The average atomic mass of an element shown in a periodic table or listed in a periodic table of elements is a weighted average mass of all the isotopes present in a naturally occurring sample of that element. The average mass is equal to the sum of each individual isotope's mass multiplied by its fractional abundance.

2. **Classification of nuclides**

a. *Nuclides:* Families of nuclides (isotopes, isobars, isotones, and isomers) can be characterized by the constituents of their nucleus have the same property, Table 2-2.

**TABLE 2-2 NUCLEAR FAMILIES: ISOTOPES, ISOBARS, ISOTONES, AND ISOMERS**

| FAMILY | NUCLIDES WITH SAME | EXAMPLE |
|---|---|---|
| Isoto**p**es | Atomic number (*Z*) (# of **p**rotons) | I-131 and I-125: *Z* = 53 |
| Isobars | Mass number (*A*) | Mo-99 and Tc-99: *A* = 99 |
| Isoto**n**es | Number of **n**eutrons (*A* − *Z*) | $_{53}$I-131: 131 − 53 = 78 |
|  |  | $_{54}$Xe-132: 132 − 54 = 78 |
| Isomers | Atomic and mass numbers but different **e**nergy states in the nucleus | Tc-99m and Tc-99: *Z* = 43 |
|  |  | *A* = 99 |
|  |  | Energy of Tc-99m > Tc-99: $\Delta E$ = 142 keV |

*Note:* See text for description of the bold and italicized letters in the nuclear family terms.

3. **Nuclear forces and energy levels** (Fig. 2-9)

| Forces acting within the Atom | Relative Strength | Representations | Range | Particle Mediator (mass) | Examples |
|---|---|---|---|---|---|
| **Strong Force:** The repulsive Coulomb force of protons within a nucleus is overcome by the *strong* but short-range nuclear force that provides transformations among nucleons through meson exchange. | 1 | 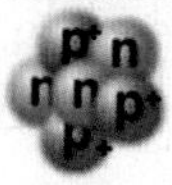  | Diameter of the nucleus ≈$10^{-14}$–$10^{-15}$ m | Mesons (≈0.135–9.5 GeV/C²) | Holds the atom's nucleus together |
| **Electromagnetic Force:** Electrons are bound to nuclei through the *coulombic* (electrostatic) attractive forces. | $10^{-2}$ | $F_{\bar{q}} = \dfrac{k\,q_1\,q_2}{r^2}$ | Infinite | Photons (0) | Holds atoms together and provides for formation of chemical bonds |
| **Weak Force:** Neutrons can decay into protons nuclei through *weak* nuclear force, emitting an electron or beta minus (β⁻) particle and an anti-neutrino (v̄). | $10^{-4}$ | $n \longrightarrow p^+ + \beta^- + \bar{v}$ | 0.1% diameter of a proton ≈$10^{-18}$ m | W & Z bosons (≈86 & ≈97 amu) | Exchange force in radioactive decay and triggers nuclear fusion in stars |
| **Gravity:** Strong planetary force, but very weak at the subatomic atomic level. | $10^{-38}$ | $F_G = \dfrac{G\,m_1\,m_2}{r^2}$ | Infinite | Graviton (< ≈10–22 eV/C²) | Holds your feet on the ground and the universe together |

■ **FIGURE 2-9** The four classical forces of nature.

a. The *electromagnetic* and *strong force* act in opposite directions on protons in the nucleus to maintain the incredibly small and ultra-dense center of the atom.

b. The *weak-force* is composed of "exchange forces," which allow for the conversion of neutrons into protons and vice-versa during the process of radioactive decay.

(i) *Ground state* is the lowest energy state of an atomic nucleus

(ii) *Excited state:* nuclei with energy in excess of the ground state

(iii) *Metastable nuclei* have excited states with half-lives 100 to 1,000 times longer than typical excited nuclear states, which transition to more stable states in typically less than $10^{-12}s$

c. *Gravitational forces* are proportional to mass and thus are insignificant on the atomic scale.

## 2.10   NUCLEAR STABILITY AND RADIOACTIVITY

On a plot of *Z* versus *N*, stable (nonradioactive) nuclides fall along a **"line of stability"** for which the *N/Z* ratio is approximately 1 for low Z nuclides and gradually increases with Z to approximately 1.5 for heaviest element with stable isotopes (Bismuth Z = 83 $^{209}$Bi) (Fig. 2-10).

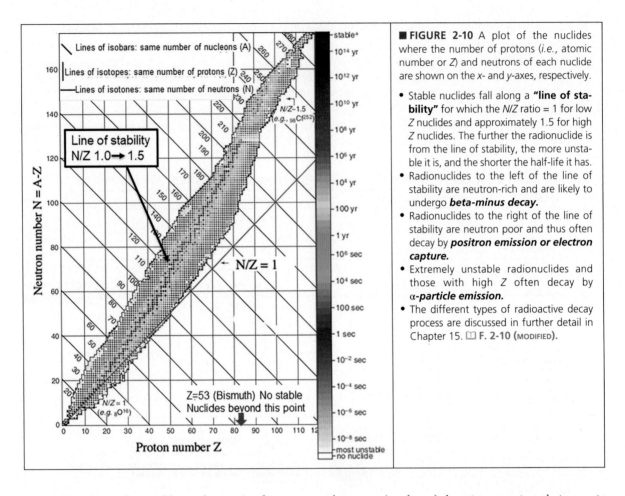

**■ FIGURE 2-10** A plot of the nuclides where the number of protons (*i.e.*, atomic number or *Z*) and neutrons of each nuclide are shown on the *x*- and *y*-axes, respectively.

- Stable nuclides fall along a **"line of stability"** for which the *N*/*Z* ratio = 1 for low *Z* nuclides and approximately 1.5 for high *Z* nuclides. The further the radionuclide is from the line of stability, the more unstable it is, and the shorter the half-life it has.
- Radionuclides to the left of the line of stability are neutron-rich and are likely to undergo **beta-minus decay**.
- Radionuclides to the right of the line of stability are neutron poor and thus often decay by **positron emission or electron capture**.
- Extremely unstable radionuclides and those with high *Z* often decay by **α-particle emission**.
- The different types of radioactive decay process are discussed in further detail in Chapter 15. ▢ **F. 2-10** (MODIFIED).

1. While atoms with unstable combinations of neutrons and protons (nucleons) do exist, over time their atomic nuclei will undergo periodic spontaneous transformations rendering them less unstable or stable.
2. **Nuclear instability** can be due to either **neutron excess** or **neutron deficiency** (*i.e.*, proton excess).
3. *Radioactive decay:* The transformative process where ***radioactive*** nuclides decay to more stable nuclei.
   a. *Parent:* radionuclide at the beginning of a particular decay sequence.
   b. *Daughter:* decay products (progeny) of radionuclides that are stable/less radioactive.
   c. *Half-life:* characteristic constant of a radionuclide indicating the time required for a quantity of radioactive atoms to decay to the point where the number of radioactive atoms remaining are equal to one-half of their initial value.
4. **Gamma rays (γ):** The EMR emitted from the nucleus as the excited state transitions to a lower (more stable) energy state.
   a. Emanate from the nucleus, much more energetic than characteristic x-rays
   b. *Isomeric transition:* when nuclear de-excitation takes place in an isomer, and the energy state of the nucleus is reduced without affecting *A* or *Z*, for example, $^{99m}Tc/^{99}Tc$
5. **Internal conversion electrons:** An alternative form of de-excitation in which the de-excitation energy is completely transferred to an orbital electron.
   a. Conversion electron is ejected from the atom with a kinetic energy equal to the difference between the γ-ray and the electron binding energy.
   b. Vacancy will be filled by electron cascade process previously discussed.
6. **Nuclear spin, angular momentum, and nuclear magnetic moment**
   a. **Protons and neutrons that make up a nucleus have a quantum property called "spin"**
      (i)   The term "spin" is used to indicate the intrinsic **angular momentum** of elementary particles and nucleons in even though none of the particles are actually spinning or rotating).
      (ii)  Spin is a fundamental property of nature and does not arise from more basic mechanisms.
      (iii) Protons, neutrons, and electrons all have spin = ½.
   b. **Nuclear magnetic moment:**

(i)   Protons and neutrons are composed of elementary particles that have spin and orbital angular momentum. This contributes toward the overall "spin" angular momentum of the nucleus as a whole. Pairs of protons and neutrons align in such a way that their spins cancel.

(ii)  Like the angular momentum of a gyroscope, spin has both magnitude and direction (vector); however, unlike angular momentum in classical mechanics, this spin is quantized.

(iii) The value of the spin angular momentum is expressed by the nuclear spin quantum number (I) whose value can only be discrete integers or half-integer units (0, 1/2, 1, 3/2, 2, 5/2, …).

(iv)  However, when there is an odd number of protons or neutrons (odd mass numbers), some of the spins will not be canceled and the total nucleus will have a **net spin** characteristic that behaves like a singular particle with its own spin angular momentum.

(v)   It is this process that creates the magnetic property known as the nuclear magnetic moment.

c. **Nuclear magnetic properties of isotopes**

(i)   All stable isotopes that contain an odd number of protons and/or of neutrons have an intrinsic magnetic moment and spin angular momentum, in other words a nonzero spin. However, all nuclides with even numbers of both protons and neutrons have net spin = 0.

(ii)  Only nuclei with nonzero spins ($I \neq 0$) can absorb and emit EMR and undergo "resonance" when placed in a magnetic field. As you will see in Chapter 12, only some of these nuclides have the proper characteristics to be useful for MRI. The number of stable nuclides with different odd and even combinations of neutrons and protons is shown in Table 2-3.

### TABLE 2-3 DISTRIBUTION OF STABLE NUCLIDES AS A FUNCTION OF NEUTRON AND PROTON NUMBER

| NUMBER OF PROTONS (Z) | NUMBER OF NEUTRONS (N) | NUMBER OF STABLE NUCLIDES |
|---|---|---|
| Even | Even | 165 |
| Even | Odd | 57 (NMR signal) |
| Odd | Even | 53 (NMR signal) |
| Odd | Odd | 4 (NMR signal) |
| | Total | 279 |

NMR, nuclear magnetic resonance.

## 2.11    NUCLEAR BINDING ENERGY AND MASS

1. The term binding energy refers to the quantity of energy necessary to disassemble a system of particles into individual parts or to remove a particle from a system of particles.

   a. Atomic binding energy: The energy required to separate an atom into free electrons and its nucleus and thus is equal to the sum of the orbital electron-binding energies.

   b. Nuclear binding energy: The energy needed to dissociate a nucleus into free protons and neutrons and thus is equal to the sum of the strong force acting between nucleons.

   (i)   Nuclear particle experiments have demonstrated that the total mass of a nucleus is less than the sum of the masses of its constituent nucleons (protons and neutrons).

   (ii)  This mass difference, or **mass defect**, is the result of the action of the attractive strong nuclear force acting between nucleons to overcome the electrostatic repulsive force of the protons.

   (iii) This is an exothermic reaction in which the resulting loss of energy is emitted in the form of radiation.

   (iv)  The energy emitted is calculated by subtracting the mass of the atom from the total mass of its constituent protons, neutrons, and electrons. According to Einstein's special theory of relativity, this difference in mass is a measure of the total energy lost by the system and is equal to $E = mc^2$.

   (v)   The total binding energy of the nucleus can be divided by the mass number A to obtain the average binding energy per nucleon.

2. **Nuclear Fission and Fusion**

   a. *Nuclear fission*: when a nucleus with a large atomic mass captures a thermal (low kinetic energy) neutron and splits into two (usually unequal) parts (*fission fragments*), each has an average binding energy per nucleon greater than that of the original nucleus (Fig. 2-11). As a consequence:

   **(i)**   Total nuclear binding energy increases (*i.e.*, more stable nuclei are formed although they will likely still be radioactive).

   **(ii)**  The difference in binding energy is released as EMR and particulate radiation (including several energetic neutrons and as kinetic energy of the fission fragments (two new nuclides).

   **(iii)** Probability of fission increases with neutron flux (the number of neutrons per cm²/s).

**b.** *Nuclear reactors:* device that can maintain a self-sustaining nuclear fission chain reaction.

   **(i)**   Fission is used in nuclear-powered electrical generating plants where the reactor core consists of sealed metal fuel rods in which uranium pellets (enriched in U-235) fuel have been placed. The vast majority of the heat in a nuclear reactor comes from kinetic energy of fission products that are converted to thermal energy when these nuclei collide with nearby atoms. This heat is transferred the water surrounding the fuel rods and the water is eventually turned into steam which run a steam turbine to produce electricity. U-235 releases approximately three million times more energy via nuclear fission than an equal mass of coal.

   **(ii)**  Fission was also the process used in the development of the first "atomic" or A-bombs.

**c.** *Fusion*: combining of two light atomic nuclei into one heavier nuclei; the resulting nuclei has an average binding energy per nucleon greater than that of the original nuclei that were fused together, thus energy is released.

   **(i)**   *Hydrogen "H"-bomb*: uses fission device (A-bomb) to generate the temperature and pressure needed for fusion (are also known as "thermonuclear" weapons)

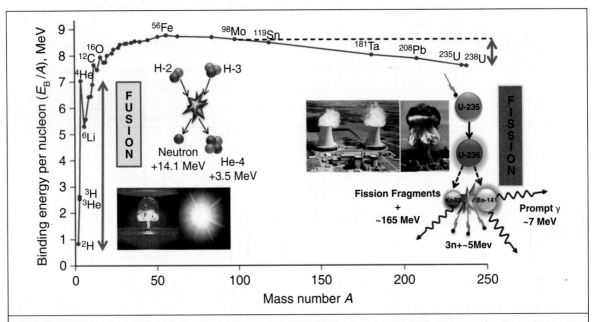

■ **FIGURE 2-11** Graph of average binding energy per nucleon as a function of mass number. The curve reaches its maximum near the middle of the elements and decreases at either end, this predicts that large quantities of energy can be released from a small amount of matter. This can occur by two processes: ***nuclear fission*** and ***nuclear fusion.*** The absorption of a single thermal neutron by the nucleus of a U-235 atom can result in the instantaneous fission of U-236 into two fission fragments (*e.g.*, Kr-82 and Ba-141 or Sn-131 and Mo-102) and two or three neutrons with large kinetic energies. The fusion of deuterium ($_2$H) and tritium ($_3$He) nuclei results in the production of $_4$He and a neutron. The $_4$He atom has a much higher average binding energy per nucleon than either tritium ($_3$H) or deuterium ($_2$H).

# Section II Questions and Answers

1. All of the following are properties of electromagnetic radiation *except*:
   A. Zero mass
   B. Velocity of approximately $3 \times 10^8$ m/s in all media
   C. Energies greater than 13 eV are capable of producing ionization
   D. Certain frequencies can be perceived by the eye
   E. Frequencies in the RF spectral region can stimulate hydrogen nuclei in a 1.5T magnetic field

2. What parameter indicates the distance between any two identical points on adjacent cycles of EM waves?
   A. Wavelength
   B. Frequency
   C. Amplitude
   D. Period

3. What is the frequency of red light with a wavelength of 700 nm in a vacuum?
   A. $7.5 \times 10^{14}$ Hz
   B. $4.3 \times 10^{14}$ Hz
   C. $3.0 \times 10^{14}$ Hz
   D. $2.5 \times 10^{14}$ Hz

4. Wave characteristics are more apparent when the EMR interacts with objects having dimensions:
   A. Much greater than the photon's $\lambda$
   B. Much smaller than the photon's $\lambda$
   C. Similar to the photon's $\lambda$
   D. Equal to the square root of the photon's $\lambda$

5. The minimum energies required to remove the outermost electron of an atom in its ground state is referred to as the:
   A. Transition energy
   B. Strong force
   C. Weak force
   D. Ionization energy

6. Which of the following consists of two protons and two neutrons and has a 2+ charge?
   A. Alpha particle
   B. Beta-minus particle
   C. Positron
   D. Beta-plus particle

7. Circle all following statements that are true regarding Auger electron emission:
   A. Predominates in elements where mass number is less than 99.
   B. Predominates in low Z elements.
   C. Energy released is transferred to an orbital electron, typically in the same shell as the cascading electron.
   D. Auger electron is ejected with kinetic energy equal to the difference in binding energy between origin shell of the cascading electron and its destination shell, minus the binding energy of the ejected Auger electron.

8. Regarding transmission of EMR through tissue (circle all correct statements):
   A. Nonionizing radiation is completely absorbed in tissues regardless of thickness.
   B. Most ionizing radiation incident on the patient from CT scans is transported through the patient where a small fraction is recorded on an image receptor.
   C. Optimum x-ray energy is a balance between sufficient energy to reach the target of interest and too much energy that may not interact with the target or image receptor.
   D. 64 MHz RF radiation can be transmitted into but not received from the body.

9. Which of the following will cause an increase in orbital electron binding energy?
   A. Increase in number of protons.
   B. Decrease in number of protons.
   C. Closer proximity of electrons to the positively charged nucleus.
   D. Answers a and c are both correct.

10. Which of the following refers to EMR emissions following an electron transition from the M shell to the K shell of an atom?
    A. Kα characteristic x-ray
    B. Kβ characteristic x-ray
    C. Lβ characteristic x-ray
    D. Kβ gamma ray

11. Calculate the energy equivalent of an electron with a mass of $9.109 \times 10^{-31}$ kg where $E$ is in joules. (c = $2.998 \times 10^8$ m/s):
    A. $3.038 \times 10^{-23}$ J
    B. $8.187 \times 10^{-14}$ J
    C. $2.723 \times 10^{-22}$ J
    D. $1.010 \times 10^{-47}$ J

12. Which of the following forces holds the nucleus together and is a contact force that operates only over very short (nuclear) distances (less than $10^{-15}$ m), beyond which it rapidly drops to zero?
    A. Gravity
    B. Electromagnetic force
    C. Weak force
    D. Strong force

13. On a plot of $Z$ versus $N$, stable nuclides fall along a "line of stability" for which the $N/Z$ ratio is approximately:
    A. 1.5 for low $Z$ nuclides and 1 for high $Z$ nuclides
    B. 1 for low $Z$ nuclides and 1.5 for high $Z$ nuclides
    C. 1 for both low and high $Z$ nuclides
    D. 1.5 for both low and high $Z$ nuclides

14. Following radioactive decay, which type EMR is emitted from the nucleus in an excited state which then transitions to lower (more stable) energy state?
    A. Gamma-rays
    B. X-rays
    C. Radio waves
    D. Infrared radiation

15. What is the process by which a nucleus with a large atomic mass captures a thermal neutron (low kinetic energy) and splits into two usually unequal parts, each with an average binding energy per nucleon greater than that of the original nucleus?
    A. Nuclear fusion
    B. Nuclear transformation
    C. Internal conversion
    D. Nuclear fission

16. What gives rise to the magnetic properties of the nucleus of an atom?
    A. Nuclides with excessive numbers of neutrons
    B. Nuclides with excessive numbers of protons
    C. Nuclides with an odd number of nucleons
    D. Nuclides with an even number of nucleons

# Answers

1.  **B**  Velocity ($v$) of EMR in a medium other than a vacuum is described by $v = c/n$ where a $n$ is the refractive index of the medium being traversed. *(Pg. 23)*

2.  **A**  Wavelength is the distance between any two identical points on adjacent cycles. Amplitude is the height (intensity) of the wave, frequency is the number of periods that occur per second, and period is the time required to complete once cycle (time for wave of $\lambda$ to pass a fixed point). *(Pg. 23)*

3.  **B**  $v = c/\lambda = (3 \times 10^8$ m/s$)(10^9$ nm/m$)/700$ nm$= 4.28 \times 10^{14}$ Hz. *(Pg. 23)*

4.  **C**  Wave characteristics are more apparent when EMR interacts with objects having dimensions similar to the photon's wavelength. For example, light photons with wavelengths of approximately $4$–$7 \times 10^{-7}$ m are separated into colors by a diffraction grating of tracks on a compact disc (CD) where the track separation ($1.6 \times 10^{-6}$ m) is of the same order of magnitude as the wavelength of light. *(Pg. 27)*

5.  **D**  The minimum energies required to remove the outermost electron of an atom in its ground state is referred to as the *ionization energy*. EMR with higher frequency of photons than the far UV region of spectrum (*e.g.*, x-rays and $\gamma$-rays) are called *ionizing radiation*. EMR with photon energies in and below the UV region (*e.g.*, visible, infrared, terahertz, microwave, and radio waves) are types of and referred to collectively as *non-ionizing radiation*. Without additional qualification, the *transition energy* is a nonspecific term. The *strong force* binds elementary particles together in clusters to form familiar subatomic particles, such as protons and neutrons. It is also responsible for holding the nucleus together. *Weak force* is responsible for radioactive decay, especially during beta decay. *(Pg. 28)*

6.  **A**  An alpha particle ($\alpha$) consists of two protons and two neutrons, giving it a $+2$ charge and is thus identical to the nucleus of a helium atom ($^4$He$^{2+}$). Many radioactive elements with large atomic numbers, such as uranium, thorium, and radium, emit $\alpha$ particles. *Beta-minus particles* are electrons emitted by the nuclei of radioactive atoms and are negatively charged. *Positrons,* also known as *beta-plus particles,* are positively charged electrons. *(Pg. 29)*

7.  **B,C,D**  B, C, and D are correct regarding *Auger electron emission*. A is incorrect because this would not be a low Z radionuclide. *(Pg. 34)*

8.  **C**  (A) Is not correct as RF energy can penetrate tissue as exemplified by the return signal in MRI. (B) Is not correct as typically less than 1% of the radiation incident on the entrance side of the patient emerges to be recorded on the image receptor. (C) Is correct because at the extremes (*e.g.*, energy too low), the photons will be completely absorbed in the body and thus never reach the image receptor or be too high such that the probability that they interact with either the anatomy of interest or the image receptor will be too low. (D) False, this is RF output signal is picked up by the RF receive coil and transmitted to an RF amplifier for the reconstruction of the image in the main computer. *(Pg. 26)*

9.  **D**  Due to the closer proximity of the electrons to the positively charged nucleus, the binding energy of the K shell is greater than that of outer shells. For a particular electron shell, binding energy also increases with the number of protons in the nucleus (*i.e.*, atomic number). The energy necessary to separate electrons (ionize) in particular orbits from the atom (not drawn to scale) increases with $Z$ and decreases with distance from the nucleus. *(Pg. 32)*

10. **B**  If the vacancy in one shell is filled by the adjacent shell, it is identified by a subscript $\alpha$ *for example, $L \rightarrow K$* transition $= K\alpha$, $M \rightarrow L$ transition $= L\alpha$. If the electron vacancy is filled from a nonadjacent shell, as described in the question, the subscript beta is used, so $M \rightarrow K$ transition $= K\beta$. *(Pg. 33)*

11. **B**   $E = mc^2 = (9.109 \times 10^{-31}\text{ kg}) (2.998 \times 10^8\text{ m/s})^2 = 8.187 \times 10^{-14}\text{ kg ms}^{-1}$ or $8.187 \times 10^{-14}$ J where 1 kg ms$^{-1}$ = 1 J. (*Pg. 30*)

12. **D**   *Strong forces (D)* act between nucleons (n-p, n-n, and p-p) through the exchange of mesons (quark/anti-quark pairs with opposite color charge) and is one of the strongest known force in the universe. It only operates over extremely short (subatomic) distances. The strong force binds elementary particles together in clusters to make more familiar subatomic particles, such as protons and neutrons. The strong force is also responsible for holding the nucleus together by overcoming the substantial electrostatic repulsive forces between protons held together in an unimaginably small volume. *Gravity (A)* is a strong planetary force but very weak at the subatomic atomic level. For example, it holds your feet on the ground and the universe together. *Electromagnetic forces (B)* hold atoms together and provides formation of chemical bonds. *Weak forces (C)* are responsible for radioactive decay, for example, beta decay, where a neutron within the nucleus is transformed into a proton and an electron (beta-minus particle) and an antineutrino that are ejected from the nucleus. (*Pg. 36*)

13. **B**   On a plot of *Z* versus *N*, stable nuclides fall along a "line of stability" for which the *N/Z* ratio is approximately 1 for low *Z* nuclides and approximately 1.5 for high *Z* nuclide. Only four nuclides with odd numbers of neutrons and odd numbers of protons are stable, whereas many more nuclides with even numbers of neutrons and even numbers of protons are stable. (*Pg. 37*)

14. **A**   The EMR emitted from the nucleus as the excited state transitions to a lower (more stable) energy state is referred to as *gamma rays*. This energy transition is analogous to the emission of characteristic x-rays following electron transitions; however, γ-rays (by definition) emanate from the nucleus. (*Pg. 37*)

15. **D**   *Nuclear fission (D)* is the process by which a nucleus with a large atomic mass captures a neutron and splits into two usually unequal parts called *fission fragments*, each with an average binding energy per nucleon greater than that of the original nucleus. *Nuclear fusion (A)*, on the other hand, is the release of energy by combining (fusing) light atomic nuclei. *Internal conversion (C)* is a form of de-excitation in which the de-excitation energy is completely transferred to an orbital electron. The conversion electron is ejected from the atom, with a kinetic energy equal to the difference between the γ-ray and the electron binding energy. During *nuclear transformation (B)*, simply refers to a process by which the nucleons within unstable nuclei of radioactive atoms transform into more stable energy states. (*Pg. 40*)

16. **C**   The nuclear magnetic characteristics are determined by the number of nucleons (protons and neutrons) in the nucleus. For an odd number of protons (or neutrons) and even number of neutrons (or protons) a noninteger spin will be exhibited, which is an odd number of nucleons. This generates a magnetic moment that is used in MRI. Note that nuclei with an odd number of protons and odd number of neutrons (only 4 stable nuclides in this category) also generate a magnetic moment. (*Pg. 37, Table 2-3*)

# Section III Key Equations and Symbols

| QUANTITY | EQUATION | EQ NO./PAGE/COMMENTS |
|---|---|---|
| Energy | $E = h\nu$ | Where $h$ is Planck's constant ($6.62607004 \times 10^{-34}$ kg m²s⁻¹). $\nu$ = frequency. |
| Speed $(c)$ of EM wave in a vacuum | $c = \lambda\nu$ | Eq. 2-1/Pg. 23/Relates the speed $(c)$, wavelength, and frequency of all EM waves in a vacuum |
| Speed $(v)$ of any wave in a medium with refractive index $(n)$ | $v = c/n$ | Eq. 2-2/Pg. 23 |
| Energy of a photon | $E = h\nu = \dfrac{hc}{\lambda}$ | Eq. 2-3/Pg. 27/Where Planck's constant $(h)$ = $6.626 \times 10^{-34}$ J-s = $4.136 \times 10^{-18}$ keV-s |
| When $E$ is expressed in keV and $\lambda$ in nanometers (nm) | $E\,(\text{keV}) = \dfrac{1.24}{\lambda(\text{nm})}$ | Eq. 2-4/Pg. 27/Based on values from Eq. 2-3 |
| Relationship between the mass and the energy in any system | $E = mc^2$ | Eq. 2-5/Pg. 30/Energy $E$ in joules (J) (where 1 kg m²s⁻² = 1 J) represents the energy equivalent to mass $m$ at rest and $c$ is the speed of light in a vacuum ($2.998 \times 10^8$ m/s) |

| SYMBOL | QUANTITY | UNITS |
|---|---|---|
| $A$ | Number of protons and neutrons | Mass number |
| $Z$ | Number of protons | Atomic number |
| eV | Used to express energies of photons | Electron volts: multiples of eV common to medical imaging are keV (1,000 eV) and MeV (1,000,000 eV) |
| $\lambda$ | Measures the distance between any two identical points on adjacent cycles | Wavelength |
| $\nu$ | The number of periods per second | Frequency |
| Hz | Expresses frequency | Hertz, 1 Hz= 1 cycle/s; MHz |
| J | Energy | Joules |
| $E$ | Energy | Where 1 kg m²s⁻²= 1 J |
| $\tau$ | Time required to complete one cycle | Period |
| $n$ | Refractive index | Unitless |
| T | Magnetic (B-field) strength (also, magnetic flux density) | Tesla |
| $h$ | $6.626 \times 10^{-34}$ J-s = $4.136 \times 10^{-18}$ keV-s | Planck's constant |
| $\alpha$ | Alpha particle | Unitless |
| $\beta^+$ | Beta-plus particle | Unitless |
| $\beta^-$ | Beta-minus particle | Unitless |
| $m$ | Mass | kg; amu |
| $c$ | Speed of light in a vacuum | $2.998 \times 10^8$ m s⁻¹ |
| $v$ | Speed | m s⁻¹ |

# CHAPTER 3

# Interaction of Radiation with Matter

## 3.0 INTRODUCTION

This chapter introduces the concepts and principles that govern x- and γ-ray photon interactions with matter and the energetic electrons those interactions set into motion. It considers the fate of these electrons as they subsequently transfer and distribute their kinetic energy in the material they traverse. The photons with energy typical of diagnostic imaging are either completely absorbed by or scattered by electrons in the medium they traverse. Having absorbed this additional energy, the electrons are either elevated to an "excited" energy state within the atom or ejected from it creating a positive ion from a neutral atom. Ejected electrons with sufficient kinetic energy undergo multiple interactions with surrounding electrons during which their energy is transferred to the surrounding medium via excitation, ionization, and radiative emissions.

## 3.1 PARTICLE INTERACTIONS

Particles of ionizing radiation include charged particles, such as alpha particles ($\alpha^{+2}$), protons ($p^+$), beta particles ($\beta^-$), positrons ($\beta^+$), and energetic extranuclear electrons ($e^-$), and uncharged particles, such as neutrons. The behavior of heavy charged particles (*e.g.*, alpha particles and protons) is different than that of lighter charged particles such as electrons and positrons.

1. **Excitation, ionization, and radiative losses:** Energetic charged particles interact with matter by electrical (*i.e.*, coulombic) forces and lose kinetic energy via excitation, ionization, and radiative losses. Excitation and ionization occur when charged particles lose energy by interacting with orbital electrons in the medium. These interactional, or collisional, losses occur due to the coulombic forces exerted on charged particles when they pass in proximity to the electric field generated by the atom's electrons and protons.
2. **Excitation:**
   a. Occurs when energy transferred to an electron does not exceed its binding energy
   b. Following excitation (Fig. 3-1A), de-excitation occurs as the electron returns to a lower energy level releasing energy by either:
      (i) Emitting it in the form of electromagnetic radiation (Fig. 3-1B) or
      (ii) Transferring the energy to a weakly bound orbital electron which is ejected as an "Auger" electron (Fig. 3-1C)

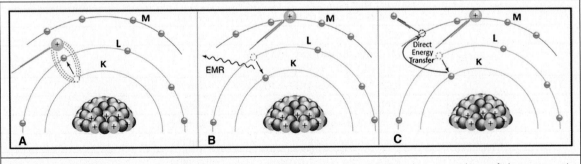

■ **FIGURE 3-1 A.** Excitation of a K-shell electron to the L-shell. **B.** De-excitation with the subsequent release of electromagnetic radiation (EMR). **C.** Auger electron emission resulting from EMR interacting with M-shell electron. 📖 **F. 3-1A** (MODIFIED)

**3. Ionization:**
  **a.** Occurs when transferred energy exceeds the binding energy (Fig. 3-2)
  **b.** Electron is ejected from the atom
  **c.** Results in an ion pair consisting of an ejected electron and a positively charged atom
  **d.** Secondary ionization occurs when the ejected electron has sufficient energy to produce further ionization, these electrons are called delta rays

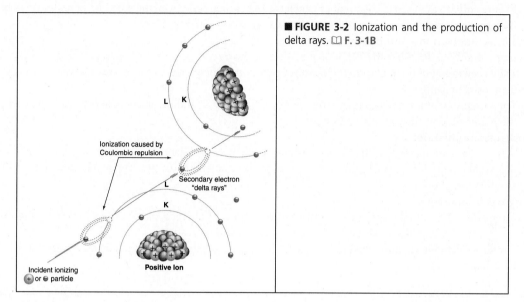

■ **FIGURE 3-2** Ionization and the production of delta rays. 📖 **F. 3-1B**

**4. Radiative losses:**
  **a.** As electron energy decreases, the probability of energy loss via excitation increases
**5. Specific ionization:**
  **a.** The average number of primary and secondary ion pairs produced per unit length of a charged particle's path
  **b.** Specific ionization (SI) $\propto \dfrac{Q^2}{v^2}$, where $Q$ is the electrical charge and $v$ is the velocity of the incident particle
  **c.** The maximum specific ionization is referred to as the *Bragg peak*
    **(i)** Beyond the peak there is a rapid decrease in SI as the particle acquires electrons, becoming electrically neutral, and losing its capacity for further ionization (Fig. 3-3)
**6. Charged particle tracks:**
  **a.** Electrons follow tortuous paths as the result of multiple scattering events caused by coulombic deflections (repulsion, and/or attraction), Fig. 3-4A.
  **b.** Heavy charged particles have dense and usually linear ionization tracks (Fig. 3-4B).
  **c.** Path-length of a particle is defined as the distance the particle travels.
  **d.** Range is the depth of penetration of the particle in matter.

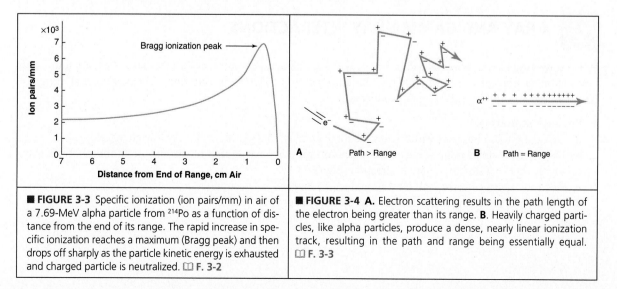

■ **FIGURE 3-3** Specific ionization (ion pairs/mm) in air of a 7.69-MeV alpha particle from $^{214}$Po as a function of distance from the end of its range. The rapid increase in specific ionization reaches a maximum (Bragg peak) and then drops off sharply as the particle kinetic energy is exhausted and charged particle is neutralized. 📖 **F. 3-2**

■ **FIGURE 3-4 A.** Electron scattering results in the path length of the electron being greater than its range. **B.** Heavily charged particles, like alpha particles, produce a dense, nearly linear ionization track, resulting in the path and range being essentially equal. 📖 **F. 3-3**

7. **Linear energy transfer (LET):**
    a. A measure of the average amount of energy deposited locally in the absorber per unit path length.
    b. For charged particles LET $\propto Q^2/E_k$, where $Q$ is the charge and $E_k$ is the particle kinetic energy
        (i)   High LET: dense short-range ionization tracks that are much more damaging
        (ii)  Low LET: sparse ionization patterns and produce less damage to cells
8. **Scattering:** an interaction that deflects a particle or photon from its original trajectory
    a. **Elastic collisions:** A scattering event in which the total kinetic energy of the colliding particles is unchanged
    b. **Inelastic collisions:** When scattering occurs with a loss of kinetic energy
9. **Radiative interactions—bremsstrahlung:**
    a. Bremsstrahlung describes the radiation emission accompanying electron deceleration (Fig. 3-5).
    b. The deceleration of the high-speed electrons in an x-ray tube produces the bremsstrahlung x-rays used in diagnostic imaging.
    c. Total bremsstrahlung emission per atom is proportional to $Z^2$ and inversely proportional to the square of the mass of the incident particle, $Z^2/m^2$.
10. **Positron annihilation:**
    a. When a positron interacts with an electron, resulting in the annihilation of an electron-positron pair, resulting in the complete conversion of their rest mass into the energy of two oppositely directed 0.511 MeV annihilation photons
11. **Neutron interactions:**
    a. Interaction with atomic nuclei can result in the ejection of charged particles (*e.g.*, protons, Fig. 3-6) or nuclear fission fragments that directly cause excitation and ionization
    b. Particles ejected from atomic nuclei and fission fragments created following neutron absorption have very high kinetic energies

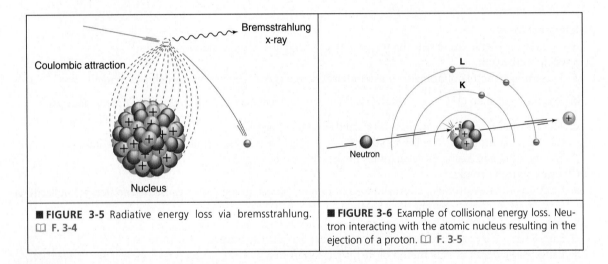

■ **FIGURE 3-5** Radiative energy loss via bremsstrahlung. 📖 **F. 3-4**

■ **FIGURE 3-6** Example of collisional energy loss. Neutron interacting with the atomic nucleus resulting in the ejection of a proton. 📖 **F. 3-5**

## 3.2   X-RAY AND GAMMA-RAY INTERACTIONS

When traversing matter, photons will penetrate without interaction, scatter, or be absorbed. There are four major types of interactions of x-ray and γ-ray photons with matter: (1) Rayleigh scattering, (2) Compton scattering, (3) photoelectric absorption, and (4) pair production.

1. **Rayleigh scattering:**
    a. Incident photon interacts with/excites the total atom, occurs mainly with very low energy x-rays.
    b. The electron cloud immediately emits a photon proportional to that of the change in the photon's wave energy, but in a slightly different direction (Fig. 3-7).
    c. Electrons are not ejected, and ionization does not occur.
    d. The average scattering angle decreases as the x-ray energy increases.

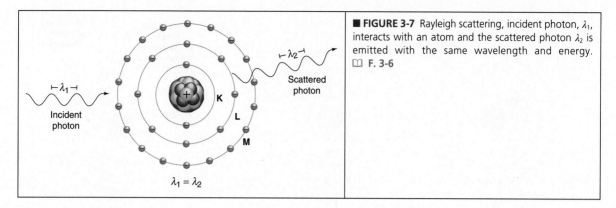

■ **FIGURE 3-7** Rayleigh scattering, incident photon, $\lambda_1$, interacts with an atom and the scattered photon $\lambda_2$ is emitted with the same wavelength and energy. 📖 **F. 3-6**

2. **Compton scattering**:
   a. Predominant interaction of x-ray and γ-ray photons in the diagnostic energy range with soft tissue.
   b. Occurs between photons and valence-shell electrons (Fig. 3-8), the electron is ejected from the atom, and the scattered photon is emitted with some reduction in energy.
   c. The ejected electron loses kinetic energy via excitation and ionization.
   d. The energy of the incident photon ($E_o$) is equal to the sum of the energy of the scattered photon ($E_{sc}$) and the kinetic energy of the ejected electron ($E_{e^-}$), (Eq. 3-1)

$$E_o = E_{sc} + E_{e^-}$$

   [3-1]

   e. The energy of the scattered photon can be calculated using Equation 3-2, where $E_{sc}$ = energy of the scattered photon, $E_o$ = incident photon energy, and θ = angle of the scattered photon

$$E_{sc} = \frac{E_o}{1 + \frac{E_o}{511 \text{ keV}}(1 - \cos\theta)}$$

   [3-2]

   f. As incident photon energy increases, the fraction of energy transferred to the scattered photon decreases and the photon and electrons are preferentially scattered in the forward direction (Fig. 3-9).

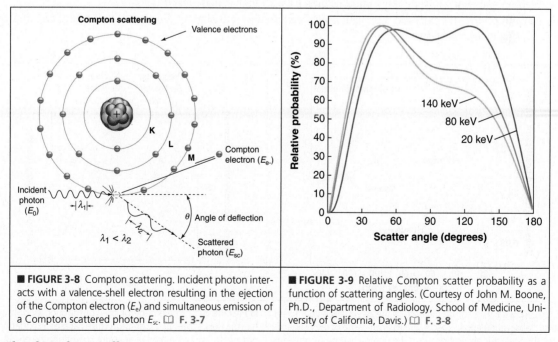

■ **FIGURE 3-8** Compton scattering. Incident photon interacts with a valence-shell electron resulting in the ejection of the Compton electron ($E_e$) and simultaneous emission of a Compton scattered photon $E_{sc}$. 📖 **F. 3-7**

■ **FIGURE 3-9** Relative Compton scatter probability as a function of scattering angles. (Courtesy of John M. Boone, Ph.D., Department of Radiology, School of Medicine, University of California, Davis.) 📖 **F. 3-8**

3. **The photoelectric effect**:
   a. Occurs when the incident photon energy is greater than or equal to the binding energy of the ejected electron.
   b. All of the incident photon energy is transferred to an electron, which is ejected from the atom.
   c. The kinetic energy of the ejected photoelectron ($E_{pe}$) is equal to the incident photon energy ($E_o$) minus the binding energy of the orbital electron ($E_b$) (Eq. 3-3) (Fig. 3-10A)

$$E_{pe} = E_o + E_b$$

   [3-3]

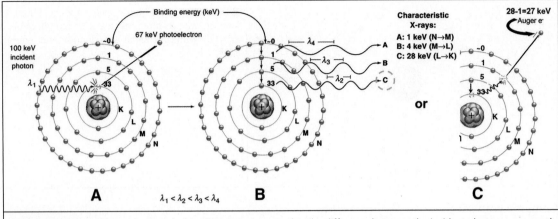

**■ FIGURE 3-10 A**. Electron is ejected with a kinetic energy equal to the difference between the incident photon energy and binding energy. **B**. Electron cascade created from the vacancy previously created, this will continue until the production of characteristic x-ray. **C**. Auger electron emission is an alternative process in which the difference in binding energy (transition energy), which would otherwise have been emitted as a characteristic x-ray, is instantaneously transferred to an electron in the same atom whose binding energy is less than the transition energy. Since the L → K characteristic x-ray is 28 keV, the Auger electron energy is 28 keV − 1 keV = 27 keV. 📖 **F. 3-9**

   **d.** Following a photoelectric interaction, the atom is ionized, with an inner-shell electron vacancy. Creating a cascade of vacancies to be filled with electrons from a shell with lower binding energies.

   **e.** The difference in binding energy is released as either characteristic x-rays or Auger electrons (see Chapter 2).

   **f.** The probability of photoelectric absorption $\propto Z^3/E^3$, where $Z$ is the atomic number, and $E$ is the energy of the incident photon.

   **g.** Optimal for x-ray imaging as there are no scattered photons to degrade the image.

      **(i)** Probability is $\propto Z^3/E^3$ which explains why the image contrast decreases when higher x-ray energies are used in the imaging process (see Chapters 4 and 7)

   **h.** For every element, the probability of the photoelectric effect, as a function of photon energy, exhibits sharp discontinuities called absorption edges (see Fig. 3-11).

   **i.** Predominate when lower energy photons interact with high $Z$ materials (Fig. 3-12)

      **(i)** Amplifies differences in attenuation between tissues with slightly different atomic numbers, improving image contrast

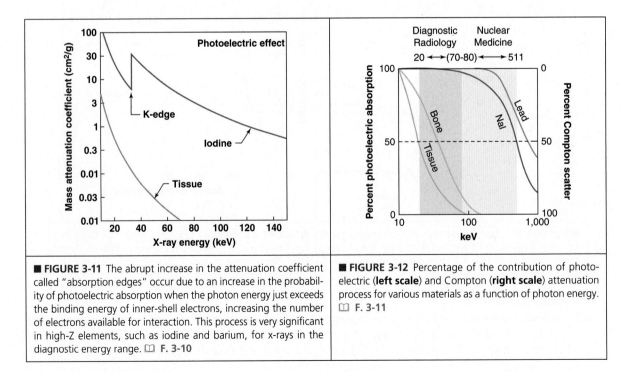

**■ FIGURE 3-11** The abrupt increase in the attenuation coefficient called "absorption edges" occur due to an increase in the probability of photoelectric absorption when the photon energy just exceeds the binding energy of inner-shell electrons, increasing the number of electrons available for interaction. This process is very significant in high-Z elements, such as iodine and barium, for x-rays in the diagnostic energy range. 📖 **F. 3-10**

**■ FIGURE 3-12** Percentage of the contribution of photoelectric (**left scale**) and Compton (**right scale**) attenuation process for various materials as a function of photon energy. 📖 **F. 3-11**

4. **Pair production:**
   a. Only occurs when the energies of x-rays and γ-rays exceed 1.02 MeV.
   b. An x-ray or γ-rays interacts with the electric field, the photon's energy is transformed into an electron-positron pair (Fig. 3-13A).
   c. The rest mass energy equivalent of each electron is 0.511 MeV, thus the energy threshold for this reaction is 1.02 MeV.
   d. The electron and positron lose their kinetic energy via excitation and ionization. When the positron comes to rest, it interacts with a negatively charged electron, resulting in the formation of two oppositely directed 0.511-MeV annihilation photons (Fig. 3-13B).

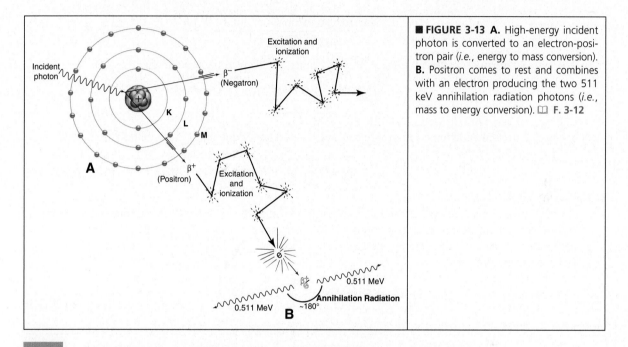

■ **FIGURE 3-13 A.** High-energy incident photon is converted to an electron-positron pair (*i.e.*, energy to mass conversion). **B.** Positron comes to rest and combines with an electron producing the two 511 keV annihilation radiation photons (*i.e.*, mass to energy conversion). F. 3-12

## 3.3  ATTENUATION OF X-RAYS AND GAMMA RAYS

Attenuation is the removal of photons from a beam of x-rays or γ-rays as it passes through matter, caused by absorption and scattering of primary photons. At low photon energies (less than 26 keV), the photoelectric effect dominates the attenuation processes in soft tissue. The probability of photoelectric absorption is highly dependent on photon energy and the atomic number of the absorber. When higher energy photons interact with low $Z$ materials (*e.g.*, soft tissue), Compton scattering dominates (Fig. 3-14).

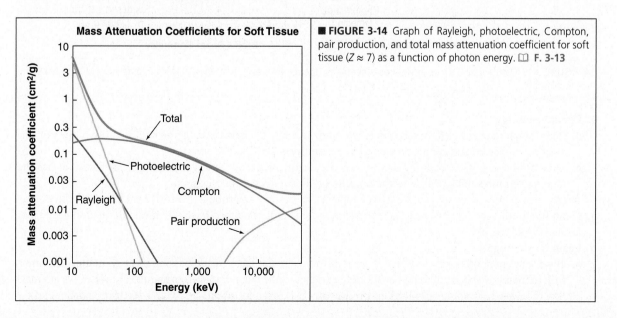

■ **FIGURE 3-14** Graph of Rayleigh, photoelectric, Compton, pair production, and total mass attenuation coefficient for soft tissue ($Z \approx 7$) as a function of photon energy. F. 3-13

1. **Linear attenuation coefficient:**
   a. The fraction of photons removed from a monoenergetic beam of x-rays or γ-rays per extremely thin unit thickness of material is called the linear attenuation coefficient (μ).
   b. The number of photons removed ($n$) from the beam of ($N_o$) photons traversing a very extremely thin $\Delta x$, (Eq. 3-4)

$$n = \mu N_o \Delta x \qquad [3\text{-}4]$$

2. **Mass attenuation coefficient:**
   a. The mass attenuation coefficient (Eq. 3-5) is the linear attenuation coefficient normalized to unit density, mathematically expressed as:

$$\frac{\mu}{\rho} = \frac{\text{Linear Attenuation Coefficient}}{\text{Density of Material}} \qquad [3\text{-}5] \quad \text{📖 E. 3-7}$$

   b. The mass attenuation coefficient is *independent of density*. For a given photon energy,

$$\frac{\mu_{\text{water}}}{\rho_{\text{water}}} = \frac{\mu_{\text{ice}}}{\rho_{\text{ice}}} = \frac{\mu_{\text{water vapor}}}{\rho_{\text{water vapor}}}$$

   c. To use the mass attenuation coefficient to compute attenuation, Equation 3-5 can be rewritten as:

$$N = N_o e^{-\left(\frac{\mu}{\rho}\right)\rho x} \qquad [3\text{-}6] \quad \text{📖 E. 3-8}$$

3. **Half-value layer (HVL):**
   a. The thickness of material required to reduce the intensity of an x-ray or γ-ray beam to one-half of its initial value (Eq. 3-7); measured under conditions of "narrow-beam geometry" (Fig. 3-15).
   b. This indirect measure of the photon energies is sometimes referred to as the beam quality.
   c. For a monoenergetic beam,

$$\text{HVL} = \frac{N_o}{2} = N_o e^{-\mu(\text{HVL})}; \text{HVL} = \frac{0.693}{\mu} \qquad [3\text{-}7] \quad \text{📖 E. 3-9}$$

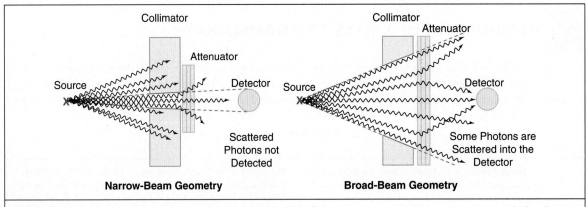

**■ FIGURE 3-15** Narrow-beam versus broad-beam geometry, the differences in scattered photons interacting with the detector are highlighted.

4. **Effective energy:**
   a. Determination of the HVL in diagnostic radiology is a way of characterizing the penetrability of the polyenergetic x-ray beam and can be converted to a quantity called *effective energy*.
   b. The effective energy of an x-ray spectrum is the energy of a mono-energetic beam of photons that has the same penetrating ability (HVL) as the polyenergetic spectrum of photons.
   c. Effective energy of an x-ray beam from a typical diagnostic x-ray tube is 1/3 to 1/2 the maximal value.
5. **Mean free path**—average distance traveled before interaction, calculated from the linear attenuation coefficient or the HVL of the beam
6. **Beam hardening:**
   a. Lower energy photons of x-ray beams are removed from the beam while passing through matter, causing a shift of the x-ray spectrum to higher effective energies as the beam transverses matter. This selective attenuation of lower (soft) energy photons is also referred to as beam filtration. (See Fig. 3-16, text, and Chapter 6.)

   b. X-ray machines remove most of this soft radiation with filters made of various materials inherent to the x-ray tube (inherent filtration) and additional metals depending on the application.
   c. Molybdenum is commonly used in mammography (which uses low-energy photons). Other types of x-ray imaging systems generally use aluminum, copper, or tin.
   d. Regardless of the actual material used, in most cases, the extent of the filtration is expressed as the equivalent thickness of aluminum that would produce the same attenuation.
   e. Added filtration will result in an x-ray beam with higher effective energy and a greater HVL.
   f. FDA regulations require a minimum total filtration of 2.5 mm of aluminum equivalent for x-ray tubes operating above 70 kV.

## 3.4   ABSORPTION OF ENERGY FROM X-RAYS AND GAMMA RAYS

1. **Fluence ($\Phi$):** The number of photons/particles passing through a unit cross-sectional area is referred to as the fluence (Eq. 3-8)

$$\Phi = \frac{\text{Photons}}{\text{Area}}$$                [3-8]   📖 E. 3-11

2. **Flux ($\dot{\phi}$):** Defined as fluence per unit time (Eq. 3-9). The flux is useful in situations in which a photon beam is on for extended durations, such as in fluoroscopy.

$$\dot{\Phi} = \frac{\text{Photons}}{\text{Area} \times \text{Time}}$$                [3-9]   📖 E. 3-12

3. **Energy fluence ($\Psi$):** The amount of energy passing through a unit cross-sectional area is referred to as energy fluence (Eq. 3-10)
   a. For monoenergetic beams of photons the energy fluence

$$\Psi = \text{fluence}\ (\Phi) \times \text{energy per photon}\ (E)$$                [3-10]   📖 E. 3-13

   b. For polyenergetic spectrums, the total energy in the beam is calculated by multiplying the number of photons at each energy by that energy and adding the products.
4. **Mass energy transfer coefficient:** The mass attenuation coefficient multiplied by the fraction of the energy of interacting photons transferred to charged particles as kinetic energy.
   a. Energy in scattered photons that escape the interaction site is not transferred to charged particles in the volume of interest.
   b. When pair production occurs, 1.02 MeV of the incident photon's energy is required to produce the electron-positron pair and the remaining energy is given to the electron and positron as kinetic energy.
5. **Kerma ($K$):** Kinetic energy transferred to charged particles by indirectly ionizing radiation (x-rays & $\gamma$-rays) per unit mass (Eq. 3-11)
   a. Energy is deposited in the medium in a two-step process:
      **(i)** Step 1: Energy carried by the indirectly ionizing radiation is transformed into kinetic energy of charged particles
         **1.** For x-rays and $\gamma$-rays, transfer is via Compton scattering or photoelectric absorption
         **2.** For very high energy photons, energy is transferred via pair production
      **(ii)** Step 2: Directly ionizing particles deposit their energy locally by excitation and ionization
6. **Calculation of kerma**
   a. The mass energy-transfer coefficient $(\mu_{tr}/\rho)_E$ multiplied by the photon energy fluence, $\Psi$, gives the dosimetric quantity *kerma* (note: $\Psi = \Phi E$, where $\Phi$ is the photon fluence and $E$ the photon energy)

$$K = \Psi \left( \frac{\mu_{tr}}{\rho} \right)_E$$                [3-11]   📖 E. 3-14 corrected.

   where $\left( \dfrac{\mu_{tr}}{\rho} \right)_E$ is the mass-energy transfer coefficient of the absorber at energy $E$

   b. Kerma can be expressed in either energy unity per mass (J/kg) or the special name specific to the energy deposited by ionizing radiation, the *gray* (Gy) where 1 Gy = 1 J/kg

7. **Mass-energy absorption coefficient** $\left(\dfrac{\mu_{en}}{\rho}\right)$
   a. The same as the mass-energy transfer coefficient when all transferred energy is absorbed locally
   b. When diagnostic x-rays interact with low-Z absorbers, the radiative losses are minimal and thus

   $$\left(\frac{\mu_{en}}{\rho}\right) \cong \left(\frac{\mu_{tr}}{\rho}\right)$$

8. **Absorbed dose (D):**
   a. Absorbed dose is defined for all types of ionizing radiation (Eq. 3-12).
   b. The energy (E) imparted by ionizing radiation per unit mass (m):

   $$D = \frac{E}{m} \qquad\qquad \text{[3-11]} \quad \text{E. 3-15}$$

   c. Charged particles deposit imparted energy locally, when bremsstrahlung production is negligible, kerma will be equal to the absorbed dose.
   d. For X-rays and $\gamma$-rays, the absorbed dose, D (Eq. 3-13), is calculated from the mass-energy absorption coefficient and the energy fluence at photon energy E

   $$D = \psi\left(\frac{\mu_{en}}{\rho}\right)_E \qquad\qquad \text{[3-13]} \quad \text{E. 3-16 CORRECTED}$$

   e. The absorbed dose is expressed in either energ unit per mass (J/kg) or in units of Gy gray (Gy).

9. **Exposure:** The amount of electrical charge (Q) produced by ionizing electromagnetic radiation per mass (m) of air is called exposure, X (Eq. 3-14):

   $$X = \frac{Q}{m_{air}} \qquad\qquad \text{[3-14]} \quad \text{E. 3-17}$$

   The historical unit of exposure is the Roentgen (R), where 1 R = $2.58 \times 10^{-4}$ C/kg air and coulomb (C) is the unit of charge
   a. X is nearly proportional to dose in soft tissue over the range of photon energies used in radiology.
   b. The average energy deposited per ion pair in air (W) is approximately constant as a function of photon energy (33.97 eV/ion pair or 33.97 J/C).
   c. W is calculated from the dose to air (Eq. 3-15). Using dose to air ($D_{air}$), and the exposure ($X_{air}$) in air

   $$W = \frac{D_{air}}{X_{air}} = \frac{E}{Q} \qquad\qquad \text{[3-15]} \quad \text{E. 3-18}$$

## 3.5    IMPARTED ENERGY, EQUIVALENT DOSE, AND EFFECTIVE DOSE

1. **Imparted energy:**
   a. Total amount of energy deposited in a given amount of matter
   b. Product of the absorbed dose and the mass over which the energy was imparted
2. **Modality-specific dosimetric quantities** specific to CT and fluoroscopy are discussed in Chapter 11, mammography in Chapter 8, dose metrics defined for radiation protection by regulatory agencies are discussed further in Chapter 21.
3. **Equivalent dose:**
   a. Not a "real" dose but rather a dose-weighted radiation protection quantity incorporating the biological variability of potential long term adverse effects of radiations with significantly different LETs.

   Equivalent dose to tissue $T\left(H_T\right)$

   = Absorbed Dose to tissue $T\left(D_T\right) \times$ Radiation Weighting Factor $\left(w_R\right)$    [3-16]    E. 3-23 modified

   (i)  $w_R$ = 1.0 for x- and $\gamma$-rays and electrons including beta particles.

**a.** $w_R$ is greater than 1 for protons, neutrons, alpha because they produce more dense ionization tracks that have a greater capacity to cause biological damage. See Section III for specific $w_R$ values.

**b.** The product of the absorbed dose (Gy) of the organ/tissue irradiated and the $w_R$ (unitless) of the radiation is given the special radiation protection name, *equivalent dose*, ($H_T$) and is expressed in units of *sieverts* (Sv).

**c.** The previous (non-SI) unit for equivalent dose was the **rad** (radiation absorbed dose), where 100 rad = 1 Gy

4. **Effective dose:**

  **a.** Not a real "dose" but rather an equivalent dose tissue-weighted radiation protection quantity incorporating relative inherent differences in organ system sensitivity to potential long term adverse effects of radiation exposure

  **b.** Biological tissues vary in their sensitivity to induction of long-term effects (like cancer) from exposure to ionizing radiation

  **(i)** Tissue weighting factors ($w_T$), assigned to a particular organ or tissue corresponding to the fraction of the total risk ($x/1.0$) that would have come from that organ or tissue if the whole body was irradiated. See Section III for specific $w_T$ values.

  **(ii)** The sum of the products of the equivalent dose to each organ/tissue irradiated ($H_T$) and its corresponding tissue weighting factor ($w_T$) is given the special radiation protection name, *effective dose*, (E) and is also expressed in units of sievert (Sv)

$$E(\text{Sv}) = \sum_T \left[ w_T \times H_T (\text{Sv}) \right]$$

[3-17]    📖 **E. 3-25**

  **(iii)** Effective dose should not be used as a substitute for (or as part of an estimate of) individual patient, public, or worker risk from radiation exposure. Only absorbed dose and the appropriate age, gender, and other potential qualifying factors associated with a specific dose-response risk metrics should be used for such purposes.

  **c.** The previous (non-SI) unit for effective dose was the **rem** (radiation equivalent in man), where 100 rem = 1 Sv

# Section II Questions and Answers

1. What is the ratio of mass attenuation coefficients, $\mu/\rho$, in calcium deposits ($Z_{eff} \sim 11$; $\rho \sim 1.92$ g/cm$^3$) compared to that of normal breast tissue ($Z_{eff} \sim 7$; $P \cong 1.02$ g/cm$^3$) for 20 keV x-rays?
   A. 0.8                  D. 4.1
   B. 1.4                  E. 5.9
   C. 2.6

2. The traditional unit of absorbed dose is the rad. One rad is equal to
   A. 1.0 mGy              C. 0.1 mGy
   B. 10 J/kg              D. 0.01 J/kg

3. The incident energy of a photon that undergoes Compton scattering is 250 keV and scatters at an angle of 180°. What is the energy of the scattered photon?
   A. 12.6 keV             C. 126.4 keV
   B. 12.6 MeV             D. 126.4 MeV

4. For monoenergetic photons under narrow-beam geometry conditions, how many HVLs are needed to attenuate 97% of photons?
   A. 3                    D. 7
   B. 4                    E. 9
   C. 5

5. The mean free path (MFP) can be calculated using which of the following?
   A. The linear attenuation coefficient
   B. The energy of the beam
   C. The half value layer (HVL) of the beam
   D. Both A and C
   E. All of the above

6. Electrons ejected from their atoms as a result of the interaction with a photoelectron in matter are referred to as?
   A. Characteristic particles
   B. Delta rays
   C. Incident ionizing particle
   D. Energetic extranuclear electrons ($e^-$)
   E. Beta particle ($\beta^+$)

7. The depth of penetration of a particle in matter is the definition of:
   A. Mean free path (MFP)
   B. Path length
   C. Linear ionization track
   D. Range

8. Total bremsstrahlung emission is proportional to:
   A. $Z/M$                C. $Z^2M^2$
   B. $M/Z$                D. $M^2/Z^2$

9. Given an HVL of 5.6 mm for a monoenergetic beam, find the linear attenuation coefficient.
   A. 0.12 cm$^{-1}$       C. 2.6 cm$^{-1}$
   B. 1.2 cm$^{-1}$        D. 3.8 cm$^{-1}$

10. Compared to high linear energy transfer (LET) radiation, low LET radiation of the same energy has:
    A. Dense ionization tracks, and short ranges
    B. Short ionization range, and more damage
    C. Sparse ionization tracks, and short ranges
    D. Longer path length, and less damage
    E. Dense ionization tracks, and more damage

11. An incident photon interacting with and exciting the total atom describes which of the following:
    A. Rayleigh scattering
    B. The photoelectric effect
    C. Compton scattering
    D. Pair production

12. The energy ($E$) imparted by ionizing radiation per unit mass of irradiated material ($m$) best describes:
    A. Effective dose       D. Kerma
    B. Exposure             E. Equivalent dose
    C. Absorbed dose

13. The photon energy necessary to produce the photoelectric effect in a given inner shell electron, corresponding to a particular absorption edge increases with the _____ of an element:
    A. Density ($\rho$)
    B. Number of valence electrons
    C. Atomic number ($Z$)
    D. Binding energy
    E. Stopping power

14. Which of the following is the correct mathematical expression for the probability of interaction for incident monoenergetic photons traversing a defined thickness $x$:

    A. $N = N_o e^{-\mu^x}$
    
    B. $(x) = 1 - e^{-\mu^x}$
    
    C. $(x) = e^{-N\mu^x}$
    
    D. $I(x) = I(0)e^{-N\mu^x}$

15. Photoelectric absorption results in the production of which of the following?

    A. A photoelectron, negative ion, and delta rays
    
    B. A photoelectron, negative ion, and characteristic x-rays/Auger electrons
    
    C. A positive ion, characteristic x-rays/Auger electrons, and delta rays
    
    D. A negative ion, characteristic x-rays/Auger electrons, and gamma rays
    
    E. A photoelectron, positive ion, and/or characteristic x-rays/Auger electrons

16. What x and γ-ray interactions predominant in the diagnostic energy range with soft tissue?

    A. Compton scattering
    
    B. Pair production
    
    C. Rayleigh scattering
    
    D. Photoelectric effect

17. What is the quantity that reflects the sum of the products of the equivalent dose to each organ ($H_T$) and the corresponding weighting factor ($w_T$) for the organ?

    A. Effective dose
    
    B. Kerma
    
    C. Absorbed dose
    
    D. Imparted energy
    
    E. Exposure

18. What is the nature of the risk expressed in the quantity *effective dose*?

    A. Cancer incidence
    
    B. Cancer mortality
    
    C. Detriment from cancer and heritable mutations
    
    D. Tissue reactions
    
    E. Heritable mutations

# Answers

1. **C** The probability of photoelectric absorption per unit mass approximately proportional to $Z^3/E^3$, where $Z$ is the atomic number, and $E$ is the energy of the incident photon. Using this relationship, you would take the ratio of the two given energies to obtain an answer of 2.6. *(Pg. 52)*

2. **D** The SI unit of absorbed dose and kerma is the same (gray), where 1 Gy = 1 J/kg. The traditional unit of absorbed dose is the rad, an acronym for radiation absorption. One rad is equal to 0.01 J/kg. Thus, there are 100 rad in a gray, and 1 rad = 10 mGy. *(Pg. 63)*

3. **C** In Compton scattering, the ejected electron will lose its kinetic energy via excitation, and ionization of the atoms in the surrounding material. The energy of the scattered fountain can be calculated from the energy of the incident photon and the angle of the scattered photon, mathematically expressed as Equation 3-2. *(Pg. 49)*

4. **C** For monoenergetic photons under narrow-beam geometry conditions, the probability of attenuation remains the same for each additional HVL thickness placed in the beam. Reduction in the beam intensity can be expressed as $(1/2)^n$, or $n$ equals the number of HVLs. Thus $(1/2)^5 = 3.1\%$ of photons are transmitted. 100 − 3.1 = 97% of photons are attenuated. *(Pg. 58)*

5. **D** The mean free path can be calculated from the linear attenuation coefficient or the HVL of the beam. This can be seen in the definition for mean free path. *(Pg. 60)*

6. **B** Delta rays are electrons set into motion following their interaction with a primary electron (*e.g.*, photo-electron) as it traverses matter losing kinetic energy via excitation and ionization (delta rays). When electrons are ejected from atoms, they are considered secondary ionizations. *(Pg. 43)*

7. **D** The range of a particle is defined as the depth of penetration of a particle of matter. This is illustrated in Figure 3-3 or path length and range are displayed. *(Pg. 45)*

8. **C** Total bremsstrahlung emission per atom is proportional to the $Z^2$, where $Z$ is the atomic number of the absorber, and inversely proportional to the square of the mass of the incident particle, that is, $Z^2/M^2$. *(Pg. 46)*

9. **B** For monoenergetic incident photon beam, the HVL can be easily calculated from the linear attenuation coefficient, and vice versa. For example, given an HVL of 5.6 mm, $\mu = 0.693/\text{HVL}$. *(Pg. 59)*

10. **D** High LET radiation, such as alpha particles, protons, etc., produce dense ionization tracks over their path, producing biological damage that is more difficult to repair correctly compared to the sparse more tortuous ionization pattern that is associated with low LET radiation. *(Pg. 45)*

11. **A** Rayleigh scattering occurs when the incident photon interacts with and excites the total atom. This contrasts with Compton scattering in which the photons interact with outer shell electrons. In the photoelectric effect, all incident photon energy is transferred to an inner shell electron, which is subsequently ejected from the atom. The previous three interactions are entirely different from pair production, which occurs when a high energy (must be greater than 1.02 MeV) x-ray or γ-ray interacts with the electric field of the nucleus of an atom and undergoes a change of state as it is transformed into two particles, one electron and one positron (essentially creating matter from energy). *(Pg. 48)*

12. **C** Absorbed dose can be described as the energy ($E$) **deposited (*locally*)** by ionizing radiation per unit mass of irradiated material. Effective dose is the sum of the products of the equivalent dose to each organ/tissue irradiated ($H_T$) and its corresponding tissue weighting factor ($w_T$), while the term exposure refers to the amount of electrical charge ($Q$) produced by ionizing electromagnetic radiation per mass ($m$) of air. Kerma ($K$): Kinetic energy transferred to charged particles by indirectly ionizing radiation (x-rays and γ-rays) per unit mass. Equivalent dose to tissue $T(H_T)$ = Absorbed dose to tissue $T(D_T)$ × Radiation weighting factor ($w_R$) *(Pg. 63–67)*

**13.** **C**   Photon energy corresponds to particular absorption edge increase with the atomic number (Z) of the element. It is also important to note that the photoelectric process predominates when lower energy photons interact with high Z materials. This can be seen in Figure 3-11. *(Pg. 53)*

**14.** **B**   The mathematical expression shown in A shows number of photons transmitted after traversing thickness *x*. B takes the total probability (1.0) and subtracts the probability that photons will be transmitted through a previously defined thickness *x*, leaving the probability of photon interaction. *(Pg. 55)*

**15.** **E**   Photoelectric absorption results in the production of a photoelectron, a positive ion (ionized atom), characteristic x-rays and/or Auger electrons. *(Pg. 52)*

**16.** **A**   Compton scattering is the predominant reaction of x-rays and γ-ray in the diagnostic energy range with soft tissue. Compton scattering that only predominates in the diagnostic energy range above 26 keV in soft tissue but also continues to predominant will be on diagnostic energies to approximately 30 MeV. *(Pg. 48)*

**17.** **A**   This is the definition of effective dose. *(Pg. 67, Eq. 3-25)*

**18.** **C**   Effective dose is expressed as the total harm to health experienced by an exposed group and its descendants as a result of the group's exposure to a radiation source. Detriment is a multidimensional concept. Its principal components are the stochastic quantities: probability of attributable fatal cancer, weighted probability of attributable nonfatal cancer, weighted probability of severe heritable effects, and length of life lost if the harm occurs. *(Pg. 67–70)*

# Section III Key Equations and Symbols

| QUANTITY | EQUATION | EQ NO./PAGE/COMMENTS |
|---|---|---|
| Incident photon energy | $E_o = E_{sc} + E_{e^-}$ | Eq. 3-1/Pg. 49/An incident photon with energy $E_o$ will interact with a valence-shell electron resulting in the ejection of a Compton electron ($E_{e^-}$) (Fig. 3-7). As the incident photon energy increases, both scattered photons and electrons are scattered more toward the forward direction (Fig. 3-8). |
| Scattered photon energy | $E_{sc} = \dfrac{E_o}{1 + \dfrac{E_o}{511 \text{ keV}}(1 - \cos\theta)}$ | Eq. 3-2/Pg. 49/The energy for the scattered photon is dependent on the incident photon energy and the angle of the scatter photon. |
| Kinetic energy of the ejected photoelectron | $E_{pe} = E_o - E_b$ | Eq. 3-3/Pg. 51/Where $E_b$ is the binding energy of the orbital electron (Fig. 3-9). |
| Number of monoenergetic photons transmitted through a thickness $x$ from a beam of $N_o$ photons | $N = N_0 e^{-\mu x}$ | Eq. 3-5/Pg. 55/The linear attenuation coefficient ($\mu$) is a constant describing the fraction of photons removed from a monochromatic photon beam by a homogeneous absorber per unit thickness is and is typically expressed in units of inverse centimeters (cm$^{-1}$). |
| Mass attenuation coefficient ($\mu/\rho$)<br><br>The fraction of photons removed from a monochromatic x-ray beam by a homogeneous absorber per unit mass. Note: $\rho x$ = mass thickness in (g/cm$^2$) | $\dfrac{\mu}{\rho} = \dfrac{\text{Linear Attenuation Coefficient}}{\text{Density of Material}}$<br><br>$N = N_o e^{-(\mu/\rho)\rho x}$ | Eq. 3-7/Pg. 56/The linear attenuation coefficient, normalized to unit density, is called the mass attenuation coefficient, measured in cm$^2$/g. Also known as the mass absorption coefficient, it is a constant describing the fraction of photons removed from a monochromatic photon beam by a homogeneous absorber per unit mass. |
| Half-value layer | $\text{HVL} = \dfrac{0.693}{\mu}$ | Eq. 3-9/Pg. 58/Defined as the thickness of the material required to reduce the intensity of an x-ray or $\gamma$-ray beam to one half of its initial value. See Tables 3-2 and 3-3 for HVL's commonly used in nuclear medicine and radiography, respectively |
| Energy fluence | $\Psi = \Phi\left(\dfrac{\text{Photons}}{\text{Area}}\right) \times E\left(\dfrac{\text{Energy}}{\text{Photon}}\right)$ | Eq. 3-13/Pg. 62/Energy fluence refers to the amount of energy passing through a unit cross-sectional area. |
| Kerma | $K = \Psi\left(\dfrac{\mu_{tr}}{\rho}\right)_E$ | Kerma measures the amount of energy that is transferred from photons to electrons (in the form of their kinetic energy) per unit mass at a certain location. Absorbed dose, on the other hand, measures the energy deposited in a unit mass at a certain location. |

| QUANTITY | EQUATION | EQ NO./PAGE/COMMENTS | | |
|---|---|---|---|---|
| Equivalent dose | $H_T = (D_T) \times (w_R)$ | A radiation protection term where the absorbed dose to tissue $D_T$ is multiplied by a tissue weighting factor ($w_R$) established by ICRP. Values >1 (up to ~20) to reflect increased potential for biological damage from higher LET radiations (*e.g.*, alpha particles; protons and neutrons) relative to that of low LET radiation like x- and $\gamma$-rays which are assigned a $w_R = 1$ | | |
| Effective dose | $E(\text{Sv}) = \sum_T \left[ w_T \times H_T(\text{Sv}) \right]$ | A radiation protection term. Eq. 3-25/Pg. 67/$w_T$ is the tissue weighting factor established by ICRP, $H_T$ is the sum of products of the equivalent dose to each organ or tissue irradiated. Note: Sum of $w_T = 1$ | | |
| **SYMBOL** | **QUANTITY** | **S.I. UNITS** | | **SPECIAL NAME** |
| $X$ | Exposure | C/kg | | |
| $D$ | Absorbed dose | J/kg | | Gray (G) |
| $K$ | Kerma | J/kg | | Gray (G) |
| $K_{air}$ | Air kerma | J/kg | | Gray (G) |
| $E$ | Imparted energy | J | | |
| $H_T$ | Equivalent dose to tissue $T$ | J/kg | | Sievert (Sv) |
| $E$ | Effective dose | J/kg | | Sievert (Sv) |
| $w_R$ | Radiation weighting factor | 1.0 for x- and $\gamma$-ray: 2–20 for high LET radiation | | |
| $w_T$ | Tissue weighting factor | 0.01–0.12 | | |
| **$w_T$ Values: 0.12** | **0.08** | **0.04** | **0.01** | |
| Breast; bone marrow; colon; lung; stomach; remainder | Gonads | Bladder; esophagus; liver; thyroid | Bone surface; brain; salivary gland; skin | |

# Image Quality

## 4.0 INTRODUCTION

At a fundamental level, image quality is about diagnostic accuracy, which is a difficult quantity to measure. Because of this, most image quality measures are based on surrogate measures that are linked, by assumption, to task performance. Optimal image quality typically requires balancing image resolution, contrast, and noise along with other considerations such as dose or cost. The results of image quality assessments are typically a ratio measure (CNR or SNR) or a performance curve (contrast-detail or ROC).

## 4.1 SPATIAL RESOLUTION

Spatial resolution describes the level of detail that can be seen on an image with low-resolution images appearing "blurry" and high-resolution images appearing "sharp."

1. **Physical mechanisms of blurring**
   a. X-ray focal spot blur
   b. Positron diffusion
   c. Optical diffusion in a phosphor-based detector
   d. Image processing for noise control—smoothing operations that employ averaging
2. **Convolution—a mathematical way to describe blurring**
   a. Involves a blurring kernel that integrates over position (Fig. 4-1)
   b. Assumes that the blurring operation is shift-invariant
   c. Can be used to smooth noisy data (Fig. 4-2)
   d. Smoothing can reduce the effects of noise but can also blur fine structure in images
   e. Convolution formula (see Fig. 4-1 caption for description of equation variables):

$$G(x) = \int_{-\infty}^{\infty} H(x')k(x - x')\mathrm{d}x' = H(x) \otimes k(x)$$

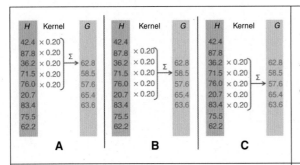

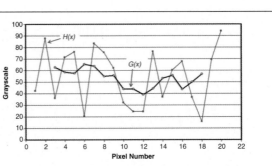

■ **FIGURE 4-1** The basic operation of discrete convolution is illustrated. In the three panes **(A–C)**, the input array H is convolved with a five-element boxcar kernel, k, resulting in the output array, G. The different panes show the convolution kernel, and the output value, advancing by one index element at a time. The entire convolution is performed over the complete length of H.

■ **FIGURE 4-2** A plot of the noisy input data in H(x), and of the smoothed function G(x), where x is the pixel number (x = 1, 2, 3, …). The first few elements in the data shown on this plot correspond to the data illustrated in Figure 4-1. The input function H(x) is random noise distributed around a mean value of 50. The convolution process with the boxcar average results in substantial smoothing, and this is evident by the much smoother G(x) function that is closer to this mean value.

## 3. The spatial domain: spread functions

**a.** Blurring can be characterized by a point-spread function (PSF) (Fig. 4-3), a line-spread function (LSF) (Fig. 4-4), or an edge-spread function (ESF), as compared in Figure 4-5.

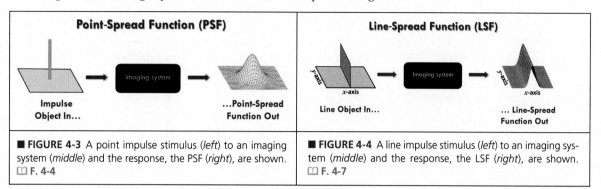

**FIGURE 4-3** A point impulse stimulus (*left*) to an imaging system (*middle*) and the response, the PSF (*right*), are shown. F. 4-4

**FIGURE 4-4** A line impulse stimulus (*left*) to an imaging system (*middle*) and the response, the LSF (*right*), are shown. F. 4-7

**b.** These are generated by imaging a point, a slit (line), or an edge (Fig. 4-5).

**c.** Integral relationships exist between each of these spread functions.

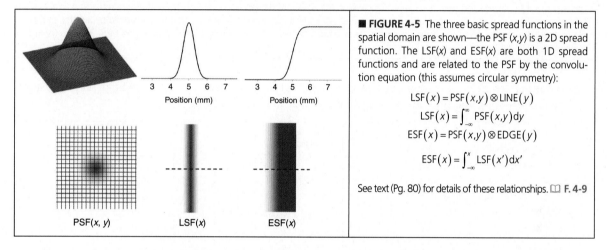

**FIGURE 4-5** The three basic spread functions in the spatial domain are shown—the PSF $(x,y)$ is a 2D spread function. The LSF$(x)$ and ESF$(x)$ are both 1D spread functions and are related to the PSF by the convolution equation (this assumes circular symmetry):

$$LSF(x) = PSF(x,y) \otimes LINE(y)$$
$$LSF(x) = \int_{-\infty}^{\infty} PSF(x,y)\,dy$$
$$ESF(x) = PSF(x,y) \otimes EDGE(y)$$
$$ESF(x) = \int_{-\infty}^{x} LSF(x')\,dx'$$

See text (Pg. 80) for details of these relationships. F. 4-9

## 4. The frequency domain: modulation transfer function

**a.** Fourier analysis describes how a signal variation in the spatial domain can be approximated by sine waves assembled with a spatial frequency, phase, and amplitude as shown in Figure 4-6.

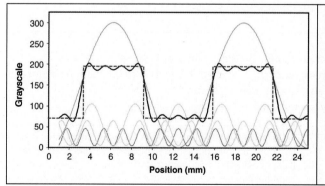

**FIGURE 4-6** The basic concept of Fourier analysis demonstrates how a spatial domain object (the *dashed line* rectangle [RECT] functions) can be estimated by the summation of sine waves. The *solid black lines* are the sum of the four sets of sine waves (shown toward the *bottom* of the plot) and approximate the two RECT functions (*dashed lines*). With higher frequency waves, the RECT functions could be better matched. The Fourier transform breaks any arbitrary signal down into the sum of a set of sine waves of different phase, frequency, and amplitude. F. 4-10

**b.** The Fourier transform converts an image from the spatial domain to the frequency domain.

**c.** The Fourier transform of a sinusoidal wave function is an impulse at the wave frequency.

**d.** The *period* of a wave is the distance of one cycle; *for example, period* (mm)= 1/ *frequency* (cycles/mm).

**e.** Fine-scale image structure is typically reflected by high frequency content in the Fourier transform.

**f.** The modulation transfer function (MTF) describes how sine-wave components are modulated by an imaging system (Fig. 4-7).

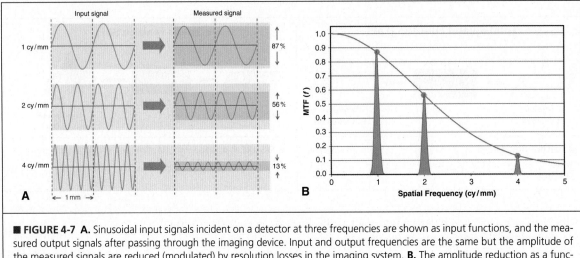

■ **FIGURE 4-7  A.** Sinusoidal input signals incident on a detector at three frequencies are shown as input functions, and the measured output signals after passing through the imaging device. Input and output frequencies are the same but the amplitude of the measured signals are reduced (modulated) by resolution losses in the imaging system. **B.** The amplitude reduction as a function of spatial frequency is the modulation transfer function (MTF($f$)). System resolution is often characterized by an MTF threshold (*e.g.*, MTF = 10%) called the **limiting spatial resolution**. In this MTF, the limiting resolution would be 4.3 cycles (or line pairs/mm). 📖 **F. 4-11**

**g. Sampling** describes the mathematical process of going from a continuous function to finite set of measured values; **sampling aperture, a,** and **sampling pitch, Δ,** are described (Fig. 4-8).

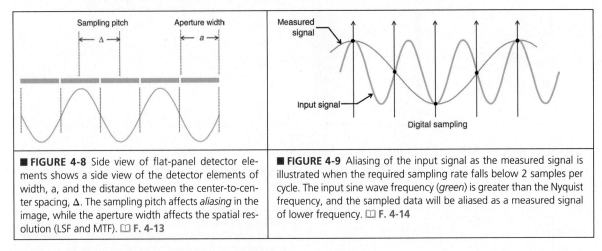

■ **FIGURE 4-8** Side view of flat-panel detector elements shows a side view of the detector elements of width, a, and the distance between the center-to-center spacing, Δ. The sampling pitch affects *aliasing* in the image, while the aperture width affects the spatial resolution (LSF and MTF). 📖 **F. 4-13**

■ **FIGURE 4-9** Aliasing of the input signal as the measured signal is illustrated when the required sampling rate falls below 2 samples per cycle. The input sine wave frequency (*green*) is greater than the Nyquist frequency, and the sampled data will be aliased as a measured signal of lower frequency. 📖 **F. 4-14**

**h.** Sampling at a fixed pixel pitch leads to fundamental limits on the resolution of the sampled signal.
**i. Nyquist frequency** $= 1/2\Delta$ (at least two samples per cycle of the input signal) is the maximum frequency that can accurately rendered in the image; when violated, aliasing occurs (Fig. 4-9).
**j.** Frequencies larger than the Nyquist frequency are reflected as lower frequencies (Fig. 4-10).

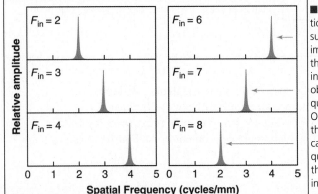

■ **FIGURE 4-10** For a single-frequency sinusoidal input function to an imaging system (sinusoidally varying intensity versus position), the Fourier transform of the image results in an impulse at the measured frequency. The Nyquist frequency in this example is 5 cycles/mm. For the three input frequencies in the *left panel*, all are below the Nyquist frequency and obey the Nyquist criterion, and the measured (recorded) frequencies are exactly what was input into the imaging system. On the *right panel*, the input frequencies were higher than the Nyquist frequency, and the recorded frequencies in all cases were aliased—they wrapped around the Nyquist frequency—that is, the measured frequencies were lower than the Nyquist frequency by the same amount by which the input frequencies exceeded the Nyquist frequency. 📖 **F. 4-15**

## 4.2 CONTRAST RESOLUTION

Contrast resolution refers to the ability to render subtle differences in displayed image grayscale. Contrast, $C_S$, is defined in terms of a background intensity, $S_0$, and a target intensity, $S_1$:

$$C_S = \frac{(S_0 - S_1)}{S_0}$$

Contrast is evaluated at multiple stages during imaging (subject contrast, detector contrast and image contrast)

1. **Subject contrast is** the contrast in the signal after interacting with the patient (Fig. 4-11).

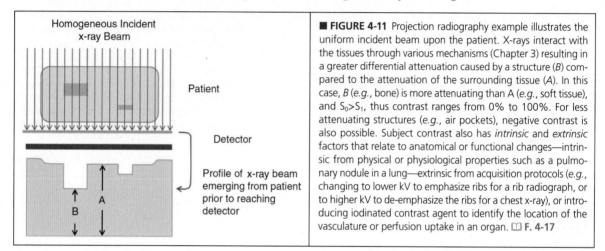

■ **FIGURE 4-11** Projection radiography example illustrates the uniform incident beam upon the patient. X-rays interact with the tissues through various mechanisms (Chapter 3) resulting in a greater differential attenuation caused by a structure (*B*) compared to the attenuation of the surrounding tissue (*A*). In this case, *B* (*e.g.*, bone) is more attenuating than A (*e.g.*, soft tissue), and $S_0 > S_1$, thus contrast ranges from 0% to 100%. For less attenuating structures (*e.g.*, air pockets), negative contrast is also possible. Subject contrast also has *intrinsic* and *extrinsic* factors that relate to anatomical or functional changes—intrinsic from physical or physiological properties such as a pulmonary nodule in a lung—extrinsic from acquisition protocols (*e.g.*, changing to lower kV to emphasize the ribs for a rib radiograph, or to higher kV to de-emphasize the ribs for a chest x-ray), or introducing iodinated contrast agent to identify the location of the vasculature or perfusion uptake in an organ. 📖 **F. 4-17**

2. **Detector contrast** transduces the incident signal through many possible processes that impact the contrast of structures of interest (Fig. 4-12).

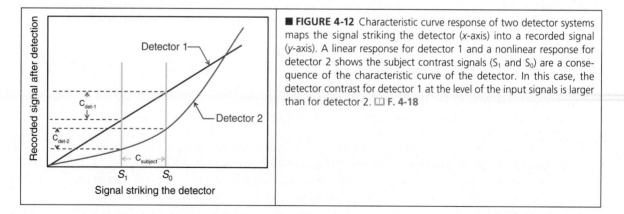

■ **FIGURE 4-12** Characteristic curve response of two detector systems maps the signal striking the detector (*x*-axis) into a recorded signal (*y*-axis). A linear response for detector 1 and a nonlinear response for detector 2 shows the subject contrast signals ($S_1$ and $S_0$) are a consequence of the characteristic curve of the detector. In this case, the detector contrast for detector 1 at the level of the input signals is larger than for detector 2. 📖 **F. 4-18**

3. Image contrast
   a. Capture of digital image data allows for interactive adjustment of image contrast through window/level manipulation and lookup table (LUT) conversion (Fig. 4-13).
   b. Medical images have bit depths of 8, 10, 12, and 14 bits, representing possible shades of gray equal to $2^{\#bits}$, delivering 256, 1,024, 4,096, to 16,384 levels.
   c. Display monitors typically render 8 or 10 bits of luminance resolution (256 to 1,024 shades).

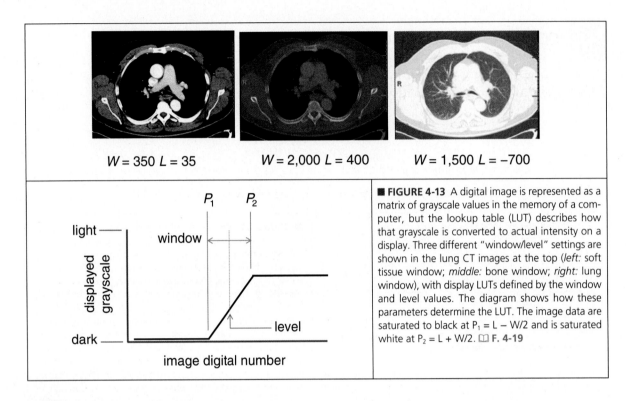

$W = 350\ L = 35$      $W = 2,000\ L = 400$      $W = 1,500\ L = -700$

■ **FIGURE 4-13** A digital image is represented as a matrix of grayscale values in the memory of a computer, but the lookup table (LUT) describes how that grayscale is converted to actual intensity on a display. Three different "window/level" settings are shown in the lung CT images at the top (*left:* soft tissue window; *middle:* bone window; *right:* lung window), with display LUTs defined by the window and level values. The diagram shows how these parameters determine the LUT. The image data are saturated to black at $P_1 = L - W/2$ and is saturated white at $P_2 = L + W/2$. 📖 **F. 4-19**

## 4.3 NOISE AND NOISE TEXTURE

Noise in images arises from various random processes in the process of generating an image (*e.g.*, quantum noise, anatomical noise, electronic noise, structured noise).

1. **Sources of image noise**
   a. Quantum noise describes randomness in a signal arising from randomness in the number of photons.
      i. Poisson distribution (*e.g.*, counts) for an expectation of Q counts is characterized by mean value of $y$, $\mu_y$, and variance in $y$, where $\sigma_y^2 = \mu_y = Q$.
      ii. Standard deviation, $\sigma_y$, is the square root of the variance.
      iii. Coefficient of variation, the mean divided by std. dev. $= \sigma_y/\mu_y = 1/\sqrt{Q}$.
      iv. Fluctuations in the randomness are larger when fewer photons are generated.
      v. Lower dose procedures, therefore, have greater quantum noise.
      vi. Alternatively, signal to noise ratio (SNR) $= \mu_y/\sigma_y = \sqrt{Q}$; thus, SNR is lower in low-count regimes and the coefficient of variation is larger.
   b. Anatomic noise describes contrast generated by patient anatomy not important for diagnosis.
      i. Processing such as dual-energy subtraction can selectively remove interfering anatomy.
   c. Electronic noise describes analog or digital signals in the imaging chain that contaminate signals.
      i. Cooling detectors can reduce detector thermal noise, as can double-correlated sampling.
   d. Structured noise describes a reproducible pattern that reflects differences in the local gain or offset of digital detector components—"flat-field" correction algorithms remove structured noise.
2. **Mathematical characterizations of noise**
   a. Noise magnitude is typically quantified by the variance ($\sigma^2$) or standard deviation ($\sigma$).
   b. Noise texture is typically quantified by the noise power spectrum, based on autocovariance function.
   c. Autocovariance function represents the covariance between two pixels. For pixels that are the same, the covariance is the variance.
   d. Noise texture and differences in the autocovariance function are shown (Figs. 4-14 and 4-15).
   e. Noise power spectrum (NPS) is the Fourier transform of the autocovariance function; it describes the contribution of different spatial frequencies to the image noise (Fig. 4-16).

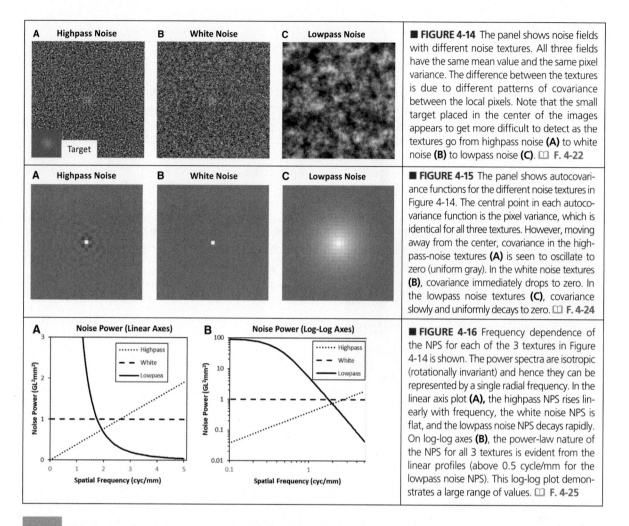

■ **FIGURE 4-14** The panel shows noise fields with different noise textures. All three fields have the same mean value and the same pixel variance. The difference between the textures is due to different patterns of covariance between the local pixels. Note that the small target placed in the center of the images appears to get more difficult to detect as the textures go from highpass noise **(A)** to white noise **(B)** to lowpass noise **(C)**. 📖 F. 4-22

■ **FIGURE 4-15** The panel shows autocovariance functions for the different noise textures in Figure 4-14. The central point in each autocovariance function is the pixel variance, which is identical for all three textures. However, moving away from the center, covariance in the highpass-noise textures **(A)** is seen to oscillate to zero (uniform gray). In the white noise textures **(B)**, covariance immediately drops to zero. In the lowpass noise textures **(C)**, covariance slowly and uniformly decays to zero. 📖 F. 4-24

■ **FIGURE 4-16** Frequency dependence of the NPS for each of the 3 textures in Figure 4-14 is shown. The power spectra are isotropic (rotationally invariant) and hence they can be represented by a single radial frequency. In the linear axis plot **(A)**, the highpass NPS rises linearly with frequency, the white noise NPS is flat, and the lowpass noise NPS decays rapidly. On log-log axes **(B)**, the power-law nature of the NPS for all 3 textures is evident from the linear profiles (above 0.5 cycle/mm for the lowpass noise NPS). This log-log plot demonstrates a large range of values. 📖 F. 4-25

## 4.4 RATIO MEASURES OF IMAGE QUALITY

A balance of some measure of signal with some measure of noise

1. **Contrast to noise ratio**
   a. An object *size-independent* measure of the signal level in the presence of noise.
   b. Describes the signal amplitude relative to the magnitude of noise in an image.
   c. Metric is most applicable when test objects generate homogeneous signal levels.
   d. In this condition, a region of interest (ROI) placed in the object is representative of the entire object, and the background noise can be similarly measured adjacent to the object (Fig. 4-17).

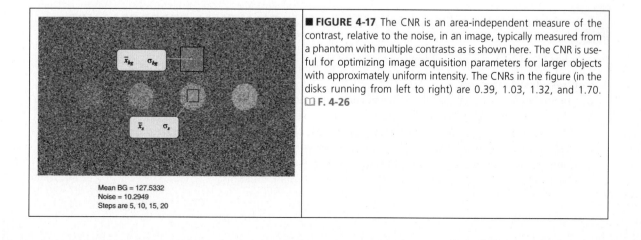

■ **FIGURE 4-17** The CNR is an area-independent measure of the contrast, relative to the noise, in an image, typically measured from a phantom with multiple contrasts as is shown here. The CNR is useful for optimizing image acquisition parameters for larger objects with approximately uniform intensity. The CNRs in the figure (in the disks running from left to right) are 0.39, 1.03, 1.32, and 1.70. 📖 F. 4-26

**e.** Uses: optimizing kV to maximize bone contrast at a fixed dose level; computing dose to achieve a given CNR for a given object; computing the minimum contrast agent concentration for confident visualization at a fixed radiation dose.

**2. Signal-to-noise ratio**

  **a.** Can be defined in a variety of ways dependent on how signal and noise are quantified.

  **b.** In some cases, it is reported as the mean value of a uniform ROI divided by the standard deviation.

  **c.** For measures of detectability, it is defined as the integrated difference of the target and the average background squared relative to the standard deviation of the noise; does not require a homogeneous signal; however, the background should be homogeneous in principle (Fig. 4-18).

  **d.** SNR as a measure of conspicuity is specified as the **Rose criterion**; when SNR ≥ 5, an object is likely be detected by an observer.

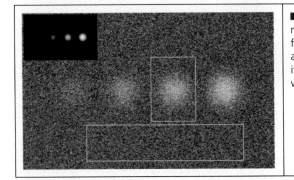

■ **FIGURE 4-18** For nondisk signals, the SNR can be a more useful measure than CNR, since it accommodates nonuniform signal profiles as shown here. Signal regions with Gaussian-based intensities are shown. The SNR has a fundamental relationship with detectability, and the Rose criterion states that if SNR ≥ 5, the signal region will be detectable by an observer in most situations. ▥ **F. 4-27**

**3. SNR in the frequency domain**: noise equivalent quanta (NEQ)

  **a.** NEQ represents the number of quanta needed to achieve the observed SNR, $SNR^2$

$$NEQ(f) = SNR^2(f), \text{ the SNR in the frequency domain, where } SNR(f) = g\frac{MTF(f)}{\sqrt{NPS(f)}}$$

**4. Detective quantum efficiency (DQE)**

  **a.** DQE($f$) is a measure of the information transfer efficiency of an imaging system that determines the impact of the detector on image quality in a frequency-dependent manner.

  **b.** $DQE(f) = \dfrac{SNR_{OUT}^2(f)}{SNR_{IN}^2}$; $SNR_{IN}^2$ is the incident photon fluence $q$, while $SNR_{OUT}^2$ is a measure of the *noise equivalent quanta* measured in the image. Thus, DQE($f$)= NEQ($f$)/$q$, where the measured equivalent noise through the detector response is normalized by the actual number of quanta incident on the detector (mean fluence).

  **c.** At zero spatial frequency, the DQE(0) converges to quantum detection efficiency (QDE), a measure of the absorption efficiency of the detector, linking the evaluation of image quality and information transfer to material properties of the detector.

## 4.5   IMAGE QUALITY MEASURES BASED ON VISUAL PERFORMANCE

**Reader-based evaluations of performance**

**1. Contrast-detail diagrams**

  **a.** Combines the effects of spatial resolution and contrast resolution on detectability

  **b.** Measures the impact of signal area relative to background noise

  **c.** Plots the size of object (detail) on *x*-axis and contrast of object on *y*-axis

  **d.** Determines visibility of objects of various size and contrast in the presence of noise (Fig. 4-19)

  **e.** Compares the performance of imaging systems (Fig. 4-20)

  **f.** Unites the concepts of spatial resolution, contrast resolution and noise

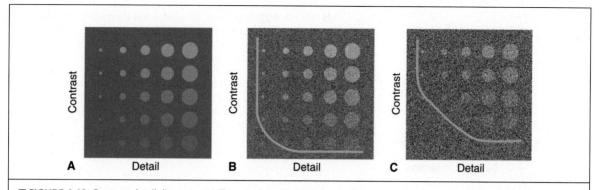

■ **FIGURE 4-19** Contrast detail diagrams are illustrated. **A.** The noiseless CD phantom—disks are smaller to the left and less contrast to the bottom. **B.** Loss of resolution and added noise causes objects to become less visible—the line separates objects detected (*upper right*) with objects not detected (*lower left*). **C.** In an imaging situation with higher noise and less resolution, fewer objects become detectable, and the line moves to the *upper right*. ▱ **F. 4-28**

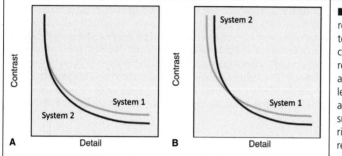

■ **FIGURE 4-20** Contrast-detail diagrams depict the response of two imaging systems. **A.** System 1 and system 2 exhibit similar detail (limiting resolution) of high-contrast objects, but system 2 has superior low-contrast resolution; one explanation is that system 2 response is a result of higher dose and less noise. **B.** System 2 has less detail than system 1, but better contrast resolution; an explanation is that system 2 corresponds to a smoothed image relative to that of system 1, since blurring reduces resolution (detail) and reduces noise, resulting in improved contrast resolution. ▱ **F. 4-29**

2. **Receiver operating characteristic (ROC) curves**
   **a.** ROC analysis: an objective evaluation of detection performance for a *binary* task—normal and abnormal decisions based upon presentation of diagnostic information such as a radiological image.
   **b.** Starting point is the 2 × 2 decision matrix (truth table) (Fig. 4-21).

|  |  | Truth | |
|---|---|---|---|
|  |  | actually normal | actually abnormal |
| Observer Response | normal | TN | FN |
|  | abnormal | FP | TP |

■ **FIGURE 4-21** A 2 × 2 decision matrix (truth table) for a patient outcome using a medical test. The patient either has the suspected disease (actually abnormal) or not (actually normal)—considered the "truth" shown in the columns of the matrix. The diagnostician makes a binary decision—whether the patient is normal or abnormal based upon review of the information shown in the rows of the matrix. The cross section of the observer response and the truth generates four possible outcomes: *true positive* (TP), *true negative* (TN), *false positive* (FP), and *false negative* (FN). Most of the work in performing patient-based ROC analysis is the independent confirmation of the truth, which may require biopsy confirmation, long-term patient follow-up, or other methods to verify the actual condition of the patient. ▱ **F. 4-30**

   **c.** The ability of a diagnostician to render a correct diagnosis (outcome) is dependent on a test (*e.g.*, imaging exam) and the ability to separate the "normal" from abnormal findings, where an overlap of the distributions (normal versus abnormal) overlap (Fig. 4-22).
   **d.** From the values of the truth table, the following can be computed:
   ■ True-positive fraction (TPF) = sensitivity = TP/(TP + FN); a true abnormal finding
   ■ True-negative fraction (TNF) = specificity = TN/(TN + FP); a true normal finding
   ■ False-positive fraction (FPF) = FP/(TN + FP) = 1−TNF = 1−specificity
   **e.** The ROC curve is a plot of the TPF (sensitivity) as a function of FPF (1−specificity), where any point on the curve is associated with a given decision threshold, T (Fig. 4-23).
   **f.** The ROC curve describes the performance of a skilled observer, operating at a given point on the curve for a given threshold response, T (Fig. 4-24).

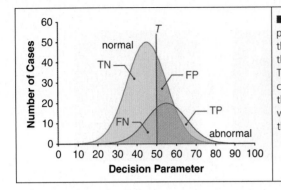

■ **FIGURE 4-22** Histograms of normal and abnormal populations of patients are illustrated as a function of underlying level of suspicion, but the observer needs to see a decision threshold (vertical line, *T*) such that the cases to the right of T are called abnormal, and cases to the left of T are called normal. These data are not always observable, but the concept informs the analysis of decision-making. The two populations and the single threshold value define the TP, FN, TN, and TP fractions. These values are used to compute the sensitivity and specificity outcomes of the observations from the values in the truth table. 📖 **F. 4-31A**

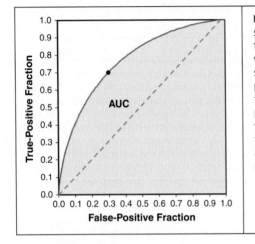

■ **FIGURE 4-23** The underlying model for ROC analysis is based on a decision parameter that is not directly observable for human readers. The assumption is that normal and abnormal cases have distributions of the decision variable, and that a decision is made for any once case by comparing its decision variable to a threshold. The ROC curve is generated by considering all possible thresholds, which sweeps out a curve from (0,0) to (1,1) as the threshold goes from high to low. Each point on the ROC curve represents a possible operating point for some given threshold. The ROC curve associated with perfect performance goes up the *y*-axis to the point (0,1) and then over to the point (1,1). Chance performance is represented by a *diagonal line*. The area under the ROC curve is used as a general measure of detection (normal/abnormal) or discrimination (benign/malignant) performance. 📖 **F. 4-31B**

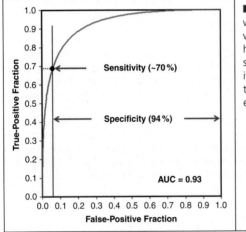

■ **FIGURE 4-24** From a given ROC curve, it is relatively straight-forward to work out the sensitivity for a given false-positive rate or specificity, and vice versa. On an ROC curve, an operating point with a higher sensitivity and higher false-positive rate (low specificity) represents more aggressive decision-making with a lower decision threshold. Lower sensitivity and false-positive rates represent more conservative decision making with a higher decision threshold. For a given operating threshold, sensitivity can be improved at the expense of specificity, and vice-versa. 📖 **F. 4-32**

g. Prevalence-dependent measures include **accuracy, positive predictive value (PPV)**, and **negative predictive value (NPV)**
   (i) Accuracy = (TP + TN)/(TP + TN + FP + FN), the fraction of correct responses
   (ii) PPV = TP/(TP + FP), the fraction of positive decisions that are actually positive
   (iii) NPV = TN/(TN + FN), the fraction of negative decisions that are actually negative
h. Accuracy is rarely used as a metric for performance of a diagnostic test.
i. The PPV and NPV of a diagnostic test (such as an imaging exam with radiologist interpretation) are useful metrics for referring physicians as they weigh the information from a number of diagnostic tests (some of which may be contradictory) for a given patient in the process of determining the specific diagnosis.

# Section II Questions and Answers

1. How can blurring in an imaging system be modeled?
   A. The interaction of x-rays with tissue
   B. Convolution with a kernel of equal weighting
   C. Covariance with neighboring pixels
   D. Fourier transform of the noisy data

2. Which of the following is a source of blur in an imaging system?
   A. Photon diffusion in a detector
   B. Convolution with a kernel of equal weighting
   C. Covariance with neighboring pixels
   D. The presence of normal anatomy in the image

3. How does the point spread function represent blurring?
   A. A reflection of the high frequency information about the Nyquist frequency
   B. Multiplication in the frequency domain
   C. The image of a slit over the detector at an angle of 2°
   D. The intensity obtained from a point impulse

4. Why are the line-spread function and edge-spread function preferred over the point spread function?
   A. They have a closer relation to the MTF.
   B. They are less susceptible to shift-variant effects.
   C. They do not require the assumption of rotational symmetry.
   D. They are easier to acquire in practice.

5. The modulation transfer function is defined as:
   A. The number of quanta produced by an x-ray generator
   B. The ratio of disk target intensity to background noise
   C. The frequency-dependent relative change in the amplitude of an input sine wave
   D. The Fourier transform of the autocovariance function

Figure for questions 6 and 7:

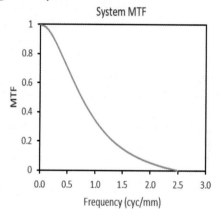

6. For the MTF shown, how much modulation is expected for an input sine wave with a *period* of 2.5 mm?
   A. Output amplitude = 0% of input amplitude
   B. Output amplitude = 10% of input amplitude
   C. Output amplitude = 50% of input amplitude
   D. Output amplitude = 80% of input amplitude
   E. Output amplitude = 100% of input amplitude

7. If the system MTF is a *presampled* MTF, what is the largest pixel pitch the system will support without aliasing?
   A. 0.1 mm
   B. 0.2 mm
   C. 0.4 mm
   D. 0.8 mm

8. An input signal of 1.5 cycles/mm is sampled with a pitch of 0.4 mm by a digital detector. Which one of the following is true?
   A. Frequency impulse at 0.25 mm$^{-1}$, with aliasing
   B. Frequency impulse at 0.75 mm$^{-1}$, no aliasing
   C. Frequency impulse at 1.0 mm$^{-1}$, with aliasing
   D. Frequency impulse at 1.5 mm$^{-1}$, no aliasing
   E. Frequency impulse at 1.75 mm$^{-1}$, with aliasing

9. For this coarse resolution phantom sampled with a 0.1 mm pitch, what is the estimate of limiting resolution?
   A. 1 cycle/mm
   B. 2 cycle/mm
   C. 4 cycle/mm
   D. 5 cycle/mm

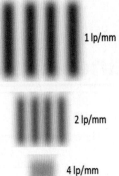

1 lp/mm

2 lp/mm

4 lp/mm

10. Which of the following can be described as an intrinsic source of subject contrast?
    A. The presence of calcifications in intracranial arteries
    B. Improved visualization of breast tissue from scatter correction
    C. Coronary artery visualization from iodine contrast
    D. Use of a soft tissue window on fatty regions of the liver

11. In x-ray imaging, when will electronic noise dominate quantum noise?
    A. There is little attenuating material between the source and the detector.
    B. There is a lot of attenuating material between the source and the detector.
    C. Few photons interact with the detector.
    D. Many photons interact with the detector.

Figure for question 12:

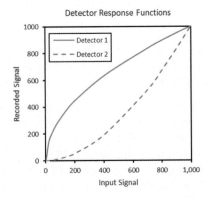

12. For the two detector response functions shown in the plots, which detector yields the higher detector contrast for input signals near 200, and which is higher for signals near 800?
    A. Detector 1 is better for both signals.
    B. Detector 1 for signals near 200 and detector 2 for signals near 800.
    C. Detector 2 is better for both signals.
    D. Detector 2 for signals near 200 and detector 1 for signals near 800.

Figure for question 13:

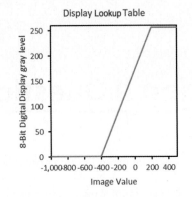

13. The window and level parameters for the display lookup table at the left are:
    A. Window = 200 and level −400
    B. Window = 600 and level −400
    C. Window = −400 and level 600
    D. Window = 600 and level −100
    E. Window = −100 and level 600

14. So-called anatomical noise and structured noise are considered random effects over the populations of:
    A. Thermal electrons and patients, respectively
    B. Patients and detectors, respectively
    C. Photon counts and thermal electrons, respectively
    D. Detectors and photon counts, respectively

15. An image has a pixel standard deviation of 5% of the mean value. When quantum mottle dominates, what is the expected number of quanta for the pixel value?
    A. 400
    B. 200
    C. 40
    D. 20

16. A negative covariance between two image pixels means which of the following?
    A. As the noise pushes one pixel higher, it tends to push the other pixel higher.
    B. As the noise pushes one pixel lower, it tends to push the other pixel higher.
    C. As the noise pushes one pixel lower, it tends to push the other pixel lower.
    D. There is no relation between pixels.

17. An autocovariance function that falls off to zero for every pair of adjacent pixels is called which one of the following?
    A. Poisson noise
    B. Highpass noise
    C. White noise
    D. Lowpass noise
    E. Correlated noise

Figure for question 18:

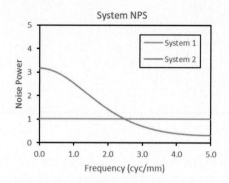

18. Two identical imaging systems (except for noise) have the measured NPS plots. Which is best for fine structure (0.25 mm) and coarse structure (2 mm)?
    A. System 1 is best for both.
    B. System 1 is best for fine and system 2 for coarse.
    C. System 2 is best for fine and system 1 for coarse.
    D. System 2 is best for both.

19. An imaging system is being optimized for contrast between fat and soft tissues, and another for contrast of small focal lesions. Which metric, SNR or CNR?
    A. SNR is most appropriate for both situations.
    B. SNR for first situation and CNR for the second situation.
    C. CNR is most appropriate for both situations.
    D. CNR for first situation and SNR for the second situation.

20. When noise in an imaging system is characterized by white noise, what is the noise equivalent quanta [NEQ($f$)] proportional to?
    A. Frequency SNR
    B. $MTF^2$ of the system
    C. MTF of the system
    D. A constant

Figure for questions 21, 22, and 23

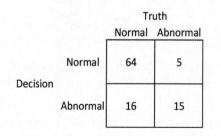

21. Which of the following is true for the 2 × 2 decision table?
    A. Sensitivity 75% and specificity 20%
    B. Sensitivity 80% and false-positive fraction 20%
    C. Sensitivity 75% and false-positive fraction 20%
    D. Sensitivity 80% and specificity 80%
    E. Sensitivity 75% and false-positive fraction 80%

22. Which of the following is true for the 2 × 2 table?
    A. PPV = 48% and NPV = 93%
    B. PPV = 75% and NPV = 80%
    C. PPV = 7% and NPV = 52%
    D. PPV = 80% and NPV = 25%

23. Which of the following is true for the 2 × 2 table?
    A. Accuracy is 80% and disease prevalence is 50%
    B. Accuracy is 75% and disease prevalence is 20%
    C. Accuracy is 75% and disease prevalence is 50%
    D. Accuracy is 79% and disease prevalence is 20%
    E. Accuracy is 79% and disease prevalence is 80%

24. For the contrast-detail curves shown of a noisy imaging system, smoothing is represented by which CD curve?
    A. Curve labeled A
    B. Curve labeled B
    C. Curve labeled C
    D. Curve labeled D

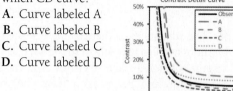

25. For the ROC curve shown, the sensitivity at a specificity of 90% is
    A. ~95%
    B. ~90%
    C. ~80%
    D. ~70%
    E. ~60%

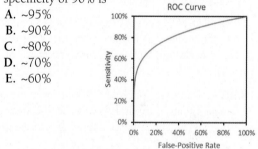

Figure for question 26:

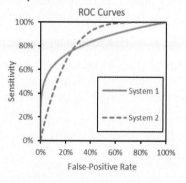

26. Which one of the following statements is true?
    A. Equal AUC represents equivalent performance.
    B. System 1 is preferred in tasks where a high false-positive rate is tolerable.
    C. System 1 is preferred in tasks where high specificity is required.
    D. System 2 is preferred in tasks where high specificity is required.

# Answers

1. **B** Convolution with a blurring kernel is the most common model of blurring. It assumes that the blurred output is a weighted sum of the input function, where the blurring kernel is the weights. *(Pg. 73–75)*

2. **A** Photon diffusion in a detector is a source of blur in real images. *(Pg. 73)*

3. **D** The point spread function represents the system response to an impulse. *(Pg. 76–77)*

4. **D** The advantages of the LSF and ESF are that they are less difficult to acquire, even though it takes a little bit more work to relate them to the MTF, they are more susceptible to shift variance effects, and they usually assume rotational symmetry. However, the PSF phantoms (*e.g.*, pinhole camera) are often more difficult to manufacture and the images of them often suffer from photon starvation. *(Pg. 77–80)*

5. **C** The MTF maps the modulation of sinusoidal inputs as a function of their frequency. *(Pg. 81–83)*

6. **D** A period of 2.5 mm corresponds to a frequency of 0.4 cycle/mm, calculated as 1/(2.5 mm/cycle) = 0.4 cycle/mm. At that frequency, the plotted MTF is approximately 80%. *(Pg. 83–85)*

7. **B** The MTF goes to zero at 2.5 cycle/mm, which is the smallest frequency that can be the Nyquist frequency without aliasing. The pixel size that supports this value of the Nyquist frequency is 0.2 mm, calculated as 1/(2.5 cycle/mm $\times$ 2) = 0.2 mm (the factor of 2 is part of the Nyquist equation, 2 samples needed per cycle). *(Pg. 83–85)*

8. **C** A sampling pitch of 0.4 mm results in a Nyquist frequency of 1/(0.4 mm $\times$ 2) = 1.25 cycle/mm. This means that an input sine wave with a frequency of 1.5 cycle/mm (0.25 cycle/mm beyond the Nyquist frequency) will be reflected about the Nyquist frequency, giving 1.25 − 0.25 cycle/mm = 1 cycle/mm. *(Pg. 83–85)*

9. **B** The bars at 2 line-pairs/mm are the last ones where the individual bars are visible. While it is likely that there is a higher frequency where the bars are visible (*e.g.*, 3 lp/mm), this is not shown. Therefore, 2 cycle/mm is specified as the limiting resolution since line-pairs/mm is equivalent to spatial frequency. *(Pg. 85–86)*

10. **A** Calcifications are anatomical changes in the patient's tissues that give rise to contrast. *(Pg. 87–88)*

11. **C** Few photons interacting with the detector means that the electronic noise of the detector will be larger relative to the signal. Both attenuating material and low DQE can lead to this situation, but both of these can be rectified by turning up the source intensity. *(Pg. 88–92)*

12. **B** Detector contrast for signals near a given value is based on how steep the curve is near that value. Near a value of 200 the curve for detector 1 is steeper, and near 800 the curve for detector 2 is steeper. *(Pg. 88)*

13. **D** The window is defined as the input image intensity that goes from the min to the max of the displayed image. Here the range is from −400 to 200, which gives a range of 600. The level is defined as the middle of the window, which is readily seen to be −100. *(Pg. 88–89)*

14. **B** Anatomical noise is a random effect across patients since it describes variability in the arrangement of patient anatomy. Structured noise is randomness in the manufacturing of the detector, so it can be thought of as representing a population of detectors. *(Pg. 90–92)*

15. **A** Recall that the standard deviation over the mean is 1 divided by the square-root of Q for quantum noise limited (Poisson) observations. So, if $0.05 = 1/\sqrt{Q}$, then Q = 400. *(Pg. 92–94)*

16. **B** Negative covariance means that the noise tends to have the opposite effect on two pixels. So, if one goes up, the other one will tend to go down. *(Pg. 94–96)*

17. **C**  White noise has the property that every pixel is uncorrelated with every other pixel, meaning that the covariance between them is zero. *(Pg. 94–96)*

18. **C**  Fine structure on the scale of 0.25 mm indicates that the important frequencies will be near 4 cycle/mm, and coarse structure on the scale of 2.0 mm indicates that the important frequencies will be near 0.5 cycle/mm. System 1 has lower noise at 0.5 cycle/mm and system 2 has lower noise at 4 cycle/mm. So system 2 is better for the fine structure, and system 1 is better for the coarse structure. *(Pg. 102–103)*

19. **D**  The fat and soft tissue contrast consists of two levels of intensity without any specific size indicated. This makes it more appropriate for the CNR for optimizing imaging. For small focal lesions, the lesion profile and size will likely be important features, and so the SNR is more appropriate. *(Pg. 98–100)*

20. **B**  NEQ($f$) is basically MTF($f$)$^2$/NPS($f$). So when the NPS is constant, NEQ is proportional to the MTF($f$)$^2$. *(Pg. 100–101)*

21. **C**  Sensitivity is 15/(15 + 5) = 75% and the false-positive fraction is 16/(16 + 64) = 20%. Note that the specificity is 1 − FPF = 80%. *(Pg. 103–107)*

22. **A**  The positive predictive value is 15/(15 + 16) = 48%. The negative predictive value is 64/(64 + 5) = 93%. *(Pg. 103–107)*

23. **D**  The decision accuracy is (64 + 15)/(64 + 5 + 16 + 15) = 79/100 = 79%. The prevalence is (5 + 15)/100 = 20%. *(Pg. 103–107)*

24. **B**  Smoothing will lower the resolution of the images which will tend to impact the visibility of small disks, so the curve will tend to go up faster as the *x*-axis approaches zero. But for larger disks, the smoothing will tend to reduce the masking effects of noise, and so the visibility of the larger disks will improve. This means that the curve will get lower than the observer CD curve for larger disks. Curve B is the only curve consistent with these two trends. *(Pg. 102–103)*

25. **E**  A specificity of 90% translates to a false-positive rate of 10%, and at an *x* value of 10%, the ROC curve indicates a sensitivity of approximately 60%. *(Pg. 103–107)*

26. **C**  A high required specificity means that a low false-positive rate is required, and the ROC curve for system 1 is clearly higher at low false-positive rates. *(Pg. 103–107)*

# Section III Key Equations and Symbols

| QUANTITY | EQUATION | EQ NO./PAGE (TXT)/COMMENTS |
|---|---|---|
| Convolution integral (1D) | $$G(x) = \int_{-\infty}^{\infty} H(x')k(x-x')dx' \;,$$ | Eq. 4-1/Pg. 74/This forms the basis for shift-invariant transformations. |
| Relation of line-spread function and point-spread function | $$LSF(x) = \int_{y=-\infty}^{\infty} PSF(x,y)dy$$ | Eq. 4-3/Pg. 80/This equation relates the commonly measured line-spread function to the more fundamental point-spread function. |
| Relation of line-spread function and point-spread function | $$ESF(x) = \int_{x'=-\infty}^{x} LSF(x')dx'$$ | Eq. 4-5, Pg. 80/This equation relates another commonly measured quantity to the LSF (and to the PSF by Eq. 4-3). |
| Convolution in the frequency domain | $$G(x) = FT^{-1}\{FT(H(x)) \times FT(k(x))\}$$ | Eq. 4-7/Pg. 81/This shows how the Fourier transform can be implemented in the frequency domain as multiplication at each frequency. |
| Definition of contrast | $$C = \frac{S_0 - S_1}{S_0}$$ | Eq. 4-8/Pg. 86/Defines contrast as a difference in signal intensity relative to a background. Note that in some situations the numerator is defined as $S_1 - S_0$. |
| Pixel mean | $$\hat{\mu}_y = \frac{1}{N}\sum_{n=1}^{N} y_n$$ | Eq. 4-14/Pg. 94/The $y_n$ is the pixel value in $N$ repeated measurements. The caret on $\hat{\mu}$ indicates that this is an estimate of the mean pixel value. |
| Pixel variance | $$\hat{\sigma}_y^2 = \frac{1}{N-1}\sum_{n=1}^{N}\left(y_n - \hat{\mu}_y\right)^2$$ | Eq. 4-15/Pg. 94/The caret on $\hat{\sigma}_y^2$ indicates that this is an estimate of the pixel variance. |
| Pixel covariance | $$\hat{\Sigma}_{yz} = \frac{1}{N-1}\sum_{n=1}^{N}\left(y_n - \hat{\mu}_y\right)\left(z_n - \hat{\mu}_z\right)$$ | Eq. 4-17/Pg. 95/The covariance between two pixels ($y$ and $z$) in $N$ repeated measurements. Note that if $y = z$, the equation simplifies to the variance estimate. |
| Contrast to noise ratio | $$CNR = \frac{\left(\hat{\mu}_s - \hat{\mu}_{bg}\right)}{\hat{\sigma}_{bg}}$$ | Eq. 4-18/Pg. 98/Note that the denominator is the standard deviation, not the variance. The numerator represents a measure of signal strength and the denominator represents a measure of noise strength. |
| Signal to noise ratio | $$SNR = \frac{\sqrt{\sum_{i,j}\left(I[i,j] - \hat{\mu}_{bg}\right)^2}}{\hat{\sigma}_{bg}}$$ | Eq. 4-19/Pg. 100/$I[i,j]$ represents the image intensity in pixel $[i,j]$. |
| Frequency SNR | $$SNR(f) = g\frac{MTF(f)}{\sqrt{NPS(f)}}$$ | Eq. 4-20/Pg. 100/Note that $g$ is a gain factor determined by the average regional intensity. Also note that the noise-equivalent quanta is defined as $NEQ(f) = SNR^2(f)$. |
| Detective quantum efficiency | $$DQE(f) = \frac{NEQ(f)}{q}$$ | Eq. 4-22/Pg. 101/Note that $q$ is the photon fluence on the detector. |
| Quantum detection efficiency | $$QDE = \frac{\int_E \phi(E)\left(1 - e^{\mu(E)T}\right)dE}{\int_E \phi(E)dE}$$ | Eq. 4-23/Pg. 101/$\phi(E)$ is x-ray energy spectrum, $\mu(E)$ is the attenuation spectrum of the detector material, and $T$ is the thickness of the detector material. The QDE reflects the global efficiency of x-ray detection in a detector. |

*(Continued)*

| QUANTITY | EQUATION | EQ NO./PAGE (TXT)/COMMENTS |
|---|---|---|
| True-positive fraction (sensitivity) | $TPF = \dfrac{TP}{TP+FN}$ | Eq. 4-24/Pg. 105/TP and FN are the number of true-positive and false-negative cases. TPF tells us the fraction of positive case that are correctly identified as positive. |
| False-positive fraction (1−specificity) | $FPF = \dfrac{FP}{FP+TN}$ | Eq. 4-26/Pg. 105/FP and TN are the number of false-positive and true-negative cases. FPF tells us the fraction of negative cases incorrectly identified as positive. |
| Accuracy | $Accuracy = \dfrac{TP+TN}{TP+FN+FP+TN}$ | Eq. 4-27/Pg. 107/Accuracy is the fraction of correct decisions across both positive and negative cases. |
| Positive predictive value | $PPV = \dfrac{TP}{TP+FP}$ | Eq. 4-28/Pg. 107/PPV tells us the fraction of cases identified as positive that are actually positive. |
| Negative predictive value (NPV) | $NPV = \dfrac{TN}{TN+FN}$ | Eq. 4-29/Pg. 107/NPV tells us the fraction of cases identified as negative that are actually negative. |

# Medical Imaging Informatics

## 5.0 INTRODUCTION

Medical informatics represents the process of collecting, analyzing, storing, and communicating information that is crucial to the provision and delivery of patient care. Medical imaging informatics is a subfield that addresses aspects of image generation, processing, management, transfer, storage, distribution, display, perception, privacy, and security. Communications ontologies and standards, computers and networking, picture archiving and communications systems, life cycle of a radiology exam from within and outside a radiology department, and business considerations are areas highlighted in this chapter.

## 5.1 ONTOLOGIES, STANDARDS, PROFILES

1. Ontologies
   a. A collection of terms and their relationships to represent concepts in this application—medicine
      (i) Common vocabularies and standardization of terms for representation of knowledge.
      (ii) Benefits include enhancing interoperability between information systems, sharing of structured content, and integrating knowledge and data.
   b. SNOMED-CT: Systematized Nomenclature of Medicine—clinical terms
      (i) Standard, multilingual vocabulary of clinical terminology used by physicians and providers
      (ii) Supported by the National Library of Medicine
      (iii) Designated as the national standard for additional categories of information in the EHR
      (iv) Enables semantic interoperability and supports exchange of validated health information between providers, researchers, and others in the healthcare environment
   c. ICD: International statistical Classification of Diseases and related health problems
      (i) ICD is in its 10th revision (ICD-10) and is sponsored by the World Health Organization.
      (ii) Manual with codes for diseases, signs, symptoms, abnormal findings, and external causes of injury.
      (iii) In the United States, ICD-10-CM (clinical modification) and ICD-10-PCS (Procedure Coding System) by Centers for Medicaid and Medicare Services (CMS) assigns codes for procedures, and diagnoses for conditions and diseases (69,000 diagnosis and 70,000 procedure codes).
   d. CPT: current procedural terminology—describes procedures performed on the patient
      (i) Manual published by the American Medical Association.
      (ii) Physicians' bill is paid for services performed in a hospital or other place of service.
      (iii) CPT codes are updated frequently; often human coding teams or automated software assist in the verification and validation of codes for specific procedures for reimbursement.
   e. RadLex: radiology lexicon—sponsored by the Radiological Society of North America
      (i) Radiology-specific terms and vocabulary for anatomy, procedures, and protocols
      (ii) RadLex playbook assigns RPID (RadLex Playbook Identifier) tags to the terms
   f. LOINC: Logical Observation Identifiers Names and Codes—sponsored by the Regenstrief Institute
      (i) A more widely adopted ontology over many medical domains.
      (ii) RadLex is being harmonized into the LOINC coding schema.

## 2. Standards Organizations

**a.** ANSI: American National Standards Institute—coordinates standards development in the United States.

    **(i)** Accredits Standards Development Organizations (SDOs) and designates technical advisory groups to the International Organization for Standardization (ISO)

**b.** In healthcare, the two most important SDOs are Health Level 7 (HL7) and the National Electrical Manufacturers Association (NEMA).

## 3. Internet Standards

**a.** The Internet Engineering Task Force (ITEF) of the Internet Society develops protocol standards.

**b.** TCP/IP: Transmission Control Protocol/Internet Protocol—links devices worldwide.

**c.** HTTP: HyperText Transfer Protocol: application protocol for distributing collaborative hypermedia information systems is the foundation for data communications for the World Wide Web.

**d.** HTML: HyperText Markup Language—standard for documents to be displayed in a web browser.

**e.** URL: Uniform Resource Locater: specifies syntax and semantics for location/access via the Internet.

**f.** NTP: Network Time Protocol; SMTP: Simple Mail Transfer Protocol; IMAP: Internet Message Access Protocol; MIME: Multipurpose Internet Message Extensions—provide standardized synchronization protocols and basis for interactive transactions on the Internet.

**g.** TLS: Transport Layer Security and SSL: Secure Socket Layer define cryptographic mechanisms.

**h.** XML: eXtensible Markup Layer encodes structured data and serializes it for communication.

## 4. DICOM—Digital Imaging and COmmunications in Medicine

**a.** Standards-based protocols for exchanging, storing, and viewing medical images.

**b.** Managed by MITA (Medical and Imaging Technical Alliance)—a division of NEMA.

**c.** The structure of the DICOM standard is divided into parts 1 to 21 (see textbook, Pg. 112, Table 5-1).

**d.** DICOM is an open, public standard defined and regulated by public communities.

**e.** DICOM Conformance Statement is a required document by vendors that specifies DICOM services and data types that the implementation can provide, but doesn't guarantee availability.

**f.** DICOMWeb: standard for web-based medical imaging using architectural styles for hypermedia systems using interfaces for simple, lightweight, and fast interactions.

## 5. HL7—Health Level 7

**a.** Standard for the exchange, integration, sharing, and retrieval of electronic health information.

**b.** HL7 International is the ANSI-accredited organization for developing standards.

**c.** Interoperability between information systems using HL7 is achieved through messages and documents.

**d.** Common message types: *ORU*—provides results; *ORM*—provides orders; *ADT*—admission, discharge, transfer interactions.

**e.** Common segment types in a message: *OBR*—observation requests; *OBX*—observation results.

**f.** HL7 version 2 and HL7 version 3 are common HL7 implementations.

**g.** HL7 *FHIR* ("Fire"—Fast Health Interoperability Resources) uses application programming interface (API) methods and file formats such as XML to interact with systems with fast, lightweight access.

## 6. IHE—Integrating the Healthcare Enterprise

**a.** Does not generate Information Technology Standards but promotes their use to ensure interoperability.

**b.** IHE International consists of over 150 member organizations.

**c.** Organized in "domains" including radiology, cardiology, pathology, etc.

**d.** Planning committee: strategize the direction and coordination of activities from stakeholders.

**e.** Technical committee: develops *Integration Profiles* (IP) to describe specific strategies, standards (*e.g.*, DICOM and HL7), and solutions used to solve informatics workflow and interoperability challenges.

**f.** Profile testing occurs in a *Connectathon*—a vendor-neutral, monitored testing environment.

**g.** IHE conformance to a specific IP can be used as a contractual obligation to achieve interoperability.

## 5.2 COMPUTERS AND NETWORKING

## 1. Computer Hardware (Workstation)

**a.** Components include the *motherboard*, the *central processing unit (CPU)*, the *graphics processing unit (GPU)*, *random access memory (RAM)*, network card, video display card, storage devices (solid-state and spinning disk drives), and peripherals (keyboard, mouse, microphone, video camera, printers).

  **b.** Configuration (typical for workstations): 32 to 64 GB RAM: multi-core CPU operating at 1 to 5 GHz clock speed: GPU processing for fast, parallel image processing; terabyte local disk storage; gigabit/s network speed; high-resolution displays (3 to 5 megapixel, large format, portrait orientation).

  **c.** *Thin client* workstations: can be less capable, depend on server-side rendering to provide services.

**2. Software and Application Programming Interface**

  **a.** Software programs consist of sequences of instructions executed by a computer.

  **b.** *Application programs* perform a specific function, for example, email, word processing, web browser..

  **c.** *System software* are the files and programs that make up the computer's operating system (OS).

   **(i)** Microsoft Windows, Mac OS, Linux Unbuntu.

   **(ii)** System files manage memory, input/output devices, system performance, and error messages.

   **(iii)** Firmware: operational software embedded in a chip to provide start-up instructions, such as a BIOS (Basic Input/Output System) on a motherboard to wake up hardware and boot the OS.

  **d.** *Programming language translators* allow software programmers to translate human understandable high-level source code (C++, Java, Python) into machine language code instructions for a CPU.

  **e.** *Utility software* sits between the OS and supplication software for diagnostic and maintenance tasks (*e.g.*, antivirus, disk partition, file compression/decompression, firewall algorithms).

  **f.** *Application Programming Interface (API)*—defines the way to request services from an application

   **(i)** Private APIs have specifications for a company's products and services that are not shared.

   **(ii)** Public (open) APIs can be used by a third party without restriction.

   **(iii)** Local APIs provide database access, memory management, security, for example, Microsoft.NET.

   **(iv)** Web APIs represent HTML resources addressed using the HTTP protocol.

   **(v)** REST (Representational State Transfer) architectural pattern for creating web services; a RESTful service implements that pattern using a set of simple, well-defined operations—FHIR and DICOMweb use the RESTful API to request and receive independent data access.

**3. Networks and Gateways**

  **a.** *Local area network (LAN)* connects computers within a department, building, or buildings.

  **b.** *Wide area network (WAN)* connects computers at large distances—consisting of multiple LANs with long-distance communications links—the largest WAN is the Internet itself.

  **c.** Networks permit transfer of information between computers using hardware and software components.

   **(i)** Hardware connections include copper wiring, coaxial cable, fiber-optic cable, and electronic, such as radiowave and microwave links used by Bluetooth and Wi-Fi.

   **(ii)** Software operates between the user application program and hardware communications link, necessitating *network protocols* for communication and provision of services.

   **(iii)** Computers and switching devices (*nodes*) share communications pathways on a network; protocols divide information into *packets* that contain header information identifying the destination, and communications pathways between the nodes are called *links*.

  **d.** Network bandwidth is the data transfer rate of a link or connection; throughput is the maximum rate.

   **(i)** Megabits/second (Mbps) or gigabits/second (Gbps); 100 Mbps to 10 Gbps are typical rates.

   **(ii)** Must also accommodate overhead from protocols (packet framing, addressing, etc.).

   **(iii)** Latency is the time delay of a transmission between two nodes.

  **e.** Network layer model: the ISO-OSI (Open Systems Interconnection) seven-layer stack (Fig. 5-1).

   **(i)** Conceptual framework to describe the functions of a network system.

   **(ii)** Communications begin at the upper (7th) layer by an applications program, passing information to the next lower layer in the stack, with each layer adding information (*e.g.*, addresses).

   **(iii)** The lowest (layer 1) is the physical layer that sends information to the destination computer.

   **(iv)** The destination computer passes information back up the stack, removing information as it moves upward and reaches the intended application.

  **f.** Model of network interconnection of medical imaging with a DICOM process (Fig. 5-2).

   **(i)** Transmission Control Protocol—Internet Protocol (TCP-IP) is the packet-based protocol used by the Internet for information transfer operating at the lower layers of the ISO-OSI stack.

   **(ii)** DICOM interactions occur at higher levels (session and presentation).

   **(iii)** Application entity (image modality or server) is at the upper layer (7) for image handling.

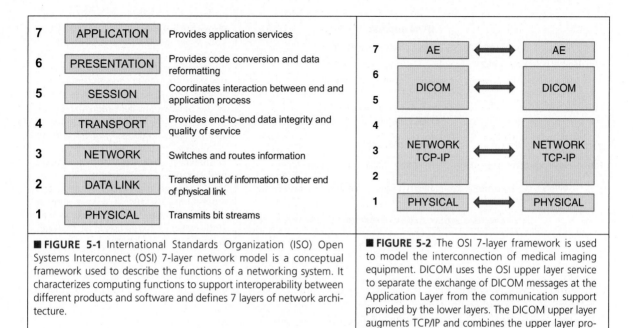

| 7 | APPLICATION | Provides application services |
|---|---|---|
| 6 | PRESENTATION | Provides code conversion and data reformatting |
| 5 | SESSION | Coordinates interaction between end and application process |
| 4 | TRANSPORT | Provides end-to-end data integrity and quality of service |
| 3 | NETWORK | Switches and routes information |
| 2 | DATA LINK | Transfers unit of information to other end of physical link |
| 1 | PHYSICAL | Transmits bit streams |

■ **FIGURE 5-1** International Standards Organization (ISO) Open Systems Interconnect (OSI) 7-layer network model is a conceptual framework used to describe the functions of a networking system. It characterizes computing functions to support interoperability between different products and software and defines 7 layers of network architecture.

■ **FIGURE 5-2** The OSI 7-layer framework is used to model the interconnection of medical imaging equipment. DICOM uses the OSI upper layer service to separate the exchange of DICOM messages at the Application Layer from the communication support provided by the lower layers. The DICOM upper layer augments TCP/IP and combines the upper layer protocols into a simple to implement single protocol on general networks.

g. LANs use Ethernet—a "connections-based" protocol.
   (i) Star topology is most often used for point-to-point connections (Fig. 5-3).
   (ii) Ethernet bandwidth specified as 100 Mbit, Gbit or 10 Gbit rates between LAN segments.
   (iii) Connections require fiberoptic, twisted pair copper, Wi-Fi, or cellular signal transmission.
h. Routers (smart switches) connect local networks using the internet protocol (IP) and operate at the network protocol stack level to route messages to the destination address.
   (i) Packet switching is performed by the router.
   (ii) Each computer and router are assigned IP addresses.
i. Network address protocols (Fig. 5-4).
   (i) IP v4 *dot-decimal*: 32-bit address with 8 bit encoding per segment, for example, 152.79.110.12.
   (ii) IP v6 *hexadecimal*: 128 bit address—larger address space.
   (iii) *Host names* are convenient ways to designate a specific computer on the network.
   (iv) Domain Name System (DNS) is an Internet service consisting of servers that translate host names into IP addresses.

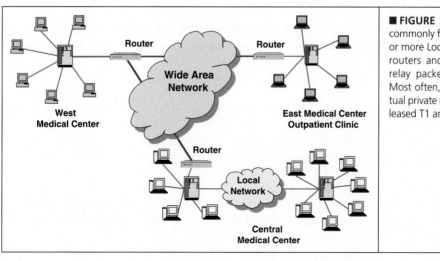

■ **FIGURE 5-3** Wide area networks are commonly formed by linking together two or more Local Area Networks (LANs) using routers and links. Routers connect and relay packets to intended destinations. Most often, the public Internet with a virtual private network is used, in lieu of older leased T1 and T3 links between LANs.

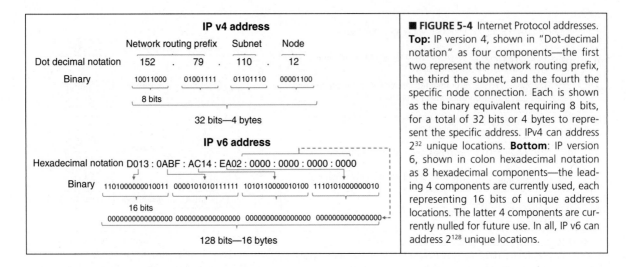

**FIGURE 5-4** Internet Protocol addresses. **Top:** IP version 4, shown in "Dot-decimal notation" as four components—the first two represent the network routing prefix, the third the subnet, and the fourth the specific node connection. Each is shown as the binary equivalent requiring 8 bits, for a total of 32 bits or 4 bytes to represent the specific address. IPv4 can address $2^{32}$ unique locations. **Bottom:** IP version 6, shown in colon hexadecimal notation as 8 hexadecimal components—the leading 4 components are currently used, each representing 16 bits of unique address locations. The latter 4 components are currently nulled for future use. In all, IP v6 can address $2^{128}$ unique locations.

    **j.** Virtual Private Network (VPN) provides encryption and authentication that allows use of the public Internet WAN in a safe and secure manner.

    **k.** MultiProtocol Label Switching (MPLS) defines the path between nodes in web-based networks.

**4. Servers**

    **a.** A computer on a network that provides a service to other computers on the network

    **b.** Applications servers, database servers, web servers, and cloud servers are commonly implemented.

    **c.** VM (virtual machine) environments house servers in a flexible environment whereby CPUs, GPUs, RAM, operating system, and file space can be allocated to meet server needs in an efficient manner.

    **d.** *Cloud server* runs in a VM environment that is hosted and delivered on a cloud-computing platform via the Internet with remote access.

    **e.** Cloud-based PACS with server-side rendering requires several computers for data extraction, DICOM conversion, image rendering, storage, and load balancing.

    **f.** Client-server relationships: *thick client* and *thin client*.

        **(i)** Thick client—the client computer provides most information processing and requires substantial CPU and GPU processing—the major function of the server is to store information.

        **(ii)** Thin client—information processing is provided by the server—the client serves to display the information only and therefore does not require much processing or storage capabilities

**5. Cloud Computing**

    **a.** Using a network of remote computers and software hosted on the Internet to deliver a service

    **b.** Examples: Google email, Dropbox storage provider, some PACS vendors

    **c.** Provisioned services: *SaaS*—software as a service; *IaaS*—infrastructure as a service; *PaaS*—platform as a service

    **d.** *Advantages*: reduced operating costs; accessibility to files and data with an Internet connection; recovery of local computer files that are lost or damaged; automated synchronization; increased layers of security; faster information deployment with flexible sizing

    **e.** *Disadvantages*: dependence on an Internet connection with restricted upload/download bandwidth; physical storage devices often needed locally for high-performance access; customer support often lacking; concern about privacy and who owns the data.

    **f.** *Major Providers*: Amazon Web Services (AWS); ServerSpace; Microsoft Azure; Google Cloud.

**6. Active Directory**

    **a.** *LDAP*—Lightweight Directory Access Protocol—accesses and maintains directory information services over an IP network

    **b.** *AD*—Active Directory—is a service developed by Microsoft for Windows domain networks and servers

    **c.** Authenticates and authorizes all users and computers, and enforces security policies on the network

**7. Internet of Things (IoT)**

    **a.** *IoT* encompasses connected devices on the Internet that have a unique identifier (UID).

    **b.** Connected devices provide information and access about their environment and the way they are used.

    **c.** In healthcare, *IoT* applications include remote monitoring of smart sensors, integration of dialysis machines, and all imaging modalities in a radiology department, as examples.

    **d.** Device use requires regular patching and updating to reduce risk from outside threats (hackers) and maintenance of security.

## 5.3  PICTURE ARCHIVING AND COMMUNICATIONS SYSTEM

**1. PACS Infrastructure**
   **a.** A collection of software, interfaces, display workstations, and databases for storage, transfer, and display of medical images (Fig. 5-5)

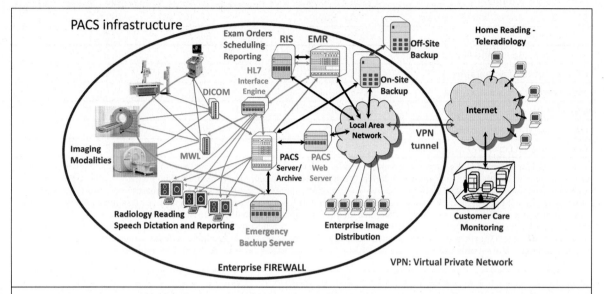

■ **FIGURE 5-5** Modern PACS infrastructure. The PACS is interconnected to the imaging modalities and information systems including the RIS (Radiology Information System) and the EMR (Electronic Medical Record). The RIS provides the patient database for scheduling and reporting of image examinations through HL7 transactions and provides modality worklists (MWLs) with patient demographic information to the modalities, allowing technologists to select patient-specific scheduled studies to ensure accuracy. After a study is performed, image information is sent to the PACS in DICOM format and reconciled with the exam-specific information (accession number). Radiologist reporting is performed at the primary diagnostic workstations and transmitted to the RIS via HL7 transactions. An emergency backup server ensures business continuity (*orange line* directly connecting the modalities) in the event of unscheduled PACS downtime. For referring physicians and remote reading radiologists (teleradiology applications), a webserver is connected to the Internet—access is protected by a Virtual Private Network (VPN) to obtain images and reports. Users within the medical enterprise have protected access through a LAN. Also depicted are an "offsite" backup archive for disaster recovery and real-time customer care monitoring to provide around the clock support. A mirror archive provides on-site backup within the enterprise firewall with immediate availability in case of failure of the primary archive.

   **b.** "Mini-PACS" provide *modality-specific* capabilities for handling images not available in a large PACS.
      **(i)**   Examples include mini-PACS for mammography, nuclear medicine, and ultrasound.
   **c.** "Federated PACS" includes independent PACS functionality at different sites and sharing of DICOM images and information through a software federation manager.
   **d.** "Web-server PACS" provides remote access to images for referring clinicians and healthcare staff.
   **e.** Emergency backup server and business continuity procedures are important infrastructure needs.
   **f.** *VPN*—virtual private network—provides security for devices and software and access by authorized users only through the implementation of an "enterprise firewall."

**2. Image Distribution**
   **a.** Networks are a key to the distribution of images and associated information in a PACS.
   **b.** Bandwidth requirements are dependent on the imaging modalities and their composite workloads.
   **c.** Network design must consider both peak and average bandwidth requirements and tolerable delays.
   **d.** Segmentation of networks with bandwidths sufficient to meet peak demand are often required.

**3. Image Size and Image Compression**
   **a.** Medical image acquisition in radiology involves massive amounts of data (Table 5-1).
   **b.** Image compression reduces image size for efficient network transmission and storage.
      **(i)**   Various compression-storage/retrieval-decompression algorithms are used.
      **(ii)**  Redundancies in data can be used to reduce the number of bytes in an image or image series.
   **c.** *Reversible* compression, also known as *lossless*, preserves the original image data after decompression.
      **(i)**   Typical compression ratios are 3:1 to 5:1 for most images.

**TABLE 5-1 TYPICAL RADIOLOGIC IMAGE FORMATS AND STORAGE REQUIREMENTS PER STUDY** ▭ T. 5-2

| MODALITY IOD—DESCRIPTION | PIXEL FORMAT (APPROXIMATE) | BITS PER PIXEL | EXAM STUDY SIZE (MB) |
|---|---|---|---|
| **CR**—Computed Radiography | $2,000 \times 2,500$ | 10–12 | 28.5 |
| **DX**—Digital Radiography | $3,000 \times 3,000$ | 12–16 | 40.5 |
| **MG**—Mammography | $3,000 \times 4,000$ | 12–16 | 65.3 |
| **BTO**—Digital Breast Tomosynthesis | $2,000 \times 3,000$ | 12–16 | 450.0 |
| **RF**—Fluoroscopy | $512^2$ or $1,024^2$ | 8–12 | 37.0 |
| **XA**—Fluoroscopy Guided Intervention | $512^2$ or $1,024^2$ | 8–12 | 34.9 |
| **CT**—Computed Tomography | $512^2$ | 12 | 235.6 |
| **MR**—Magnetic Resonance Imaging | $64^2$–$512^2$ | 12 | 151.0 |
| **US**—Ultrasound | $512^2$ to $900 \times 1,450$ | 8 | 137.8 |
| **NM**—Nuclear Medicine/SPECT | $64^2$ or $128^2$ | 8 or 16 | 116.0 |
| **PT/CT**—Positron Emission Tomography/CT | $128^2$–$512^2$ | 16 | 416.1 |

Pixel format is an estimate of the typical image matrix size for an image. Average study size is based on one calendar quarter of imaging studies at a major health group in Northern California. Mammography data represent projection radiographs of the breast. Breast tomosynthesis study sizes are from a different source where the data represent the average size of a breast tomosynthesis screening study (4 sequences) using lossless compression to store projection (BPO) and tomographic (BTO) images. Ultrasound studies (video clips) are compressed with conventional JPEG algorithms in a lossy format from the modality. PT represents PET/CT combination studies. Not shown are future systems such as Total Body PET/CT where a typical exam will have 1.9 GB of data, and high resolution CT, where matrix sizes are 4 times and 16 times larger than the conventional CT acquisition, increasing the data size by the same factor. Overall storage requirements over a given time period can be estimated by the product of the exam study size and the number of expected exams for each modality.

    **d.** *Irreversible* compression, also known as *lossy*, results in loss of information and detail fidelity.
        **(i)** Compression ratios that are "acceptable" depend on the image type (DX, MG, CT, MR…).
        **(ii)** More complex single images have less acceptable compression ratio (up to approximately 10:1).
        **(iii)** Data series and video clips (ultrasound) can get approximately 25:1 ratio with acceptable image quality.
        **(iv)** Too much compression renders images nondiagnostic (see textbook, Fig. 5-8).
    **e.** The FDA, under the Mammography Quality Standards Act (MQSA), *prohibits irreversible* compression of digital mammography images for retention, transmission, or final interpretation.
        **(i)** Exceptions to this rule include images from previous studies if deemed of acceptable quality.
        **(ii)** Digital breast tomosynthesis studies use irreversible compression with little loss of fidelity, because of similarities of image content from adjacent reconstructed slices.

**4. Archive and Storage**
    **a.** Archive is a location containing records, document, and objects of historical importance.
        **(i)** For radiology PACS, the archive is a long-term storage of medical images in DICOM format.
        **(ii)** For an enterprise PACS, the archive is a vendor neutral archive (*VNA*) that stores all documents, non-image data (*e.g.,* EKG traces), non-DICOM (*e.g.,* jpeg), and DICOM images.
        **(iii)** Vendors use reversible compression to efficiently store data; proprietary, nonstandard compression schemes require vendor-provided proprietary decompression.
    **b.** Archive protection from failures and disasters.
        **(i)** *RAID*—redundant array of independent disks (level 5)—to protect from disk failure
        **(ii)** Backup mirror copies—on site and geographically remote, to protect from environmental issues
    **c.** Archive and storage management software algorithms.
        **(i)** Central versus distributed archives.
        **(ii)** *On-demand* management provides instantly available images.
        **(iii)** *Pre-fetching* algorithms retrieve previous comparison studies to a local disk from slow media.
    **d.** Hierarchical storage management.
        **(i)** *On-line*—instantaneous access to images
        **(ii)** *Near-line*—storage on less accessible, less expensive media with electronic retrieval—used with pre-fetching algorithms
        **(iii)** *Off-line*—storage that isn't accessible without human intervention (*e.g.,* disks on shelves)
    **e.** Archives and storage in the cloud environment provide great expansion and extensibility.

**5. DICOM, HL7, and IHE**

  **a.** *DICOM*—represents *standards* that provide the ability to transfer images and related information between devices (*e.g.*, image acquisition and image storage).

    **(i)** Specifies standard formats, services, and messages between devices

    **(ii)** Specifies standards for workflow, storage of images on removable media, and consistency and presentation of displayed images

    **(iii)** Specifies standard services performed on information objects, such as storage, query and retrieve, storage commitment, and media storage

  **b.** DICOM Information Model.

    **(i)** *Information Object Definition* (*IOD*) entities include modalities (*e.g.*, CT—computed tomography; DX—digital x-radiography; MG—mammography; MR—magnetic resonance imaging; NM—nuclear medicine; PT—positron emission tomography).

    **(ii)** *Service-Object Pair* (*SOP*) is a union of an IOD and DICOM Message Service Element (*DIMSE*)—for example, "Store a CT study."

    **(iii)** *Service Class* is a collection of related SOPs with a specific definition of a service supported by cooperating devices to perform an action on a specific IOD class; for example, Service Class User (*SCU*)—invokes operations; Service Class Provider (*SCP*)—performs operations.

    **(iv)** *Unique Identifier* (*UID*) is a value (usually a long-string number segmented by periods) associated with a particular SOP class describing a DICOM transfer syntax.

  **c.** Common DICOM vocabulary terms and acronyms (Table 5-2).

  **d.** *DICOM Modality WorkList* (*MWL*)—provides patient demographics for technologist selection.

  **e.** *Performed Procedure Step* (*PPS*)—indicates the status of a procedure.

  **f.** *Gray scale Softcopy Presentation State* (*GSPS*)—captures and stores image adjustments, measurements, and notes for a specific patient.

  **g.** *Hanging protocols*: instructions on how to present images according to radiologist's preference on a workstation display; uses DICOM image metadata including anatomic laterality and projection, current versus previous studies, modality, acquisition protocols, display format, and other parameters.

**TABLE 5-2 COMMON DICOM VOCABULARY TERMS AND ACRONYMS** 📖 T. 5-3

| | |
|---|---|
| IOD: Information Object Definition | Modality-specific attributes (*e.g.*, the structure of a DICOM image) |
| AE: Application Entity<br><br>AET: Application Entity Title | Applications (programs and devices) that communicate via DICOM; title = "name" of device |
| Service | Action to perform on an object, such as: *store, get, find, echo* |
| SOP: Service-Object-Pair | Union of an IOD and a DICOM message service element (DIMSE): for example, "Store a CT study" |
| Service Class: Collection of related SOPs | Specific definition of a supported service to perform an action on a specific class of information object; for example,<br><br>SCU—Service Class User—invokes operations<br><br>SCP—Service Class Provider—performs operations |
| Conformance Statement | Associated with a specific DICOM implementation—specifies what can and can't be performed; a public document provided by the vendor |
| Association | First phase of communication between AE and SOP classes, requiring IP address, port number, and AET |
| DICOM Metadata | Data that contains information about other data, for example, patient, study, series, image data, and attributes |
| UID: Unique Identifier | Provides the capability to uniquely identify a wide variety of items. For instance DICOM transfer syntax, which has a registered root of "1.2.840.10008" followed by a suffix unique to the item |

**h.** *HL7* is the standard for messaging contextual data between the various information systems (EMR, RIS, LIS) (Laboratory Information System) and PACS for patient demographics, scheduling, reporting, etc.

    **(i)** The modality worklist (MWL) broker is the translation device for HL7 messages (patient demographics, etc.) to transfer to the PACS and modalities using DICOM.

**i.** *IHE* provides *integration profiles* that use DICOM and HL7 standards to ensure interoperability among different systems and enhance functionality for improved/efficient patient care.

6. **Downtime Procedures, Data Integrity, Other Policies**

  **a.** PACS is a critical part of medical management of patients that rely on availability of images.

    **(i)** A well-established set of policies and procedures are necessary to ensure *business continuity*.

  **b.** Downtime procedures must account for scheduled and unscheduled events.

    **(i)** Planned downtime: software upgrades, bug fixes, security patches, and preventive maintenance—schedule more time than needed, and have a roll-back plan in an unsuccessful attempt

    **(ii)** Unplanned downtime: mitigated by redundancy for critical systems and assessing system architecture for points of failure, having built-in fault tolerance

  **c.** Data integrity procedures should be in place—for example, when MWL is unavailable, entry of patient demographic data should be indicated, and if images fail to send from modality, manual send to PACS

7. **PACS Quality Control**

  **a.** PACS maintenance and quality control challenges

    **(i)** Verification of automated subsystem components—MWL, radiologist worklist, speed of image access and display, hanging protocols, GSPS, image manipulation, digital speech recognition, prompt transmission of diagnostic reports, accuracy of data and measurements

    **(ii)** Ensuring adequate display capabilities and appropriate environmental viewing conditions

  **b.** Image display technical considerations

    **(i)** Considers the human visual system and optimization of information transfer to the viewer.

    **(ii)** Medical diagnostic display types: liquid crystal display (*LCD*) with backlight or organic light emitting diode (*OLED*)—most displays are color LCD at the present time.

    **(iii)** Display bit depth—most medical grade monitors provide 10 to 12 bits of gray scale (1,024 to 4,096 shades of gray) per pixel; consumer grade displays typically 8 bits per pixel—determined by the video card hardware and firmware.

    **(iv)** Display size: medical diagnosis—54 cm diagonal (21.3 inch) with 1,536 pixels (horizontal) and 2048 pixels (vertical) portrait mode, with pixel dimension of ~0.2 mm—"3-megapixel" (MP) monitor that optimizes human visual acuity at a distance of 50 to 60 cm (arms length).

    **(v)** Mammography display: 5 MP monitor (2,000 × 2,500 pixels) with pixel dimension ~0.16 mm.

    **(vi)** Large format displays—76 cm diagonal (30 inch) provide "seamless" virtual portrait displays.

    **(vii)** *Luminance* is the rate of light energy emitted or reflected from a surface per unit area per solid angle, measured in candela/$m^2$ ($cd/m^2$); perceived brightness is not proportional to luminance.

    **(viii)** Display luminance: medical diagnostic displays—350 $cd/m^2$ or higher; mammography 450 $cd/m^2$ or higher (often up to 1,000 to 1,200 $cd/m^2$).

    **(ix)** Other display categories: modality, clinical specialist, EHR applications—with decreasing specifications (*e.g.*, 2 MP, lower luminance less than 200 $cd/m^2$) and cost, respectively.

  **c.** Image perception and viewing conditions.

    **(i)** Assessment of perceived contrast and spatial resolution of the human viewer.

    **(ii)** Determined respectively by experiments of contrast signals at a fixed spatial frequency, and high contrast signals at variable spatial frequencies (detail) that are just detectable.

    **(iii)** *Illuminance* is environmental light impinging on a surface, units of *lux*; 20 to 50 lux is optimal.

    **(iv)** Human perception of contrast signals are nonlinear with luminance and have a limited range of fixed visual adaptation for a given luminance level (Fig. 5-6).

    **(v)** *Luminance ratio* is the detection range of threshold contrast—depends on contrast generated in the display as determined by digital driving levels (DDL) and just-noticeable differences (JND) detected by the viewer; to optimize contrast across gray scale, luminance ratio is approximately 250 to 350:1.

    **(vi)** *Display function* describes the display luminance produced as a function of the digital signal, often called a *digital driving level* (DDL).

  **d.** DICOM GSDF—*gray scale standard display function*, DICOM part 14

    **(i)** Standardizes the display of image contrast for gray scale images

    **(ii)** Provides *perceptual linearization*, where equal differences in pixel values received by the display system are perceived as equal by the human visualization system

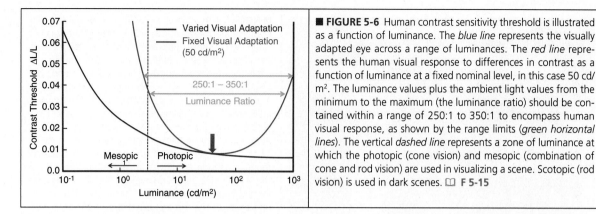

**FIGURE 5-6** Human contrast sensitivity threshold is illustrated as a function of luminance. The *blue line* represents the visually adapted eye across a range of luminances. The *red line* represents the human visual response to differences in contrast as a function of luminance at a fixed nominal level, in this case 50 cd/m². The luminance values plus the ambient light values from the minimum to the maximum (the luminance ratio) should be contained within a range of 250:1 to 350:1 to encompass human visual response, as shown by the range limits (*green horizontal lines*). The vertical *dashed line* represents a zone of luminance at which the photopic (cone vision) and mesopic (combination of cone and rod vision) are used in visualizing a scene. Scotopic (rod vision) is used in dark scenes. ◻ **F 5-15**

**(iii)** *Just-noticeable differences (JND)* and *JND index*—DICOM GSDF defines the JND index as the input value to the GSDF such that one step in the JND index results in a luminance difference that is a just-noticeable difference, as described by the Barten curve (Fig. 5-7).

**(iv)** Measured display function is modified to the "Barten curve" using a Look-Up-Table (LUT) that is used by the video card connected to the display to achieve conformance.

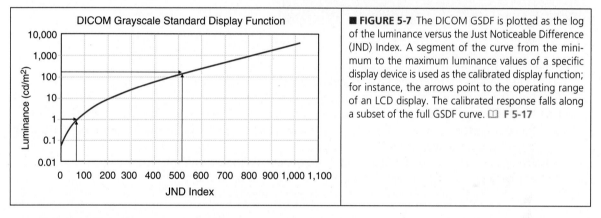

**FIGURE 5-7** The DICOM GSDF is plotted as the log of the luminance versus the Just Noticeable Difference (JND) Index. A segment of the curve from the minimum to the maximum luminance values of a specific display device is used as the calibrated display function; for instance, the arrows point to the operating range of an LCD display. The calibrated response falls along a subset of the full GSDF curve. ◻ **F 5-17**

**e.** Display calibration

**(i)** A calibrated photometer and software are used for display measurement—the software generates DDLs to produce the display luminance, which is measured by the photometer.

**(ii)** The luminance values are recorded in a stepwise fashion for the display function measurement.

**(iii)** Software calculates values in a LUT that causes the display system to conform to the GSDF.

**(iv)** The LUT is downloaded to the display card so that DDLs will be translated (Figs. 5-8).

**(v)** Annual evaluation (minimum) for GSDF, luminance, and luminance ratio are recommended.

**(vi)** Qualitative evaluation using SMPTE (Society of Motion Picture and Television Engineers) or AAPM OIQ (overall image quality) patterns for 5% contrast in darkest and brightest areas (Fig. 5-9).

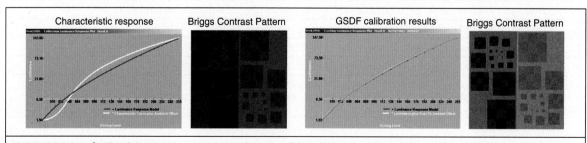

**FIGURE 5-8 Left:** The characteristic response as a function of digital driving number on an uncalibrated display is shown by the *white curve*, and the DICOM GSDF is shown as the *red curve*, with a "Briggs Contrast Pattern" shown. **Right:** After calculating the adjustment Look-Up-Table and downloading to the video display driver, the subsequent conformance measurement indicates performance matching the GSDF, with the corresponding "Briggs" test pattern demonstrating improvement in perceived contrast for the patterns in the darker areas of the image for the calibrated display. ◻ **F 5-19**

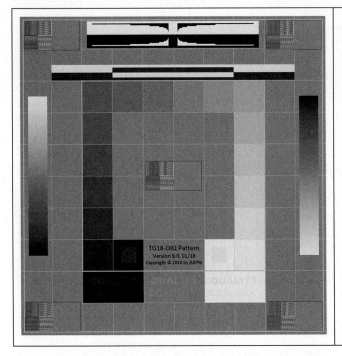

TG18-OIQ Pattern
Version 9.0, 01/18
Copyright © 2018 by AAPM

■ **FIGURE 5-9** Qualitative verification of display calibration. The AAPM TG18 OIQ (overall image quality) video test pattern (Reprinted with permission from American Association of Physicists in Medicine) has 18 luminance regions from 0 to 100%. At the ends are 0%/5% and 95%/100% contrast patches representing a difference of 13 digital numbers for an 8-bit display (256 gray levels). On the row below in the dark, mid-range, and bright luminance areas are the letters "Quality Control" with a background contrast difference of 14 to 1 gray levels (1 level per letter). Spatial resolution modules of high and low contrast in the corners and the center, linear ramps on the sides for evaluating contouring and bit-depth artifacts, and dark-bright transition zones at the top are included in the test pattern. An alternate, simpler video test pattern is the Society of Motion Picture Television Engineers (SMPTE) pattern (not shown). ▭ F 5-20

   **f.** Validating patient demographics with acquired images
     **(i)** Relies on many information systems and databases: PACS, RIS, EHR, MWL.
     **(ii)** Proper association is critical for patient safety, privacy, security, and care.
     **(iii)** IHE Scheduled Workflow (*SWF*) integration profile ensures data availability and consistency.
     **(iv)** Processes detect errors (*e.g.*, incorrect MRN) and create *exceptions* and require reconciliation, typically requiring human intervention.
     **(v)** IHE Patient Information Reconciliation (*PIR*) integration profile supports nonstandard workflow (*e.g.*, emergency "Doe" patients) for subsequent automated reconciliation.
   **g.** Interoperability assessment of medical imaging acquisition systems (Table 5-3)

## TABLE 5-3 INTEROPERABILITY ASSESSMENT TESTS ▭ T. 5-4

| | |
|---|---|
| 1. | DICOM Modality Worklist configuration and Information Display is accurate |
| 2. | Procedure or RIS Code Mapping is properly loaded into the imaging modality |
| 3. | Images appear in a timely fashion and are associated with the correct worklist |
| 4. | Exams and image labeling have appropriate appearance |
| 5. | Quantitative measurement consistency is validated between systems and viewers |
| 6. | Patient demographics are correct and editing (if allowed) is validated downstream |
| 7. | Image orientation and laterality are properly encoded in the DICOM metadata |
| 8. | Fidelity of information in the DICOM header is maintained with information exchange |
| 9. | DICOM structured reports (SR) are accurate and mapped correctly |
| 10. | Postprocessing functionality is consistent across systems and reproducible |
| 11. | Downtime procedures and alternative connectivity channels are validated |

*Source: Interoperability Assessment for the Commissioning of Medical Imaging Acquisition Systems, Report of AAPM Task Group 248.* American Association of Physicists in Medicine; 2019b. https://www.aapm.org/pubs/reports/detail.asp?docid_180. Accessed August 10, 2020.

# LIFE CYCLE OF A RADIOLOGY EXAMINATION

The radiology examination requires the orchestration of a number of messages and interactions between various software and information systems for patient registration, scheduling, acquisition, diagnosis, reporting, and care (Fig. 5-10)

**1. Registration and Order Entry**
    **a.** The EHR contains the master record and provides registration events, with messaging via HL7
        **(i)** HL7 has several message types—*ADT*—Admit, Discharge, Transfer A04 message is used initially.
        **(ii)** The A04 message contains patient identification (medical record number) and other information about the patient (*e.g.*, address, allergies, initial diagnosis, insurance, etc.).
        **(iii)** Referring physician places orders through the EHR, an HL7 order message (*ORM-O01*).
        **(iv)** The ORM is sent to the appropriate information system (*e.g.*, lab work to the LIS, radiology request to the RIS) specifying the type of request through *OBR* (observation request) element.

**2. RIS and Scheduling**
    **a.** RIS manages orders, protocols, exam scheduling, and technologist workflow.
    **b.** Once an HL7 ORM message is received, the RIS sends an HL7 ORM message to speech recognition (SR), EHR, and PACS/MWL interfaces to schedule the patient, location, and time.

**3. Modalities and Modality Worklist**
    **a.** RIS interfaces via the interface engine to the PACS and modality worklist broker (Fig. 5-11).
    **b.** MWL presents a list of patients to be selected by the technologist for demographics.
    **c.** Patient information is transferred to the DICOM metadata at the modality.

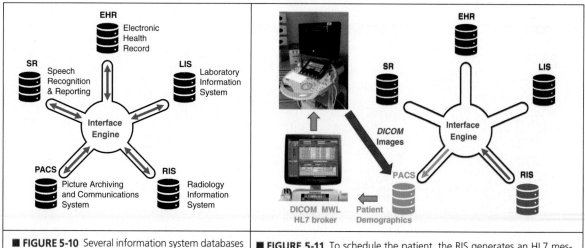

■ **FIGURE 5-10** Several information system databases are necessary to deliver timely assistance and care for a patient undergoing an imaging examination. These systems communicate on the Local Area Network bidirectionally with HL7 messaging through an interface engine, which routes HL7 messages based upon internal content to specific target databases. Each database system plays a role in the life cycle of a radiology encounter with a patient for an imaging examination by creating, sending, using, and storing information useful for the care of the patient. ▢ **F 5-23**

■ **FIGURE 5-11** To schedule the patient, the RIS generates an HL7 message routed to the PACS indicating the availability of the patient to be imaged. The imaging modality does not use HL7 messaging for handling image acquisition and archiving events. A PACS "HL7-DICOM broker" interface generates a DICOM Modality Worklist on the modality. The technologist identifies the patient and selects the name from the list, ensuring reproducible demographic information appended to the DICOM metadata associated with the patient images at the modality (*green arrows*). The study is performed, and the DICOM images are sent to the PACS for review and storage (*red arrow*). ▢ **F 5-26**

**4. Exam Acquisition and Storage**
    **a.** Modality device on the network—each unique network node is composed of application entity (*AE*) title, IP address, and port number for communication with the PACS, which has its own node.
    **b.** Images acquired on the modality are sent to the PACS via negotiated transfer syntax SOP—the union of an IOD (*e.g.*, US) and a DICOM message service element (DIMSE)—for example, "store the ultrasound study."
    **c.** The modality is the storage service class user (SSCU) and the PACS (archive) is the storage service class provider (SSCP) using the DICOM standard for image transfer (red arrow, Fig. 5-11).

**5. Radiologist Worklist, Speech Recognition, and Report Generation**
   **a.** Images on the PACS are assigned or selected with a *radiologist worklist* generated by the PACS or RIS.
   **b.** Worklist filters allow selectivity of exam types, subspecialty sections, modalities, anatomic sites, etc.
   **c.** Once selected, the PACS "hangs" the images according to radiologist-specific *hanging protocols*.
   **d.** Contemporaneously, the radiologist reviews patient history and other information from the EHR.
   **e.** Initiation of the speech recognition system allows the radiologist to dictate findings after review.
   **f.** Once the dictation is completed, an HL7 observation return (*ORU*) R01 message with the composed diagnosis in an observation result (*OBX*) segment is sent to the PACS, EHR, and RIS (Figs. 5-12 and 5-13).
   **g.** The patient diagnosis is appended to the patient record for consumption by the referring physician.
   **h.** The referring physician treats the patient based on information and images accessible by the EHR.

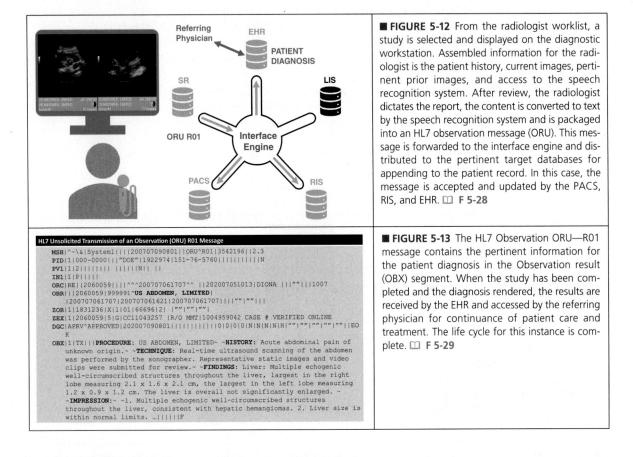

■ **FIGURE 5-12** From the radiologist worklist, a study is selected and displayed on the diagnostic workstation. Assembled information for the radiologist is the patient history, current images, pertinent prior images, and access to the speech recognition system. After review, the radiologist dictates the report, the content is converted to text by the speech recognition system and is packaged into an HL7 observation message (ORU). This message is forwarded to the interface engine and distributed to the pertinent target databases for appending to the patient record. In this case, the message is accepted and updated by the PACS, RIS, and EHR. ▢ F 5-28

■ **FIGURE 5-13** The HL7 Observation ORU—R01 message contains the pertinent information for the patient diagnosis in the Observation result (OBX) segment. When the study has been completed and the diagnosis rendered, the results are received by the EHR and accessed by the referring physician for continuance of patient care and treatment. The life cycle for this instance is complete. ▢ F 5-29

**6. Structured Reporting**
   **a.** Structured reporting has several different meanings in the context of a radiology report.
      **(i)** Presence of lists and hierarchical relationships
      **(ii)** Use of coded/numerical content and plain text
      **(iii)** Use of relationships between concepts
      **(iv)** Presence of embedded references to images and other objects
   **b.** DICOM SR is defined more by its construction than by what it contains—a structured document.
   **c.** Capabilities of SR are just being realized for increasing accuracy and efficiency.
   **d.** Principal uses currently include radiation dose SR (RDSR) and ultrasound measurements.

**7. Billing**
   **a.** Payment for imaging exams is initiated by HL7 message to the EHR and RIS from the reporting system.
   **b.** Human coders, billers, or automated methods assign CPT or ICD-10 codes and modifiers, as needed.
   **c.** Most radiology services are composed of a technical (equipment and infrastructure used) and professional component (radiologist supervision, interpretation, and reporting).

**8. Report Distribution—Completion of the Exam Life Cycle**
   **a.** Workflow steps diagrammed in Figure 5-14.

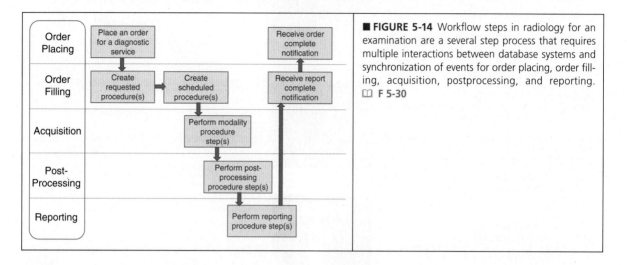

■ **FIGURE 5-14** Workflow steps in radiology for an examination are a several step process that requires multiple interactions between database systems and synchronization of events for order placing, order filling, acquisition, postprocessing, and reporting. 📖 **F 5-30**

## 5.5  RADIOLOGY FROM OUTSIDE THE DEPARTMENT

**1. Clinical Decision Support and Computerized Provider Order Entry**
   **a.** Appropriate ordering and use of imaging examinations requires clinical decision support (*CDS*).
   **b.** Appropriate use criteria (*AUC*) has been mandated by the Protecting Access to Medicare Act (*PAMA*) of 2014, which requires physicians ordering advanced diagnostic imaging services to consult AUC.
   **c.** A Clinical Decision Support Mechanism (*CDSM*) is an interactive, electronic tool communicating AUC considering a patient's clinical condition by scoring the choice of an examination according to the AUC.
   **d.** AUC is evidence-based criteria developed or endorsed by a provider led entity (*PLE*) that must be qualified by CMS to become a *QPLE* through specific requirements including peer-review, literature review, and assessment of evidence.
   **e.** Goals are to assist providers in their computerized provider order entry (*CPOE*) to select the most appropriate examination based on AUC guidance with the CDSM software.
**2. Reporting**
   **a.** Assisting the referring physician with multimedia-enhanced radiology reports (*MERR*) beyond plain text.
   **b.** Reference links to images or annotations are built into the report using the IHE *Key Image Notes (KIN)* integration profile as well as structured exchange and storage integration profile, *Simple Image and Numeric Report (SINR)* (Fig. 5-15).
**3. Reading Room**
   **a.** Historical concepts of the "Reading Room" are changing rapidly, with more reading performed remotely in individual offices and in radiologists' homes.
   **b.** Enabling technologies.
      **(i)**  Availability of high-performance CPU, GPU, memory, and graphics components
      **(ii)**  Decreased cost of diagnostic displays: "prosumer" grade close to "medical grade" performance
      **(iii)**  Higher bandwidth through a standard home or remote office Internet service provider (ISP)
      **(iv)**  High-performance virtual private networks (VPNs) enabling fully secure remote reading
      **(v)**  Development of wide-scale virtual radiology practices disassociated and independent of hospital enterprises or healthcare organizations (*e.g.*, "NightHawk" services)
   **c.** "Teleradiology" as a definition is losing meaning, being supplanted by virtual radiology services.
**4. Social Media**
   **a.** Concept in the context of informatics needs to be considered more widely.
   **b.** Shared Wikis, virtual conferences and presentations, online messages, video teleconferencing.
   **c.** Pandemic (COVID-19) and other factors are additional drivers to the virtualization of collaboration.

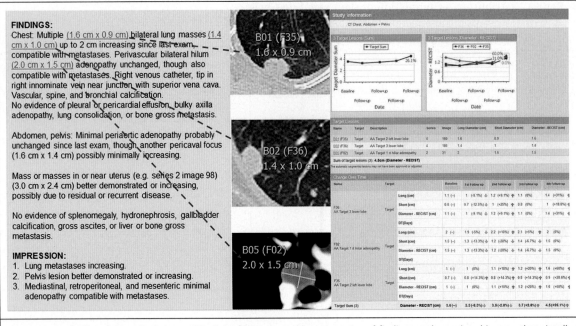

**FIGURE 5-15** The Multimedia Enhanced Radiology Report provides a narrative of findings and associated images that visually show the details as well as quantitative content to demonstrate longitudinal outcomes through measurements and graphs—in this case a continuing evaluation of lung metastases and patterns of evolving size. 📖 **F 5-31** (Reproduced by permission from Folio LR, Machado LB, Dwyer AJ. Multimedia-enhanced radiology reports; concept, components, and challenges. *Radiographics* 2018;38(2):462–482. Copyright Radiological Society of North America. doi: 10.1148/rg. 2071170047.)

## 5.6    SECURITY AND PRIVACY

Security and privacy for the patient requires data integrity, authentication, nonrepudiation, and availability.

1. **Layers of Security**
   a. Safeguards: *Physical, Technical, and Administrative* (Fig. 5-16)
2. **Security Threats**
   a. Loss of information through mechanical or unintentional deletion of data on storage disks

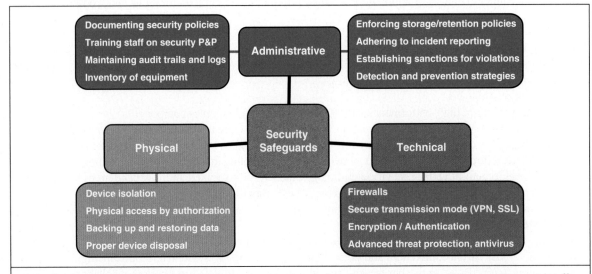

**FIGURE 5-16** Security safeguards entail a three-pronged approach, including administrative (policies, procedures, and staffing processes), physical (prevent or limit access to protected information), and technical (implementation of firewalls, virtual private networks, encryption, antivirus) components with a summary of key points. 📖 **F 5-32**

     **b.** *Ransomware*—hacker-encrypted critical information

     **c.** Software "*viruses*" loaded via programs from other infected disks that can cause harm

     **d.** *Trojan horses* (programs of being of interest—but with hidden purposes); *worms*—malicious programs spreading over networks; *time bombs*—programs or program segments to do something on a future date

     **e.** *Key loggers*—programs that record keystrokes; *password grabbers*—asking users to log in to get info

     **f.** *Denial of service*—attacks to overload networks from "bots"—multiple computers controlled by hackers

     **g.** *Phishing*—fraudulent practice of sending emails purporting to be from reputable sources in order to induce individuals to reveal personal information, passwords, etc.

     **h.** *Spear phishing*—email designed to get a single recipient to respond, modified to specifically address that victim, purportedly coming from an entity of familiarity that contains personal information

**3. Security Considerations**

     **a.** Deny unauthorized users' access to all enterprise systems.

     **b.** Ensure business continuity with fault tolerance and backup protection—part of PACS standard operations.

     **c.** Account for probability and consequences of risk, such as human error.

     **d.** Provide access to valid users using 2 factor authentication to provide appropriate patient care.

     **e.** Review strategies for a PACS and enterprise imaging security plan.

          **(i)** Perform a risk analysis.

          **(ii)** Establish written policies and procedures for information security—train staff accordingly.

          **(iii)** Backups—maintain copies of programs and information—stored in a remote, secure location.

          **(iv)** Installation of antivirus software, with periodic updates.

          **(v)** Forbid loading of removable media—USB drives, optical disks—and unknown programs.

          **(vi)** Authenticate users by passwords and two-factor authentication (*e.g.*, biometric, cell phone).

          **(vii)** Promptly terminate access privileges of former employees.

          **(viii)** Log off workstations when not in use, particularly in nonsecure areas.

          **(ix)** Grant each user only sufficient privileges and access required to accomplish needed tasks.

          **(x)** Encrypt information over networks (in flight) and on storage media (at rest).

          **(xi)** Physically secure media via encryption; destroy removable media and disks no longer needed.

          **(xii)** Routinely install "patches" to the OS and software programs.

          **(xiii)** Install firewalls at nodes where LANs are connected to other LANs and WANs (the Internet).

          **(xiv)** Implement and record audit trails to protected healthcare information.

          **(xv)** Establish emergency operations and disaster recovery plans.

**4. Privacy: HIPAA and HITECH**

     **a.** Health Insurance Portability and Accountability Act (*HIPAA*) of 1996.

          **(i)** Standards for electronic protected healthcare information (*PHI*)

          **(ii)** Covered entities: healthcare providers, health plans, clearinghouses, and business associates

          **(iii)** *Business Associate Agreement* (*BAA*) specifies each party's responsibilities for PHI

     **b.** The privacy rule attempts to strike a balance that permits important use of information (the "portability") while protecting privacy of patients (the "accountability") seeking care.

     **c.** Electronic PHI—*ePHI*—and compliance with the security rule

          **(i)** Ensure confidentiality, integrity, and availability of all ePHI.

          **(ii)** Detect and safeguard against anticipated threats to the security of information.

          **(iii)** Protect against reasonably anticipated impermissible uses or disclosures.

          **(iv)** Certify compliance by the workforce.

     **d.** Health Information Technology for Economic and Clinical Health (*HITECH*) Act

          **(i)** Created in 2009 to motivate the implementation of EHRs.

          **(ii)** Expanded the scope of privacy and security protections available under HIPAA for ePHI.

          **(iii)** Increased the potential legal liability for noncompliance and for more stringent enforcement.

          **(iv)** Substantial fines are assessed when breaches of ePHI occur.

**5. De-Identification of Protected Health Information**

     **a.** HIPAA privacy rule provides the standard for de-identification of PHI.

     **b.** Removing patient ePHI is required for performing research on clinical information and images.

     **c.** De-identification is defined as being one of two methods.

          **(i)** *Statistical method* requires an "expert" statistician to document that there is a small likelihood that a given record could be traced back to the patient.

          **(ii)** *Safe Harbor method* details 18 features that must be removed from electronic information (Table 5-4); for specialized uses, fewer or more than 18 elements need to be removed.

     **d.** Researchers must request and receive permission from the local Institutional Review Board (IRB) to gain access to properly de-identified data prior to initiation of investigations.

**TABLE 5-4 IDENTIFIERS TO BE REMOVED FROM ePHI TO BE DESIGNATED AS DE-IDENTIFIED BY THE SAFE HARBOR METHOD** 📖 T. 5-5

| | |
|---|---|
| 1. Names (the individual and his or her relatives, employers, or household members) | 10. Account numbers |
| 2. Geographic subdivisions smaller than a state, with exceptions for the use of part of the zip code | 11. Certificate or license numbers |
| 3. All dates, except year, and all ages over 89 | 12. Vehicle identifiers and license plate numbers |
| 4. Telephone numbers | 13. Device identifiers and serial numbers |
| 5. Fax numbers | 14. URLs |
| 6. Email addresses | 15. IP addresses |
| 7. Social Security numbers | 16. Biometric identifiers |
| 8. Medical Record numbers | 17. Full-face photographs and any comparable images |
| 9. Health plan beneficiary numbers | 18. Any other unique identifying characteristic or code |

## 5.7 "BIG DATA" AND DATA PLUMBING

1. **Data: Data Types and Locations—"Big Data"**
   a. Imaging is increasingly becoming a part of machine learning (*ML*) and advanced analytic tools, requiring access to very large data sets beyond traditional processes and methods that cannot scale effectively to the requirements of new use cases.
   b. Access to 100,000s of images—many terabytes—might be required to build ML algorithms, beyond the scope of traditional PACS, which are chiefly built to support a linear processing pipeline.
      (i) Scaling up requires massive parallel processing capabilities not currently in place.
   c. DICOM standard for image transfer and storage does not align well with protocols for Big Data analytics.
      (i) Access to DICOM data requires intermediate processing to facilitate efficient access.
      (ii) One resolution is to create a separate representation of metadata in formats such as JSON (JavaScript Object Notation) that is more amenable to enterprise analytics.
   d. Most PACS are based on standard relational databases (RDMS, Relational Database Management Systems) and typically accessible by SQL (Structured Query Language) that do not scale into Big Data
      (i) Newer data models, "NoSQL" or "NewSQL," can support the enterprise analytics and cloud-specific protocols, for example, Amazon DocumentDB, Microsoft Azure Storage Services
2. **Data Plumbing**
   a. Classic DIMSE-based DICOM is not well suited for massive parallel access and extraction of data.
      (i) Indexed data curation and annotation of image findings are not well suited to current PACS.
   b. Existing DICOM pipelines are not effectively scalable to "getting the right image to the right algorithm and presented in the right context" for ML algorithms.
   c. Opportunities exist for web-based access, represented by the DICOMweb suite of services.
      (i) Can be supported by RESTful web services by the characteristics of REST (statelessness, cacheability, and ability to dynamically code on demand on the client side)
   d. Opportunity to apply more sophisticated rules engine capability and intelligence to PACS image management is necessary for predictive series-level routing based on feature recognition.
   e. New and emerging functional requirements for data plumbing are the key to successful application of ML and implementation of artificial intelligence algorithms.

## 5.8 ALGORITHMS FOR IMAGE AND NONIMAGE ANALYTICS

1. **Basic Image Processing**
   a. Conversion of pixel values into display luminance
      (i) Look-Up-Table (*LUT*) transformation adjusts image contrast and brightness (window and level)
      (ii) Optimizes human visualization of the content with interactive adjustments (Fig. 5-17)
   b. Other image processing: edge enhancement, smoothing, temporal subtraction (see examples in Chapter 4)

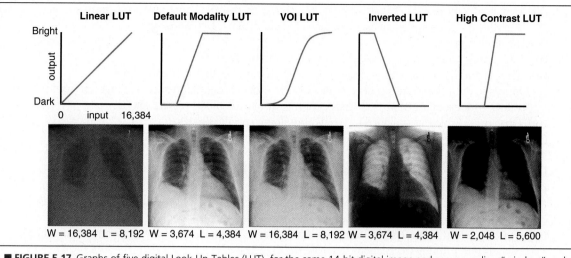

**FIGURE 5-17** Graphs of five digital Look-Up-Tables (LUT), for the same 14-bit digital image and corresponding "window" and "level" settings. From **left** to **right**, the first is a linear LUT that preserves the way the image was originally acquired. Typically, the useful image data occupies only a small range of values for this 14-bit image, and thus, contrast is low. The second is the "default modality LUT" that is assigned by the modality, based upon an optimized gray scale range. Note that a large fraction of the range of the image is set to zero (*dark*) or largest output (*maximal brightness*) and that a small range of values is mapped from the dark to the bright values on the display. The third is the "Value of Interest" LUT (VOILUT), which encompasses the full range of input values and maps the output according to the capabilities of the display. Typically, this LUT is a sigmoidally shaped curve, which softens the appearance of the image in the dark and bright regions. The fourth LUT inverts image contrast. Shown here is the inverted second image. The fifth image demonstrates windowing to enhance contrast in underpenetrated parts of the image by increasing the slope of the LUT. Note that this causes the loss of all contrast in the highly penetrated regions of the lung. 📖 **F 5-36**

2. **Advanced 3D Visualization and Printing**
   a. Multiplanar reconstruction (*MPR*)
      (i)   Reformatting of tomographic images (usually axial) and data into sagittal and coronal planes.
      (ii)  Isotropic resolution is achieved with thin slices equal to the x-y plane dimensions (Fig. 5-18).
      (iii) Slab (thicker sections), curved, and oblique MPR slices are commonly produced.
      (iv)  Maximum Intensity Projection (*MIP*) is a method of forming projection images by casting rays through the volume dataset and selecting the maximum pixel value along each ray
      (v)   Variations of MIP include thin and thick slab and minimum Intensity projection (*minIP*), the latter useful for visualizing low-intensity structures such as the trachea and lungs.

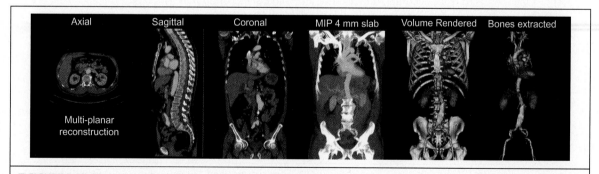

**FIGURE 5-18** CT angiography and data reformatting. **Left to Right**: the native *axial slices* from the top of the shoulder to the bottom of the pelvis (one image shown); *sagittal* reformat from the axial data; *coronal* reformat; *4 mm slab coronal Maximum Intensity Projection* image reformat; *volume-rendered* data set, showing bone and contrast-filled vessel anatomy; *selective bone removal* to show contrast-filled vessels. 📖 **F 5-37**

   b. Viewing in three dimensions
      (i)  A stack of 2D images is viewed as a 3D object using a shaded surface display (*SSD*) approach, also known as surface rendering, or a volume rendering (*VR*) approach.
      (ii) In SSD, surfaces are identified by marking individual voxels as belonging or not belonging to the surface by using simple thresholding methods.

(iii) Observed light intensity is calculated by the computer by calculating reflections from simulated direct and diffuse light sources; an example using SSD is virtual CT colonoscopy.

c. Volume rendering
   (i) Uses a more complete set of voxels within the volume than SSD.
   (ii) The produced VR image set uses an opacity range from 0% to 100% and colors.
   (iii) Voxels in the volume are segmented into various tissues based upon specific ranges of pixel (voxel) values—for example, bone, soft tissue, contrast enhanced blood vessels, air, fat.
   (iv) Opacity and color are assigned to voxels containing specific tissues.
   (v) VR provides a robust view of the anatomy and depth relationships (Fig. 5-18).

d. Three-dimensional printing
   (i) Creation of 3D physical models from acquired CT or MRI datasets.
   (ii) Process of making an object by depositing materials (plastic, metals) one small layer at a time.
   (iii) A 3D blueprint from the tomographic datasets renders the surface geometry into triangular tiles, a process known as *tessellation*, to create a file format (*e.g.*, STL).
   (iv) The STL (or other similar files) is opened in a "slicer" 3D printer software that converts digital 3D models into printing instructions to create the object.
   (v) User-configured settings control the quality and time of the output.

3. **Radiomics**
   a. Describes the process of the conversion of digital medical images into mineable high-dimensional data that can potentially reveal information (biomarkers) for underlying pathophysiology or other findings.
   b. Steps to achieve quantitative image analysis.
      (i) Acquiring images under known conditions
      (ii) Identifying areas or volumes in the images that may contain prognostic value
      (iii) Segmenting volumes by delineating borders manually or by computer-assisted AI algorithms
      (iv) Extracting and qualifying descriptive features from the volume in a relational database
      (v) Mining the data to develop classifier models to predict outcomes
   c. Challenges include reproducibility, adequate image quality, using similar tools for analysis, and transparency in the methods and benchmarks used in collecting the information.
   d. Compliance with HIPAA and restricted PHI could hinder or limit such investigations.
   e. Radiomic analysis is likely to advance the precision in diagnosis, assessment of prognosis, and prediction of therapy response.

4. **Artificial Intelligence**
   AI is a wide-ranging branch of computer science concerned with building smart algorithms capable of performing tasks that typically require human intelligence
   a. Natural language processing (*NLP*)
      (i) Objective is to read, decipher, understand, and make sense of human language.
      (ii) NLP techniques often rely on machine learning and AI to derive meaning.
   b. Machine learning and deep learning
      (i) ML allows computers to "learn" in an supervised or unsupervised environment.
      (ii) *Supervised learning* uses large numbers of inputs such as curated image sets with annotations, markups with known outputs based upon outcome data.
      (iii) *Unsupervised learning* uses datasets without any specified structure.
      (iv) One widely used method of learning is based upon a neural network composed of an input layer, one or more "hidden" layers, and an output layer, connected by "weighting" (Fig. 5-19).

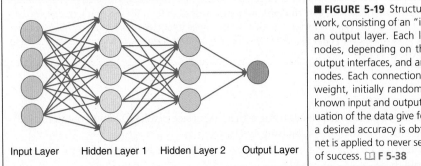

Input Layer   Hidden Layer 1   Hidden Layer 2   Output Layer

■ **FIGURE 5-19** Structure of a convolutional neural network, consisting of an "input layer," "hidden layer(s)," and an output layer. Each layer can consist of one or many nodes, depending on the task and number of input and output interfaces, and are interconnected to adjacent layer nodes. Each connection is assigned a positive or negative weight, initially randomized but with a "training set" of known input and output layers. Iterations based upon evaluation of the data give feedback to adjust the weights until a desired accuracy is obtained. Once "trained," the neural net is applied to never seen cases for testing and evaluation of success. 📖 **F 5-38**

**(v)** A challenge is to determine the number of hidden layers and number of nodes on each layer.

**(vi)** Limitations of AI include (1) a lack of generalizability; (2) extensive effort to mark up and curate data sets for training; and (3) access to large enough data sets for training that can function in a sensitive, specific, and accurate way on unknown cases.

**(vii)** The benefits of AI for radiologists is to provide a "value-add" to the practice, not replacement.

## 5.9   THE BUSINESS OF INFORMATICS

1. **Revenue Cycle**
   a. Required revenue to sustain operations is formalized by using CPT codes and further refined by CMS as the Healthcare Common Procedure Coding System (HPCPS) for Medicare and Medicaid funding.
      **(i)** The relative value unit (*RVU*) provides a relative workload weight for each procedure.
      **(ii)** The RVU for a chest CT is greater than a chest radiograph, reflecting radiologist effort and technology costs (interpretation of several hundred tomograph images versus 1 or 2 radiographs).
   b. Revenue cycle management (RCM) aligns procedures to be performed and interpreted to the metrics used to assign value to them is termed the revenue cycle (orders, procedures, billing, reimbursement).
      **(i)** Decision support, structured reporting, and use of templates for completeness have a value impact.
2. **Impact of Regulations on Informatics**
   a. Office of the National Coordinator for Health Information Technology (*ONC*) is a key resource for various federal initiatives and regulations as they relate to technology.
   b. HIPAA and PHI protections
      **(i)** Distinction between anonymization (elimination of links to the originating source) and de-identification (ability to reference the original data through indexing with an honest broker)
      **(ii)** Safe harbor method (Table 5-4)—18 data elements that are removed to meet HIPAA security
   c. HITECH Act—key concept, meaningful use (MU) with promotional incentives to implement technology and penalties for failure to adopt as well as for breaches of patient security and privacy
   d. PAMA, AUC, CDS, and CPOE are important aspects in driving ordering appropriateness (see Section 5.5)

## 5.10   BEYOND IMAGING INFORMATICS

Imaging informatics resides as a discipline of medical informatics—"The science of how to use data, information, and knowledge to improve human health and the delivery of healthcare services"

1. **EMR and EHR**
   a. Terms are used interchangeably but are distinct: EHR focus is on the total health of the patient, while the EMR is considered the digital version of the medical chart contained in one practice (ONC definition).
   b. EHRs are built to share information with other healthcare providers such as laboratories and specialists.
2. **HIEs**
   a. Health information exchange—attaining interoperability and still maintaining patient information security among vendors and organizations through "brokers"—ONC and CMS models.
      **(i)** Directed exchange—from provider/organization to provider/organization as a "push" model
      **(ii)** Query-based exchange—facilitates *find and retrieve* mechanisms between organizations
      **(iii)** Consumer-mediated exchange—facilitates patients to retrieve and transmit health records
   b. Regional Health Information Organizations (RHIOs) have been implemented statewide or in a region for providing limited geographic interoperability.
3. **Image Sharing**
   a. DICOM is the lexicon for medical imaging, both internally and externally; image exchange is being facilitated by efforts such as RSNA Image Share and Sequoia Project to ensure interoperability.
4. **Clinical Informatics**
   a. Imaging informatics is a specialty of clinical and medical informatics, and increasingly as an integrated part of the larger discipline—as such, PACS and RIS can no longer operate independently, but as an essential part of the community-wide interoperative and image-enabled EHR.

# Section II Questions and Answers

1. Which one of the following is not a standard or standards body but uses standards in developing a framework of integration profiles?
   A. Digital Imaging and COmmunications in Medicine
   B. Health Level 7
   C. Internet Engineering Task Force
   D. Integrating the Healthcare Enterprise
   E. International Organization for Standardization

2. Communication between the EHR, RIS, and PACS to deliver *patient demographic information* uses which protocol standard?
   A. DICOM
   B. HL7
   C. IHE
   D. SNOMED-CT
   E. ICD-10

3. What method provides a set of instructions on how to lay out a class of images at a PACS workstation?
   A. Grayscale softcopy presentation state
   B. Grayscale standard display function
   C. Modality worklist
   D. Hanging protocol

4. What is the recommended *Luminance Ratio* for a diagnostic display that optimizes the fixed visual adaptation of the human eye?
   A. 50
   B. 150
   C. 350
   D. 850

5. Where would you look to find the specific parameters regarding the modality acquisition details for an imaging study on the PACS?
   A. DICOM metadata
   B. IHE profile for scheduled workflow
   C. HL7 ADT message
   D. Modality worklist

6. Which one of the following is an example of a *technical security safeguard*?
   A. Audit trail and logging
   B. Device disposal
   C. Sanctions for Violations
   D. Virtual Private Network

7. What is the typical factor for reversible (*lossless*) image compression of radiographic images?
   A. 3
   B. 10
   C. 30
   D. 60
   E. 100

8. What is the DICOM information object descriptor that specifies how annotations and image manipulations implemented by a viewer are stored?
   A. GSDF—grayscale standard display function
   B. GSPS—grayscale softcopy presentation state
   C. PPS—performed procedure step
   D. MWL—modality work list
   E. AET—application entity title

9. In an active-matrix liquid crystal display monitor, what changes are implemented to modulate the intensity of the light from individual pixels?
   A. Current in an electron beam
   B. Intensity of the backlight
   C. Polarity of the light
   D. Voltages applied to individual light emitting diodes
   E. Voltage between the electron gun and the anode

10. A main goal of the DICOM gray scale standard display function is to
    A. Prevent adjustment of image contrast by the user
    B. Make adjustments of image contrast by windowing and leveling unnecessary
    C. Change the image contrast on monitors of different maximal luminances
    D. Provide a predictable transformation of digital presentation values to luminance
    E. compensate for differences in spatial resolution

11. Which of the following best describes IHE?
    A. A Local Area Network protocol
    B. A wide area network protocol
    C. An image transfer standard that replaces DICOM
    D. A guide for the use of standards such as DICOM
    E. An upper-level communications protocol used in healthcare information systems

12. Which act specifies legal liability and penalties for noncompliance of ePHI security and privacy?
    A. HIPAA
    B. HITECH
    C. PAMA
    D. MIPS

13. Which of the following represents the federal law specifying security measures for PHI?
    A. MQSA
    B. PAMA
    C. NEMA
    D. HIPAA

14. Of the following, what modality *on average* produces the largest uncompressed study size?
    A. Digital mammography (MG)
    B. Computed tomography (CT)
    C. Fluoroscopy-guided intervention (XA)
    D. Magnetic resonance imaging (MR)
    E. Digital radiography (DX)

15. What security threat is posed by hackers when using e-mail purported to be from reputable sources?
    A. Time bomb
    B. Ransomware
    C. Phishing
    D. Denial of service

16. In the ISO-OSI 7 layer framework for network interconnections, at what layer does the software application function?
    A. Layer 1
    B. Layer 3
    C. Layer 5
    D. Layer 7

17. What is the approximate pixel dimension of a display monitor that optimizes human visual acuity when viewing at arms length?
    A. 5 μm
    B. 20 μm
    C. 50 μm
    D. 200 μm
    E. 500 μm

18. Why is a luminance ratio of 350:1 recommended when calibrating a diagnostic display monitor?
    A. To match human contrast sensitivity threshold range
    B. To achieve better display color balance accuracy
    C. To allow for higher background illuminance levels
    D. To accurately calibrate the darkest and brightest levels

19. The Protecting Access to Medicare Act (PAMA) mandates a QPLE to create which of the following?
    A. Multimedia enhanced radiology report (MERR)
    B. Computerized provider order entry (CPOE)
    C. Meaningful use (MU)
    D. Appropriate use criteria (AUC)

20. What is the protocol that accesses and maintains directory information services over an IP network?
    A. SMTP
    B. LDAP
    C. TLS
    D. HTML

21. What is necessary and required to allow sharing of PHI between healthcare entities for patient care?
    A. BAA
    B. IRB
    C. SSL
    D. VNA
    E. VPN

22. What is the required maximum luminance (cd/m²) capability for a mammography display used for primary diagnosis?
    A. 150
    B. 250
    C. 350
    D. 450
    E. 550

23. Regarding electronic access and use of medical imaging systems, who is ultimately responsible for ensuring security and privacy of patient image data?
    A. Manufacturer
    B. Food and Drug Administration
    C. Medical Imaging & Technology Alliance
    D. International Electrotechnical Commission
    E. Healthcare organization

24. In multiplanar reconstruction (MPR) from a CT scan of the upper torso, which plane generates a frontal view of the lungs?
    A. Axial
    B. Coronal
    C. Sagittal
    D. Oblique

25. What is the term for the process of extracting imaging biomarkers from medical images?
    A. Deep learning
    B. Radiomics
    C. Artificial intelligence
    D. Data plumbing

26. In hierarchical storage management, which of the following algorithms are used in ensuring pertinent older comparison studies are available for diagnosis?
    A. Image compression
    B. RAID
    C. Vendor neutral archive
    D. Prefetching

# Answers

1. **D**  Standards do not confer the ability to interoperate between systems. The Integrating the Healthcare Enterprise effort develops relevant "use cases" and describes how standards such as HL7 and DICOM can be used in "integration profiles." Manufacturers that claim to be compliant to a specific IHE profile validate their implementations in a "connectathon" process that allows purchasers to use the IHE profiles as request for proposal (RFP) shorthand in describing interoperability requirements. *(Pg. 114–115 and 149–150)*

2. **B**  Health Level 7 (HL7) is the standard used for textural communications between information systems. This standard provides information on patient demographics and a lot more, such as admission, transfer, and discharge messages, diagnostic reports, and a lot more. *(Pg. 113–114, and Section 5.4, "Lifecycle of a Radiology Exam")*

3. **D**  "Hanging" protocols are software instructions on how to arrange images in a picture archiving and communications system (PACS). This word originates from the practice of "hanging" films on an alternator in a way that could help the radiologist do their job more efficiently. Hanging protocols are not specific to a patient but to the examination type, patient laterality, longitudinal studies over time, and pertinent other image types. *(Pg. 134–135)*

4. **C**  The luminance ratio is the minimum to the maximum brightness (luminance) emanating from a display, including ambient illuminance, taking into account the accommodation and adaptation that a human viewer can achieve at a fixed average luminance value. This is typically a range of 250:1 to 350:1. If the luminance ratio is too large, information in the darkest or brightest areas of the image will not be perceived appropriately by the human viewer at the same time. *(Pg. 142–148)*

5. **A**  Digital Imaging and COmmunications in Medicine (DICOM) standard provides a way for manufacturers to specify acquisition parameters of a study in the metadata of the image DICOM "header." This metadata contains patient demographic information, information about the study, series, and images, and many other parameters in DICOM "tags" composed of a group number and element number, as specified in a DICOM conformance statement. *(Pg. 112–114 and 132–136)*

6. **D**  Security safeguards are based on administrative, technical, and physical considerations. Physical safeguards prevent or limit access to protected information; administrative safeguards represent policies and procedures and staffing processes to ensure security. Technical safeguards are usually software-based programs such as authentication, passwords, anti-malware, encryption, 2-factor authentication, and virtual private network access as examples. *(Pg. 161–165)*

7. **A**  Reversible image compression, in which the uncompressed image is identical to the initial image, typically permits compression ratios of 2 to 3. *(Pg. 128–130 and Figure 5-8)*

8. **B**  The Grayscale Softcopy Presentation State specifies how the images in a study are manipulated. Note: GSDF describes how a display monitor can be calibrated; PPS is an action to indicate a procedure has been completed; MWL is the interface between the HL7 messages containing patient information and the modalities using DICOM for the technologist to choose the patient to be imaged; AET is the "name" of a device used for communication on the network in conjunction with the port # and the IP address. *(Pg. 132–135 and Figure 5-10)*

9. **C**  In an active-matrix liquid crystal display monitor, the intensity of the light from an individual pixel or subpixel is modulated by changing the polarity of the light that passes through a pair of polarizing filters. A layer of liquid crystal material is between a pair of polarizing filters in each pixel or subpixel. A voltage applied

to that pixel or subpixel causes the LCD molecules to twist, changing the polarization of the light, and modifying the amount of light that passes through the second polarizing filter. *(Pg. 138–140 and Figure 5-12)*

10. **D**  A main goal of the DICOM Grayscale Standard Display Function (GSDF) is to provide a predictable transformation of digital presentation values from an application to luminance on a video monitor. Another goal is to provide *similar* displays of contrast on different monitors. The displays of contrast on two different video monitors would be nearly identical only if both monitors had the same minimal and maximal luminances. The user can adjust image contrast, for example, by windowing and leveling, when the GSDF is implemented. The GSDF affects the display of contrast and does not affect spatial resolution, although it certainly may affect the conspicuity of small objects by improving the display of contrast. *(Pg. 145–148 and Figures 5-16, 5-17, 5-19)*

11. **D**  IHE is a guide for the use of standards such as HL7 and DICOM to improve interoperability between informatics systems to achieve better patient care. *(Pg. 114–115, 149–150)*

12. **B**  The HITECH Act, enacted in 2009, is an addition to the 1996 HIPAA (Health Insurance Portability and Accountability Act) that specifies legal liabilities and penalties for loss of electronic Protected Health Information by the United States Government. (Note: PAMA is the Protecting Access to Medicare Act that describes the need for computerized decision support tools based on Appropriate Use Criteria (AUC); MIPS is the Medicare Incentive Payment System). *(Pg. 165–167)*

13. **D**  HIPAA is the Health Insurance Portability and Accountability Act of 1996 that regulates electronic protected healthcare information (ePHI), describes covered entities and business associate agreement (BAA) requirements, and attempts to strike a balance between information sharing and patient privacy. *(Pg. 165–167)*

14. **B**  Of the modalities listed, CT has the largest study size. This is subject to change with new technologies and clinical operations. *(Pg. 128–130, Table 5-2)*

15. **C**  Phishing is an e-mail scheme perpetrated by hackers posing as a reputable source to induce individuals who receive "convincing" emails to reveal personal information, passwords, etc. Spear Phishing is to a single recipient (victim) to specifically address personal information coming from a (false) entity of familiarity. *(Pg. 161–162)*

16. **D**  The application software interacts at the top of the stack, Layer 7. Lower layers provide code conversion (Layer 6), coordinating between the end and application process (Layer 5), ensuring end to end data integrity (Layer 4); switching and routing information (Layer 3), transferring units of information to other end of the physical link (Layer 2), and transmitting bit streams (Layer 1). *(Pg. 117–119, Figures 5-1 and 5-2)*

17. **D**  The human visual system has visual acuity that is maximized at about five cycles per visual degree. At a approximately 60 cm viewing distance (approximately arms length), a visual degree is equivalent to 60 cm $\times$ tan 1° = 10.5 mm; thus, the best pixel dimension is about five cycles/10.5 mm = 0.5 mm$^{-1}$. In terms of spatial dimension, this is 1/0.5 mm$^{-1}$ = 0.2 mm = 200 µm. This size is approximately what a 3 MP display monitor of 54 cm diagonal dimension provides. *(Pg. 142–145 and Figure 5-14)*

18. **A**  The human visual response to differences in contrast for a fixed nominal luminance is limited. The luminance ratio is the luminance values plus the ambient light values from the minimum to the maximum. This value ranges from 250:1 to 350:1. Beyond this range, the contrast differences and detection are lost at the extremes. *(Pg. 144–145 and Figure 5-15)*

19. **D**  The PAMA act of 2014 requires physicians ordering advanced diagnostic imaging services to consult *Appropriate Use Criteria (AUC)*. The QPLE—Qualified Provider Led Entity—qualified by the Centers for Medicare and Medicaid Services, is responsible for developing and modifying AUC through outcomes research, peer review, and assessment of evidence. *(Pg. 158 and 177)*

20. **B**  Lightweight Directory Access Protocol, LDAP provides for accessing and maintaining directory information services over an IP network. In the Microsoft Windows domain, this is known as *Active Directory (AD)* to authenticate and authorize users for all computers on the network that have AD installed. The other acronyms are *SMTP—Simple Mail Transport Protocol, TLS—Transport Layer Security,* and *HTML—HyperText Markup Language. (Pg. 125)*

21. **A**   A Business Associate Agreement, BAA between two healthcare entities, is a legal document that specifies each party's responsibilities when it comes to PHI. The distractors in the possible answers, spelled out, include *IRB—institutional Review Board, SSL—Secure Socket Layer, VNA—Vendor Neutral Archive,* and *VPN—Virtual Private Network. (Pg. 165)*

22. **D**   Mammography displays used for diagnosis are specified to have a luminance of at least 420 to 450 cd/m$^2$ when driven at the maximum Digital Driving Level for a pixel in a digital mammography image. *(Pg. 145)*

23. **E**   The healthcare organization is ultimately responsible for protecting and maintaining imaging and health records acquired as a part of delivering patient care, as described in HIPAA and HITECH acts. *(Pg. 176–177)*

24. **B**   A CT scan typically produces tomographic images in the axial plane, creating a large number of thin slices representing the patient volume of the area scanned. By rearranging and reformatting the voxels (represented by pixel data), other planes can be displayed, most often orthogonal. Sagittal and coronal planes are commonly evaluated by the radiologist to visualize the anatomy. For this question, the frontal view of the lungs are generated in the coronal plane. *(Pg. 170–172 and Figure 5-37)*

25. **B**   Radiomics is the term given to the process of the conversion of digital medical images into mineable high-dimensional data that can reveal information (biomarkers) of underlying pathophysiology or other findings using quantitative methods of data extraction. *(Pg. 173)*

26. **D**   Hierarchical storage (and retrieval) management uses on-line (immediate access) storage media for recent studies to allow fast access without delays, with older images and studies on slower, but more capacious and cost effective storage media. Often, for thick client workstations, the ability to have older studies on the local disk without having to be transmitted through network infrastructure is also a key to time efficiency. Prefetching is the process of moving pertinent older studies from slower disks or from a server archive to local disks for immediate access by the radiologist. This is very important for longitudinal evaluations such as in mammography, where 3 to 5 years of previous studies may be needed to evaluate anatomical changes over the time course. *(Pg. 130–132)*

# Section III Key Equations and Symbols

| SYMBOL | QUANTITY | UNITS |
|---|---|---|
| *Illuminance* | Environmental light impinging on a surface | lux |
| *Luminance* | Rate of light energy emitted from a surface | cd/m² |

## ACRONYM TABLE

| ACRONYM | DESCRIPTION | ACRONYM | DESCRIPTION |
|---|---|---|---|
| AD | Active Directory | US | DICOM IOD—Ultrasound |
| AWS | Amazon Web Services | DIMSE | Dicom Message Service Element |
| ANSI | American National Standards Institute | DDL | Digital Driving Level |
| AE | Application Entity | DICOM | Digital Imaging COmmunications in Medicine |
| AET | Application Entity Title | EHR | Electronic Health Record |
| API | Application Programming Interface | EMR | Electronic Medical Record |
| AUC | Appropriate Use Criteria | ePHI | Electronic Protected Health Information |
| AI | Artificial Intelligence | FDA | Food and Drug Administration |
| BIOS | Basic Input Output System (firmware) | GPU | Graphics Processing Unit |
| CMS | Centers for Medicare and Medicaid Services | GSPS | Grayscale Softcopy Presentation State |
| CPU | Central Processing Unit | GSDF | Grayscale Standard Display Function |
| CDS | Clinical Decision Support | HIE | Health Information Exchange |
| CDSM | Clinical Decision Support Mechanism | HITECH | Health Information Technology for Economic and Clinical Health |
| CPOE | Computerized Order Entry | HIPAA | Health Insurance Portability and Accountability Act |
| CPT | Current Procedural Terminology | HL7 | Health Level 7 |
| DL | Deep Learning | FHIR | HL7—Fast Health Interoperability Resources |
| CR | DICOM IOD—Computed Radiography | ADT | HL7 Admission, Discharge, Transfer interactions |
| CT | DICOM IOD—Computed Tomography | ORM | HL7 message that provides orders |
| BTO | DICOM IOD—Digital Breast Tomosynthesis | ORU | HL7 message that provides results |
| RF | DICOM IOD—Digital Fluoroscopy | OBR | HL7 observation requests segment |
| MG | DICOM IOD—Digital Mammography | OBX | HL7 observation results segment |
| DX | DICOM IOD—Digital Radiography | HTML | HyperText Markup Language |
| XA | DICOM IOD—Fluoroscopy-Guided Intervention | HTTP | HyperText Transfer Protocol |
| MR | DICOM IOD—Magnetic Resonance Imaging | IOD | Information Object Descriptor |
| NM | DICOM IOD—Nuclear Medicine | IHE | Integrating the Healthcare Enterprise |
| PET | DICOM IOD—Positron Emission Tomography | IP | Integration Profile (based on IHE) |
| PT/CT | DICOM IOD—Positron Emission Tomography/Computed Tomography | ISO | International Organization for Standardization |

*(Continued)*

**ACRONYM TABLE (*Continued*)**

| ACRONYM | DESCRIPTION | ACRONYM | DESCRIPTION |
|---------|-------------|---------|-------------|
| ICD | International statistical Classification of Diseases | RIS | Radiology Information System |
| ITEF | Internet Engineering Task Force | RadLex | Radiology Lexicon |
| IMAP | Internet Message Access Protocol | RAM | Random Access Memory |
| IoT | Internet of Things | RAID | Redundant Array of Independent Disks |
| IP | Internet Protocol | RHIO | Regional Health Information Organization |
| ISP | Internet Service Provider | RVU | Relative Value Unit |
| JND | Just Noticeable Difference | REST | REpresentational State Transfer |
| LIS | Laboratory Information System | RCM | Revenue Cycle Management |
| LDAP | Lightweight Directory Access Protocol | SSL | Secure Socket Layer |
| LCD | Liquid Crystal Display | SCP | Service Class Provider |
| LAN | Local Area Network | SCU | Service Class User |
| LOINC | Logical Observation Identifier Names and Codes | SOP | Service Object Pair |
| LUT | Look-Up-Table | SSD | Shaded Surface Display |
| ML | Machine Learning | SMTP | Simple Mail Transfer Protocol |
| MQSA | Mammography Quality Standards Act | SMPTE | Society of Motion Picture Television Engineers |
| MU | Meaningful Use | SR (VR) | Speech Recognition (Voice Recognition) |
| MWL | Modality WorkList | SDO | Standards Development Organization |
| MIME | Multipurpose Internet Message Extensions | SR | Structured Report (DICOM) |
| NEMA | National Electrical Manufacturers Association | SNOMED-CT | Systematized Nomenclature of Medicine-Clinical Terms |
| NLP | Natural Language Processing | TCP/IP | Transmission Control Protocol/Internet Protocol |
| NTP | Network Time Protocol | TLS | Transport Layer Security |
| ONC | Office of the National Coordinator for Health Information Technology | URL | Uniform Resource Locator |
| OSI | Open Systems Interconnection | UID | Unique IDentifier |
| OLED | Organic Light Emitting Diode | USB | Universal Serial Bus |
| PPS | Performed Procedure Step | VM | Virtual Machine |
| PHI | Protected Health Information | VPN | Virtual Private Network |
| PAMA | Protecting Access to Medicare Act | VR | Volume Rendering; Value Representation |
| PLE | Provider Led Entity | WAN | Wide Area Network |
| QPLE | Qualified Provider Led Entity | XML | Xtensible Markup Layer |
| RDSR | Radiation Dose Structured Report | | |

Note: this table is sorted alphabetically by description.

SECTION

II

# Diagnostic Radiology

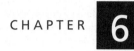

CHAPTER **6**

# X-Ray Production, Tubes, and Generators

## 6.0 INTRODUCTION

This chapter describes the x-ray production process, characteristics of the x-ray beam, x-ray tube design x-ray generator components, and factors that affect exposure and exposure rate.

## 6.1 PRODUCTION OF X-RAYS

1. **Bremsstrahlung spectrum**
   **a.** Conversion of kinetic energy of electrons into electromagnetic radiation (x-rays).
   **b.** An environment and requirements to produce x-rays are shown in Figure 6-1.
   **c.** Voltage applied to the cathode and anode accelerates electrons to a kinetic energy = voltage.
   **d.** Electrons interact with other electrons to produce heat; electrons that interact with the nucleus of the tungsten target are decelerated through coulombic interactions as illustrated in Figure 6-2.
   **e.** X-ray energies produced have a distribution described by the bremsstrahlung spectrum (Fig. 6-3).
   **f.** Efficiency of x-ray production relative to heat production is typically less than 1%.

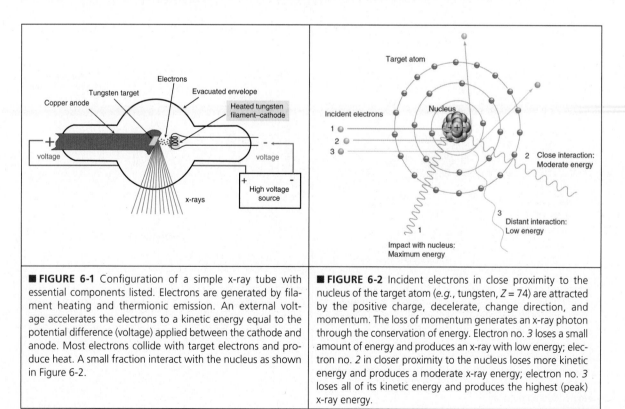

■ **FIGURE 6-1** Configuration of a simple x-ray tube with essential components listed. Electrons are generated by filament heating and thermionic emission. An external voltage accelerates the electrons to a kinetic energy equal to the potential difference (voltage) applied between the cathode and anode. Most electrons collide with target electrons and produce heat. A small fraction interact with the nucleus as shown in Figure 6-2.

■ **FIGURE 6-2** Incident electrons in close proximity to the nucleus of the target atom (*e.g.*, tungsten, *Z* = 74) are attracted by the positive charge, decelerate, change direction, and momentum. The loss of momentum generates an x-ray photon through the conservation of energy. Electron no. *3* loses a small amount of energy and produces an x-ray with low energy; electron no. *2* in closer proximity to the nucleus loses more kinetic energy and produces a moderate x-ray energy; electron no. *3* loses all of its kinetic energy and produces the highest (peak) x-ray energy.

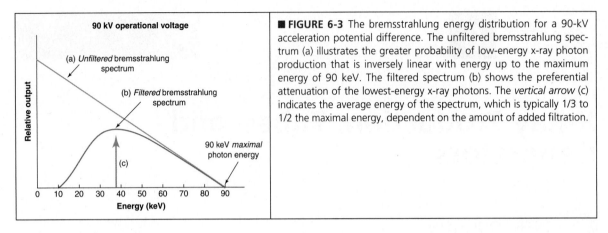

■ **FIGURE 6-3** The bremsstrahlung energy distribution for a 90-kV acceleration potential difference. The unfiltered bremsstrahlung spectrum (a) illustrates the greater probability of low-energy x-ray photon production that is inversely linear with energy up to the maximum energy of 90 keV. The filtered spectrum (b) shows the preferential attenuation of the lowest-energy x-ray photons. The *vertical arrow* (c) indicates the average energy of the spectrum, which is typically 1/3 to 1/2 the maximal energy, dependent on the amount of added filtration.

2. **Characteristic X-rays**
   a. Incident electrons can interact with inner orbital electrons of the target atom.
   b. Requires incident electron kinetic energy greater than binding energy of the electron in the atomic orbital.
   c. Vacant shell via ejected electron from the target atom is immediately filled with electrons of lower binding energy, generating a "characteristic x-ray" of discrete energy equal to energy difference.
   d. Electron binding energies of pertinent target materials are listed in Table 6-1.
   e. Characteristic x-ray formation is illustrated in Figure 6-4 and resultant spectrum in Figure 6-5.
   f. $K_A$ and $K_B$ characteristic x-ray energies result from adjacent shell and nonadjacent shell transitions.

**TABLE 6-1 ELECTRON BINDING ENERGIES (keV) OF COMMON X-RAY TUBE TARGET MATERIALS**

| ELECTRON SHELL | TUNGSTEN | MOLYBDENUM | RHODIUM |
|---|---|---|---|
| K | 69.5 | 20.0 | 23.2 |
| L | 12.1/11.5/10.2 | 2.8/2.6/2.5 | 3.4/3.1/3.0 |
| M | 2.8–1.9 | 0.5–0.4 | 0.6–0.2 |

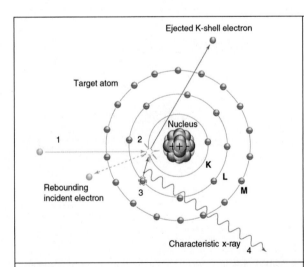

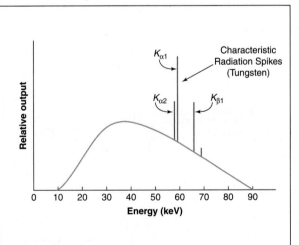

■ **FIGURE 6-4** Generation of a characteristic x-ray in a target atom: *(1)* The incident electron interacts with the **K**-shell electron. *(2)* The **K**-shell electron is removed (only if the energy of the incident electron is greater than the **K**-shell binding energy), leaving a vacancy in the **K**-shell. *(3)* An electron from the adjacent **L**-shell fills the vacancy. *(4)* A **K**α characteristic x-ray photon is emitted with energy equal to the difference between the binding energies of the two shells, for example, 69.5 to 10.2 = 59.3 keV photon is emitted for tungsten target.

■ **FIGURE 6-5** The filtered spectrum of bremsstrahlung and characteristic radiation from a tungsten target with a potential difference of 90 kV illustrates specific characteristic radiation energies from $K\alpha$ and $K\beta$ transitions. Filtration (the preferential removal of low-energy photons as they traverse matter) is discussed in Section 6.5.

## 6.2  X-RAY TUBES

X-ray tube cross-sectional diagram (Fig. 6-6) and actual tube insert/housing (Fig. 6-7)

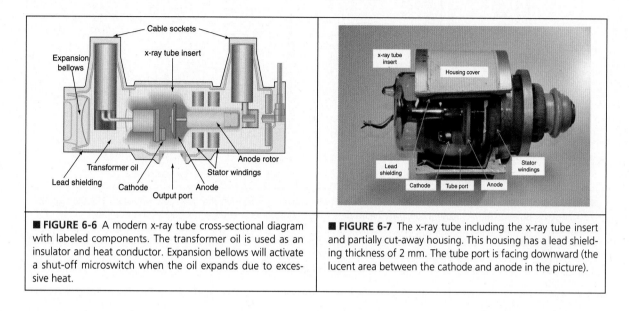

■ **FIGURE 6-6** A modern x-ray tube cross-sectional diagram with labeled components. The transformer oil is used as an insulator and heat conductor. Expansion bellows will activate a shut-off microswitch when the oil expands due to excessive heat.

■ **FIGURE 6-7** The x-ray tube including the x-ray tube insert and partially cut-away housing. This housing has a lead shielding thickness of 2 mm. The tube port is facing downward (the lucent area between the cathode and anode in the picture).

1. **Cathode**
   a. The negative electrode comprised of electron emitters (filaments) and focusing cup; filament length provides small and large focal spot selections (Fig. 6-8).
   b. Filament circuit activates filament to release electrons due to thermionic emission. A flow of electrons occurs when a voltage is applied; note difference of filament and tube current (Fig. 6-9).
   c. Focusing cup shapes the electron distribution accelerated toward the anode; biased cups (more negative) can produce smaller distributions; grid biased focusing cups can stop flow (Fig. 6-10).

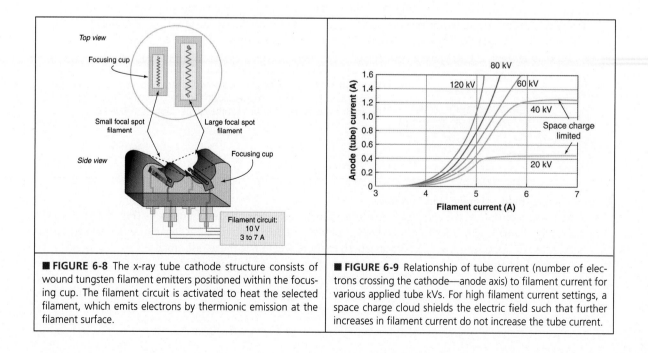

■ **FIGURE 6-8** The x-ray tube cathode structure consists of wound tungsten filament emitters positioned within the focusing cup. The filament circuit is activated to heat the selected filament, which emits electrons by thermionic emission at the filament surface.

■ **FIGURE 6-9** Relationship of tube current (number of electrons crossing the cathode—anode axis) to filament current for various applied tube kVs. For high filament current settings, a space charge cloud shields the electric field such that further increases in filament current do not increase the tube current.

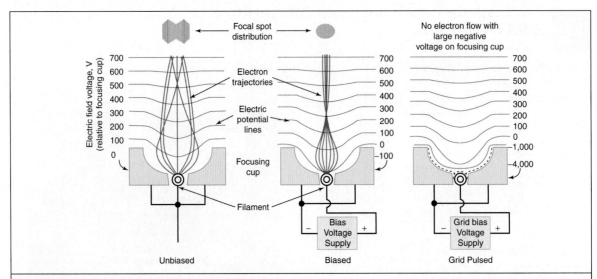

■ **FIGURE 6-10** The focusing cup shapes the electron distribution when it is at the same voltage ("unbiased") as the filament (*left*). Electrical Isolation of the focusing cup from the filament and application of a negative "biased" voltage (approximately −100 V) reduces the distribution of emerging electrons by increasing the repelling electric fields surrounding the filament (note the 0 V electric field potential line) and modifying the electron trajectories (*middle*). At the top are typical electron distributions incident on the target anode (the focal spot) for the unbiased and biased focusing cups. Application of −4,000 V on an electrically isolated focusing cup completely stops electron flow, even with high voltage applied on the tube; this is known as a grid-biased or "grid pulsed" tube (*right*).

2. **Anode**
   a. The target electrode maintained at positive potential difference with respect to the cathode.
   b. Tungsten (W), Z = 74, has a high melting point—used for most diagnostic systems.
   c. Molybdenum (Mo), Z = 42, and rhodium (Rh), Z = 45, produce characteristic x-rays beneficial for mammography imaging (see Chapter 8).
3. **Anode configurations**
   a. Stationary tungsten target embedded in a copper block (copper efficiently conducts heat) (Fig. 6-11)
      (i)   Used in low-power applications such as dental x-ray and handheld fluoro units
   b. Rotating anode—higher heat-loading capability achieved by spreading out area of power deposition
      (i)   Requires induction motor (stator-rotor design) to rotate at 3,000 to 10,000 rpm (Fig. 6-12)
      (ii)  Focal track increased by circumference of anode (2πr) for radius r (Fig. 6-13)

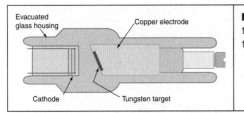

■ **FIGURE 6-11** The anode of a fixed anode x-ray tube consists of a tungsten target insert mounted in a copper block. Generated heat is removed from the tungsten target by conduction into the copper block. ▭ **F. 6-12**

4. **Anode angle, field coverage, focal spot size**
   a. Anode angle: surface of the focal track to the perpendicular of the anode-cathode axis (Fig. 6-13).
   b. Actual focal area length is foreshortened when projected down central axis according to the *line focus principle:* Effective focal length = Actual focal length × sin θ, where θ is the anode angle.
   c. Focal spot effective size: width (determined by the focusing cup) × length (filament length).
   d. Field coverage: dependent on anode angle and source to image distance (Fig. 6-14).
   e. Effective focal spot varies in size along cathode-anode direction of the projection beam (Fig. 6-15).

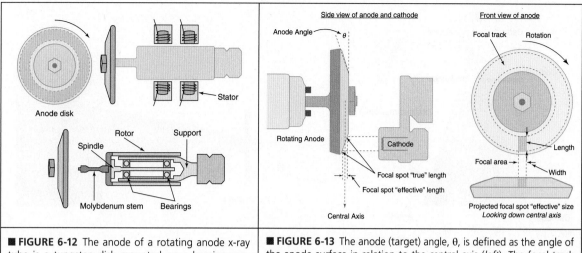

**■ FIGURE 6-12** The anode of a rotating anode x-ray tube is a tungsten disk mounted on a bearing-supported rotor assembly (front view, *top left*; side view, *top right*). The rotor consists of a copper and iron laminated core and forms part of an induction motor. The other component is the stator, which exists outside of the insert, *top right*. A molybdenum stem reduces heat transfer to the rotor bearings (*bottom*). 📖 **F. 6-13**

**■ FIGURE 6-13** The anode (target) angle, θ, is defined as the angle of the anode surface in relation to the central axis (*left*). The focal track represents the total area over which heat is distributed during the x-ray exposure as the anode rotates. The actual focal area is characterized by a length and width (*right*). The focal spot length, as projected down the central axis, is foreshortened, according to the line focus principle (*lower right*). 📖 **F. 6-14**

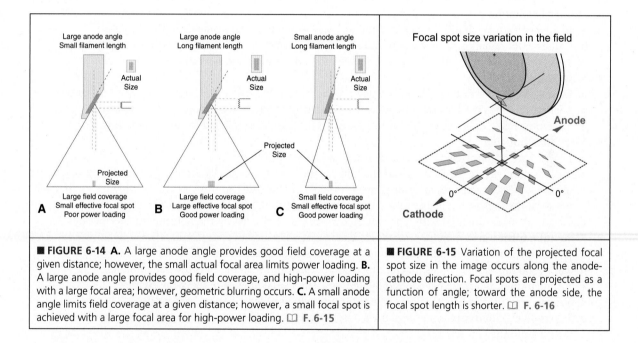

**■ FIGURE 6-14 A.** A large anode angle provides good field coverage at a given distance; however, the small actual focal area limits power loading. **B.** A large anode angle provides good field coverage, and high-power loading with a large focal area; however, geometric blurring occurs. **C.** A small anode angle limits field coverage at a given distance; however, a small focal spot is achieved with a large focal area for high-power loading. 📖 **F. 6-15**

**■ FIGURE 6-15** Variation of the projected focal spot size in the image occurs along the anode-cathode direction. Focal spots are projected as a function of angle; toward the anode side, the focal spot length is shorter. 📖 **F. 6-16**

    **f.** Measurement of focal spot size can be achieved by a pinhole camera, slit camera, star pattern, or resolution bar patterns (see Figs. 6-17, 6-18, and 6-19 in the textbook).

    **g.** Nominal focal spot sizes are specified by the International Electrotechnical Commission (see Table 6-3 in the textbook).

**5. Heel effect**

    **a.** Reduction in beam fluence on the anode side of the projected field caused by anode self-attenuation.

    **b.** Heel effect is more prominent at short source-image distances (Fig. 6-16).

    **c.** Orientation of the x-ray tube is important for equalizing transmitted x-ray fluence (Fig. 6-17).

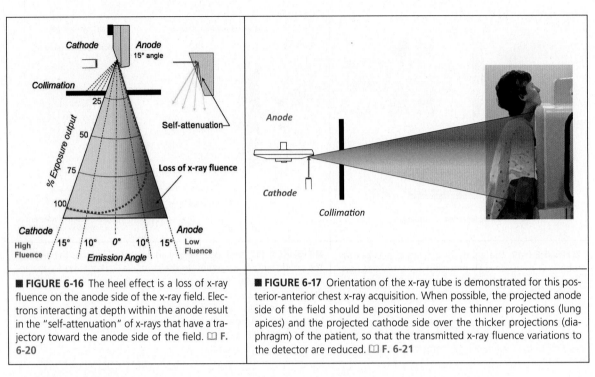

**■ FIGURE 6-16** The heel effect is a loss of x-ray fluence on the anode side of the x-ray field. Electrons interacting at depth within the anode result in the "self-attenuation" of x-rays that have a trajectory toward the anode side of the field. 📖 **F. 6-20**

**■ FIGURE 6-17** Orientation of the x-ray tube is demonstrated for this posterior-anterior chest x-ray acquisition. When possible, the projected anode side of the field should be positioned over the thinner projections (lung apices) and the projected cathode side over the thicker projections (diaphragm) of the patient, so that the transmitted x-ray fluence variations to the detector are reduced. 📖 **F. 6-21**

6. **Off-focal radiation**
   a. Incident electrons elastically rebound and impact the anode at areas outside of the focal spot.
   b. Causes extra radiation dose, background signal, and geometric blurring (see textbook Fig. 6-22).
   c. This effect is reduced with a grounded anode and hooded structure next to the anode focal area.
7. **X-ray tube insert**
   a. Evacuated glass or metal enclosure containing the x-ray tube structures (see Figs. 6-6 and 6-7 above).
   b. "Getter" circuit is used for trapping released outgassing of internal x-ray tube components.
   c. Tube port made of beryllium (Be) is necessary for x-ray tubes employed for mammography.
8. **X-ray tube housing**
   a. Provides mechanical, electrical, thermal, and radiation protection.
   b. "Leakage x-rays" are reduced by lead shielding in the housing (typically 2 mm or more thick) to radiation levels no greater than 0.88 mGy air kerma (100 mR) per hour at 1 m from focal spot when using the highest kV at the highest *continuous* tube current (typically 125 to 150 kV and 3 to 5 mA).
   c. Heat exchangers are used with high-power x-ray tubes by circulating the housing transformer oil.
9. **X-ray tube filtration**
   a. Added metal filters (typically aluminum or copper sheets) placed near the tube port in the beam.
   b. Tube total filtration includes inherent filtration of the insert material plus the added filters.
   c. Compensation filters are used to modify the incident spatial fluence of the x-ray beam.
   d. Wedge, trough, and bow-tie filters (the latter typically used for CT tubes) are used.
   e. Filters chiefly modify the x-ray spectrum to selectively remove low-energy x-ray photons and lower radiation dose to the patient.
10. **Collimators**
    a. User-adjustable high-attenuation blades positioned in the collimator assembly.
    b. Automatic aperture sizing for fluoroscopy magnification applications.
    c. Positive beam limitation (PBL) shutters: max opening to detector in cassette-sensing systems.
    d. X-ray field-light field congruence: position of light in collimator assembly mimics x-ray beam projected area (Fig. 6-18). Alignment of x-ray field to light field must be within 2% of SID.
11. **X-ray tube designs**
    a. Designs are engineered for specific use. Radiography, mammography, cardiovascular angiography, and CT applications use widely different kV and energy per patient encounter (Fig. 6-19).
    b. Considerations include anode instantaneous power loading, cooling, and focal spot size.
    c. Advanced x-ray tube technologies include liquid metal bearings for CT and angiography tubes (see textbook Fig. 6-25) and multi-source x-ray tube assemblies (see textbook Fig. 6-26).

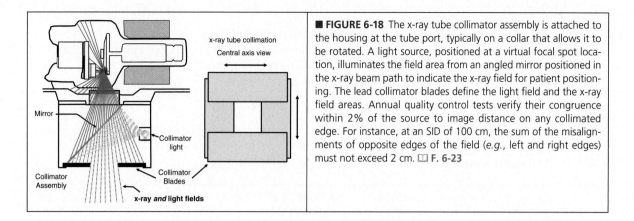

■ **FIGURE 6-18** The x-ray tube collimator assembly is attached to the housing at the tube port, typically on a collar that allows it to be rotated. A light source, positioned at a virtual focal spot location, illuminates the field area from an angled mirror positioned in the x-ray beam path to indicate the x-ray field for patient positioning. The lead collimator blades define the light field and the x-ray field areas. Annual quality control tests verify their congruence within 2% of the source to image distance on any collimated edge. For instance, at an SID of 100 cm, the sum of the misalignments of opposite edges of the field (*e.g.*, left and right edges) must not exceed 2 cm. ⌑ **F. 6-23**

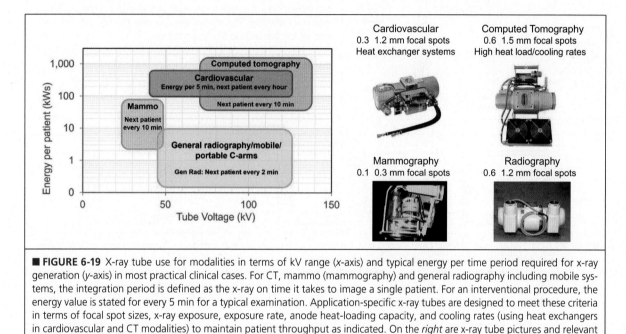

■ **FIGURE 6-19** X-ray tube use for modalities in terms of kV range (*x*-axis) and typical energy per time period required for x-ray generation (*y*-axis) in most practical clinical cases. For CT, mammo (mammography) and general radiography including mobile systems, the integration period is defined as the x-ray on time it takes to image a single patient. For an interventional procedure, the energy value is stated for every 5 min for a typical examination. Application-specific x-ray tubes are designed to meet these criteria in terms of focal spot sizes, x-ray exposure, exposure rate, anode heat-loading capacity, and cooling rates (using heat exchangers in cardiovascular and CT modalities) to maintain patient throughput as indicated. On the *right* are x-ray tube pictures and relevant focal spot size ranges for four categories of x-ray tubes indicated in the figure on the *left*. ⌑ **F. 6-24**

12. **Maximizing x-ray tube life**
    a. Minimize filament boost prep time—the time the filament current is at a maximum.
    b. Use lower tube current with longer exposure times for a given mAs (not for moving anatomy).
    c. Avoid extended or repeated operation of the x-ray tube with high kV and mAs.
    d. Use manufacturer warm-up procedures to get the anode at a reasonable temperature.
    e. Limit rotor start and stop times.

## 6.3  X-RAY GENERATORS

1. **Electromagnetic induction and voltage transformation**
    a. A changing magnetic field induces an electromotive force in a conductive wire with electron flow.
    b. Electron flow in a wire creates an associated magnetic field.
       (i)  A constant magnetic field is generated by direct current.
       (ii) A changing magnetic field is generated by alternating current.
    c. Magnitude of the magnetic field strength is proportional to the current.
    d. Magnetic fields pass through electrical insulators.
    e. Insulated wires wrapped in a coil geometry will generate summed magnetic fields.

### 2. Transformers

**a.** Principles of electromagnetic induction are the foundation of transformers

**b.** Using an iron core as a conduit of magnetic fields, alternating current sources can transform voltage and power through wire-wrapped primary and secondary windings (Fig. 6-20).

**c.** Law of transformers equates voltage changes on the number of primary and secondary winding "turns:"

$$V_P/N_P = V_S/N_S \text{ or } V_P/V_S = N_P/N_S.$$

**d.** For an "ideal" transformer, the input power (primary) = output power (secondary); power is the product of voltage ($V$) and current ($I$): $V_P I_P = V_S I_S$ so an increase in $V_S$ results in a decrease in $I_S$.

**e.** Generic transformer designs are illustrated in Figure 6-21.

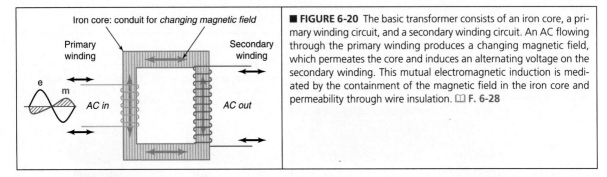

■ **FIGURE 6-20** The basic transformer consists of an iron core, a primary winding circuit, and a secondary winding circuit. An AC flowing through the primary winding produces a changing magnetic field, which permeates the core and induces an alternating voltage on the secondary winding. This mutual electromagnetic induction is mediated by the containment of the magnetic field in the iron core and permeability through wire insulation. ⫏ **F. 6-28**

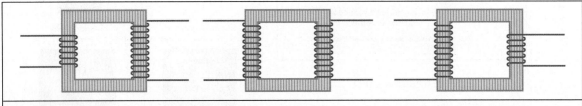

■ **FIGURE 6-21** Transformer designs: **Left:** "Step-up" transformer where $N_P < N_S$, and voltage on the secondary side is increased. An application is the high-voltage transformer in an x-ray generator, where the primary to secondary turns ratio is typically 1:1,000, so an input of 50 V results in an output of 50 kV. **Middle:** "Isolation" transformer, where $N_P = N_S$; this transformer effectively isolates circuits for safety purposes; **Right:** "Step-down" transformer, where $N_P < N_S$; an application is for the filament circuit where lower voltage (*e.g.*, 10 V) and high current (greater than 5,000 A) is needed to heat up the x-ray tube filament for thermionic emission to create tube current. ⫏ **F. 6-29**

### 3. X-ray generator modules

**a.** Provide functions to control the acquisition factors for x-ray system operation; major components are illustrated in Figure 6-22, **right**.

### 4. Operator console

**a.** Provides the interface and settings for the technologist to control the system shown in Figure 6-22, **left**.

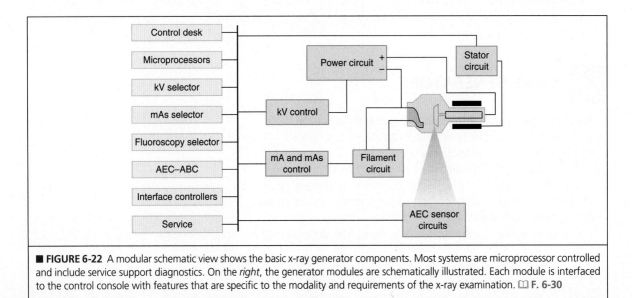

■ **FIGURE 6-22** A modular schematic view shows the basic x-ray generator components. Most systems are microprocessor controlled and include service support diagnostics. On the *right*, the generator modules are schematically illustrated. Each module is interfaced to the control console with features that are specific to the modality and requirements of the x-ray examination. ⫏ **F. 6-30**

5. **High-frequency generator**
   a. Converts input AC into DC waveform and then converted into a high-frequency AC waveform.
   b. Transformer efficiency is improved, and the rectified high-voltage output has low-voltage ripple.
   c. See textbook Figures 6-31 and 6-32 for more details.
6. **Voltage ripple**
   a. Represents the variation during high-voltage transformation, where average V is less than peak V.
   b. Single-phase (60 Hz) AC has the greatest ripple (100%), for example, applied voltage ranges from 0 V to peak V; three-phase and high-frequency generators have lower-voltage ripple of 3% to 15%.
   c. Constant potential generators have voltage ripple less than 2% (see textbook Fig. 6-33).
   d. Because voltage ripple is low in modern generators, the "p" in kVp is now often simply kV.
7. **Timers**
   a. Control of the x-ray exposure time requires millisecond accuracy, provided by digital electronics.
   b. Automatic Exposure Control Feedback circuits (see item 9 below) measure radiation to time the acquisition.
   c. "Back-up" timers represent a countdown timer of prescribed duration should the electronics fail.
8. **Switches**
   a. Timers determine the length of exposure by controlling switches in the high-voltage circuit.
   b. Switches can be placed on the primary or secondary high-voltage circuits—typically, for high-frequency generators, exposures down to 2 ms are possible for primary switching; switching on the secondary circuits requires "triode" or "tetrode" devices to control the on-off status of the circuit.
   c. "Grid-controlled" x-ray tubes can be used for extremely fast switching at the tube focusing cup, but circuit insulation at high-voltage operation adds complexity and cost (see Section 6.2.1 and Fig. 6-10).
9. **Automatic exposure control**
   a. Components and electrical circuits are used for measuring residual x-rays incident on the detector.
   b. In radiography, transparent ionization chambers are positioned in front of the detector (Fig. 6-23).
   c. Signals from the chambers are amplified and accumulated into one input of a voltage comparator.
   d. A calibrated AEC selector reference voltage is the other comparator input.
   e. When the comparator voltages are equal, a termination signal is sent to the generator.
   f. In the event of circuit failure, a backup timer initiates a termination signal after an elapsed time.

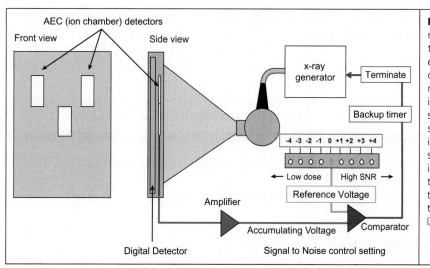

■ **FIGURE 6-23** AEC detectors measure the radiation incident on the detector and terminate the exposure according to a preset optical density or signal-to-noise ratio achieved in the analog or digital image. A front view (*left*) and side view (*middle*) of a chest cassette stand and the locations of ionization chamber detectors are shown. The desired signal to the image receptor and thus the signal-to-noise ratio may be selected at the operator's console with respect to a normalized reference voltage. ⬚ F. 6-34

## 6.4  POWER RATINGS, ANODE LOADING AND COOLING

1. **Power ratings**
   a. Generator: maximum power available for 100 kV at the maximum tube current for 0.1-s exposure
      (i) Power (kilowatt, kW) = 100 kV × A$_{max}$ for 0.1 s; for example, 800 mA$_{max}$ = 100 kV × 0.8A = 80 kW
      (ii) 80 to 120 kW generators: interventional radiology, cardiology, and high-end CT
      (iii) 30 to 80 kW generators: general radiographic and/or fluoroscopic systems
      (iv) 5 to 30 kW generators: mobile radiography, fluoroscopy, dental units
      (v) Generator power maximum should be approximately equal to large focal spot power rating

   b. Focal spot: maximum power deposition at 100 kV and maximum tube current for 0.1-s exposure
      (i) Determined by anode angle, anode diameter, rotation speed, mass, and focal spot size
      (ii) 50 to 120 kW focal spot: 1.0 to 1.5 mm and larger; large diameter, heavy mass anode, shallow anode angle, mechanism for active tube cooling
      (iii) 20 to 50 kW focal spot: 0.4 to 1.0 mm (medium focal spot size)
      (iv) 5 to 15 kW focal spot: 0.1 to 0.4 mm (small focal spot size) for mammography, fixed anode tubes, magnification studies for interventional neuroangiography
   c. X-ray generators have lock-out mechanisms to prohibit combinations of kV, mA, and exposure time that could exceed the power deposition tolerance of the focal spot.
2. **Anode heating and cooling:** Inefficiency of x-ray production requires a limitation of power deposition that must take heating and cooling into consideration (Fig. 6-24). A new definition by the IEC is explained in the textbook on Page 217, Section 6.4.1, which uses a new paradigm to classify x-ray anode heating and cooling.

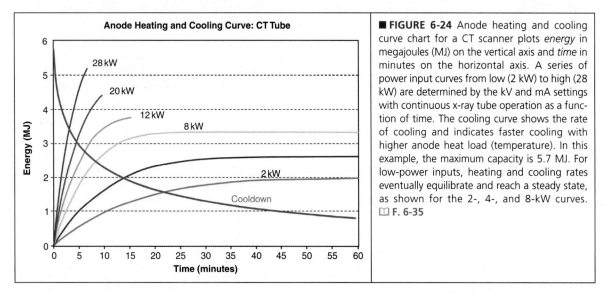

■ **FIGURE 6-24** Anode heating and cooling curve chart for a CT scanner plots *energy* in megajoules (MJ) on the vertical axis and *time* in minutes on the horizontal axis. A series of power input curves from low (2 kW) to high (28 kW) are determined by the kV and mA settings with continuous x-ray tube operation as a function of time. The cooling curve shows the rate of cooling and indicates faster cooling with higher anode heat load (temperature). In this example, the maximum capacity is 5.7 MJ. For low-power inputs, heating and cooling rates eventually equilibrate and reach a steady state, as shown for the 2-, 4-, and 8-kW curves. □ F. 6-35

3. **Historical definitions: the heat unit and the joule**
   a. Heat unit (HU) is the legacy traditional unit describing energy deposition (heating) on the anode
   b. HU = $\alpha$ × peak voltage (kVp) × tube current (mA) × exposure time (s)
      (i) The constant $\alpha$ is a function of the kV waveform; 1 for single phase, 1.35 for 3 phase.
      (ii) Three-phase and high-frequency generators have average voltage approximately equal to the peak voltage, whereas single-phase generator average voltage is approximately 70% of the peak voltage.
   c. Continuous x-ray production uses HU/s = kV × mA.
   d. Joule is the SI unit of energy, where 1 joule is equal to a power of 1 watt for 1 s.
   e. Energy (J) heat input = root-mean-square voltage ($V_{RMS}$) × tube current (A) × exposure time (s).
      (i) For a single-phase generator, $V_{RMS}$ = 0.71.
      (ii) Comparison to HU (above): Energy (HU) $\cong$ 1.4 × Heat Input (J).

## 6.5 FACTORS AFFECTING X-RAY EMISSION

There are four major factors that affect x-ray emission (output) of an x-ray tube, including the anode target material, the tube voltage, the tube current, and the beam filtration. The x-ray output is described in terms of quality (penetrability), quantity (number), and exposure (energy fluence—the energy weighted photon number).

1. **Anode target material**
   a. Efficiency of x-ray production is proportional to Z (*e.g.*, a W target is 74/42 more efficient than a Mo target in producing x-rays, all other parameters constant).
   b. Characteristic x-rays are of higher quality (energy) with higher Z anodes (see Section 6.1.2 above).
2. **Tube voltage (kV)**
   a. In general, exposure $\propto kV^2$, as electrons of higher energy have a higher probability of bremsstrahlung.
   b. Predictions of output for changes in kV are the ratio of the kV values squared: for example, going from 60 to 80 kV, with other parameters fixed will result in an exposure output of $(80/60)^2 = 1.78$ times greater for free-in-air exposure measurements (Fig. 6-25).

c. For equal transmission through an object, the ratio of the kV values increase from a squared term to an exponent value of approximately 4 to 5, because of higher attenuation of the lower-energy beam. For example, comparing 60 to 80 kV through 20 cm of tissue is calculated as: $(60/80)^5 = 0.24$; for the same transmitted exposure, therefore, the mAs at 80 kV will be approximately 1/4th that at 60 kV.

3. **Tube current (mA)**

   a. Output is proportional to the tube current for a fixed kV (Fig. 6-26).

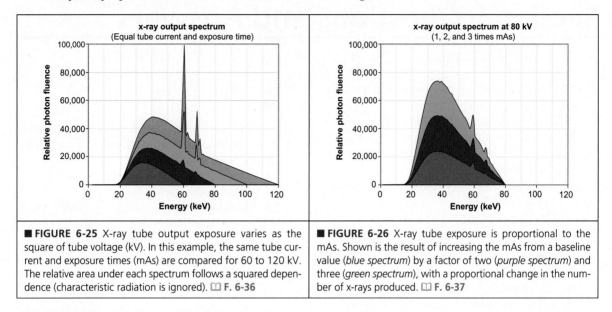

■ **FIGURE 6-25** X-ray tube output exposure varies as the square of tube voltage (kV). In this example, the same tube current and exposure times (mAs) are compared for 60 to 120 kV. The relative area under each spectrum follows a squared dependence (characteristic radiation is ignored). ▢ **F. 6-36**

■ **FIGURE 6-26** X-ray tube exposure is proportional to the mAs. Shown is the result of increasing the mAs from a baseline value (*blue spectrum*) by a factor of two (*purple spectrum*) and three (*green spectrum*), with a proportional change in the number of x-rays produced. ▢ **F. 6-37**

4. **Beam filtration**

   a. Added metal filtration (aluminum, copper) selectively remove lower x-ray energies in the spectrum.

   b. Spectral shift to higher effective energy results (Fig. 6-27).

   c. Typical added Al thicknesses: 1 to 2 mm; Cu thicknesses: 0.1 to 0.9 mm in 0.1 mm increments.

   d. A minimum half-value layer (HVL) at a given kV is required (see textbook Table 6-4).

   e. X-ray beam filtration results in decreased patient dose for a given entrance dose (Fig. 6-28).

   f. Technique factors (kV, mAs) *must* also indicate HVL in technique charts (see textbook Table 6-5 for specific examples explaining the information presented in Fig. 6-28).

5. **Summary**: X-ray beam *quantity* (fluence) is proportional to $Z_{target} \times kV^2 \times mAs$

   X-ray beam *quality* (penetrability) depends on kV, generator waveform, and tube filtration.

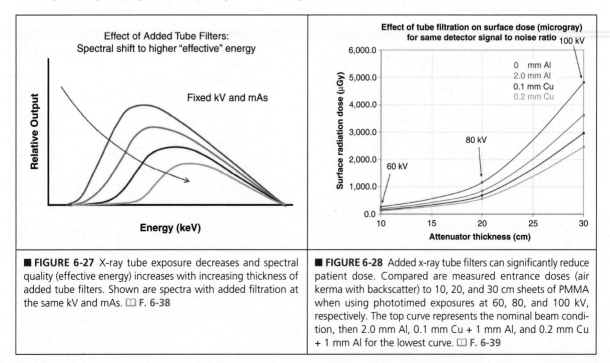

■ **FIGURE 6-27** X-ray tube exposure decreases and spectral quality (effective energy) increases with increasing thickness of added tube filters. Shown are spectra with added filtration at the same kV and mAs. ▢ **F. 6-38**

■ **FIGURE 6-28** Added x-ray tube filters can significantly reduce patient dose. Compared are measured entrance doses (air kerma with backscatter) to 10, 20, and 30 cm sheets of PMMA when using phototimed exposures at 60, 80, and 100 kV, respectively. The top curve represents the nominal beam condition, then 2.0 mm Al, 0.1 mm Cu + 1 mm Al, and 0.2 mm Cu + 1 mm Al for the lowest curve. ▢ **F. 6-39**

# Section II Questions and Answers

1. How is the continuous bremsstrahlung spectrum obtained from an x-ray tube?
   A. Target anode heating by electrons
   B. Gamma-ray emissions from the target nuclei
   C. Transitions of atomic electrons from higher to lower binding energies
   D. Conversion of all electron kinetic energy into x-rays
   E. Deceleration of electrons in the target

2. What determines the maximum *characteristic* x-ray energy emitted from an x-ray tube operating at 100 kV?
   A. The elemental composition of the target
   B. The x-ray generator phase and average kV
   C. The rectification of the high-voltage circuit
   D. The x-ray tube current and filament current
   E. The space charge compensation circuit

3. What is the purpose of the x-ray tube filament?
   A. Conversion of electron kinetic energy to x-ray photons
   B. Electrical/radiation safety
   C. Electron beam shaping
   D. Source of electrons
   E. X-ray field visible light for positioning

4. What is the difference between kV and keV?
   A. Exposure and dose
   B. Monoenergetic and polyenergetic x-ray photon beams
   C. Potential difference and energy
   D. Gamma-rays and x-rays
   E. Ionizing and nonionizing radiation

5. What factor of x-ray production efficiency is achieved by replacing a Mo (Z = 42) target with a W (Z = 74) target?
   A. 3.2
   B. 1.8
   C. 1 (no difference)
   D. 0.6
   E. 0.3

6. Which device in the x-ray tube assembly rotates the anode through electromagnetic induction?
   A. Bearings
   B. Getter circuit

C. Spindle
D. Stator

7. The fastest switching of an x-ray tube/generator assembly is accomplished by which of the following devices?
   A. Mechanical contactor switch on the primary side of the circuit
   B. Electronic timer connected to a tetrode switch on the secondary circuit
   C. Phototimer switch directly integrated into the x-ray generator
   D. Grid-biased focusing cup with −2,000 V bias potential

8. Which letter points to the cathode in this x-ray tube diagram?

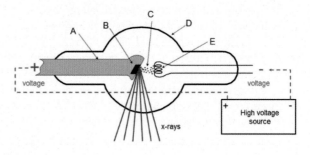

9. What is the major role of the cathode cup in an x-ray tube?
   A. Electron acceleration
   B. Electron bremsstrahlung
   C. Electron capture
   D. Electron focus
   E. Electron source

10. In what position in the x-ray field does the projected effective x-ray tube focal spot size become larger than that projected down the central axis?
    A. Toward the perpendicular axis to the anode side of the field
    B. Toward the perpendicular axis to the cathode side of the field
    C. Toward the cathode side of the field
    D. Toward the anode side of the field

11. Referring to the schematic, which one of the modules contains the filament circuit?

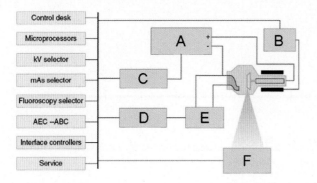

12. At a fixed source-image distance, which x-ray tube parameter will result in the largest heel effect variations across the x-ray field?
    A. Small anode angle
    B. Large anode angle
    C. Small focal spot
    D. Large focal spot

13. If any one of the HVL, mA, kV, or exposure time values *are increased by 20%* and all other parameters remain the same, the x-ray intensity output will be highest with which one of the following?
    A. HVL
    B. mA
    C. Exposure time
    D. kV

14. Which of the following focal spot measurement tools is used for measurement of the focal spot line-spread function (LSF)?

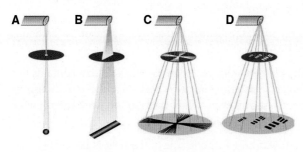

15. What is the purpose of a "backup timer" circuit in an x-ray generator?
    A. To determine the minimum exposure pulse duration
    B. To stop the anode from spinning after the exposure

C. To compare the set time to the actual exposure time
D. To achieve the correct exposure to the detector
E. To shut off of the x-ray beam if the AEC fails

16. What is the typical HVL of a calibrated x-ray tube operating at 80 kV?
    A. 1 mm Al          D. 7 mm Al
    B. 3 mm Al          E. 10 mm A
    C. 5 mm Al

17. To determine x-ray exposure for radiography, the automatic exposure control (AEC) ion chambers are located at which physical position in the x-ray system?
    A. In the x-ray tube collimator assembly
    B. In the x-ray generator circuit
    C. In front of the image receptor
    D. In the technologist control panel

18. For a conventional fluoroscopy rotating anode tube insert, which of the following will have the greatest impact on tube output and heat loading limitations?
    A. Anode diameter
    B. Anode rotation speed
    C. Focal spot size
    D. Housing heat exchanger

19. When acquiring a chest radiograph, which one of the following depictions results in the most balanced outcome in terms of transmitted x-rays to the detector?

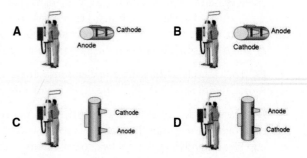

20. Select the application requiring the x-ray tube with the highest heat load capacity during typical clinical operation.
    A. Interventional radiology
    B. Computed tomography
    C. Dedicated chest radiography
    D. Mammography

# Answers

1. **E**  The *deceleration* of the electrons as they impact the target produces a spectrum of photon energies known as the bremsstrahlung ("braking radiation") spectrum. *(Pg. 186–187)*

2. **A**  The photon energies of the characteristic radiation are solely determined by the target material. If the energy of the electrons does not exceed the binding energy of the target electrons, characteristic radiation will not be produced. *(Pg. 188–189)*

3. **D**  The filament is the source of electrons, caused by resistive heating; electrons are emitted from the cathode filament by "thermionic emission." *(Pg. 190–191)*

4. **C**  kV is kilovoltage, a potential difference that accelerates electrons to a specific kinetic energy; keV is kilo electron volts, a unit of energy. *(Pg. 185)*

5. **B**  X-ray production efficiency is proportional to the atomic number Z of the anode. For Mo, Z = 42; for W, Z = 74. To achieve the same production efficiency for fixed kV, the ratio of Z's is taken: 74/42 = 1.76 $\cong$ 1.8. *(Pg. 187–188)*

6. **D**  The stator exists outside of the x-ray tube insert and contains the windings that produce a rotating magnetic field to "drag" the rotor, which is made of an alternating iron/copper core mounted on heat-resistant bearings inside of the x-ray tube insert. The anode is attached to the rotor with a molybdenum spindle. Heat in the anode is not efficiently conducted to the bearings, as Mo is a poor heat conductor. *(Pg. 195)*

7. **D**  Grid-biased focusing cups can instantaneously pinch off the flow of electrons emerging from the cathode with a negative voltage of about 2,000 volts. This is the fastest way to turn on and off the x-ray beam and is often used by "pulsed fluoroscopy" systems. Mechanical contactor switches are only used in single-phase x-ray generators; electronic timers are very fast; however, there is a small delay in turning on/off the power to the x-ray generator due to cable capacitance effects. Automatic exposure control sensors measure the amount of x-rays transmitted through the patient but are relatively slow. *(Pg. 193)*

8. **E**  The cathode is the source of electrons; for the x-ray tube, the filament structure is part of the cathode. Although not shown in this diagram, it is surrounded by a focusing cup. *(Pg. 186 and 191)*

9. **D**  The cathode cup is the structure that surrounds the filament and creates an electric field that contains the electrons emitted from the filament structure and prevents spreading apart. A biased cathode (or focusing) cup has a slightly negative voltage to contain the electrons into an even tighter distribution, with the result of producing a smaller focal spot. *(Pg. 191–193)*

10. **C**  The size of the effective focal spot when projected toward the cathode side of the field is larger, because the "effective" projection angle is larger, and vice versa for the effective focal size when projected toward the anode size of the x-ray field. *(Pg. 197–198)*

11. **E**  The filament circuit is a closed-loop circuit that heats up the filament and therefore must be part of the cathode structure of the x-ray tube. The filament circuit is characterized by having a high current (approximately 5 to 10 A) and low voltage (tens of volts) to heat up the filament and allow electrons to be released by a process known as thermionic emission. *(Pg. 211–212)*

12. **A**  Heel effect is caused by the self-filtration of x-rays that are produced at a depth within the anode materials that are projected toward the anode side of the field. These photons must propagate through more anode material to emerge, the intensity of the x-rays are reduced, and the average energy is increased (the latter resulting from the preferential absorption of the lower-energy x-rays). A smaller anode angle will manifest a

greater variation in heel effect intensity for a given field dimension, as the x-rays emerging toward the anode side (emission angle) must go through even more anode material to the point of anode (field) cutoff. *(Pg. 201)*

13. **D** X-ray output increases linearly with mA, linearly with time, and by approximately a power of 2 with kV (kV²). If the HVL of the beam is increased, the x-ray output intensity will be lower. *(Pg. 219–220)*

14. **B** The line-spread function is measured with a slit camera, which can be depicted as a series of point sources along a line. The useful attribute of the LSF is the determination of the MTF through Fourier transformation. *(Pg. 198–200)*

15. **E** The "backup timer" is preset to a maximum exposure time (typically for about 1 second for conventional radiography) and terminates the exposure in the event that the phototimer detector fails. This is a safety mechanism required for all phototiming systems. *(Pg. 215–216)*

16. **B** According to Federal Regulations, the HVL at 80 kV must be 2.9 mm Al (as of June 2006). A higher HVL beam is more penetrable and for a given entrance exposure will result in a lower dose to the patient when the same exposure to the detector is achieved. *(Pg. 221–222)*

17. **C** The AEC ion chambers are positioned prior to the image receptor (whether screen-film or digital detectors) to measure the radiation fluence transmitted through the patient. In a properly calibrated AEC system, the radiation dose will be continuously measured and turned off when a predetermined energy fluence exposes the detector that results in an adequate image quality and low (optimal) patient dose. *(Pg. 215–216)*

18. **C** Heating limits are most affected by the area of electron bombardment, known as the focal spot. Rotation speed and anode diameter also have a substantial impact but definitely less than the focal spot. *(Pg. 216–217)*

19. **D** The body habitus for a PA chest x-ray is typically thinner at the apices of the lung and neck area and thicker at the base of the lungs and the diaphragm. The heel effect, which describes the lower x-ray beam intensity due to self-filtration of the bremsstrahlung beam on the anode side of the beam, should thus be positioned over the thinner parts of the anatomy when acquiring a 2D projection radiograph and the higher-intensity beam positioned over the thicker parts of the anatomy.

20. **B** Computed tomography on average generates the most energy per patient examination and thus requires the highest anode heating and cooling capabilities of all x-ray tubes used in diagnostic radiology. *(Pg. 205–206)*

# Section III Key Equations and Symbols

| QUANTITY | EQUATION | EQ NO./PAGE/COMMENTS |
|---|---|---|
| Efficiency of x-ray production | $\dfrac{\text{Radiative energy loss}}{\text{Collisional energy loss}} \cong \dfrac{E_{K}Z}{820{,}000}$ | Eq. 6-1/Pg. 187/This equation is for diagnostic imaging operation where electron kinetic energy $E_K$ < 150 keV |
| Energy and potential difference | Energy (keV); voltage (kV) | Pg. 185/Electron kinetic energy accelerated under a voltage. 1 eV = $1.6022 \times 10^{-19}$ joules |
| Characteristic x-rays | Prominent peaks: $K\alpha$ and $K\beta$ | Pg. 187 and Fig. 6-5; represents adjacent ($\alpha$) and nonadjacent ($\beta$) discrete orbital energy transitions |
| Tube current (mA) | 1 mA = $6.24 \times 10^{15}$ electrons | Pg. 190/Electrons passing from cathode to anode in x-ray tube |
| Line focus principle | Effective focal length = actual focal length × sin $\theta$ | Eq. 6-2/Fig. 6-14/Pg. 196/$\theta$ is the anode angle relative to central axis |
| Law of transformers | $\dfrac{V_{P}}{V_{S}} = \dfrac{N_{P}}{N_{S}}$ | Eq. 6-3/Pg. 209/$V_p$ = input voltage; $V_s$ = output voltage; $N_p$ = # primary turns, $N_s$ = # secondary turns |
| Transformer power law | $V_P I_P = V_S I_S$ | Eq. 6-5/Pg. 210/Describes power on primary side of transformer = power on secondary side; power = $V \times I$, where $I$ is current |
| Power rating of x-ray generator or focal spot power deposition | Power (kW) = 100 kV × I ($A_{max}$) for a 0.1-s exposure time | Eq. 6-6/Pg. 216/Describes max power delivered by a generator or received by a focal spot |
| Energy deposition to anode expressed in *Heat Unit* | Energy (HU) = $\alpha$ × kVp × mA × s | Eq. 6-7/Pg. 217/Anode energy deposition; s = exposure time in seconds. $\alpha$ = 1 for single-phase and $\alpha$ = 1.35 for three-phase or high-frequency generator |
| Energy deposition to anode expressed in *Joule* | Energy (J) = $V_{RMS} \times A \times$ s | Eq. 6-9/Pg. 218/$V_{RMS}$ = Root mean square voltage; $A$ = tube current in amperes; s = exposure time in seconds. Does not depend on generator waveform |
| Tube output as a function of kV | Exposure $\propto$ kV$^2$ | Eq. 6-11/Pg. 219/Expresses energy fluence (exposure) free-in-air for a fixed mA for a ratio of kV selections to be compared |
| X-ray transmission through an attenuator as function of kV; transmitted exposure $\propto$ kV$\alpha$, where $\alpha$ (2–6) depends on thickness | $\left(\dfrac{kVp_1}{kVp_2}\right)^5 \times mAs_1 = mAs_2$ | Eq. 6-12/Pg. 219/Expresses the x-ray tube output adjustment of mA for equal transmission through an attenuator with kV. The exponent varies with thickness, and is ~5 for 20 cm |

# CHAPTER 7

# Radiography

## INTRODUCTION

This chapter explains how the technology described in Chapter 6 is used to project the shadows of a three-dimensional object onto a two-dimensional detector to produce a clinical radiographic image (Fig. 7-1). Understanding the fundamentals of radiography is important because many of these principles also apply to other imaging modalities such as mammography, fluoroscopy, and computed tomography. The geometry of the examination, scattered radiation and methods of control, and selection of exposure technique settings are discussed including their effects on the resulting image. Methods for converting x-rays that exit the patient into a digital image are described in detail. Patient safety aspects include the need for derived quantities for feedback of appropriate exposure factor selection and the meaning of these exposure index values, as well as special considerations for pediatric digital radiography. Artifacts in digital radiographic images and their underlying causes are discussed because they may limit the clinical value of the examination or result in additional patient radiation exposure in the event of repeated imaging. Dual energy subtraction, a specialized method for isolating high-density and low-density features from radiographic projections, is explained.

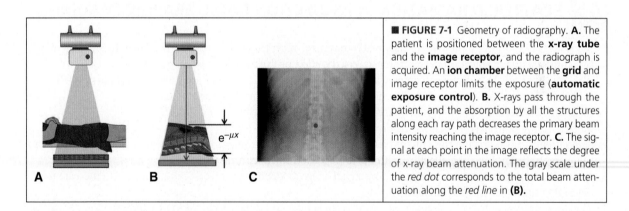

■ **FIGURE 7-1** Geometry of radiography. **A.** The patient is positioned between the **x-ray tube** and the **image receptor**, and the radiograph is acquired. An **ion chamber** between the **grid** and image receptor limits the exposure (**automatic exposure control**). **B.** X-rays pass through the patient, and the absorption by all the structures along each ray path decreases the primary beam intensity reaching the image receptor. **C.** The signal at each point in the image reflects the degree of x-ray beam attenuation. The gray scale under the *red dot* corresponds to the total beam attenuation along the *red line* in **(B).**

## GEOMETRY OF X-RAY PROJECTION

1. *Magnification*: divergence of the x-ray beam from the focal spot (Fig. **7-2**).
   **a.** Magnification of features depend on distance from the image receptor, depth in the patient, and lateral distance from the *central ray* of the x-ray beam.
   **b.** *Geometric distortion* of features is worse for large body parts and short *source to image distance*.
2. Magnification aggravates *blurring* or *unsharpness* (Fig. 7-3).

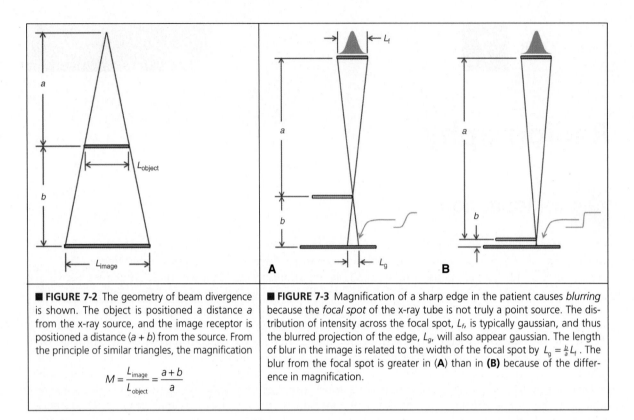

■ **FIGURE 7-2** The geometry of beam divergence is shown. The object is positioned a distance *a* from the x-ray source, and the image receptor is positioned a distance (*a* + *b*) from the source. From the principle of similar triangles, the magnification

$$M = \frac{L_{\text{image}}}{L_{\text{object}}} = \frac{a+b}{a}$$

■ **FIGURE 7-3** Magnification of a sharp edge in the patient causes *blurring* because the *focal spot* of the x-ray tube is not truly a point source. The distribution of intensity across the focal spot, $L_f$, is typically gaussian, and thus the blurred projection of the edge, $L_g$, will also appear gaussian. The length of blur in the image is related to the width of the focal spot by $L_g = \frac{b}{a} L_f$. The blur from the focal spot is greater in (**A**) than in (**B**) because of the difference in magnification.

## 7.2   SCATTERED RADIATION IN PROJECTION RADIOGRAPHIC IMAGING

1. X-rays traveling through the patient may reach the image receptor unimpeded, or they may interact by one of two fundamental physical processes, the *photoelectric effect* or *Compton scatter*.
   a. X-rays that reach the image receptor without interacting with the patient are called *primary x-rays* (*P*).
   b. X-rays that interact via the photoelectric effect are removed from the primary beam.
   c. X-rays that interact via Compton scatter are usually deflected from their path (Fig. 7-4).
   d. Depending on trajectory, *scatter* may reach the image receptor (*S*).
2. *Subject contrast* is related to the ratio of primary x-rays reaching the image receptor versus those removed from the primary beam; thus, the effect of scatter is to degrade subject contrast.
3. In a *digital image*, contrast can be adjusted by *digital image processing*; however, scatter still acts to increase *noise*, degrading the *signal-to-noise ratio* (*SNR*).
4. The amount of scatter (*S*) in an image is given by the *scatter-to-primary ratio* (*SPR*) or *scatter fraction* (*F*).

$$\text{SPR} = \frac{S}{P} \qquad F = \frac{S}{P+S} \qquad F \text{ in terms of SPR}: F = \frac{\text{SPR}}{\text{SPR}+1}$$

   a. SPR increases with the volume of tissue in the beam, which increases with the thickness of the anatomy in the *field of view* (*FOV*) and the dimensions of the FOV (Fig. 7-5).
   b. Example: For a typical abdominal radiograph of thickness = 25 cm and FOV = 30 cm × 30 cm, SPR = 4.5 and *F* = 82%; thus, most of the captured image is useless information (*noise*).
5. Scatter rejection methods are required for large FOV images of thick body parts.
6. Antiscatter grids are used to selectively transmit primary radiation and prevent scattered radiation from reaching the detector (Fig. 7-6).
7. Perpendicular and lateral alignment of the grid with the central ray of the x-ray beam is critical for proper scatter removal; misalignment can cause *artifacts* in the image.

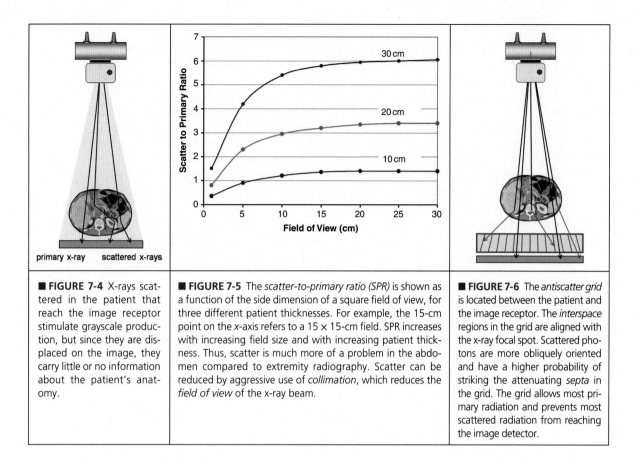

■ **FIGURE 7-4** X-rays scattered in the patient that reach the image receptor stimulate grayscale production, but since they are displaced on the image, they carry little or no information about the patient's anatomy.

■ **FIGURE 7-5** The *scatter-to-primary ratio (SPR)* is shown as a function of the side dimension of a square field of view, for three different patient thicknesses. For example, the 15-cm point on the *x*-axis refers to a 15 × 15-cm field. SPR increases with increasing field size and with increasing patient thickness. Thus, scatter is much more of a problem in the abdomen compared to extremity radiography. Scatter can be reduced by aggressive use of *collimation*, which reduces the *field of view* of the x-ray beam.

■ **FIGURE 7-6** The *antiscatter grid* is located between the patient and the image receptor. The *interspace* regions in the grid are aligned with the x-ray focal spot. Scattered photons are more obliquely oriented and have a higher probability of striking the attenuating *septa* in the grid. The grid allows most primary radiation and prevents most scattered radiation from reaching the image detector.

8. Characterization of grids by features of their construction (Fig. 7-7).
   a. *Grid types*: linear, focused, crossed.
   b. *Grid ratio* = interspace height versus interspace width with ratios of 8:1, 10:1 and 12:1 common; 6:1 and 14:1 less common.
   c. *Interspace* material: aluminum (low cost) or carbon fiber (high transmission of primary).
   d. *Grid frequency* = # grid septa/cm; in Figure 7-7, the frequency is 60 lines/cm; 70 to 80 lines/cm grids are available but are more expensive; typically used for digital receptors with high resolution.
   e. *Focal length* = intended SID range—typical source-image distances are 100 and 183 cm; lower ratio grids have less crucial focusing range.
   f. *Grid cutoff* occurs when the primary beam is attenuated and occurs with the wrong SID; other sources include laterally shifted or tilted grid (nonperpendicular) with respect to the central axis, or upside-down focused grid.

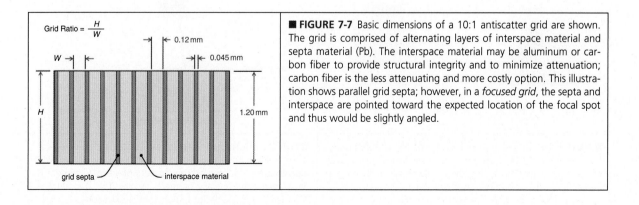

■ **FIGURE 7-7** Basic dimensions of a 10:1 antiscatter grid are shown. The grid is comprised of alternating layers of interspace material and septa material (Pb). The interspace material may be aluminum or carbon fiber to provide structural integrity and to minimize attenuation; carbon fiber is the less attenuating and more costly option. This illustration shows parallel grid septa; however, in a *focused grid*, the septa and interspace are pointed toward the expected location of the focal spot and thus would be slightly angled.

9. Grids can be stationary or moving.
    a. A stationary grid produces regularly spaced image shadows (grid lines) that are routinely ignored by radiologists; high frequency fixed grids have unresolvable lines relative to the detector resolution, but low frequency aliasing patterns can result in image nonuniformity.
    b. A *Bucky grid* moves perpendicular to the linear septa during the x-ray exposure to blur the grid lines.
10. The *Bucky factor* is the relative increase in x-ray output that must be used to compensate for using the grid.
    a. Primary x-rays falling on septa and scattered x-rays are prevented from reaching the receptor.
    b. For fixed speed receptors, the ratio of the mAs with grid versus without grid is the Bucky factor.
    c. For variable speed digital receptors, lower signal with grid is adjusted by amplification.
    d. Loss of primary radiation considers grid *primary transmission factor* for compensation.
    e. The Bucky factor for variable speed receptor is typically less than for a fixed speed receptor.
11. Other metrics describing grid performance:
    a. *Primary transmission factor*, $T_p$ = the fraction of primary x-rays penetrating the grid
        (i) The septa in Figure 7.7 above cover 27% of the grid, so $T_p$ must be $\leq 0.73$.
        (ii) In digital radiography, $1/T_p$ is a reasonable replacement for the Bucky factor.
    b. *Scatter transmission factor*, $T_s$ = the fraction of scattered x-rays penetrating the grid—ideally this is 0, but typical values of $T_s$ are between 0.05 and 0.20
    c. *Selectivity*, $\Sigma$ = the ratio of primary transmission to scattered transmission $\Sigma = \dfrac{T_p}{T_s}$
    d. *Contrast degradation factor*, *CDF* = the reduction of contrast from scatter $CDF = \dfrac{1}{1+SPR}$
12. Alternate scatter rejection methods: *air gap technique, slot-scan technique, scatter processing*
    a. The air gap technique (Fig. 7-8) involves moving the patient away from the image receptor.
        (i) X-rays scattered in the patient are less likely to reach the image receptor.
        (ii) Introduces magnification, decreases the anatomy within the FOV, increases blur from the focal spot, and requires higher exposure technique with increased SID.
    b. The slot-scan technique (Fig. 7-9) works by exposing only a small part of the anatomy at a time and translating across the FOV to create the composite image.
        (i) The amount of scatter is reduced because of the narrow FOV of the slot.
        (ii) The slot-scanner does not require a grid.
        (iii) Dose efficiency depends on alignment of prepatient slit and postpatient slot.
        (iv) Higher mAs and higher tube loading, with opportunity for patient motion.
    c. Digital image processing for a physical antiscatter grid—"virtual grid."
        (i) Useful where grid alignment is difficult (*e.g.*, bedside radiography) and cutoff likely.
        (ii) Requires estimate of patient thickness, amount of scatter reaching detector.

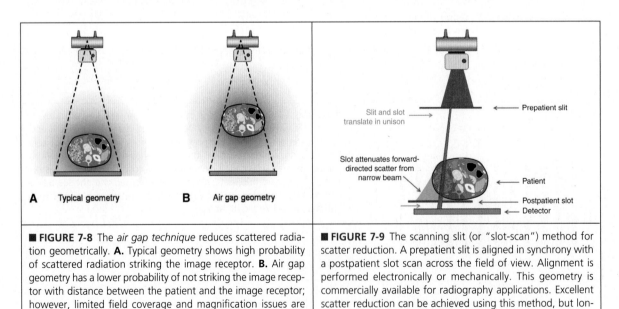

**■ FIGURE 7-8** The *air gap technique* reduces scattered radiation geometrically. **A.** Typical geometry shows high probability of scattered radiation striking the image receptor. **B.** Air gap geometry has a lower probability of not striking the image receptor with distance between the patient and the image receptor; however, limited field coverage and magnification issues are concerns and is used only rarely in diagnostic imaging.

**■ FIGURE 7-9** The scanning slit (or "slot-scan") method for scatter reduction. A prepatient slit is aligned in synchrony with a postpatient slot scan across the field of view. Alignment is performed electronically or mechanically. This geometry is commercially available for radiography applications. Excellent scatter reduction can be achieved using this method, but longer exposure times and patient motion can be a drawback.

(iii) Scatter is nonuniform and depends on collimation; anatomy is variable.
(iv) Noise and signal indistinguishable, and possibly compromising for low contrast signals.
(v) Uses lower kV and similar mAs as technique required for grid study.

## 7.3 TECHNIQUE FACTORS IN RADIOGRAPHY

1. Primary technique factors include *tube voltage* (kV), *tube current* (mA), *exposure time* (s), and *source to image distance* (SID); added filtration must also be considered (Fig. 7-10).
   a. SID usually 100 cm, 183 cm for upright chest examination
   b. kV adjusted for examination type
   c. Product of tube current (mA) and time (s) as *mAs* to adjust fluence for kV, SID, and filtration

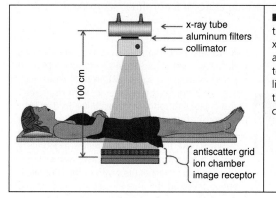

■ **FIGURE 7-10** The standard configuration for radiography is illustrated. Most table-based radiographic systems use a *SID* of 100 cm. The x-ray *collimator* has a light bulb and mirror assembly in it, and, when activated, casts a light beam onto the patient allowing the technologist to position the x-ray beam with respect to the patient's anatomy. The light beam is congruent with the x-ray beam. X-rays that pass through the patient must also pass through the *antiscatter grid* and the *ion chamber* (part of the *AEC* system) in order to reach the *image receptor*.

2. *kV selection* involves compromises based on fundamental interactions of x-rays.
   a. Lower kV emphasizes contrast based on photoelectric effect (PE) for bone/barium contrast and appropriate for thin body parts.
   b. Higher kV generally produces lower patient dose, is needed for thick body parts, is used to decrease rib contrast in chest examinations, and can reduce exposure time.
3. *Current time product* (mAs) controls x-ray fluence, where output fluence is linear with mAs.
   a. High mA allows shorter exposure time for constant mAs, but requires large focal spot.
   b. Deliberately long exposure times are selected to blur anatomic features (*breathing techniques*).
4. *Technique chart* (see textbook Table 7-1, pg. 237) specifies control settings for each radiographic view, including:
   a. kV, mAs, focal spot selection (large/small), SID, filtration (if filter-selectable system), and grid
   b. May include modifications for patient thickness
5. The *protocol book* defines views that comprise an examination, typically consisting of multiple views.
   a. Anteroposterior (AP) or posteroanterior (PA), lateral (LAT), and unique positions such as oblique
6. *Manual techniques* require the technologist to set the kV and mAs, typically based on previous exposures.
   a. Prevalent in pediatric radiology, bedside radiography and certain views
7. *Automatic exposure control* (AEC) regulates the radiation delivered to the image receptor.
   a. Ion chamber(s) measure the radiation passing through the patient incident on the receptor.
   b. Some digital image receptors can measure and integrate signal with time.
   c. Circuits measure the transmitted radiation fluence and a proportional voltage signal is produced.
   d. Signals are compared to a calibrated value, and when reached, the exposure is terminated.
   e. Proper positioning of ion chambers or active areas on a flat-panel receptor are crucial.
   f. Acquisition optimization includes patient size selection, appropriate kV, mA, SID, grid/no grid.
8. *Ideal technique guide* considers all aspects of the imaging chain, including generator output, beam quality, SID, collimation, patient thickness, grid attenuation, image receptor sensitivity, image processing, and patient dose commensurate with exam requirements in terms of SNR and CNR.

## 7.4   SCINTILLATORS AND INTENSIFYING SCREENS

1. *Scintillators* for converting x-rays to visible light (called indirect detectors) use amorphous and structured phosphors.
   a. *Amorphous scintillators* are fine-grain phosphor powders held together by binder material.
      (i) X-ray produced light spread is diffuse with mutiple scattting events.
      (ii) Spatial resolution decreases with thickness; absorption efficiency increases with thickness, with a trade-off of resolution versus dose efficiency (Fig. 7-11).
   b. *Strucured* scintillators have a crystalline structure that act as light pipes.
      (i) Internal reflection of light at crystal interfaces reduce light spread.
      (ii) Resolution is preserved with thicker material that increases absorption efficiency.
      (iii) CsI (cesium iodide) is a structured phosphor widely used in x-ray flat-panel receptors.
      (iv) Structured phosphors are fragile, hygroscopic (absorb water and must be sealed), and expensive.
      (v) Spatial resolution is better compared to an equal absorption efficient amorphous scintillator.

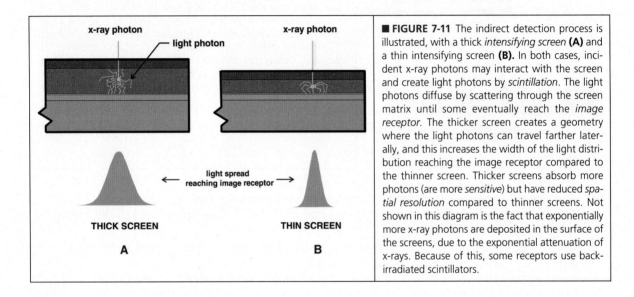

■ **FIGURE 7-11** The indirect detection process is illustrated, with a thick *intensifying screen* **(A)** and a thin intensifying screen **(B).** In both cases, incident x-ray photons may interact with the screen and create light photons by *scintillation*. The light photons diffuse by scattering through the screen matrix until some eventually reach the *image receptor*. The thicker screen creates a geometry where the light photons can travel farther laterally, and this increases the width of the light distribution reaching the image receptor compared to the thinner screen. Thicker screens absorb more photons (are more *sensitive*) but have reduced *spatial resolution* compared to thinner screens. Not shown in this diagram is the fact that exponentially more x-ray photons are deposited in the surface of the screens, due to the exponential attenuation of x-rays. Because of this, some receptors use back-irradiated scintillators.

## 7.5   ABSORPTION EFFICIENCY AND CONVERSION EFFICIENCY

1. *Absorption efficiency (AE)* and *conversion efficiency (CE)* are important factors for indirect x-ray detectors.
2. Absorption efficiency depends on effective $Z$, density ($\rho$), thickness, and x-ray beam energy.
   a. *Quantum detection efficiency (QDE)* describes how well detectors capture x-rays, but does not consider *fluorescence*, where energy is re-emitted from the detector.
   b. *Energy absorption efficiency* is a better metric because most x-ray detectors are *energy integrators*, not *photon counters*.
3. *Conversion efficiency* describes how efficiently the optical signal is transferred from the scintillator to the photodetector through amplification and conversion into a digital signal.
   a. Examples: X-ray-to-light conversion in scintillator, light-to-charge conversion in photodetector, light-gain in digital detectors, geometry and lens efficiency in optically coupled detectors
   b. Directly relates to radiation dose needed to produce a given signal level
4. Absorption efficiency and conversion efficiency consequences on image quality (Fig. 7-12).
   a. Conversion efficiency increase of $G$ (gain) allows x-ray fluence reduction by $G$ for same signal, which increases the relative quantum noise by $\sqrt{G}$, since $1/G$ photons are recorded.
   b. Absorption efficiency increase of $G$ allows x-ray fluence reduction by $G$ for same signal, but the reduction of photons by $1/G$ is balanced by absorption efficiency of $G$, so quantum noise is unchanged.
5. Thicker, denser conversion layers increase absorption efficiency but also increase blurring and decrease spatial resolution; structured phosphors overcome resolution loss.

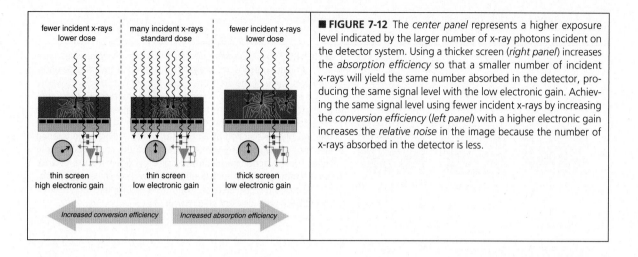

■ **FIGURE 7-12** The *center panel* represents a higher exposure level indicated by the larger number of x-ray photons incident on the detector system. Using a thicker screen (*right panel*) increases the *absorption efficiency* so that a smaller number of incident x-rays will yield the same number absorbed in the detector, producing the same signal level with the low electronic gain. Achieving the same signal level using fewer incident x-rays by increasing the *conversion efficiency* (*left panel*) with a higher electronic gain increases the *relative noise* in the image because the number of x-rays absorbed in the detector is less.

## 7.6  COMPUTED RADIOGRAPHY

**1.** *Computed radiography (CR)* = systems that use *photostimulable phosphor (PSP)* image receptors
  **a.** PSP screens, typically comprised of barium fluorobromide (BaFBr), are passive receptors manufactured in sizes similar to screen-film receptors.
  **b.** Incident x-rays generate fluorescence and elevate excited electrons into energy traps in the PSP.
  **c.** The exposed imaging plate with latent image is processed by a CR reader with an optical stage, plate translation mechanics, scanning laser beam, optical light guide, and photomultiplier tube (Fig. 7-13).
  **d.** Stored energy is released by laser light by *photostimulated luminescence (PSL)*.
  **e.** Laser excitation energy (red) is lower than stimulation luminescence (indigo); (Fig. 7-14).

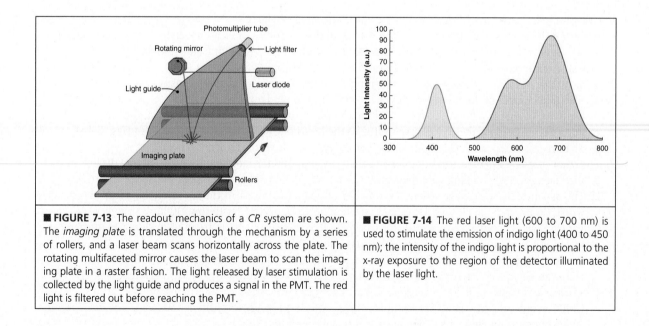

■ **FIGURE 7-13** The readout mechanics of a *CR* system are shown. The *imaging plate* is translated through the mechanism by a series of rollers, and a laser beam scans horizontally across the plate. The rotating multifaceted mirror causes the laser beam to scan the imaging plate in a raster fashion. The light released by laser stimulation is collected by the light guide and produces a signal in the PMT. The red light is filtered out before reaching the PMT.

■ **FIGURE 7-14** The red laser light (600 to 700 nm) is used to stimulate the emission of indigo light (400 to 450 nm); the intensity of the indigo light is proportional to the x-ray exposure to the region of the detector illuminated by the laser light.

**f.** Excitation models describe the production of PSL (Fig. 7-15).

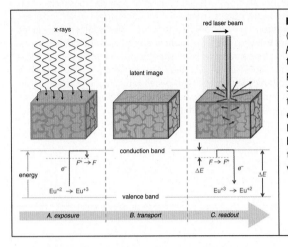

■ **FIGURE 7-15** *Takahashi model* for *photostimulated luminescence (PSL)*. **A.** During exposure, x-rays are absorbed in the *storage phosphor* and some of the electrons reach the conduction band, where they may interact with an *F-center*, causing the reduction of europium (Eu) ions. **B.** Electrons trapped in this high-energy, metastable state can remain there for minutes to months. **C.** During readout, the phosphor is scanned by a red laser, which provides the trapped electrons enough energy to be excited into the conduction band. Here, some fraction of electrons will drop down to the valence band, emitting indigo light during the transition. When the F-center releases a trapped electron, the trivalent europium ($Eu^{+3}$) is converted back to its divalent state ($Eu^{+2}$).

2. Laser scanning of the IP does not release all of the trapped electrons.
    a. The same IP can be scanned a second or third time with little loss of signal.
    b. The IP must be exposed to bright white light to remove residual signal.
    c. Without thorough erasure, a "ghost" image will appear on the next radiographic exposure.
3. CR technology enabled the all-digital radiology operation-in clinical practice for more than two decades.
    a. Limited reimbursement, higher handling, and less DQE have disincentivized use of CR.

## 7.7 CHARGE-COUPLED DEVICE AND COMPLEMENTARY METAL-OXIDE SEMICONDUCTOR DEVICES

1. *Charge-coupled device (CCD)* detectors make images from visible light.
    a. CCD chip is a Si integrated circuit with an array of discrete detector elements etched into its surface.
        (i)   Linear array—one or more rows; $1 \times 2048$ or $96 \times 4096$ dexels for a slot scanner
        (ii)  Area array—$2.5 \times 2.5$ cm with $1024 \times 1024$ or $2048 \times 2048$ dexels
    b. Si surface of CCD is photosensitive, liberating electrons linearly with light intensity.
    c. Electrons remain in dexel because of voltage barrier on boundary.
    d. Read-out of charge pattern occurs by shifting charges in parallel by voltage changes at the barrier.
    e. For a 2D CCD array, the charges are shifted to the bottom row, with horizontal readout (Fig. 7-16).
    f. The process is repeated one row at a time for complete readout of the array.
2. The small size of CCD detectors compared to the FOV required for radiography have led to a decline in use.
    a. Inefficient optical coupling with demagnification leads to loss of light and large statistical uncertainty.
    b. The *quantum sink*, the stage where the number of quanta is lowest in the imaging chain and statistics are worst, occurs in large FOV CCD systems (see text book Fig. 7-18A) with low DQE.
3. Linear CCD arrays coupled to a scintillator by tapered fiber-optic channels are used in slot-scan imagers
    a. Major advantage is scatter rejection of the slot-scan; no antiscatter grid is required.
    b. Readout by *time delay and integration (TDI)* yields high-dose efficiency and good SNR (Fig. 7-17).
    c. Slot-scan devices and systems are clinically useful for chest and full body trauma examinations.
4. *Complementary metal-oxide semiconductor (CMOS)* light-sensitive arrays are alternative to CCD arrays.
    a. CMOS arrays are random access memory "chips" with built-in photosensitive detectors, storage capacitors, and active readout electronics, operating at low voltage (3 to 5 volts).
    b. *Any* dexel on the chip can be addressed in read or read-and-erase mode, useful for "built-in" AEC.
    c. Large area CMOS detectors with up to 75 μm dexel size are being used (see Chapter 8—Mammography).
    d. CMOS detectors are also used as a replacement for image intensifiers (see Chapter 9—Fluoroscopy).

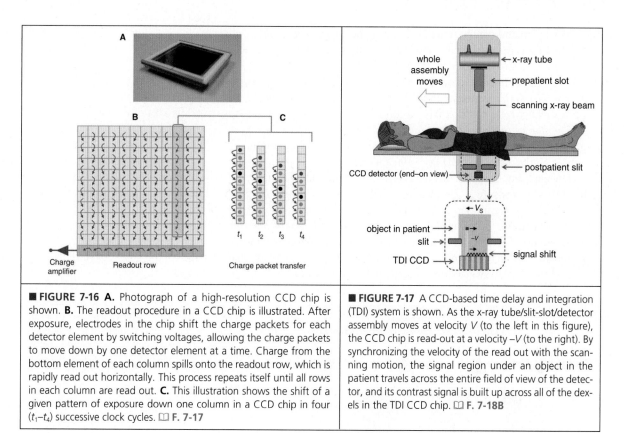

**■ FIGURE 7-16 A.** Photograph of a high-resolution CCD chip is shown. **B.** The readout procedure in a CCD chip is illustrated. After exposure, electrodes in the chip shift the charge packets for each detector element by switching voltages, allowing the charge packets to move down by one detector element at a time. Charge from the bottom element of each column spills onto the readout row, which is rapidly read out horizontally. This process repeats itself until all rows in each column are read out. **C.** This illustration shows the shift of a given pattern of exposure down one column in a CCD chip in four ($t_1$–$t_4$) successive clock cycles. 📖 **F. 7-17**

**■ FIGURE 7-17** A CCD-based time delay and integration (TDI) system is shown. As the x-ray tube/slit-slot/detector assembly moves at velocity $V$ (to the left in this figure), the CCD chip is read-out at a velocity $-V$ (to the right). By synchronizing the velocity of the read out with the scanning motion, the signal region under an object in the patient travels across the entire field of view of the detector, and its contrast signal is built up across all of the dexels in the TDI CCD chip. 📖 **F. 7-18B**

## 7.8  FLAT PANEL THIN-FILM TRANSISTOR ARRAY DETECTORS

1. Technology most widely used for radiography in 2021 (and fluoroscopy—see Chapter 8).
2. Based on large-area amorphous silicon substrate (note: CCD and CMOS use crystalline silicon substrates).
3. The lithography process etches the basic electronic components including *gate* and *drain* lines, *transistor switch*, *charge capture electrode*, and *storage capacitor* on the substrate layer (Fig. 7-18).

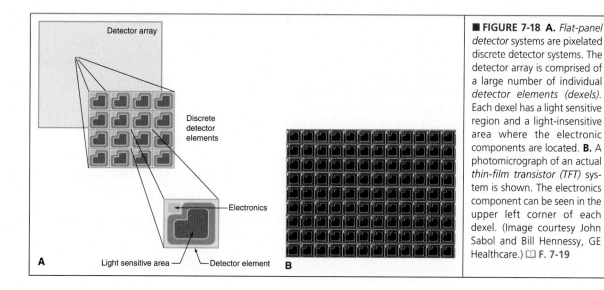

**■ FIGURE 7-18 A.** *Flat-panel detector* systems are pixelated discrete detector systems. The detector array is comprised of a large number of individual *detector elements (dexels)*. Each dexel has a light sensitive region and a light-insensitive area where the electronic components are located. **B.** A photomicrograph of an actual *thin-film transistor (TFT)* system is shown. The electronics component can be seen in the upper left corner of each dexel. (Image courtesy John Sabol and Bill Hennessy, GE Healthcare.) 📖 **F. 7-19**

4. Construction and components of the flat-panel array (Fig. 7-19):
   a. The *TFT* is the electronic on/off switch with three conductor lines.
   b. The TFT *source* is connected to the storage capacitor.
   c. The TFT *drain* is attached to the drain conductor line along each column.
   d. The TFT *switch* is attached to the gate lines of the TFT array.
   e. The *charge collection electrode* captures the charge produced by x-rays over the area of the dexel.
   f. The *storage capacitor* stores the local charge.
   g. Gate and drain lines connect each dexel along rows and columns.
5. Acquiring the x-ray image (Fig. 7-19 caption)
   a. During x-ray exposure, the TFT switch is closed, allowing each dexel to accumulate charge.
   b. After the exposure is complete, the TFT sequentially turns on the gate line to every dexel in the row.
   c. The charge accumulated in each dexel capacitor flows through the transistor to the drain line, and subsequently to the charge amplifier to complete the readout of one row in the array.
   d. After complete readout of the array, any residual charge is removed prior to the next exposure.
   e. Readout speed (milliseconds to seconds) depends on electronic characteristics of the x-ray converter material and the TFT array electronics. Many flat panels can provide real-time rates (30 images/s).

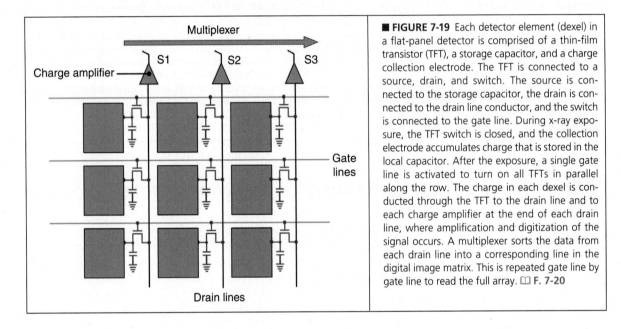

■ **FIGURE 7-19** Each detector element (dexel) in a flat-panel detector is comprised of a thin-film transistor (TFT), a storage capacitor, and a charge collection electrode. The TFT is connected to a source, drain, and switch. The source is connected to the storage capacitor, the drain is connected to the drain line conductor, and the switch is connected to the gate line. During x-ray exposure, the TFT switch is closed, and the collection electrode accumulates charge that is stored in the local capacitor. After the exposure, a single gate line is activated to turn on all TFTs in parallel along the row. The charge in each dexel is conducted through the TFT to the drain line and to each charge amplifier at the end of each drain line, where amplification and digitization of the signal occurs. A multiplexer sorts the data from each drain line into a corresponding line in the digital image matrix. This is repeated gate line by gate line to read the full array. ▢ **F. 7-20**

6. *Fill factor* represents the fraction of the dexel area occupied by electronics insensitive to incident x-rays.
   a. Efficiency is typically about 80% for dexels of 200 × 200 μm, and much less for smaller dexels; for example, 40% to 50% for 100 to 150 μm dimension.
   b. Fill factor limits the minimum size of dexel dimensions.
7. TFT *indirect x-ray conversion* (Fig. 7-20A).
   a. A photodiode layer on the TFT array is required to convert light photons to charge.
   b. A scintillator (cesium iodide, CsI or gadolinium oxysulfide, $Gd_2O_2S$) converts x-rays to light.
   c. Light spread in the scintillator reduces spatial resolution—CsI as a "structured phosphor" limits spread.
   d. Detective quantum efficiency in the lower frequency spectrum is high for CsI but more fragile than $Gd_2O_2S$.
   e. Configuration is most widely used for radiography.
8. TFT *direct x-ray conversion* (Fig. 7-20B).
   a. A semiconductor material is layered on the TFT array; x-rays produce electron-hole pairs.
      (i) Amorphous selenium (*a*-Se) is layered between two surface-area electrodes connected to a bias voltage and a dielectric layer.
      (ii) Dielectric layer prevents overcharging dexels, which could damage the TFT array.

b. Ion pairs are collected under applied voltage across the converter (10 to 50 V/μm of thickness).

c. The electric field almost completely eliminates lateral spreading, resulting in high spatial resolution.

d. Fill factor penalties are reduced, as electrical potential field lines bend and direct charge carriers to the collection electrode, avoiding insensitive regions of the dexel.

e. Se has a relatively low Z and low absorption efficiency but can be made thick (0.5 to 1.0 mm) with minor impact on preservation of spatial resolution.

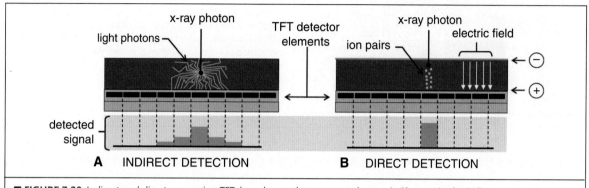

■ **FIGURE 7-20** Indirect and direct conversion TFT–based x-ray detectors are shown. **A.** Photons in the indirect system propagate laterally, compromising resolution. The detected signal shown for the indirect detector shows this lateral spread in the signal from one x-ray photon interaction. **B.** For the direct detector system, the ion pairs liberated by x-ray interaction follow the electric field lines (electron holes travel upward, electrons travel downward) with negligible lateral spread. Here, the detected electronic signal from one x-ray photon interaction is collected almost entirely in one detector element, and therefore, spatial resolution is better.
📖 F. 7-21

## 7.9 OTHER CONSIDERATIONS

1. Selection of a DR system requires assessment of facility needs.
2. CR is often the first DR system installed in a hospital.
    a. CR directly replaces screen-film cassettes in existing radiography units and in bedside examinations.
    b. The relatively expensive CR reader is stationary, but the CR IPs are relatively inexpensive, several dozen plates may be used in different radiographic rooms simultaneously.
    c. One CR reader can serve several rooms depending on room type, workload, and proximity.
        (i)   Typically, one multi-cassette CR reader can handle the workload of three radiographic rooms.
3. The cost of an individual flat panel detector is high: it can only be in one place at one time.
    a. Flat panel detectors are ideal for suites with high patient throughput, such as a dedicated chest room.
        (i)   Throughput in a single room using flat panel detectors is higher than for CR.
        (ii)  TFT flat panel cassettes with wireless technology offer an alternative to CR IPs in bedside radiography and are now the detector of choice despite higher fragility and cost.
4. Reduced reimbursement for CR detectors has led to a substantial decrease in CR receptor use.

## 7.10 RADIOGRAPHIC DETECTORS, PATIENT DOSE, AND EXPOSURE INDEX

1. In traditional screen-film radiography, film OD was the indicator of exposure (Fig. 7-21 left).
    a. Direct feedback was provided by inspection of the processed film image.
2. CR and DR detectors have wide exposure latitude.
    a. Postacquisition processing produces consistent image gray scale even with underexposed and overexposed images.
3. Automatic adjustment of the gray scale of digital radiographic images disables the traditional method of exposure factor control provided to the technologist by film density (Fig. 7-21 right).
    a. Underexposed DR images absorb fewer x-rays, which cause increased image noise.
    b. Overexposed images can easily go unnoticed, causing unnecessary patient exposure.
    c. Underexposed images are likely to be criticized by radiologists for excessive image noise.
    d. Overexposed images are likely to be high quality.

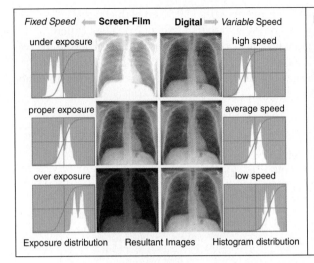

*Fixed Speed* ⟸ **Screen-Film** **Digital** ⟹ *Variable* Speed

under exposure — high speed

proper exposure — average speed

over exposure — low speed

Exposure distribution — Resultant Images — Histogram distribution

■ **FIGURE 7-21** Response of a screen-film system with fixed radiographic speed and a digital system with variable radiographic speed to underexposure, correct exposure, and overexposure are shown. For screen-film, to the left of each radiograph is a distribution representing the x-ray exposure absorbed by the screen and converted to OD on the film. Note that the characteristic curve translating exposure to OD is fixed on the exposure axis. For digital systems, to the right of each radiograph is a distribution representing the frequency of digital values (a *histogram*) linear with exposure absorbed by the image receptor and converted to a digital value. Note that the lookup table curve translating the digital values to brightness and contrast on a display monitor is variable and adjusts to the histogram to achieve optimal rendering of image contrast. ▭ F. 7-22

4. *Dose creep* describes the situation where technologists tend to use unnecessarily high exposures most likely to occur in bedside radiography where manual technique factors are used to avoid potentially noisy images.

5. Identifying the relevant areas in an x-ray acquisition.
   a. The distribution of grayscale values represents a *histogram*, which can be used to identify high exposure regions without patient attenuation, and low exposure regions outside the collimated FOV.
   b. The remaining *region of interest* contains relevant patient anatomy.

6. Segmentation is known as "*exposure recognition.*"
   a. A histogram generated from the relevant image area is compared to a histogram shape specific to the anatomic view (chest, forearm, head, etc.).
   b. The grayscale values in the raw image are then digitally transformed using a *lookup table (LUT)* providing contrast desired in the "for presentation" image.
   c. Histogram analysis accomplishes four specific tasks: (1) exposure compensation; (2) latitude compensation; (3) contrast adjustment for the values of interest (VOI); and (4) exposure index calculation.

7. The median value of the histogram is used to determine a *proprietary exposure index* (EI) value.
   a. Depend on manufacturer's algorithm and image receptor calibration method.
   b. Exposure index indicates the amount of radiation reaching the image receptor but is **not** a *direct* indicator of dose to the patient.
   c. Widely different methods to calculate the EI value have evolved (Table 7-1).

## TABLE 7-1 MANUFACTURER, CORRESPONDING SYMBOL FOR EI, AND CALCULATED EI FOR THREE INCIDENT EXPOSURES TO THE DETECTOR

| MANUFACTURER | SYMBOL | 5 μGy | 10 μGy | 20 μGy |
|---|---|---|---|---|
| Canon (brightness = 16, contrast = 10) | REX | 50 | 100 | 200 |
| Fuji, Konica | S | 400 | 200 | 100 |
| Kodak (CR, STD) | EI | 1,700 | 2,000 | 2,300 |
| IDC (ST = 200) | F# | −1 | 0 | 1 |
| Philips | EI | 200 | 100 | 50 |
| Siemens | EI | 500 | 1,000 | 2,000 |

8. An international standard for an exposure index for digital radiographic systems has been published by the *International Electrotechnical Commission (IEC)*, IEC 62494–1.

9. The standard describes "*Exposure Indices*" and "*Deviation Indices*" and a method for placing these values in the DICOM header of each radiographic image.

10. The manufacturer's responsibility is
    a. To calibrate the imaging detector according to a detector-specific procedure
    b. To provide segmentation of anatomical information in the relevant image region
    c. To generate an EI proportional to detector exposure from histogram data

11. The dose index standard for radiography requires staff to establish *target exposure index (EI$_T$)* values for each digital radiographic system and for each type of exam.
    a. The EI$_T$ for a skull radiograph will be different for a chest radiograph.
12. Feedback whether an "appropriate" exposure has been achieved is given by the *deviation index (DI)*.
    a. $DI = 10\ log_{10}\ (EI/EI_T)$.
    b. DI provides a value of 0 (zero) when the intended exposure to the detector is achieved (*i.e.*, EI = EI$_T$).
    c. A positive number indicates an overexposure has occurred.
    d. A negative number indicates an underexposure has occurred.
        (i)  DI of +1 indicates an overexposure of about 26%.
        (ii) DI of −1 indicates an underexposure of 20% less than desired.
13. The value of DI depends on
    a. Proper calibration and configuration of DR systems
    b. Proper selection of EI$_T$ values
    c. Compliance of technologists with technique guidance
    d. Proper calibration of AEC
    e. Correct selection of the examination and view by the technologist
    f. Appropriate collimation of the radiation field which has a major effect on image segmentation
14. When the DI is in the desired range, the radiographic system is considered to be working well and is able to deliver the EI$_T$ values set up by the institution.
    a. Tracking DI values with respect to equipment and technologist can be useful for QC/QA.
15. EI reports the exposure to the detector for a standard x-ray beam that may not represent the beam exiting the patient in a clinical examination.
16. Regardless of the DI or EI value, the radiologist must answer the question:
    a. *Does the image have sufficient quality to answer the clinical question?*

## 7.11 ARTIFACTS IN DIGITAL RADIOGRAPHY

1. Artifacts are undesired features in an image that mimic or mask clinical features.
   a. Artifacts may be serious or merely cosmetic in nature depending on their magnitude, location, and pattern.
   b. An artifact in the periphery of the FOV may not jeopardize the clinical value of the image.
   c. A periodic artifact, such as prominent grid lines, may pose only a distraction to the radiologist.
2. Other artifacts, such as a wispy shadow from long hair that reaches to the level of the lung apices, can mimic the appearance of a pneumothorax, a significant clinical finding.
3. The visual appearance of an artifact may not provide an unambiguous clue to its underlying cause.
4. Consider the ideal conditions of projection radiography: anything that interferes can produce an artifact.
   a. High-Z particles in the x-ray tube and collimator assembly
   b. Defects in prepatient filters
   c. Clothing, jewelry, and bedding material
   d. Metallic implants in the patient
   e. Lead aprons and shielding blankets
   f. Lead markers used to indicate laterality
   g. Physical defects in the patient support or anti-scatter grid
   h. Misalignment of the anti-scatter grid
   i. Improper calibration of the digital image receptor
   j. Defects in the x-ray conversion layer
   k. Defective dexels
   l. Errors in automatic segmentation of the digital image
   m. Incorrect digital image processing
   n. In a bedside setting, backscatter can superimpose the image of electronic or structural components on the projected image
5. Digital detector artifact causes.
   a. Gain and offset differences; nonfunctional dexels.
   b. Performance of dexels over time requires periodic calibration.
   c. In the case that calibration cannot correct nonuniformities, replacement is necessary.

6. Calibration of the image receptor is accomplished by exposing it to a uniform field of x-rays (Fig. 7-22).
   a. The exposure from an x-ray tube varies in intensity across the FOV along the anode-cathode (A-C) axis because of the heel effect; large SID is used to reduce magnitude of heel effect.
   b. Calibration of the image receptor compensates for exposure nonuniformity with gain compensation.

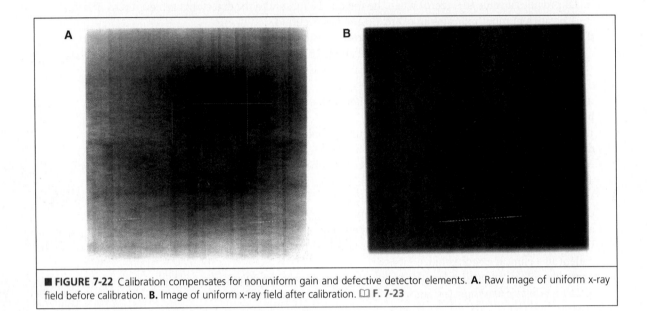

■ **FIGURE 7-22** Calibration compensates for nonuniform gain and defective detector elements. **A.** Raw image of uniform x-ray field before calibration. **B.** Image of uniform x-ray field after calibration. ▭ **F. 7-23**

7. The shadow of anything in the x-ray path at the time of calibration will be corrected by the gain calibration causing an inverse (positive) image present in all subsequent images.
8. The x-ray conversion layer is subject to degradation over time.
   a. CsI is hygroscopic (tends to absorb water); when exposed to ambient humidity, the crystalline structure breaks down losing its ability to restrict lateral spread of light.
   b. Leads to a loss of spatial resolution but also creates artifacts when the crystalline structure is disrupted.
   c. Damage to the x-ray conversion layer requires replacement of the image receptor.
9. Quality control measures ensure the proper functioning of a digital receptor (Fig. 7-23).
   a. Image phantoms can be used to establish quantitative measurements.
   b. Defines confidence limits for appropriate clinical operation.
   c. Assists in defining causes for poor performance.

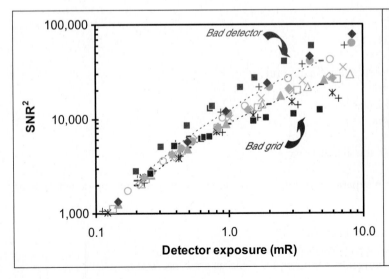

■ **FIGURE 7-23** Variation in exposure-dependent SNR is improved by gain and offset calibration. SNR at the central axis of the image of a phantom is shown for 14 identical DR systems. After calibration, 12 systems performed within confidence limits. One discrepant system required detector replacement. One discrepant system required replacement of its antiscatter grid. $SNR^2$ is a surrogate for NEQ (see Chapter 4). ▭ **F. 7-24**

## 7.12  SPECIAL CONSIDERATIONS FOR PEDIATRIC DIGITAL RADIOGRAPHY

1. Radiography of children poses special challenges.
2. Children vary from neonate to adult-sized patients.
3. Children are often noncompliant, may not be able to stand unassisted, and the small size of their body parts is not consistent with the size of AEC ion chambers.
4. Children are often radiographed using shorter SID than adults in AP orientation on radiographic tables rather than using the upright exposure station using manual technique selections instead of AEC.
5. Small body parts create less scatter so antiscatter grids are often unnecessary.
6. Children are more sensitive to ionizing radiation, with more years of life to develop late effects.
7. Special attention to practices that limit radiation exposure to children is necessary.
8. High powered generators capable of exposures at high mA stations are necessary to minimize exposure time and motion artifacts from noncompliant patients—opposite of conventional wisdom that lower power systems can be used.
9. Small focal spot should be used for pediatric radiography to minimize focal spot blur with short SID.
10. Any delay between exposure actuation and x-ray production confounds the radiologic technologist's attempts to capture full inspiration for chest radiographs.
11. Restriction of the x-ray field is critical in pediatric radiography to reduce unnecessary exposure to surrounding tissue and to enable proper image processing segmentation.
    a. Inclusion of unwanted anatomy, such as the mandible, in the FOV of a chest radiograph can compromise contrast in the lungs.
    b. Convergence of collimation and the light field indicating the field is critical.
12. Traditionally, lead blankets and gonadal shields have been employed to limit exposure in pediatric radiology, but recent studies show limited benefit to this type of shielding and often causes interference with image segmentation.
13. Routine use of postacquisition digital "shutters" leads to inattention to the collimated x-ray field.
    a. Routine appearance of digital markers for orientation instead of the image of lead markers is a clue that digital shutters may also be used.
14. Necessity for manual technique in pediatric radiology requires particular attention to technique charts by radiologic technologists who need to follow it and by medical physicists who monitor the design of the chart and its compliance.
15. The smaller thickness of pediatric anatomy translates into a smaller range of exposures of the anatomy.
    a. Digital image processing for pediatric radiography is likely different from processing appropriate for adults, even for the same radiographic view.
16. The ImageGently campaign promotes judicious use of imaging for children.

## 7.13  DUAL-ENERGY SUBTRACTION RADIOGRAPHY

1. Anatomical noise can cause a loss of conspicuity in radiological imaging.
2. Dual-energy subtraction (DES) radiographic techniques reduce anatomical noise producing images with better information content.
3. Dual-energy subtraction chest radiography illustrates the concept (Fig. 7-24).
4. Attenuation characteristics of iodine, bone, and soft tissue as a function of x-ray photon energy differ.
   a. Materials with higher atomic number (*i.e.*, bone, with effective $Z \approx 13$, or iodine, with $Z = 53$) have higher photoelectric absorption than materials with lower atomic number (soft tissue effective $Z \approx 7.6$).
   b. The photoelectric interaction of the linear attenuation coefficient has an energy dependency of $E^{-3}$.
   c. Compton scatter interaction in the x-ray energy range for diagnostic imaging is less energy dependent.
5. The different energy dependencies in tissue types allow either the bone component or the soft tissue component of the image to be removed by digital image processing of radiographic images acquired at two very different effective energies (*i.e.*, different kVs).
6. The general equation for computing dual-energy subtracted images on each pixel $(x, y)$ is as follows:
   a. 
   $$DE(x,y) = \alpha + \beta \left[ \ln\{(I_{HI}(x,y)\} \; R\ln\{I_{LO}(x,y)\} \right]$$

   where        $DE(x,y)$ is the grayscale value in the dual-energy image.
                $I_{HI}(x,y)$ is the grayscale value in the high-energy image.
                $I_{LO}(x,y)$ is the grayscale value in the low-energy image.

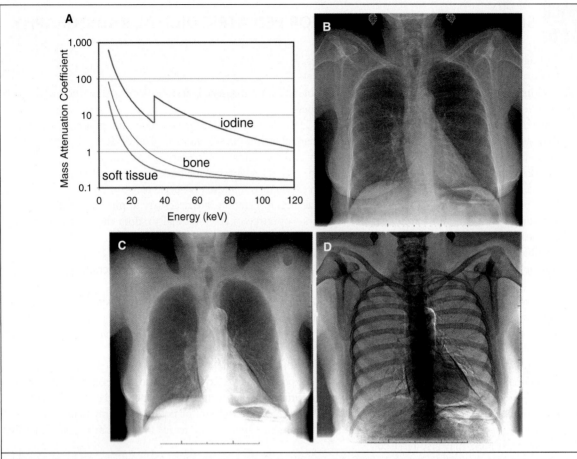

■ **FIGURE 7-24** *Dual-energy subtraction* chest radiography is illustrated. **A.** The *linear attenuation coefficients* for soft tissue, bone, and iodine are shown. **B.** The single-energy (120 kV) radiograph is shown. **C.** The bone-subtracted, *soft tissue–only* image is illustrated. This image shows the lung parenchyma and mediastinum, which are the principal organs of interest on most chest radiographs. **D.** The soft tissue–subtracted, *bone-only* image is illustrated. Note that the earrings, which are made of metal and are more similar to bone than soft tissue in terms of composition, show up on the bone-only image. □ **F. 7-25**

    **b.** The value of *R* is selected to isolate bone, iodine, or soft tissue in the subtraction.

    **c.** α and β scale the output image for brightness and contrast for optimal display.

    **d.** The equation is for weighted logarithmic subtraction.

  **7.** In the soft tissue–only image, the ribs are eliminated and the parenchyma of the lungs and mediastinum are less obscured by the ribs than in the conventional single-energy image.

  **8.** In the bone-only image, bones are better depicted than in the conventional single-energy image.

  **9.** Interestingly, one can also see the metallic earrings on this patient, whereas they are not visible on the soft tissue–only image.

    **a.** Metal earrings have attenuation properties more like bone than soft tissue.

**10.** The white area along the border of the heart and aortic arch in the soft tissue–only image is caused by cardiac motion between the first (low energy) exposure and the second (high energy) exposure.

    **a.** Misregistration of the two images is also often observed along the diaphragm, even with breath-holding by the patient.

**11.** An alternative to dual-energy subtraction is to use a specialized image processing algorithm on the single high-energy image.

    **a.** The software recognizes ribs and other bony structures and subtracts them from the original image to produce a soft tissue–only image without the dose penalty of the second low-energy exposure and without misregistration artifacts.

    **b.** The method produces remarkable images but may introduce artifacts that mimic pathology.

# Section II Questions and Answers

1. The focal spot is 1.0 mm square. The image receptor is 100 cm from the x-ray tube and the object is 25 cm from the image receptor and located on the central axis of the x-ray beam. The object width is 3.0 mm. What is the size of the edge gradient at one edge of the object?
   A. 0.33 mm
   B. 0.25 mm
   C. 0.50 mm
   D. 0.75 mm
   E. 0.20 mm

2. The SID of an imaging system is 183 cm, there is a 5 cm air gap between the patient and the image receptor, and the patient is 25 cm thick in the PA projection. The magnification factor at the patient's posterior surface is _____ and at the anterior surface it is _____.
   A. 1.2, 1.3
   B. 1.03, 1.2
   C. 1.2, 1.03
   D. 1.4, 1.2
   E. 1.2, 1.4

3. For a large field-of-view digital radiography system based on an optically coupled CCD photodetector, what is its major limitation compared to a TFT-based system?
   A. Inability to reject x-ray scatter
   B. Image readout time is too slow
   C. Overall system costs are much higher
   D. Increase noise from secondary quantum sink
   E. Less spatial resolution and detail

4. With automatic exposure control, the kV of an abdominal radiograph is increased from 75 to 90 kV. What likely impact will this have?
   A. The entrance skin exposure is reduced.
   B. The exposure time for same mA is increased.
   C. The contrast in the image is improved.
   D. The total mAs required is increased.
   E. The screen intensification factor is reduced.

5. For an indirect image receptor, with equal x-ray technique (kV and mAs) and equal electronic gain, which of the following will occur when doubling the thickness of the intensifying screen?
   A. Twice the absorption efficiency
   B. Better spatial resolution
   C. Lower perceived (relative) noise in the radiograph
   D. Increased dose to the patient
   E. Higher x-ray scatter detection

6. What is the definition of the grid ratio on an antiscatter grid?
   A. Height of the grid bars to the width of the interspaces
   B. Height of the grid bars to the sum of the width of the grid bars and interspaces
   C. Width of the interspaces to the width of the grid bars
   D. Width of the grid divided by the width of the image receptor
   E. Sum of the width of the grid bars and interspaces to the height of the grid bars

7. What is the biggest overt effect that scattered radiation has on an appropriately windowed digital radiograph?
   A. Increased exposure time due to its presence
   B. Loss of signal-to-noise ratio
   C. Loss of radiographic contrast
   D. Steeper contrast curve
   E. Aliasing of the primary signal

8. What will happen to image quality when exposing the patient to an unnecessarily large radiation dose with digital radiography?
   A. Poor image contrast
   B. Poor signal to noise ratio
   C. Excessive image intensity on a video monitor
   D. Excessive scatter fraction
   E. A high-quality image

9. A new high-resolution CR system uses a thinner imaging plate for better spatial resolution. When the cassette is scanned, the CR system increases the electronic gain by 3X to compensate for the lower absorption efficiency. What is the quantum noise in the image when compared to an image from the standard resolution cassette?
   A. 3X
   B. $\sqrt{3}X$
   C. Unchanged
   D. $\frac{1}{3}\sqrt{3}X$
   E. $\frac{1}{3}X$

10. For modern radiographic image receptors and most body imaging examinations, in which order do the patient doses range from the smallest to the largest? (DR = direct radiography, CR = computed radiography, and SF = screen film)
    A. CR, DR, SF
    B. SF, DR, CR
    C. DR, CR, SF
    D. CR, SF, DR
    E. DR, SF, CR

11. Two identical chest x-ray rooms with DR image receptors acquire chest exams performed at 120 kV and 183 cm SID using AEC with a fixed antiscatter grid. A normal-sized adult patient is imaged in room A delivers 3 mAs with $DI=0$ and $EI = 250$. In room B, 3 mAs is delivered for the same patient with $DI= 3.0$, and $EI = 250$. What most likely difference explains this?
    A. AEC calibration
    B. Image receptor calibration of $EI$
    C. $EI_T$ setting
    D. Patient positioning with AEC ion chambers
    E. X-ray tube output

12. Two technologists perform bedside chest radiography on the same portable DR machine with the same patient population. The manual technique guide calls for 90 kV and 3 mAs at 127 cm SID without an antiscatter grid. The average $DI$ for Tech A's exams is zero. The average $DI$ for Tech B's exams is 2.0. What is the most likely explanation for the discrepancy?
    A. Tech B is using too low kV
    B. Tech B is using an antiscatter grid
    C. Tech B is using too short SID
    D. Tech B is using too low mAs
    E. Tech B is using too little collimation

13. $EI_T$ for an exam is 240. $DI$ for an exposure is reported as −3.0. What should be the corresponding value of $EI$?
    A. 80
    B. 120
    C. 240
    D. 480
    E. 720

14. A technologist performs a routine chest exam on a small adult patient using AEC but selects the "large adult" menu, which uses the 630 mA station. The $DI$ value of 2.0 indicates overexposure. What is the most likely cause?
    A. AEC calibration
    B. Image receptor calibration of $EI$
    C. $EI_T$ setting
    D. Patient positioning with AEC ion chambers
    E. AEC response time

15. A series of high mAs exposures with a test instrument in the x-ray beam is acquired, but the physicist neglects to protect the image receptor by shielding it with lead. Subsequently, a uniform exposure shows a shadow of the test instrument in the image. Which of the following is the most appropriate action?
    A. Turn the DR system over to the clinic as soon as testing is complete
    B. Perform gain and offset calibration immediately
    C. Repeat the uniform exposure immediately
    D. Restrict clinical use of the DR system until testing shows shadow is no longer visible
    E. Replace DR image receptor

16. A horizontal linear artifact is observed on several clinical radiographs from a DR system. Which of the following is the most appropriate action?
    A. Continue using the DR system for clinical images until the artifact disappears
    B. Perform gain and offset calibration immediately
    C. Repeat clinical images where the artifact is visible
    D. Restrict clinical use of the DR system until artifact is no longer visible on uniform exposure
    E. Replace DR image receptor

17. A long linear artifact is observed on several clinical images from a CR system. Which of the following is the most appropriate corrective action?
    A. Clean and inspect imaging plates
    B. Replace imaging plates
    C. Perform nonuniformity calibration
    D. Clean light collection optics
    E. First D, then C

18. The adult technique for bedside DR of the medium adult abdomen (24 cm thick, 80 kV and 10 mAs at 100 cm SID with a fixed grid) is modified for pediatric abdomen (18 cm thick, 80 kV at 100 cm SID **without a grid**). Which grid performance metric would be most helpful for determining the mAs?
    A. Primary transmission factor, $T_p$
    B. Scatter transmission factor, $T_s$
    C. Selectivity, $\Sigma$
    D. Contrast degradation factor, $CDF$
    E. Bucky factor

19. A patient with a metallic hip replacement is radiographed using AEC. The mAs delivered is too high with poor image quality. The view is repeated using manual technique. The $DI$ value= −6.0, suggesting gross underexposure, with still poor quality. What is the most likely underlying problem with the repeated view?
    A. Too low mAs
    B. Too low kV
    C. $EI$ calibration of image receptor
    D. Incorrect $EI_T$ value
    E. Segmentation error

20. An antiscatter grid works by selective absorption of x-rays based on which one of the following?
    A. Energy
    B. Linear attenuation coefficient
    C. Quantity
    D. Trajectory
    E. Wavelength

21. What is the primary advantage of CsI over $Gd_2O_2S$ as an x-ray conversion layer?
    A. Cost
    B. Durability
    C. Limited lateral light spread
    D. Absorption efficiency
    E. Conversion efficiency

22. What is the primary advantage of DR over CR?
    A. Cost
    B. Durability
    C. Throughput
    D. Maintainability
    E. Spatial resolution

23. The minimum dimensions for a dexel in an indirect digital detector using a TFT array are about $100 \times 100$ μm, limited by _____.
    A. lateral light propagation in the conversion layer
    B. fill factor
    C. bias voltage
    D. dielectric layer
    E. SNR

24. What is the primary advantage of slot-scan acquisition compared to full field-of-view radiography?
    A. Speed of acquisition
    B. Mechanical simplicity
    C. X-ray tube heat loading
    D. Patient motion artifacts
    E. Scatter rejection

25. What is the primary advantage of CMOS compared to CCD detectors?
    A. Random read access of any dexel
    B. Electronic noise for storage and readout
    C. Maximum dexel size
    D. Crystalline Si material

26. In dual-energy subtraction imaging, what x-ray attenuation property is exploited?
    A. Compton scatter
    B. Rayleigh scatter
    C. Density differences
    D. Photoelectric absorption
    E. Pair production

# Answers

1. **A** Geometry of similar triangles with independent sides (focal spot blurring) $(x) / 1$ mm = 25 mm/75 mm; $x = (1/3)$ (1 mm) = 0.33 mm. *(Pg. 226; Eq. 7-3; Fig. 7-3)*

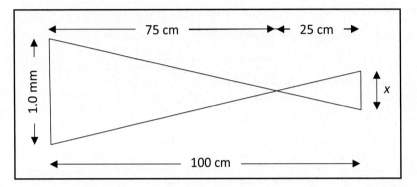

2. **C** This problem is set up with similar triangles having dependent sides, height and base. *(Pg. 224–225; Eq. 7-1, Eq. 7-2; Fig. 7-2)*

3. **D** CCD-based digital radiography systems use a small area (4 × 4 cm) high resolution (13 micron or smaller detector element with 3,000 × 3,000 matrix) charge-coupled device (CCD) photodetector to convert the light emanating from a large area fluorescent screen (43 × 43 cm) that is focused by an optical lens. The poor light collection of the lens translates into a major loss of information-carrying light photons incident on the CCD, which are statistically greater in variance than the x-rays that produced them. This is called a secondary quantum sink—a situation that is less efficient and results in noisier radiographic images compared to a similar thin-film transistor detector system when using the same acquisition parameters and geometries. Other image characteristics are similar; an advantage of CCD systems is low cost. *(Pg. 246–247; Fig. 7-18A; information on TFT detectors Pg. 248-249)*

4. **A** Automatic exposure control (AEC) provides a calibrated x-ray intensity incident on the detector to achieve an appropriate signal at the image receptor. An increase in kV will increase the penetrability of the beam through the patient, thus permitting a reduced entrance skin exposure. Answer B is incorrect because mAs is reduced; C is incorrect because increased kV reduces contrast. Answer D is incorrect because the total mAs would be reduced (same as Answer B). Answer E is incorrect because typically with higher kV, the intensification factor increases. *(Pg. 236)*

5. **C** By doubling the intensifying screen thickness, a greater absorption of x-rays occurs, and by adjusting the image receptor sensitivity to lower speed means that the image will also have lower noise (less overall conversion efficiency of light producing the signal). No change in dose will occur, because the x-ray technique is unchanged. *(Pg. 240–241; Fig. 7-12)*

6. **A** This is the definition of grid ratio. Other important criteria include grid frequency, selectivity, weight, and primary transmission factor, among others. *(Pg. 229; Fig. 7-7)*

7. **B** In digital systems, the radiographic contrast is adjustable (*e.g.*, by windowing) and can be increased to the extent that the noise does not become objectionable. The limit is thus the signal-to-noise ratio. *(Pg. 227)*

8. **E** DR and CR have wide exposure latitude, and with image processing, can compensate for under or overexposure. As long as the dynamic range is not exceeded and the system is quantum limited, an overexposure will provide a higher signal-to-noise ratio. *(Pg. 251–252; Fig. 7-22)*

9. **B** The thinner phosphor screen absorbs ⅓ as many x-rays as the standard resolution screen as evidenced by the 3X higher electronic gain applied to the image. The quantum noise in the high-resolution image will be $\sqrt{3}$ times greater than a standard resolution cassette exposure using the same radiographic technique factors. *(Pg. 240–241)*

10. **E** DR, SF, CR: This sequence is based on "typical" performance of radiographic imaging equipment and considers flat-panel detectors for DR (having a "speed class" of 400/600), a rare-earth screen-film detector of 400 speed, and a typical computed radiography imaging detector (typically within a speed class of 200 to 300 speed). Remember that the speed is inversely related to the dose to the patient for an appropriately exposed detector. *(Pg. 231)*

11. **C** $EI_T$ setting. The $DI$ value compares the $EI$ for an exposure with the $EI_T$. $EI_T$ may be set for individual DR systems or for specific radiographic views. *(Pg. 253)*

12. **C** Tech B is likely using a shorter SID than Tech A. The SID for bedside radiography is typically 100 cm (40 inches), but this technique guide specifies 127 cm (50 inches). With the same kV, mAs, and patient thickness, the air kerma at the image receptor will be higher for the shorter SID by $((127/100)^2)=1.61$. The DI will be $10\ log_{10}\ (1.61) = 2.07$. *(Pg. 253; Eq. 7-9)*

13. **B** The $DI$ value of −3.0 indicates that the $EI$ is ½ of the $EI_T$ value. $EI = EI_T \times 10\char94(3.0/10) = 120$. *(Pg. 253; Eq. 7-9)*

14. **E** AEC response time is approximately 5 ms. When a small patient is examined using a high mA station, the AEC is unable to terminate the exposure even though sufficient charge has been produced in the ion chambers. *(Pg. 236)*

15. **D** The ghost image is caused by differential residual phosphorescence in the x-ray conversion layer of the receptor. It will gradually dissipate with time (possibly days). Until then, it will show up on clinical radiographs. A gain and offset calibration at this time will burn the shadow into the calibration map, ensuring that it shows up on all subsequent images. Replacing the image receptor is an expensive alternative. *(Pg. 255)*

16. **B** Gain and offset calibration is the logical first step for correcting bad dexels and lines. DR image receptor replacement should only be considered when gain and offset calibration is unsuccessful at removing the artifact. *(Pg. 254–255; Fig. 7-23)*

17. **E** Nonlinearity calibration may mask the artifact but does not address the underlying cause. Dust on the light collection optics is a common problem in CR, but cleaning should be followed by recalibration for nonuniformity. *(Pg. 254–255)*

18. **A** For example, assuming a primary transmission factor of 0.75, the primary exiting the patient is $(1/0.75)$ = 1.3 times the amount reaching the image receptor. Without the grid, the same primary signal could be achieved with 75% of the technique for a patient of the same thickness or 7.5 mAs. The pediatric patient is 6 cm thinner for about 1.5 HVL less attenuation of the primary beam. That implies that the mAs could be reduced by another factor 1/3. $10 \times 0.75 \times 1/3 = 2.5\ mAs$ as a reasonable starting point. $EI_T$ should be modified to account for scatter: for an $18 \times 18$ cm FOV and 18 cm thickness, SPR $\approx$ 3, so that the $EI_T$ might need to be as high as $((3 \times 250) + 250) = 1,000$ to account for scatter and capture the same amount of primary signal as the adult grid case. This approach ignores the Scatter transmission factor of the grid, which would be a secondary effect on the adjustment of $EI_T$. *(Pg. 232)*

19. **E** Generation of a correct value of $EI$ depends on proper segmentation of the values of interest (VOI) within the field of view. Metallic implants can interfere with automatic segmentation by including the low exposure regions behind the dense implant in the VOI. This makes the calculation of $EI$ unusually low and has a dramatic effect on the $DI$ reported. There is usually a loss of contrast in the soft tissue regions of the default image; however, soft tissue contrast can usually be recovered by digital image processing or manual resegmentation. *(Pg. 253–254)*

20. **D** The antiscatter grid works on the principle that most scattered x-rays will have a trajectory divergent from the path of primary x-rays from the focal spot to the image receptor. *(Pg. 228–229; Fig. 7-6)*

21. **C** The columnar crystalline structure of CsI acts to direct the light photons toward the image receptor reducing lateral light spreading and preserving spatial resolution. *(Pg. 239 and Fig. 7-11)*

22. **D**  DR has many advantages over CR, but the greatest is that DR requires less frequent and less expensive maintenance. DR produces images more rapidly than CR, but this advantage is compromised by the ability for a single CR reader to support acquisition at multiple locations simultaneously. Reimbursement issues for CR may eclipse other concerns in the United States. *(Pg. 251)*

23. **B**  The limitations imposed by the physical space occupied by electronics in the TFT dexel may be overcome by advances in lithographic technology. *(Pg. 250)*

24. **E**  The slot scanner produces so little scatter that an antiscatter grid is not necessary even for imaging thick body parts. This also provides dose reduction versus full-FOV radiography. *(Pg. 233; Fig. 7-9)*

25. **A**  The random-access capability of CMOS makes possible built-in AEC. *(Pg. 248)*

26. **D**  Dual-energy radiography uses the energy dependence of photoelectric absorption to remove one tissue (*e.g.*, bone) relative to another (*e.g.*, soft tissue) by logarithmic weighting, scaling, and subtraction of the image pairs, one acquired at a low kV and one acquired at a high kV. *(Pg. 257–258)*

# Section III Key Equations and Symbols

| QUANTITY | EQUATION | EQ NO./PAGE/COMMENTS |
|---|---|---|
| Magnification | $M = \dfrac{L_{image}}{L_{object}}$ | Eq. 7-1/Pg. 224/Magnification, $M$, is the ratio of the length of a feature in the image, $L_{image}$, to the actual length of the feature, $L_{object}$. |
| Magnification | $M = \dfrac{a+b}{a}$ | Eq. 7-2/Pg. 225/Because of beam divergence, magnification, $M$, of a feature depends on the total distance from the x-ray source to the image receptor, $a + b$, divided by the distance, $a$, from the x-ray source to the feature. This can be calculated using the principle of similar triangles. |
| Blur | $L_g = L_f \dfrac{b}{a}$ | Eq. 7-3/Pg. 226/Focal spot blur also depends on the geometry of the projection. The length of the edge gradient, $L_g$, is equal to the length of the focal spot, $L_f$, times $b/a$, the ratio of the distance, $b$, from the object to the receptor to the distance, $a$, from the object to the x-ray source. In most radiography, the anatomy of interest is positioned as close as possible to the image receptor to minimize focal spot blur. Long source to image distance, $SID$, can also help to minimize focal spot blur. |
| Scatter-to-primary ratio | $SPR = \dfrac{S}{P}$ | Eq. 7-4/Pg. 228/$SPR$ is the ratio of scattered photons, $S$, to the primary, unscattered photons, $P$. If $SPR = 1$, half the photons reaching the receptor provide no information. |
| Scatter fraction | $F = \dfrac{S}{P+S}$ | Eq. 7-5/Pg. 228/Scatter fraction, $F$, is the ratio of scattered photons, $S$, to the total photons reaching the receptor, primary, $P$, plus $S$. If $S = P$, then $F = \frac{1}{2}$. |
| Scatter fraction | $F = \dfrac{SPR}{SPR+1}$ | Eq. 7-6/Pg. 228/Scatter fraction, $F$, can also be expressed in terms of $SPR$. If $SPR = 1$, then $F = \frac{1}{2}$. |
| Selectivity | $\Sigma = \dfrac{T_P}{T_s}$ | Eq. 7-7/Pg. 232/Selectivity of an antiscatter grid, $\Sigma$, is the ratio of the primary transmission factor, $T_P$, to the scatter transmission factor, $T_s$. Typical values for $\Sigma$ range from 2.5 to 15 depending on kV, scatter and grid design. |
| Contrast degradation factor | $CDF = \dfrac{1}{1+SPR}$ | Eq. 7-8/Pg. 232/$CDF$ indicates how much contrast is lost from the presence of scatter. In digital radiography, CDF is the amount of contrast that must be restored to compensate for scatter. |
| Deviation index | $DI = 10\log_{10}(EI/EI_T)$ | Eq. 7-9/Pg. 253/$DI$ provides feedback on how close the exposure index, $EI$, was to the target exposure index, $EI_T$. A value of zero indicates a perfect match. Negative values indicate underexposure; positive values indicate overexposure. ±3 is doubling or halving. ±1.5 is a range of 2×. |

*(Continued)*

*(Continued)*

| QUANTITY | EQUATION | EQ NO./PAGE/COMMENTS |
|---|---|---|
| Dual-energy subtraction grayscale value | $DE(x, y) = \alpha + \beta[\ln\{I_{HI}(x, y)\} - R \ln\{I_{LO}(x, y)\}]$ | Eq. 7-10/Pg. 257/Weighted logarithmic subtraction of grayscale values in low-energy image, $I_{LO}$, from grayscale values in the high-energy image, $I_{HI}$, produces grayscale values in the dual-energy subtracted image, *DE*. The value of R is adjusted to eliminate bone or soft tissue. Brightness and contrast are scaled by $\alpha$ and $\beta$. |

| SYMBOL | QUANTITY | UNITS |
|---|---|---|
| SID | Source to image distance | Centimeters (cm) *(or inches)* |
| $Z$ | Atomic number | Number of protons *(integer)* |
| $\rho$ | Density | Grams per centimeter cubed (g/cm³) |
| $T_P$ | Primary transmission factor | Percentage (%) |
| $T_S$ | Scatter transmission factor | Percentage (%) |
| EI | Exposure index *(IEC Standard)* | Unitless *(but proportional to air kerma at receptor for standard beam: divide by 100 to get $\mu Gy$)* |
| DI | Deviation index | Unitless *(equivalent to decibels)* |

CHAPTER  8

# Breast Imaging: Mammography

## 8.0 INTRODUCTION

Mammography is a radiographic examination that is optimized for detecting breast cancer. Breast cancer screening with mammography can catch cancers at an earlier, more treatable stage. Technological advances over the last several decades have greatly improved the diagnostic sensitivity of mammography (Fig. 8-1).

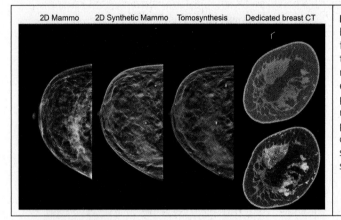

2D Mammo    2D Synthetic Mammo    Tomosynthesis    Dedicated breast CT

■ **FIGURE 8-1** Improvements in mammography and breast x-ray imaging. On the left is a 2-dimensional (2D) full-field digital mammogram (acquired after tomosynthesis study). On the middle left is a 2D synthetic mammogram created from the digital breast tomosynthesis examination on the middle right; shown is a 1-mm focal plane image of approximately 60 images. On the right are reconstructed coronal slices of the breast (of about 500) positioned at the site of the lesions from pre and post-contrast injection acquisitions using a dedicated breast CT scanner. The contrast enhanced image (**bottom**) shows significant uptake in glandular tissues.

Breast cancer *screening program*s depend on x-ray mammography as a low-cost, low-radiation dose procedure. Mammographic features include masses with irregular or "spiculated" margins, clusters of microcalcifications, and architectural distortions of breast structures.

- *Screening mammography*: detection of breast cancer in *asymptomatic* population
  - ◆ 2 views of each breast, in the mediolateral oblique and craniocaudal views
- *Diagnostic mammography*: assess lesions identified by screening mammography
  - ◆ Includes additional x-ray projections, spot compression and magnification, tomosynthesis, ultrasound, MRI, breast CT, scintigraphy, PET/CT
- X-ray attenuation between normal and cancer tissue is small, requiring low energy (Fig. 8-2)
- Requirements: high contrast sensitivity, low-dose, high spatial resolution images
- Implementation essentials: dedicated x-ray equipment (Fig. 8-3)

## 8.1 X-RAY TUBE COMPONENTS, STRUCTURES, AND OPERATION

1. **Cathode:** filament current and tube current are limited. Typical maximum tube current values: 100 to 125 mA for 0.3 mm (large focal spot); 15 to 30 mA for 0.1 mm (small focal spot).
2. **Anode:** target materials include molybdenum (Mo), rhodium (Rh), and tungsten (W).
   a. Anode angle for 65 to 70 cm SID is approximately 22° (with tube tilt) for field coverage of 24 × 30 cm (Fig. 8-4)
   b. Half field beam geometry—protects the lungs from radiation—central axis is tangent to the chest wall
   c. Heel effect—optimal orientation of x-ray tube: cathode chest wall; anode over anterior (Fig. 8-5)

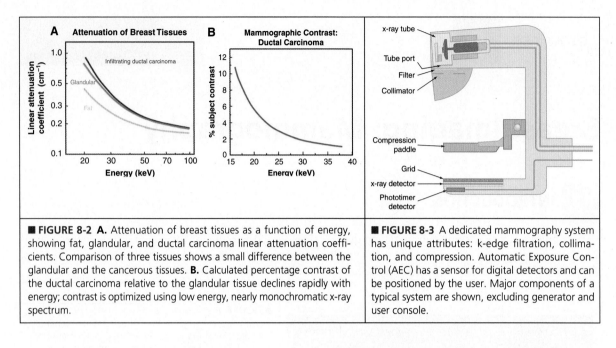

**■ FIGURE 8-2 A.** Attenuation of breast tissues as a function of energy, showing fat, glandular, and ductal carcinoma linear attenuation coefficients. Comparison of three tissues shows a small difference between the glandular and the cancerous tissues. **B.** Calculated percentage contrast of the ductal carcinoma relative to the glandular tissue declines rapidly with energy; contrast is optimized using low energy, nearly monochromatic x-ray spectrum.

**■ FIGURE 8-3** A dedicated mammography system has unique attributes: k-edge filtration, collimation, and compression. Automatic Exposure Control (AEC) has a sensor for digital detectors and can be positioned by the user. Major components of a typical system are shown, excluding generator and user console.

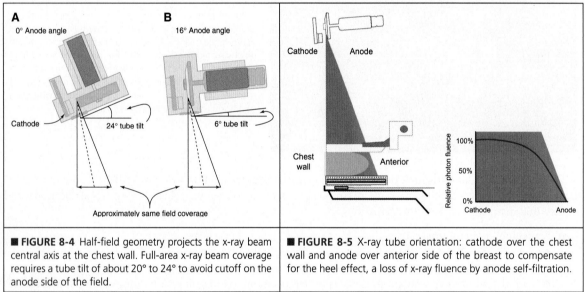

**■ FIGURE 8-4** Half-field geometry projects the x-ray beam central axis at the chest wall. Full-area x-ray beam coverage requires a tube tilt of about 20° to 24° to avoid cutoff on the anode side of the field.

**■ FIGURE 8-5** X-ray tube orientation: cathode over the chest wall and anode over anterior side of the breast to compensate for the heel effect, a loss of x-ray fluence by anode self-filtration.

3. **Focal Spot**
   a. Focal spot—0.3- and 0.1-mm spot size—for contact and magnification studies, respectively
   b. Nominal size is measured at a reference axis, halfway between chest wall and anterior dimension of the large field area
   c. Best resolution occurs on anterior side of the field per the line focus principle (Fig. 8-6A)
   d. System resolution: combination of geometric blurring and detector sampling resolution
      (i)   Measurement: line-pair bar pattern consisting of frequencies from 4 to 20-lp/mm (Fig. 8-6B)
4. **Target, Tube Port. Filtration, Beam Quality:** generate x-rays; shape the x-ray photon spectrum.
   a. Target; Mo, Rh, W.: Mo and Rh produce *useful* characteristic x-rays.
   b. Tube Port: Beryllium (Z = 4; 0.5 to 1 mm) allows high transmission of all x-ray energies.
   c. Tube filtration: Material and thickness remove low- and high-energy x-rays (Fig. 8-7).
   d. Characteristic x-rays: Mo: 17 to 19 keV; Rh: 20 to 23 keV; W: 8 to 12 keV—**L-x-rays are not useful.**
   e. Mo target filters used: 30 μm Mo; 25 μm Rh; for thin and thick breasts, respectively (Fig. 8-8)

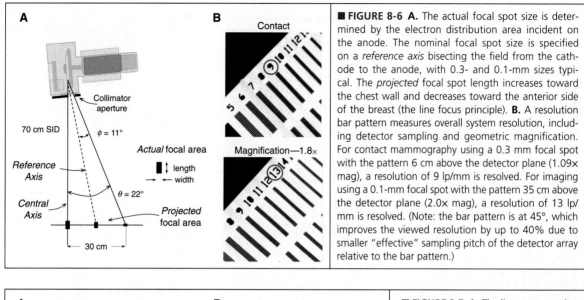

**FIGURE 8-6 A.** The actual focal spot size is determined by the electron distribution area incident on the anode. The nominal focal spot size is specified on a *reference axis* bisecting the field from the cathode to the anode, with 0.3- and 0.1-mm sizes typical. The *projected* focal spot length increases toward the chest wall and decreases toward the anterior side of the breast (the line focus principle). **B.** A resolution bar pattern measures overall system resolution, including detector sampling and geometric magnification. For contact mammography using a 0.3 mm focal spot with the pattern 6 cm above the detector plane (1.09× mag), a resolution of 9 lp/mm is resolved. For imaging using a 0.1-mm focal spot with the pattern 35 cm above the detector plane (2.0× mag), a resolution of 13 lp/mm is resolved. (Note: the bar pattern is at 45°, which improves the viewed resolution by up to 40% due to smaller "effective" sampling pitch of the detector array relative to the bar pattern.)

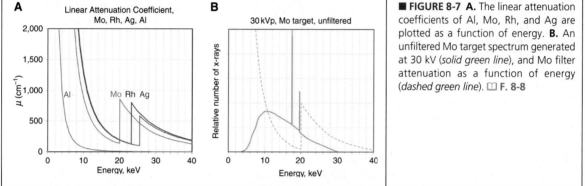

**FIGURE 8-7 A.** The linear attenuation coefficients of Al, Mo, Rh, and Ag are plotted as a function of energy. **B.** An unfiltered Mo target spectrum generated at 30 kV (*solid green line*), and Mo filter attenuation as a function of energy (*dashed green line*). F. 8-8

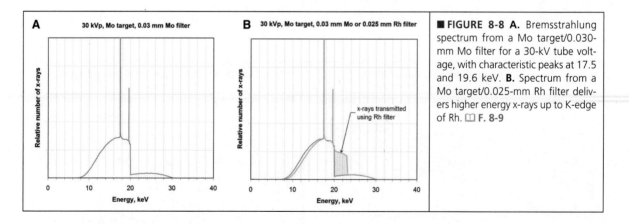

**FIGURE 8-8 A.** Bremsstrahlung spectrum from a Mo target/0.030-mm Mo filter for a 30-kV tube voltage, with characteristic peaks at 17.5 and 19.6 keV. **B.** Spectrum from a Mo target/0.025-mm Rh filter delivers higher energy x-rays up to K-edge of Rh. F. 8-9

    **f.** Rh target filters: 25 μm Rh; 25 μm Ag for thicker breasts (Fig. 8-9)
    **g.** W target filters: 50 μm Rh; 50 μm Ag; 500 to 700 μm Al. Thicker filters are required to eliminate unwanted L-x-rays in the spectrum (Fig. 8-10A); Al filter is used to achieve higher output rate with higher energy bremsstrahlung x-rays (Fig. 8-10B)
**5. Half Value Layer:** The half-value layer (HVL) of a mammography x-ray beam is the thickness in *mm* of sheets of pure Al required to reduce the x-ray beam air kerma by one-half.
    **a.** HVL depends on kV, target material (Mo, Rh, W), filter material (Mo, Rh, Ag, Al), and filter thicknesses typically used—between 0.3 and 0.7 mm Al (Fig. 8-11).

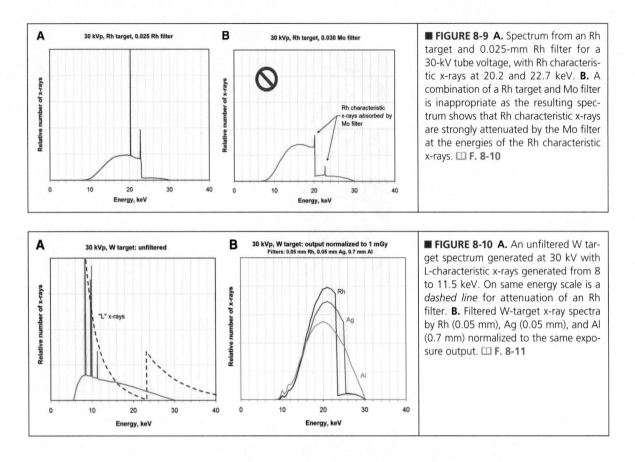

**FIGURE 8-9 A.** Spectrum from an Rh target and 0.025-mm Rh filter for a 30-kV tube voltage, with Rh characteristic x-rays at 20.2 and 22.7 keV. **B.** A combination of a Rh target and Mo filter is inappropriate as the resulting spectrum shows that Rh characteristic x-rays are strongly attenuated by the Mo filter at the energies of the Rh characteristic x-rays. **F. 8-10**

**FIGURE 8-10 A.** An unfiltered W target spectrum generated at 30 kV with L-characteristic x-rays generated from 8 to 11.5 keV. On same energy scale is a *dashed line* for attenuation of an Rh filter. **B.** Filtered W-target x-ray spectra by Rh (0.05 mm), Ag (0.05 mm), and Al (0.7 mm) normalized to the same exposure output. **F. 8-11**

**b.** Minimum HVL > kV/100 for mammography (e.g., for 30 kV beam HVL>0.3 mm Al).

**c.** HVL of breast tissue depends on breast density and kV; typically ranges from 1 to 3 cm tissue thickness.

6. **Tube output and output rate:** Air kerma in mGy normalized to 100 mAs at a specified distance from the source (focal spot); 50 cm is used in this chapter.

**a.** Mo and W target output for various filters and thicknesses are shown as a function of kV (Fig. 8-12).

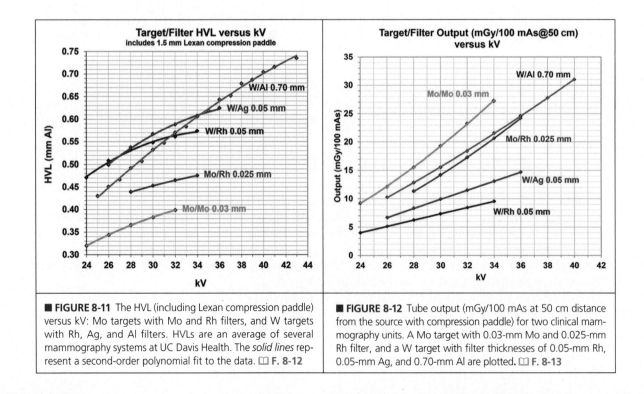

**FIGURE 8-11** The HVL (including Lexan compression paddle) versus kV: Mo targets with Mo and Rh filters, and W targets with Rh, Ag, and Al filters. HVLs are an average of several mammography systems at UC Davis Health. The *solid lines* represent a second-order polynomial fit to the data. **F. 8-12**

**FIGURE 8-12** Tube output (mGy/100 mAs at 50 cm distance from the source with compression paddle) for two clinical mammography units. A Mo target with 0.03-mm Mo and 0.025-mm Rh filter, and a W target with filter thicknesses of 0.05-mm Rh, 0.05-mm Ag, and 0.70-mm Al are plotted. **F. 8-13**

    **b.** Calibrated output values: *X* mGy (per 100 mAs at 50 cm); entrance surface air kerma, *Z* mGy, to the breast for *Y* mAs at a source-to-breast surface distance, *D* includes inverse square law distance correction:

$$Z \text{ mGy} = X \text{ mGy}(per\ 100\ mAs) \times \frac{Y \text{ mAs}}{100}\left(\frac{50 \text{ cm}}{D \text{ cm}}\right)^2 \qquad [8\text{-}1]$$

**7. X-ray tube collimation-detector-light field alignment**
    **a.** Beam-limiting devices: chest wall edge of x-ray field extends to edge of receptor
        **(i)**   X-ray field/receptor congruence: to not exceed 2% of SID
    **b.** X-ray field/light field congruence (Fig. 8-13)—misalignment (length or width) shall not exceed 2% of SID for anterior-posterior or left-right borders.
    **c.** The chest wall edge of compression paddle: shall not extend beyond the chest wall edge of receptor by greater than 1% SID; vertical edge of compression paddle shall not be visible in the image.
    **d.** Small breast imaging: left and right shift collimation accommodates MLO acquisitions to allow for positioning of the arm and shoulder at the corner of the detector (textbook Fig. 8-15).

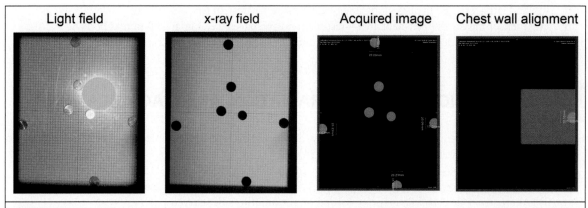

| Light field | x-ray field | Acquired image | Chest wall alignment |

■ **FIGURE 8-13** Light field to x-ray field and x-ray field to detector congruence and alignment evaluations. **Left.** Light field projected onto phosphor plate with coins placed at light field edges. **Mid left.** X-ray field phosphor image coin positions, indicating good congruence. **Mid right.** Acquired image to determine x-ray field to active detector congruence. **Right.** Compressed 40-mm attenuator thickness and coin placed at the edge of the compression paddle to evaluate paddle edge alignment and missed tissue at the chest wall in the acquired x-ray image. 📖 **F. 8-14**

## 8.2  X-RAY GENERATOR

**1. Automatic Exposure Control (AEC):** radiation sensors measure transmitted radiation
    **a.** Densest part of the breast targeted to achieve appropriate SNR
    **b.** AEC circuit assembly is detailed in Figure 8-14.

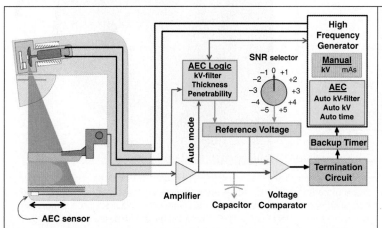

■ **FIGURE 8-14** Automatic Exposure Control (AEC) circuits use several selectable algorithms to determine the optimal exposure to the breast. The basic AEC operation uses the signal measured by the AEC sensor during the exposure in an operator positioned region that is transmitted to a comparator circuit to match a predetermined level that sends a signal to the generator to terminate the exposure. This is commonly known as "Auto-time." 📖 **F. 8-16**

    **c.** Sensors: for CR, under the detector; for flat-panel, generated by the detector electronics

      **(i)** Manual positioning by the user from posterior to anterior

      **(ii)** Automatic positioning (digital detector) at the highest attenuation in breast

    **d.** Operation: charge accumulates, is amplified, and converted to voltage; compared to reference voltage; when equal, the exposure is terminated

**2. AEC algorithms**: use compressed breast thickness, kV, tube anode selection (if available), tube filter, and AEC settings on generator control panel as inputs to determine exposure

    **a.** *Fully automatic*: 100 ms test exposure determines breast penetrability—determines kV, filtration, target (Mo and Rh anodes) to achieve an acceptable exposure time. Most often used in the clinic.

    **b.** *Automatic kV*: 100 ms test exposure, with preset target and filter

    **c.** *Automatic exposure time*: with preset target, filter, and kV

**3. AEC (SNR) exposure selector**: adjustment for increasing or decreasing reference voltage in steps of approximately 15%—"0" is baseline; 1 step increments of 1 step from, for example, −3 to +4 (vendor dependent)

**4. Overexposure and backup timer**—turns off x-ray exposure after predetermined time; protects from sensor failure, low kV, highly attenuating object in FOV—safety switch to protect patient

**5. Underexposure situations**

    **a.** Thin and fatty-replaced breasts—possible overexposure because of AEC sensor lag

    **b.** Active sensor measures open-field area—results in noisy images (see Fig. 8-16B in text book)

**6. Technique charts**: guides to determine kV, mAs, and target-filter (see Table 8-2 in text book)

## 8.3 COMPRESSION, SCATTERED RADIATION, AND MAGNIFICATION

**1. Breast compression**: reduces overlapping anatomy, decreases tissue thickness for less geometric blurring, stops inadvertent motion, lowerradiation dose (Fig. 8-15A).

    **a.** Compression paddle—Lexan plate attached to a mechanical assembly (Fig. 8-15B)

      **(i)** Right-angle edge at the chest wall produces a flat, uniform breast thickness

      **(ii)** Alternative: "flex" paddle is spring-loaded on the anterior side; curved paddle.

    **b.** Spot compression: approximately 7-cm diameter region, for aggressive compression (Fig. 8-15C)

    **c.** Compression force (optimal)—111 to 200 newtons (25 to 44 lb)

    **d.** Foot pedal motor-driven adjustment is accompanied with a mechanical adjustment knob

**2. Scattered radiation**: additive, varying distribution degrades subject contrast, adds quantum noise

    **a.** Scatter to primary ratio (SPR) is a function of breast thickness and field area (Fig. 8-16)

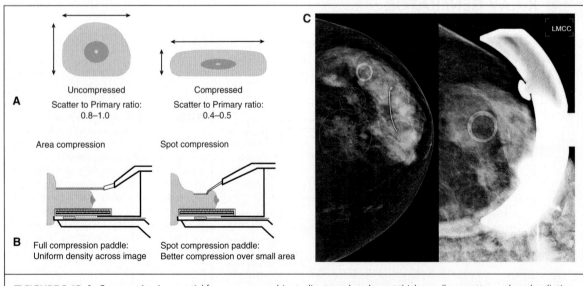

■ **FIGURE 8-15 A.** Compression is essential for mammographic studies to reduce breast thickness (less scatter, reduced radiation dose, and shorter exposure time) and to spread out superimposed anatomy. **B.** Suspicious areas often require "spot" compression to reduce superimposed anatomy by spreading the tissues over a localized area. **C.** Example image with suspicious finding (*left*). Corresponding spot compression (digitally magnified) illustrates less tissue overlap (*right*). ▢ F. 8-17

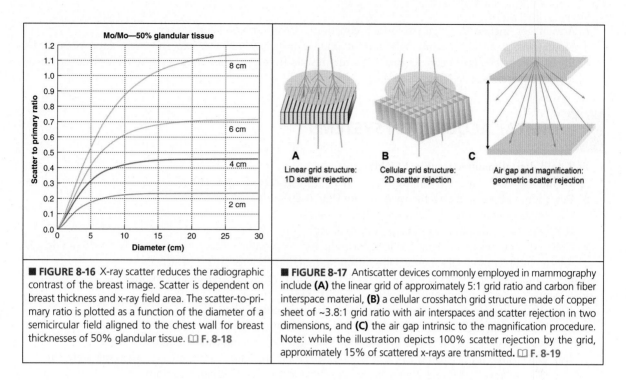

**■ FIGURE 8-16** X-ray scatter reduces the radiographic contrast of the breast image. Scatter is dependent on breast thickness and x-ray field area. The scatter-to-primary ratio is plotted as a function of the diameter of a semicircular field aligned to the chest wall for breast thicknesses of 50% glandular tissue. □ **F. 8-18**

**■ FIGURE 8-17** Antiscatter devices commonly employed in mammography include **(A)** the linear grid of approximately 5:1 grid ratio and carbon fiber interspace material, **(B)** a cellular crosshatch grid structure made of copper sheet of ~3.8:1 grid ratio with air interspaces and scatter rejection in two dimensions, and **(C)** the air gap intrinsic to the magnification procedure. Note: while the illustration depicts 100% scatter rejection by the grid, approximately 15% of scattered x-rays are transmitted. □ **F. 8-19**

    **b.** Contrast degradation factor—amount of contrast lost by detection of scatter—subject contrast without scatter—$C_0$; contrast with of scatter, $C_s$

$$\mathrm{CDF} = \frac{C_s}{C_0} = \frac{1}{1 + \mathrm{SPR}}$$

**3. Antiscatter grids**
    **a.** Transmission: 60% to 70% of primary x-rays; absorption of 75% to 85% of scattered x-rays
    **b.** Linear focused grids: ratios of 4:1 to 5:1, frequencies of 30 to 45/cm (Fig. 8-17A)
    **c.** Cellular grids: copper honeycomb with air interspace, approximately 3.8:1 ratio, achieves 2D scatter compensation (Fig. 8-17B)
    **d.** Grid motion during the exposure blurs the grid structure
    **e.** Short exposures cause most gridline artifacts due to insufficient motion.
    **f.** Increased dose for using grids is about a factor of approximately 2×.
**4. Air gap:** large fraction of scatter misses the detector.
    **a.** Achieved with magnification (Fig. 8-17C)
    **b.** Anatomic field of view (FOV) is reduced because of magnification.
**5. Magnification:** improves overall mammography system resolution
    **a.** Breast support platform (magnification stand) positions breast well above detector.
    **b.** Small (0.1 mm) focal spot is required to reduce geometric blurring.
    **c.** No antiscatter grid, compression paddles designed for magnification (Fig. 8-18)
    **d.** Typical geometric magnifications: 1.5×, 1.8×, or 2.0×

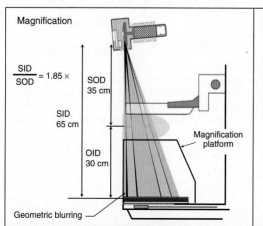

**■ FIGURE 8-18** Geometric magnification. A support platform positions the breast closer to the source focal spot, resulting in 1.5× to 2.0× image magnification. A small focal spot (0.1 to 0.15 mm nominal size) reduces geometric blurring. Effective focal spot size varies along the cathode-anode axis (large to small effective size) and is accentuated with magnification. Best spatial resolution and detail in the image exist on the anode side of the field. SID, source to image distance; SOD, source to object (midplane) distance; OID, object to image distance. □ **F. 8-20**

**e.** Advantages: Increased spatial resolution, reduction of quantum noise and scatter
**f.** Limitations: geometric blurring, tube current limit: approximately 25 mA; exposure time: approximately 4 s
**g.** Breast dose is similar to contact imaging—this results from the offset of no grid ↓(reduced dose) versus inverse square distance ↑(increased dose).

## 8.4 DIGITAL ACQUISITION SYSTEMS

1. **Full-field digital mammography (FFDM)**
   **a.** Technology: flat panel thin film transistor (TFT) array detector (Fig. 8-19)
   **b.** Detection: indirect and direct x-ray detection (Fig. 8-20)
      **(i)** Indirect—conversion of x-rays to light to charge
      **(ii)** Direct—conversion of x-rays directly to charge
   **c.** CMOS (Complementary Metal Oxide Semiconductor)—crystalline silicon approximately 50–75 μm dexels, uses an indirect mode of x-ray signal acquisition; functionally similar to TFT arrays
   **d.** Computed Radiography (CR)—cassette-based transition technology for digital mammo (no longer used)
   **e.** Benefits (over screen-film mammography)
      **(i)** Wide dynamic range with separation of acquisition and display
      **(ii)** "For Processing" (raw, corrected) images for quantitation, CAD, AI evaluation
      **(iii)** "For Presentation" enhance contrast, skin-line visibility, magnification, edges.
      **(iv)** Lower dose for flat-panel TFT and CMOS detectors; MGD for 4.2 cm breast—approximately 1 to 1.5 mGy relative to 1.8 to 2.2 mGy for screen/film and CR (see dosimetry section)
   **f.** Increased productivity (but not CR): no handling of cassettes, instant image processing
2. **Digital tomosynthesis**—a method to reduce the problem of anatomical superimposition
   **a.** Projection images acquired over a range of angles generate depth-dependent shifts.
      **(i)** Reconstruction: "shift and add" or filtered backprojection methods (Fig. 8-21)
   **b.** The x-ray tube/detector system acquires projection images over a limited angle arc.
      **(i)** Tomographic angles from ±7.5° (15°) to ±25° (50°)—larger tomographic angles provide better Z-axis resolution (Fig. 8-22).
      **(ii)** Acquisition times from approximately 5 s up to approximately 25 s dependent on tomographic angle range in continuous or "step and shoot" mode
      **(iii)** Many vendors and systems use detector binning mode (2 × 2) dexel output.
      **(iv)** DBT system design parameters are shown in Table 8-3 (in the textbook).

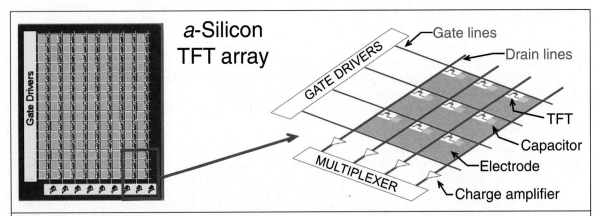

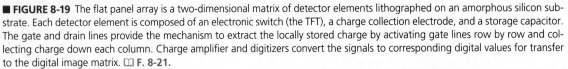

■ **FIGURE 8-19** The flat panel array is a two-dimensional matrix of detector elements lithographed on an amorphous silicon substrate. Each detector element is composed of an electronic switch (the TFT), a charge collection electrode, and a storage capacitor. The gate and drain lines provide the mechanism to extract the locally stored charge by activating gate lines row by row and collecting charge down each column. Charge amplifier and digitizers convert the signals to corresponding digital values for transfer to the digital image matrix. ▭ **F. 8-21.**

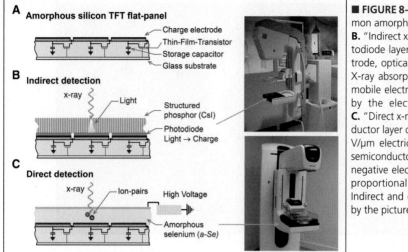

■ **FIGURE 8-20 A.** TFT flat panel arrays have a common amorphous silicon structure.
**B.** "Indirect x-ray conversion" TFT arrays have a photodiode layer placed on the charge collection electrode, optically coupled to a layer of CsI phosphor. X-ray absorption generates light, and light creates mobile electric charge in the photodiode, collected by the electrode and stored in the capacitor. **C.** "Direct x-ray conversion" TFT array uses semiconductor layer of approximately 0.5 mm thick, with 10 V/μm electric field. Hole-electron pairs created in semiconductor layer by x-rays migrate to positive and negative electrodes, with minimal lateral spread. A proportional charge is stored on the capacitor. Indirect and direct detectors appear similar, shown by the pictures on the right. 🕮 F. 8-22

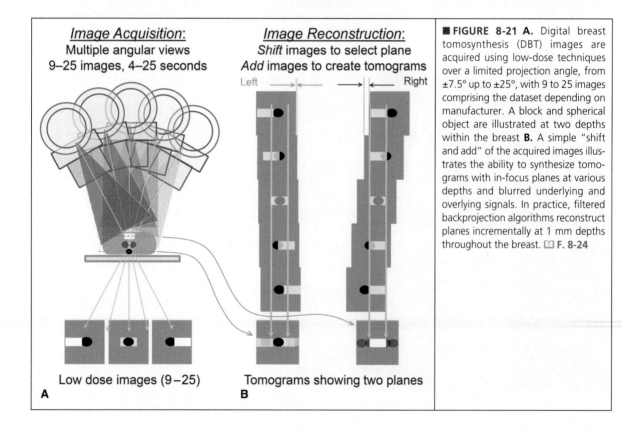

■ **FIGURE 8-21 A.** Digital breast tomosynthesis (DBT) images are acquired using low-dose techniques over a limited projection angle, from ±7.5° up to ±25°, with 9 to 25 images comprising the dataset depending on manufacturer. A block and spherical object are illustrated at two depths within the breast **B.** A simple "shift and add" of the acquired images illustrates the ability to synthesize tomograms with in-focus planes at various depths and blurred underlying and overlying signals. In practice, filtered backprojection algorithms reconstruct planes incrementally at 1 mm depths throughout the breast. 🕮 **F. 8-24**

   c. Tomosynthesis images are reconstructed approximately every 1 mm plus 2 to 3 images beyond the breast skin on each side; for example, 50 mm compressed breast thickness generates about 55 images in Z plane
   d. Image viewing: stacked mode, parallel to detector plane, with 1 mm spacing (Fig. 8-23)
   e. Image quality: number of projections affects in-plane resolution and blurring artifacts.
   f. Synthetic mammography—realign and create a projection image, like conventional 2D.
      (i)   Eliminates need for a conventional screening mammogram; reduces MGD by 50%.
      (ii)  Reduced resolution, some calcification (over) enhancement
   g. MGD: approximately 10% to 15% higher than 2D; antiscatter grid is used for some systems.
   h. Artifacts: incomplete blurring/suppression of high-density objects, with "halo" signs; anatomy close to focal plane appears larger; truncation artifacts at the reconstructed image periphery; stairstep artifacts with objects unintentionally placed in the beam, such as the shoulder

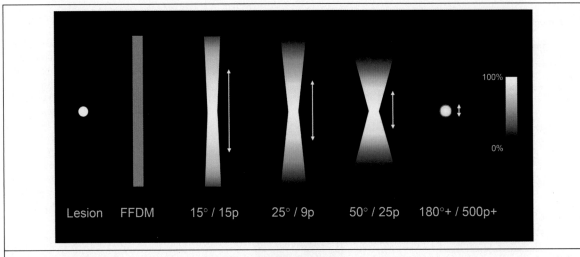

■ **FIGURE 8-22** DBT *z*-axis resolution is dependent on the x-ray tube angle and determines the amount of overlying and underlying contributions to the in-focus plane for the tomosynthesis images. A projection image (**left**) has 100% anatomical overlap. Shown are several manufacturer's implementations for progressively larger sweep angles up to 50°, with less tissue overlap and improved *z*-axis resolution (indicated by vertical *double-arrow lines*). On the right is 180°+ tube rotation achieved with dedicated breast CT, demonstrating no overlap of tissues. ▭ **F. 8-25**

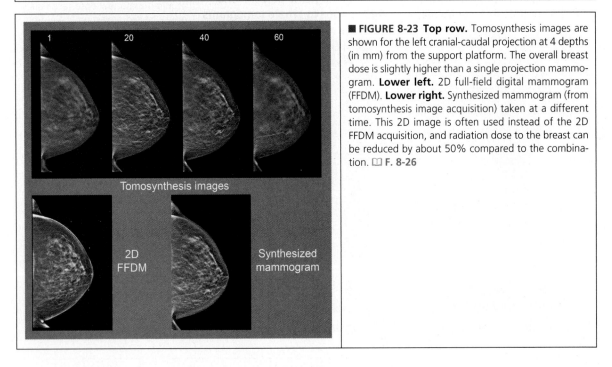

■ **FIGURE 8-23 Top row.** Tomosynthesis images are shown for the left cranial-caudal projection at 4 depths (in mm) from the support platform. The overall breast dose is slightly higher than a single projection mammogram. **Lower left.** 2D full-field digital mammogram (FFDM). **Lower right.** Synthesized mammogram (from tomosynthesis image acquisition) taken at a different time. This 2D image is often used instead of the 2D FFDM acquisition, and radiation dose to the breast can be reduced by about 50% compared to the combination. ▭ **F. 8-26**

3. **Dedicated breast CT**—true 3D volume datasets and elimination of superimposition
   a. Cone beam CT geometry in horizontal plane (Fig. 8-24) using a flat panel detector
   b. Hundreds of low-dose images acquired about the breast position without compression
   c. Reconstruction of the 2D images into nonoverlapping voxels in the breast volume
   d. Higher kV (~60 kV) permits lower radiation dose; a scatter grid is not typically used.
   e. MGD: like a two-view mammogram—for example, a 4.5 cm compressed breast ×2 = approximately 4 mGy
   f. Breast CT with contrast is thought to be largely equivalent to breast MRI.
4. **Stereotactic biopsy**—systems localize and sample breast lesions in 3D
   a. Use: biopsy of microcalcification lesions (breast mass biopsy—ultrasound or MRI)
   b. Geometry configurations
      (i) Prone table—breast placed through hole in horizontal table (Fig. 8-25)
      (ii) Standard mammography system—add-on biopsy device for lesion trajectory/depth
   c. Two images acquired ±15° (30° total) from the conventional projection (Fig. 8-26)
      (i) Objects closer to the detector shift less than objects further away (toward the focal spot)
   d. Depth and trajectory: determined by the location and shift in each image (Fig. 8-26)

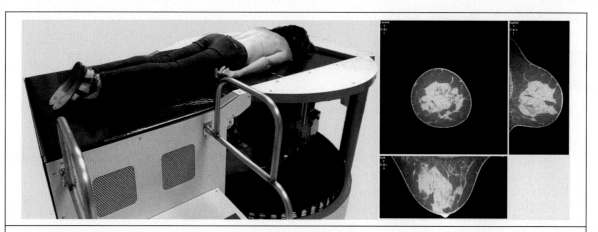

■ **FIGURE 8-24** Dedicated breast CT. **Left.** Patient is on the scanner in the prone position with one breast placed at the center of the gantry access port; about 500 projection images are acquired during a 360° rotation of the x-ray tube and detector about the breast. **Right.** CT tomographic slices are reconstructed in the coronal plane (*upper left*), with multiplanar reformatting to produce the sagittal (*right*) and axial (*lower left*) image planes. 📖 **F. 8-27**

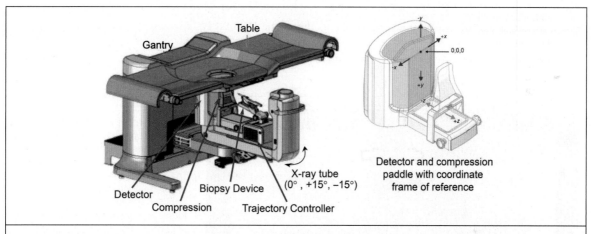

■ **FIGURE 8-25** A stereotactic biopsy system with a prone positioning system is shown. The breast is positioned through the hole onto the detector platform and compressed by an open-access paddle (close-up shown on the right, with the *x,y,z* coordinate directions indicated). The x-ray tube pivots horizontally about a fulcrum point to acquire digital images at +15° and −15° projections. 📖 **F. 8-28**

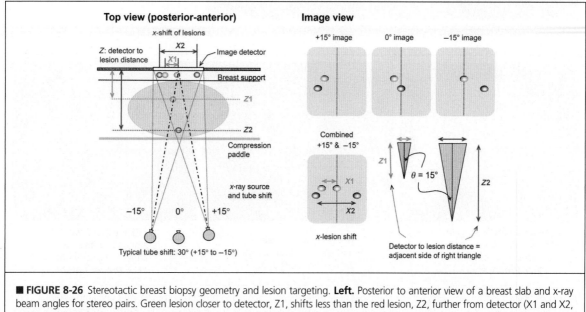

■ **FIGURE 8-26** Stereotactic breast biopsy geometry and lesion targeting. **Left.** Posterior to anterior view of a breast slab and x-ray beam angles for stereo pairs. Green lesion closer to detector, Z1, shifts less than the red lesion, Z2, further from detector (X1 and X2, respectively). **Right.** Image views and shift for each lesion. X-shift distance gives solution for Z (distance to the detector, the adjacent side of a right triangle), where tan θ = opposite/adjacent sides and ½X is the adjacent side distance. Thus, $\tan(15°) = (X/2)/Z$, and $Z = X/2\tan(15°)$. The biopsy needle trajectory controller provides the 3-D coordinate targeting to the lesion. 📖 **F. 8-29**

## 8.5 PROCESSING, VIEWING, ANALYZING BREAST MAMMOGRAM IMAGES

1. **Image preprocessing and detector corrections**
   a. Detector corrections: detector elements, column/line defects, gain variation
   b. Locations of detector flaws are determined and corrected via interpolation.
   c. *Flat-field* correction image: uniform x-ray flood field (Fig. 8-27); normalized and inverted as an inverse gain map to apply to uncorrected image
   d. Flat-field gain maps for various acquisition conditions (e.g., target/filter, tomosynthesis)
   e. DICOM *For Processing* image—quantitatively consistent for computer-aided diagnosis (CAD) and Artificial Intelligence (AI) (Fig. 8-28 Left)

2. **Image postprocessing**
   a. Wide dynamic range for digital detectors—linear with x-ray exposure levels
      (i) Screen/film detector range—25:1 (min to max "useful" signal)
      (ii) Digital detector range—greater than 1,000:1 (min to max useful signal)
   b. Linear contrast enhancement with window width/level adjustments (Fig. 8-28 Middle)
   c. Nonlinear postprocessing: skin line local area equalization (Fig. 8-28 Right)
   d. Contrast and spatial resolution enhancements create the DICOM *For-Presentation* image for viewing and diagnosis
   e. Processing is manufacturer specific with differences between vendors (Fig. 8-29).

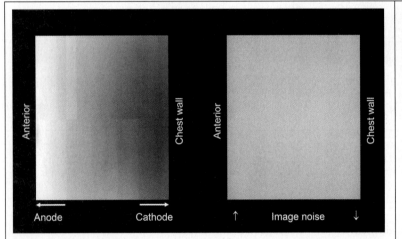

■ **FIGURE 8-27** Gain correction for flat-panel detectors for a tungsten target and rhodium filter. **Left.** Uncorrected flat-field image acquired with uniform x-ray field and 4 cm Lucite phantom. The detector modules and variable gain of this inverted grayscale image show brighter grayscale with less signal. **Right.** Gain-corrected image showing uniform response. Image noise (standard deviation of digital values) is higher on the anterior side of the x-ray image from less x-ray exposure due to the anode heel effect. ⌑ **F. 8-31**

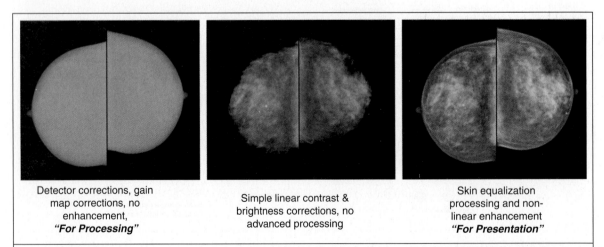

Detector corrections, gain map corrections, no enhancement, *"For Processing"*

Simple linear contrast & brightness corrections, no advanced processing

Skin equalization processing and non-linear enhancement *"For Presentation"*

■ **FIGURE 8-28 Left.** DICOM *For Processing* images have detector and gain map corrections applied with unity radiographic contrast. **Middle.** Linear contrast and brightness adjustments are applied—the skin line is not visible. **Right.** Nonlinear processing identifies the breast skin line and equalizes the response of the DICOM *For Presentation* image. ⌑ **F. 8-32**

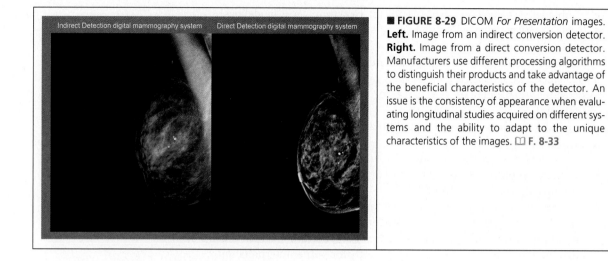

Indirect Detection digital mammography system    Direct Detection digital mammography system

■ **FIGURE 8-29** DICOM *For Presentation* images. **Left.** Image from an indirect conversion detector. **Right.** Image from a direct conversion detector. Manufacturers use different processing algorithms to distinguish their products and take advantage of the beneficial characteristics of the detector. An issue is the consistency of appearance when evaluating longitudinal studies acquired on different systems and the ability to adapt to the unique characteristics of the images. ☐ F. 8-33

3. **Image size considerations**
   **a.** System with 0.07-mm pixel, 2 bytes/pixel, and 24 × 29-cm active detector = 27 MB; 4 image study = 108 MB; with +3 years of priors = 432 MB per reading session
   **b.** Network overhead considerations important; *For Processing* image storage = 2× data size. Typical digital image sizes are listed in Table 8-1.

**TABLE 8-1 DIGITAL IMAGE SIZE FOR MAMMOGRAPHY SCREENING EXAMINATIONS** ☐ T. 8-4

| DETECTOR TYPE | FOV (cm) | PIXEL SIZE (mm) | IMAGE SIZE (MB) | EXAM SIZE (MB) | +3 Y PRIORS (MB) |
|---|---|---|---|---|---|
| Indirect TFT | 19 × 23 | 0.100 | 9 | 35 | 140 |
| Indirect TFT | 24 × 31 | 0.100 | 15 | 60 | 240 |
| Direct TFT | 18 × 24 | 0.085 | 12 | 48 | 192 |
| Direct TFT | 24 × 30 | 0.085 | 20 | 80 | 320 |
| Direct TFT | 18 × 24 | 0.070 | 18 | 70 | 280 |
| Direct TFT | 24 × 29 | 0.070 | 27 | 108 | 432 |

   **c.** DBT data: 9 to 25 projection images plus 1-mm tomographic slices = compressed breast thickness (*e.g.*, 60 mm has ~65 images). Image compression with "BTO" DICOM IOD lowers overall storage and network needs—Table 8-2.

**TABLE 8-2 DIGITAL BREAST TOMOSYNTHESIS IMAGE STORAGE REQUIREMENTS—60 cm COMPRESSED BREAST THICKNESS, 24 × 30 cm FIELD SIZE—THREE MANUFACTURER IMPLEMENTATIONS** ☐ T. 8-5

| DBT | INDIRECT DETECTOR, 0.100 mm | | | DIRECT DETECTOR, 0.085 mm | | | DIRECT DETECTOR, 0.070 mm | | |
|---|---|---|---|---|---|---|---|---|---|
| *Acquisition* | *Matrix* | *# Images* | *Size (MB)* | *Matrix* | *# Images* | *Size (MB)* | *Matrix* | *# Images* | *Size (MB)* |
| Projections | 2,394 × 2,850 | 9 | 120 | 2,816 × 3,584 | 26 | 507 | 2,560 × 4,096 | 15 | 315 |
| Planes | 2,394 × 2,850 | 145 | 1,900 | 2,816 × 3,584 | 61 | 821 | 2,560 × 3,328 | 66 | 1,120 |

*Note:* Detector element binning (2 × 2) is used by some manufacturers in the acquisition of the planar images, with reconstruction of the tomosynthesis planes at a smaller pixel pitch (*e.g.*, 140 to 100 μm).
Data from Tirada N, Li G, Dreizin D, et al. Digital breast tomosynthesis: physics, artifacts, and quality control considerations. *Radiographics.* 2019;39:413–426. doi: 10.1148/rg.2019180046.

4. **Image retention requirements**
   **a.** Per MQSA, each mammogram must be retained for at least 5 years.
   **b.** Not less than 10 years if no additional mammograms of the patient are performed at the facility, or a longer period if mandated by state or local law
5. **Image display considerations**
   **a.** MQSA requirements: FDA approved monitors with a minimum of 5 million pixels.
   **b.** Portrait display of approximately 53 cm diagonal with a pixel pitch of approximately 160 μm (2,560 × 2,048)

   c. Calibrated, sustained luminance of at least 450 cd/m² (ACR guidelines)

   d. Typical workstation configuration: two 5MP monitors or single 10 or 12 MP monitor of 76 to 80 cm diagonal for 2× virtual display areas of at least 5 MP

   e. Calibration to DICOM Grayscale Standard Display Function (see Chapter 5)

   f. *Mammography-specific hanging protocols* present the images in a useful and sequential way for review and diagnosis—dependent on view, laterality, magnification, tomosynthesis series, and prior examination comparisons.

6. **IHE mammography image and digital breast tomosynthesis profiles**

   a. Ensures optimal presentation of images at a mammography review workstation to allow adequate review of current and prior images from different vendor systems

   b. Provides complete storage and retrieval of mammography data with display functionality to allow review of current and prior images and CAD results

   c. Specifies mammography image content for optimal presentation of images:

     (i) Necessary data for identifying patients, technique acquisition parameters

     (ii) Image scaling size regardless of detector and detector element dimensions

     (iii) Orienting and justifying images correctly for proper interpretation

     (iv) Providing a clear definition of breast tissue and background air to maintain background blackness during contrast adjustments

   d. Digital Breast Tomosynthesis Extension (DBT Extension) Profile (IHE 2018)

     (i) Defines breast tomosynthesis object (BTO) and breast projection x-ray image object (BPO)

     (ii) Specifies the creation, exchange, and use of DBT images

     (iii) Defines basic display capabilities for review of DBT, 2D, and synthesized (generated 2D) mammography images

7. **Computer-aided detection and artificial intelligence**

   a. Computer-aided detection (CADe) system—marks these areas on the images, alerting the radiologist for further analysis—requires *For Processing* images

   b. Computer-assisted diagnosis (CADx) system—provides assessment of identified features and the likelihood of the presence or absence of disease or disease type

   c. Artificial intelligence (AI) and machine learning algorithms—mimic the human brain and learning process with "convolutional neural networks" (CNN) (Chapter 5).

     (i) Require a large training set of annotated and curated images associated with known outputs, including malignant and benign lesions.

     (ii) Training applied to achieve "knowledge by node weighting"

     (iii) Application to unknown cases produce detection cues.

## 8.6   RADIATION DOSIMETRY

1. *Mean Glandular Dose* (**MGD**) is the dose metric estimating dose to glandular breast tissue.

2. **Spatial tissue heterogeneity** of glandular and adipose tissue makes dose estimates nontrivial.

   a. Phantom with 50% glandular, 50% adipose tissue composition is used.

   b. Entrance surface air kerma (ESAK) is required to estimate glandular tissue dose.

   c. MGD estimates assume a homogeneous glandular tissue distribution in the breast.

   d. Dose estimates are approximately 30% lower when considering adipose tissue shielding for the heterogeneous breast as the glandular tissue is most often centrally located.

3. **Mean Glandular Dose (MGD) calculation**

   a. Method 1:

$$D_g = X_{ESAK} \times D_{gN}$$

                              [8-2]   📖 E. 8-3

where $D_g$ is the **MGD**, $X_{ESAK}$ is the entrance surface (skin) air kerma (ESAK) to the breast in mGy, and $D_{gN}$ is a conversion factor: mGy glandular dose per mGy entrance surface air kerma (Table 8-3).

**TABLE 8-3 CONVERSION FACTOR $D_{gN}$ (mGy MEAN GLANDULAR DOSE PER mGy ENTRANCE SURFACE AIR KERMA TO THE BREAST) FOR W TARGET AND Rh FILTER, 2, 4, 6, 8 cm BREAST THICKNESSES OF 50% GLANDULAR AND 50% ADIPOSE TISSUE COMPOSITION** 📖 T. 8-6

| kV | HVL (mm Al) | $D_{gN}$ (mGy MGD/mGy ENTRANCE SURFACE AIR KERMA) Compressed Breast Thickness 2 cm | 4 cm | 6 cm | 8 cm |
|---|---|---|---|---|---|
| 27 | 0.489 | 0.491 | 0.307 | 0.215 | 0.161 |
| 28 | 0.500 | 0.499 | 0.314 | 0.220 | 0.165 |
| 29 | 0.509 | 0.506 | 0.321 | 0.225 | 0.169 |
| 30 | 0.518 | 0.513 | 0.327 | 0.230 | 0.173 |
| 31 | 0.527 | 0.519 | 0.332 | 0.234 | 0.177 |
| 32 | 0.535 | 0.525 | 0.338 | 0.239 | 0.181 |

Note that HVL is determined from the Monte Carlo simulation and does not include the attenuation of the compression paddle, which increases the HVL to slightly higher values than indicated, and will thus represent a slight underestimate of the $D_{gN}$ factor for a given kV. Expanded tables include a range of HVL for each kV.

Adapted with permission from Boone JM. Glandular breast dose for monoenergetic and high-energy x-ray beams: Monte Carlo assessment. *Radiology*. 1999;213(1):23–37. Copyright © Radiological Society of North America. doi: 10.1148/radiology.213.1.r99oc3923 .

    **(i)** $D_{gN}$ values are on the order of 0.25 to 0.45 and depend on breast thickness, kV, HVL.

    **(ii)** MGDs for 50% glandular/50% adipose tissue of 2- to 8-cm tissue thicknesses using a W/Rh spectrum and AEC in auto-filter mode are shown in Fig. 8-34.

  **b.** Method 2:

$$MGD = Kgcs \qquad [8\text{-}3] \quad \text{📖 E. 8-4}$$

where $K$ is the same as $X_{ESAK}$ as above; $g$ is the fraction of $K$ absorbed by glandular tissue of 50% glandular 50% adipose composition calculated as function of HVL and breast thickness; $c$ corrects for differences in glandularity as function of beam quality and breast thickness; and $s$ accounts for x-ray spectrum target and filter combination.

*Note: Both methods 1 and 2 provide a similar estimate of MGD.*

  **c.** Digital breast tomosynthesis (DBT) dose has dose dependence on x-ray tube projection angle, with lower dose by up to 10% at steeper angles.

**4. Factors affecting breast dose**

  **a.** *Detector characteristics and detective quantum efficiency (DQE):*

    **(i)** Detector element size, x-ray conversion (direct or indirect), converter thickness, and electronic/digitization noise affect DQE.

    **(ii)** DQE is function of spatial frequency, DQE($f$); range from 100% (all information recorded) to 0% (no information recorded). Radiation dose for SNR $\propto$ DQE(0)$^{-1}$.

  **b.** *Acquisition technique factors:*

    **(i)** Target, filter, and kV affect x-ray beam HVL and beam penetrability.

    **(ii)** Higher HVL is more penetrable, lowers the MGD, but decreases subject contrast.

    **(iii)** Tube current is proportional to breast dose for other parameters fixed.

  **c.** *Antiscatter grids*: improve subject contrast but absorb a fraction of primary radiation.

    **(i)** Compensation increases MGD by approximately 2× for similar statistics.

    **(ii)** Used for contact imaging but not for magnification, where air gap reduces scatter

  **d.** *Breast thickness and tissue composition*: most impactful factor on breast dose

    **(i)** X-rays are exponentially attenuated, requiring compensation for thicker breasts with increased technique factors to ensure adequate number of transmitted photons to the detector.

  **e.** MQSA regulatory dose limits: 4.2 cm thickness and composition 50% glandular 50% adipose

    **(i)** MQSA-approved mammography phantom 3 mGy per view for contact mammography

    **(ii)** 3 mGy per view for digital breast tomosynthesis

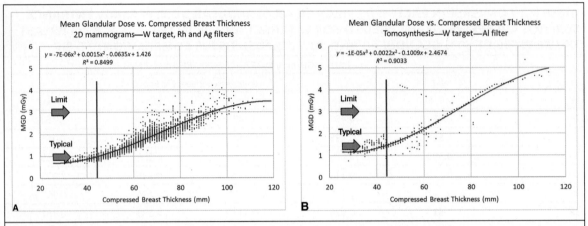

**■ FIGURE 8-30** Mean glandular dose for 2D mammograms and digital breast tomosynthesis examinations—sample of 1 month of data at UC Davis Health Mammography Clinic. **A.** MGD versus compressed breast thickness for examinations for screening mammograms using automatic exposure control (selection of kV and filter) for a system with a tungsten target and rhodium/silver filters of 0.05 mm thickness. **B.** MGD versus compressed breast thickness for digital breast tomosynthesis screening examinations using automatic exposure control (selection of kV and filter) for a system with a tungsten target and aluminium filter of 0.05 mm thickness. In both graphs, a least square fit of the data to a 3rd order polynomial is shown. The *red vertical line* represents the "standard" breast. 📖 F. 8-34

f. Above 3 mGy, the mammo system must be taken out of service for calibration. Typical MGD for flat-panel detectors (2D and tomosynthesis): accreditation phantom, 4.2 mm thickness of 50% adipose/50% glandular tissue: approximately 1.2 to 1.5 mGy for 2-D acquisition and slightly higher (1.4 to 1.6 mGy) for DBT (Fig. 8-30).

## 8.7 REGULATORY REQUIREMENTS

Mammography Quality Standards Act (MQSA) of 1992 specifies operational and technical requirements to perform mammography in the United States (Title 21 CFR, Part 900).

1. **Accreditation and Certification:** For a facility to perform mammography legally under MQSA, it must be accredited and certified.
   a. *Accreditation*: assessment of initial qualifications and continuing medical education of interpreting physicians, technologists, and physicists (15 hours every 3 years specific to mammography) and the required QC program
   b. *Accreditation body*: ACR or one of several states—personnel verifies standards set forth by the MQSA to ensure safe, high-quality mammography through annual inspections
   c. *Certification*: the approval of a facility by the US FDA to provide mammography services. Accreditation is a prerequisite.
2. **Quality Assurance and Quality Control**
   a. Quality Assurance (QA) comprises all management practices.
   b. Enhancing Quality Using the Inspection Program (EQUIP) emphasizes the responsibilities of the Lead Interpreting Radiologist in the clinical image quality process.
      (i) Ensure appropriateness and timely interpretation of every imaging procedure.
      (ii) Ensure lowest possible radiation dose, cost, and inconvenience to the patient.
      (iii) Engage in regular reviews of image quality for technologists.
      (iv) Document corrective action and review processes.
         (i) Oversee continuing education (CE) and Quality Control of equipment/peripherals.
      (v) Meet MQSA program regulations and requirements (e.g., 15 hrs CE over 3 y).
   c. Quality Control (QC)—verify reproducible, consistent, and safe operation of equipment
      (i) Optimize protocols, equipment components, radiation dose, SNR, and CNR.
      (ii) Validate image-viewing conditions, technologist, and radiologist displays.
   d. Digital imaging equipment QC testing procedures under the auspices of the FDA
      (i) QC entails following the manufacturer's specific FDA-approved QC procedures.
      (ii) Optional program by ACR for *all* digital mammography/tomosynthesis systems
   e. Harmonized program tests (Table 8-4); Accreditation phantoms (Figs. 8-31 to 8-33)

**TABLE 8-4 DIGITAL MAMMOGRAPHY (2D AND DBT) QUALITY CONTROL TESTS—ACR 2018 QUALITY CONTROL MANUAL (ACR, 2018)** 📖 T. 8-7

| Technologist Tests | | |
|---|---|---|
| 1. ACR DM Phantom Image Quality | Weekly | Before clinical use |
| 2. Computed Radiography Cassette Erasure (if applicable) | Weekly | Before clinical use |
| 3. Compression Thickness Indicator | Monthly | Within 30 days |
| 4. Visual Checklist | Monthly | Critical items: before clinical use; less critical items: within 30 days |
| 5. Acquisition Workstation Monitor QC | Monthly | Within 30 days; before clinical use for severe defects |
| 6. Radiologist Workstation Monitor QC | Monthly | Within 30 days; before clinical use for severe defects |
| 7. Film Printer QC (if applicable) | Monthly | Before clinical use |
| 8. Viewbox Cleanliness (if applicable) | Monthly | Before clinical use |
| 9. Facility QC Review | Quarterly | Not applicable |
| 10. Compression Force | Semiannual | Before clinical use |
| 11. Manufacturer Calibrations (if applicable) | Mfr. Recommendation | Before clinical use |
| Optional—Repeat Analysis | As Needed | Within 30 days after analysis |
| Optional—System QC for Radiologist | As Needed | Within 30 days; before clinical use for severe artifacts |
| Optional—Radiologist Image Quality Feedback | As Needed | Not applicable |
| **Medical Physicist Tests** | | |
| 1. Mammography Equipment Evaluation (MEE)—MQSA Requirements | MEE | Before clinical use |
| 2. ACR DM Phantom Image Quality | MEE and Annual | Before clinical use |
| 3. DBT Z Resolution | MEE and Annual | Within 30 days |
| 4. Spatial Resolution | MEE and Annual | Within 30 days |
| 5. DBT Volume Coverage | MEE and Annual | Before clinical use |
| 6. Automatic Exposure Control System Performance | MEE and Annual | Within 30 days |
| 7. Average (Mean) Glandular Dose | MEE and Annual | Before clinical use |
| 8. Unit Checklist | MEE and Annual | Critical items: before clinical use; less critical items: within 30 days |
| 9. Computed Radiography (if applicable) | MEE and Annual | Before clinical use |
| 10. Acquisition Workstation Monitor QC | MEE and Annual | Within 30 days; before clinical use for severe defects |
| 11. Radiologist Workstation Monitor QC | MEE and Annual | Within 30 days; before clinical use for severe defects |
| 12. Film Printer QC (if applicable) | MEE and Annual | Before clinical use |
| 13. Evaluation of Site's Technologist QC Program | Annual | Within 30 days |
| 14. Evaluation of Display Device Technologist QC Program | Annual | Within 30 days |
| 15. Manufacturer Calibrations (if applicable) | Mfr. Recommendation | Before clinical use |
| 16. Collimation Assessment | MEE/Troubleshooting Annual (DBT only) | Within 30 days |
| MEE or Troubleshooting—Beam Quality (Half-Value Layer) Assessment | MEE or Troubleshooting | Before clinical use |
| MEE or Troubleshooting—kVp Accuracy and Reproducibility | MEE or Troubleshooting | MEE: before clinical use; troubleshooting: within 30 days |
| Troubleshooting—Ghost Image Evaluation | Troubleshooting | Before clinical use |
| Troubleshooting—Viewbox Luminance | Troubleshooting | Not applicable |

Reproduced with permission from Digital Mammography (2D and DBT) Quality Control Tests, from ACR. *Digital Mammography Quality Control Manual.* Reston, VA: American College of Radiology; 2018.

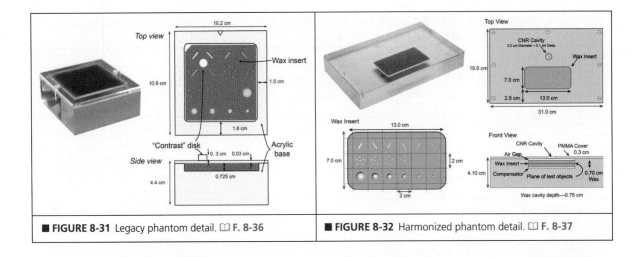

■ **FIGURE 8-31** Legacy phantom detail. ▢ F. 8-36

■ **FIGURE 8-32** Harmonized phantom detail. ▢ F. 8-37

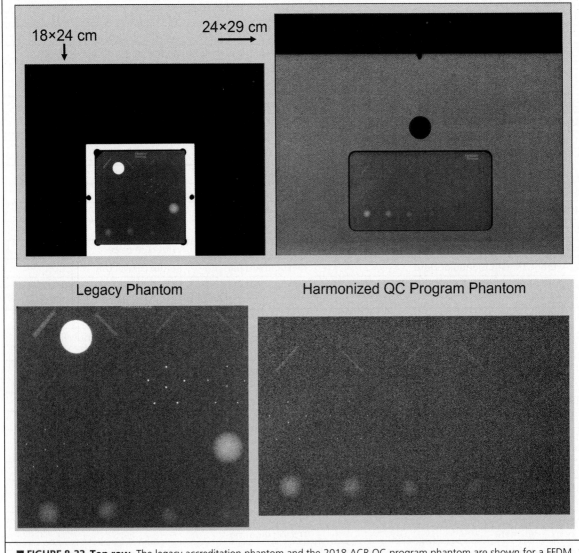

■ **FIGURE 8-33 Top row.** The legacy accreditation phantom and the 2018 ACR QC program phantom are shown for a FFDM system. The large block phantom represents a more challenging detection task, as the objects have progressively smaller dimensions than the legacy phantom and are more stringent in their size specifications. **Bottom row.** Close-up of the objects. ▢ F. 8-38

# Section II Questions and Answers

1. What is the typical mean glandular dose for a screening mammogram using a digital flat panel detector with a grid for a 4.5-cm-thick compressed breast?
   A. 0.6 mGy
   B. 1.2 mGy
   C. 2.4 mGy
   D. 5.0 mGy
   E. 7.5 mGy

2. The "back-up" timer of the AEC is reached using an "auto-time" mode, resulting in an underexposed, noisy image. The patient has thick, dense breasts. How should you instruct the technologist to repeat the examination?
   A. Increase the focal spot size.
   B. Increase the tube mA.
   C. Increase the AEC/SNR adjustment knob to "+" values.
   D. Increase the tube kV.

3. Why should grids be avoided in mammography magnification studies?
   A. Air gap reduces scatter reaching the detector.
   B. Reciprocation of the Bucky device is too slow.
   C. Small focal spot resolves the grid lines too easily.
   D. Breast stand prohibits appropriate grid focusing.

4. What is the typical overall tube shift used by stereotactic biopsy systems for geometric triangulation to determine lesion depth?
   A. 0°
   B. 30°
   C. 60°
   D. 90°
   E. 120°

5. What is the HVL of a mammography x-ray tube operated at 25 kV with a molybdenum target and tube filtration of 30 μm of molybdenum?
   A. 30 mm Al
   B. 3 mm Al
   C. 1 mm Al
   D. 0.3 mm Al
   E. 0.1 mm Al

6. The light field/x-ray field congruence of a mammography unit operating at 60 cm SID must be within what distance deviation for the left and right field edges?
   A. 1 mm
   B. 6 mm
   C. 12 mm
   D. 30 mm
   E. 60 mm

7. At which position in the projected breast image will parallax error be the least?
   A. At the geometric center of the projected field
   B. At the chest wall edge centered in the field
   C. At the anterior side edge centered in the field
   D. At the chest wall and left- or right-side edges of the field
   E. At the 0° position of the projected x-rays from the target

8. When should rhodium target and rhodium filter combinations be used clinically for breast imaging?
   A. Imaging thick, dense breasts
   B. Imaging thin, adipose breasts
   C. Achieving maximum subject contrast
   D. Achieving high spatial resolution

9. How is the mammography x-ray tube heel effect partially compensated to achieve improved uniformity for x-rays transmitted through the breast to the detector?
   A. Tilting the x-ray tube insert assembly to just eliminate field cutoff
   B. Positioning the cathode over the chest wall and anode over the nipple
   C. Using a larger field of view (24 × 30 cm) cassette
   D. Employing a variable transmission wedge filter

10. Which of the following describes radiation dose to the breast tissue at risk?
    A. Roentgen to rad conversion dose
    B. Mean glandular dose
    C. Mid-breast dose
    D. Entrance skin dose
    E. Exit skin dose

11. Of the following choices, why is firm breast compression is required in screening and diagnostic mammography?
    A. Allows the use of the small focal spot
    B. Increases the volume of breast tissue irradiated
    C. Eliminates the need for the antiscatter grid
    D. Reduces the average glandular breast dose

12. When using a 5:1 ratio, linear mammography grid, by what factor does the breast dose increase to compensate for scatter rejection and primary beam losses?
    - A. 0.3
    - B. 0.8
    - C. 1.2
    - D. 2.5
    - E. 5.0

13. Which of the following mammography target-filter combinations (with clinically relevant filter thicknesses) will have the largest HVL when operating at 32 kV?
    - A. Mo-Mo
    - B. Mo-Rh
    - C. Rh-Rh
    - D. W-Ag
    - E. W-Rh

14. To achieve a lower breast average glandular dose for a fixed detector response when using timed automatic exposure control, which parameter should be increased?
    - A. mA
    - B. kV
    - C. SNR
    - D. Focal spot size

15. For the choices below, assuming all the materials have the same physical thickness, which one would be best for transmitting the widest x-ray energy spectrum at the beam port for a mammography x-ray tube?
    - A. Aluminum
    - B. Beryllium
    - C. Rhodium
    - D. Silver
    - E. Titanium

16. Which target/filter combination should NEVER be used for mammography imaging?
    - A. Mo/Mo
    - B. Mo/Rh
    - C. Rh/Mo
    - D. Rh/Rh
    - E. W/Rh

17. To maintain accreditation status, the radiologist must document and verify Category I continuing education credits related to mammography. What is the minimum total number of hours required over 3 years?
    - A. 15
    - B. 30
    - C. 45
    - D. 60
    - E. 75

18. What breast presentation will most likely cause grid line artifacts?
    - A. A thin, fatty breast
    - B. A thick dense breast
    - C. Magnification views
    - D. A thin, dense breast
    - E. A thick, fatty breast

19. If the entrance air kerma to the accreditation phantom is 4 mGy for a 28 kV W target/0.05 mm Rh filter x-ray beam, what is the estimated average glandular dose?
    - A. 4.0 mGy
    - B. 2.9 mGy
    - C. 2.3 mGy
    - D. 1.2 mGy

20. In a dedicated mammography system, where is the x-ray beam central axis positioned?
    - A. Chest wall edge
    - B. Between the center and the chest wall edge
    - C. Middle of the field between the chest wall edge and anterior edge
    - D. Between the center and the anterior edge
    - E. Anterior edge of the detector

21. For full x-ray field coverage of a mammography system with a typical source image distance of 65 cm, what is the minimum *effective* tube anode angle? (Consider a large field area of 24 × 30 cm.)
    - A. 2°
    - B. 5°
    - C. 10°
    - D. 15°
    - E. 20°

22. According to MQSA regulations, what is the maximum allowable average glandular dose per image for a breast composed of 50% glandular/50% adipose tissue of 4.5-cm thickness (*e.g.*, the accreditation phantom)?
    - A. 0.3 mGy
    - B. 3 mGy
    - C. 30 mGy
    - D. 300 mGy
    - E. 3,000 mGy

23. Which one of the following operational descriptors represents the greatest difference between analog screen-film mammography and digital mammography?
    - A. Breast radiation dose
    - B. Sensitivity and specificity
    - C. Exposure latitude
    - D. Scattered radiation
    - E. Compression

24. Which of the following is a significant benefit of a tungsten (W) anode compared to a molybdenum (Mo) anode in a mammo x-ray tube?
    - A. Tungsten spectrum provides useful characteristic "L" x-rays.
    - B. Absorption filters are thinner for tungsten targets.
    - C. Tungsten spectra deliver increased breast contrast for the same kV.
    - D. Higher tube heat loading can be achieved with tungsten anodes.

25. What is the typical Source to Image Distance (SID) in a dedicated digital mammo system?
    - A. 50 cm
    - B. 65 cm
    - C. 80 cm
    - D. 100 cm
    - E. 180 cm

26. What is the nominal size of the small focal spot used for magnification studies in mammography?
    - A. 0.05 mm
    - B. 0.1 mm
    - C. 0.3 mm
    - D. 0.6 mm
    - E. 1.2 mm

27. A typical scatter to primary ratio for x-rays transmitted through a 6 cm compressed breast is closest to which of the following?
    A. 0.1                D. 2.1
    B. 0.7                E. 2.5
    C. 1.4

28. According to MQSA, the mammography workstation must have a monitor with a minimum number of megapixels (MP) equal to:
    A. 2 MP               D. 5 MP
    B. 3 MP               E. 6 MP
    C. 4 MP

29. What is the approximate ratio of the dose to the breast for a digital tomosynthesis study compared to a standard compressed mammogram?
    A. 1/2                D. 4
    B. 1                  E. 15
    C. 2

30. The MQSA minimum requirement for visualized objects in the ACR accreditation phantom is which of the following (for screen/film and most digital units)?
    A. 3 fibers, 3 speck groups, 3 masses
    B. 4 fibers, 3 speck groups, 3 masses
    C. 5 fibers, 4 speck groups, 4 masses
    D. 6 fibers, 5 speck groups, 5 masses

31. How many tomographic images are typically reconstructed for a breast tomosynthesis study with a compressed breast thickness of 5 cm?
    A. 5                  D. 50
    B. 10                 E. 100
    C. 25

32. To determine the typical average glandular dose, the accreditation phantom is used for Mo target and filter. Which of the following statements regarding the average glandular dose is true?
    A. It is approximately 20% to 30% of the Entrance skin air kerma.
    B. It is unaffected by tissue composition.
    C. It is independent of beam penetrability.
    D. It is typically on the order of 100 mGy.

33. What aspect of the mammography quality standards act (MQSA) does the EQUIP process mainly emphasize?
    A. Annual technical equipment performance review by the medical physicist
    B. The accreditation phantom scoring and the radiation doses delivered
    C. Daily and weekly evaluation of the mammography system by the QC technologist
    D. Responsibilities of the lead interpreting physician in overseeing the clinical image quality

34. A magnification study of the breast at 1.8× is performed using the small focal spot. Where is the detail of microcalcifications best visualized?
    A. Uniform detail is visualized over the entire image.
    B. Improved detail is visualized on the cathode side of the image.
    C. Improved detail is visualized on the anode side of the image.
    D. Improved detail is visualized at the reference axis.

35. A mammography system has a fixed detector geometry with a flat-panel TFT detector. Image acquisition of a large phantom of constant thickness is obtained, with uniformity corrections made (right). Where is the background image noise (std dev) largest in this image?

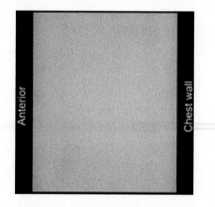

    A. Anterior side of the image
    B. Chest wall side of the image
    C. No difference across the image

# Answers

1. **C**  Average glandular doses (2020) typically range from approximately 1 to 1.5 mGy per image (4.5 cm breast) for a digital mammography system with a flat panel detector. Two images (CC and MLO) will double the dose (1.2 mGy x 2 =2.4 mGy). Thicker compressed breasts will have higher doses. *(Pg. 300)*

2. **D**  When the AEC system initiates the backup timer for a properly functioning system, this indicates that the x-ray penetrability is too low, resulting in the AEC sensor feedback not accumulating enough charge to trigger the termination switch. Thus, the penetrability of the beam must be increased by increasing the kV. Note that this would occur when in an "auto-time" mode, whereas a fully automatic mode would select the kV and filtration based upon a 100 ms test exposure. *(Pg. 275)*

3. **A**  The air gap is an effective means of reducing scatter. With magnification, a grid would not clean up as much scatter and would increase the dose by 2 or more times. *(Pg. 279)*

4. **B**  Stereotactic biopsy systems use a tube shift of +15° to −15°, for a total of 30° to produce planar images in which objects shift an amount on the detector plane dependent on the distance from the object in the breast to the detector. *(Pg. 290)*

5. **D**  The HVL should not be too high and cannot be less than kV/100; the closest answer in this group is 0.3 mm Al.*(Pg. 269)*

6. **C**  The sum of the light field/x-ray field deviations must be within 2% of the SID for the left and right edges OR for the chest wall and anterior edges (separately). For 60 cm SID, this represents 1.2 cm or 12 mm for either the left/right edges or chest wall/anterior edges. Be careful of the units!! *(Pg. 272)*

7. **B**  Parallax occurs because of beam divergence. In mammography, the x-ray beam central axis is at the chest wall, centered to the detector from left to right (mammo uses a ½ beam geometry). Therefore, the x-rays will have least parallax perpendicular to the detector at the center of the chest wall side of the detector. *(Pg. 263)*

8. **A**  Rhodium targets provide higher characteristic x-ray energies. The rhodium filter preferentially transmits the characteristic x-rays, resulting in a more penetrating x-ray beam for thick, dense breasts. *(Pg. 268)*

9. **B**  The "heel effect" describes the reduced intensity toward the anode side of the imaged area. Because the chest wall typically has the greatest thickness, the cathode is positioned over this area of the breast, and the anode over the nipple. *(Pg. 264)*

10. **B**  The mean glandular dose (also known as average glandular dose) is the benchmark, determined from the product of the measured Entrance Skin Exposure and the Roentgen to rad conversion factor, $D_{gN}$. The former is dependent on kV and HVL. *(Pg. 298)*

11. **D**  Compression helps reduce the dose by reducing the thickness of the breast, in addition to reducing scatter and spreading out the breast anatomy. While compression reduces scatter, it does not eliminate the need for a grid, however. *(Pg. 276–277)*

12. **D**  The Bucky factor for mammo grids with a 5:1 ratio is about 2 to 3. (Note: the Bucky factor is the exposure or mAs required with versus without the grid to achieve an appropriate optical density on-screen/film detectors or the same SNR on digital detectors). *(Pg. 278–279)*

13. **D**  HVL is dependent on target—filter composition and thickness, and kV. The tungsten(W) target requires a greater filter thickness (50 µm) than a corresponding Mo or Rh target (25 µm) to reduce unwanted "L" characteristic x-rays from W (Z = 74). In addition, filters with higher atomic number (at the same thickness)

will attenuate a greater number of x-rays and result in larger HVL. Therefore, W target with thicker filter (50 µm) and Silver (Ag) with high atomic number is the answer. *(Pg. 270, Fig. 8-12)*

14. **B**  Higher energies reduce subject contrast and therefore radiographic contrast; however, with digital systems, the reduced absorption of the incident x-rays in the breast reduces the average glandular dose. With the ability to increase radiographic (image) contrast with processing, the loss of subject contrast is minimized. The distractor SNR refers to the SNR control on the AEC selector. *(Pg. 275)*

15. **B**  Beryllium is used because of its extremely low Z. The low energy x-rays in the spectrum will be transmitted through the tube port, but then selectively absorbed by the added filter prior to reaching the breast. *(Pg. 266)*

16. **C**  X-ray tube targets for mammography applications consist of Mo, Rh, and W. The one target/filter combination that should never be used is Rh/Mo because the characteristic x-rays generated by the Rh target (20 to 23 keV) are readily absorbed by the Mo filter resulting from the increased attenuation just beyond the k-edge of 20 keV. *(Pg. 268, Fig. 8-10B)*

17. **A**  The required number of hours is 15 category I credits specific to mammography over 3 years. *(Pg. 303)*

18. **A**  Grid lines appear on moving grid (Bucky) units when the exposure time is short and does not give enough exposure time to blur the grid lines. Of all the choices, the thin fatty breast will result in the shortest exposure time. *(Pg. 278)*

19. **D**  The mean (average) glandular dose to the accreditation phantom (4.2 cm equivalent thickness, 50% adipose/50% glandular) for this breast composition and thickness, kV, HVL, and target/filter combination is about 0.3 mGy mean glandular dose/mGy entrance air kerma (the $D_{gN}$). Thus, the AGD is approximately 4 mGy × 0.3 mGy/mGy entrance AK = approximately 1.2 mGy. *(Pg. 299–300)*

20. **A**  The mammography acquisition geometry is that of a "half-field," extending from the chest wall side (compression paddle edge) to the anterior side of the detector plane. In this geometry, the central axis resides on the chest wall edge of the detector plane. Of note is the "reference" axis (not to be confused with the central axis), which typically bisects the FOV – distractor C. *(Pg. 263)*

21. **E**  Field cutoff occurs because of the reflection geometry of the x-ray tube target and the complete absorption of x-rays that are tangent to the anode surface. Using trigonometry, one can calculate the minimum angle as $q = \arctan(24/65) = 20°$. Usually the angle is made slightly larger (*e.g.*, 22°). The "effective anode angle" of 20° to 24° should be remembered. *(Pg. 263, Fig. 8-4)*

22. **B**  The maximum average glandular dose allowed by MQSA is 3 mGy per acquired image. Be careful of units, as 300 mrad = 3 mGy (there are 100 mrad/mGy). *(Pg. 302)*

23. **C**  The major operational difference is exposure latitude and dynamic range. This is the real benefit of digital detectors. Radiation dose is also lower, but the best answer is improved exposure latitude. *(Pg. 293)*

24. **D**  Tungsten anodes have better x-ray production efficiency and higher heat loading (higher instantaneous mA) than corresponding Molybdenum x-ray anodes. Deficits of W anodes are the lack of useful characteristic energies and a preponderance of bad "L" x-rays, which require a larger filter thickness (*e.g.*, 0.05 mm Rh), and a consequent lower output rate (mGy/mAs) compared to a Molybdenum target (0.025 mm Rh filter thickness) mammography tube. Thus, for the same tube current (mA) setting, the exposure time will be longer for a tungsten anode compared to a moly anode. *(Pg. 267–269)*

25. **B**  Most mammography systems have an SID of 60 to 70 cm, in order to allow for easy positioning of the gantry, reasonable tube output, field coverage, tolerable heel effect falloff, and an ability to achieve magnification studies of 1.5× to 1.8× by using an easy to handle magnification platform. *(Pg. 262)*

26. **B**  The small focal spot for mammography is typically 0.1 mm nominal size. This results in not only reduced geometric blurring for magnification studies but also in long exposure times due to the reduced instantaneous tube loading. *(Pg. 263)*

27. **B**  Scatter to primary ratios in mammography range from about 0.2 (2 cm breast thickness) to 1.1 (8 cm breast thickness). A 6 cm breast has an SPR of about 0.7. *(Pg. 279, Fig. 8-18)*

28. **D**  The mammography monitor used for diagnosis for digital images must have a minimum addressable matrix of 2,000 × 2,500 (5 MP) and a minimum luminance of 400 cd/m². *(Pg. 297)*

29. **B** Current state-of-the-art DBT systems are designed to acquire about 9 to 25 projections (N) from different angles to create a synthetic tomographic plane; because the images are added together with differences in shift to create an in-focal plane, each individual projection is acquired with about 1/9th to 1/25th dose (1/N per projection). In addition, a higher kV is used, such that the overall breast dose is about the same as a conventional compressed mammogram. Therefore, a conventional and tomosynthesis digital study will double the dose, but a "synthetic" mammogram produced from the tomosynthesis acquisition can replace the conventional mammogram and keep the dose approximately the same in a screening situation. *(Pg. 299, Fig. 8-34)*

30. **B** MQSA provides the oversight and rules for mammography; for screen-film imaging, the requirement is to visualize 4 fibers, 3 speck groups, and 3 masses. With digital imaging, the manufacturers are responsible for the QC program and requirements. Some digital manufacturers have a minimum of 5 fibers, 4 speck groups and 4 masses as minimum requirements. *(Pg. 304–305)*

31. **D** The "typical" reconstructed slices are reproduced every 1 millimeter, therefore the total number of slices is equal to 10 times the compressed breast thickness expressed in centimeters. *(Pg. 286–288)*

32. **A** The average glandular dose is on order of 12% to 25% of the ESAK (Mo target/filter $D_{gN}$), depending on breast composition, kV, HVL. Typical $D_{gN}$ values range from 0.12 to 0.45 mGy/mGy over a range of target/filter combinations. *(Pg. 298–299)*

33. **D** Within the clinical mammography operation, Enhancing Quality Using the Inspection Program (EQUIP) emphasizes the appropriateness, timely interpretation, and image quality of mammograms, including regular reviews to identify issues, take corrective action, document outcomes, and meet MQSA requirements (more than the technical aspects of the equipment). The goal is to ensure safe, effective, and convenient services to the patient. These goals are the responsibility of the Lead Interpreting Physician of the Mammography service. *(Pg. 303)*

34. **C** The "effective size" of focal spot varies due to the *projection* of the length of the filament along the cathode/anode direction (the line focus principle). As the "effective anode angle θ" of the projected focal spot becomes smaller toward the anode side of the field, so does the focal spot length (effective focal spot length = actual focal spot length × sin (θ)). The smaller focal spot will result in less geometric blurring and better microcalcification detail on the anode side of the field. *(Pg. 281, Fig. 8-20)*

35. **A** The orientation of the x-ray tube is with the anode side of the field projected toward the anterior, and the cathode side of the field projected toward the chest wall so that the heel effect (loss of photon fluence caused by self-filtration of x-rays projected nearly parallel to the surface of the anode) is over the thinner side of the breast. For a uniform phantom, the number of photons projected toward the anode side of the field is less than toward the cathode side of the field, and the number of photons transmitted and detected will be less; therefore, the noise (std dev) will be higher. *(Pg. 293, Fig. 8-31)*

# Section III Key Equations and Symbols

| QUANTITY | EQUATION | EQ NO./PAGE/COMMENTS |
|---|---|---|
| Focal spot effective length (line focus principle) | Effective length = actual length × sin θ is the "effective" anode angle | Eq. 6-2/Pg. 196/Focal spot length varies in the cathode-anode direction and is smaller on the anode side (Fig. 6-16) |
| Breast entrance surface dose: $Z$ (mGy) | $= X \text{ mGy(per 100 mAs)} \times \dfrac{Y \text{ mAs}}{100} \left( \dfrac{50 \text{ cm}}{D \text{ cm}} \right)^2$ | Eq. 8-1/Pg. 270/X-ray tube output, $X$, is measured at a standard distance (e.g., 50 cm) per 100 mAs. Inverse-square law correction applied for distance $D$ (source to breast surface). |
| Contrast degradation factor (CDF) | $CDF = \dfrac{C_s}{C_0} = \dfrac{1}{1 + SPR}$ | Eq. 8-2/Pg. 278/The amount of contrast achieved in the presence of scatter relative to contrast with no scatter. SPR = Scatter to Primary ratio (see Fig. 8-18) |
| Magnification, M | $M = \dfrac{\text{Image size}}{\text{object size}} = \dfrac{\text{source to image dist.}}{\text{source to object dist.}}$ | Eq. 7-2/Pg. 225/Fig. 8-20, Pg. 281. typical values run from 1.5× to 2.0× |
| Stereotactic lesion depth, Z | $Z = \dfrac{X}{2 \tan 15°}$ | Fig. 8-29 caption/Pg. 291/$X$ is lesion shift distance in stereo pair images acquired at +15° and −15° |
| Mean Glandular Dose (MGD) | $D_g = X_{ESAK} \times D_{gN}$ | Eq. 8-3/Pg. 298/$D_g$ = MGD; $X_{ESAK}$ = Entrance Surface Air Kerma; $D_{gN}$ = conversion factor, derived from Monte Carlo transport algorithm. $D_{gN}$ tables dependent on kV, HVL, target/filter, thickness, tissue composition (Table 8-6, Pg. 299.) |
| Mean Glandular Dose (MGD) | MGD = $Kgcs$ | Eq. 8-4/Pg. 299/$K$ = Entrance Surface Air Kerma; $g$ = fraction $K$ absorbed by glandular tissue; $c$ = correction for % glandularity; $s$ = factor to account for target/filter |

| SYMBOL | QUANTITY | UNITS |
|---|---|---|
| kV | Voltage applied to x-ray tube | volt, kilovolt |
| mAs | Tube current—time product | ampere-seconds |
| s | Exposure time | second |
| θ | Anode angle | degree |
| HVL | Half Value Layer | mm Aluminum |
| SPR | Scatter to Primary Ratio | unitless |
| M | Magnification | unitless |
| SID | Source-Image Distance | cm |
| SOD | Source-Object Distance | cm |
| OID | Object-Image Distance | cm |

# Fluoroscopy

## 9.0 INTRODUCTION

Fluoroscopy is a procedure that provides real-time transient x-ray imaging with permanent recording of appropriate images. Fluoroscopy is not generally intended to generally replace conventional projection radiography. The basic modes of operation of a fluoroscopic system are as follows:

*Fluoroscopy* using relatively low radiation dose rates provides real-time imaging for positioning with selective recording only when sequences contain sufficient diagnostic information for later use.

*Fluorography* (acquisition) using substantially higher radiation dose rates provides images for later use with image quality higher than that achievable using stored fluoroscopy.

Fluoroscopic systems are flexible general-purpose devices that are configurable to meet the requirements of a wide range of clinical procedures (Fig. 9-1).

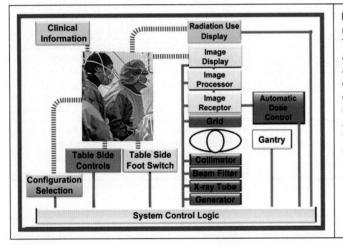

■ **FIGURE 9-1** Block diagram of an interventional fluoroscope. Key components and control loops are shown. The operator is a key element with the ability to select and modify radiation factors, imaging geometry, image acquisition parameters, and image processing; These controls include (1) x-ray generator settings (kV, mA, continuous versus pulsed fluoro operation), (2) automatic exposure rate control (AERC) dose rates, (3) acquisition modes and frame rates, (4) image-receptor field of view and collimation, and (5) image processing methods and image display adjustments.

## 9.1 FLUOROSCOPIC IMAGING CHAIN OVERVIEW

1. Principal feature of fluoroscopy over radiography is the ability to acquire real-time images.
   a. Real-time frame rates of 30 frames/s and reduced rates (15, 7.5, 3.75, 2, 1 frames/s).
   b. 20-minute fluoro "on-time" at 15 frames/s produces 18,000 individual images.
2. Images (frames) are produced with much less dose than comparable radiograph.
   a. Fluoroscopy 10 to 100 nGy/image
   b. Fluorography 100 to 1,000 nGy/image—digital acquisition (DA), digital subtraction angiography (DSA)
   c. Radiography 3,000 to 10,000 nGy/image
3. Fluoroscopic imaging chain components of a modern system (Fig. 9-2).
   a. High gain solid-state flat-panel image detector converts x-ray signal into a series of digital images.
   b. Antiscatter grid reduces scatter to achieve good subject contrast.
   c. Collimation limits the x-ray beam to the active field of view or to a clinically relevant area.
   d. X-ray tube; beam attenuation filters used to reduce dose to patient.

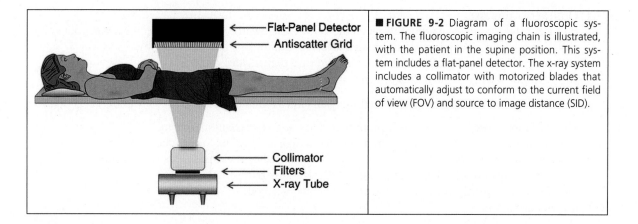

■ **FIGURE 9-2** Diagram of a fluoroscopic system. The fluoroscopic imaging chain is illustrated, with the patient in the supine position. This system includes a flat-panel detector. The x-ray system includes a collimator with motorized blades that automatically adjust to conform to the current field of view (FOV) and source to image distance (SID).

## 9.2 IMAGING CHAIN COMPONENTS

1. **X-ray image intensifier (II)**
   **a.** Key component of a fluoroscopy system from approximately 1960 to 2010; many remain in use in 2020
   **b.** Diagram of an II and its components (Fig. 9-3)

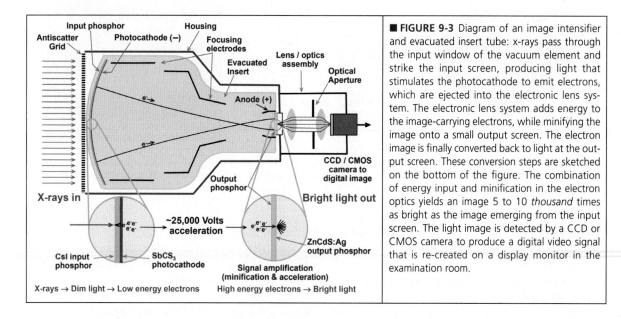

■ **FIGURE 9-3** Diagram of an image intensifier and evacuated insert tube: x-rays pass through the input window of the vacuum element and strike the input screen, producing light that stimulates the photocathode to emit electrons, which are ejected into the electronic lens system. The electronic lens system adds energy to the image-carrying electrons, while minifying the image onto a small output screen. The electron image is finally converted back to light at the output screen. These conversion steps are sketched on the bottom of the figure. The combination of energy input and minification in the electron optics yields an image 5 to 10 *thousand* times as bright as the image emerging from the input screen. The light image is detected by a CCD or CMOS camera to produce a digital video signal that is re-created on a display monitor in the examination room.

   **c.** **Input screen**
      **(i)** Includes a cesium-iodide (CsI) scintillator that converts the x-ray image into a visible light image and a photocathode that converts the light image into an electron image
      **(ii)** Curved to meet the needs of the II's electron optics, resulting in pincushion distortion of the image
   **d.** **Electron optics**
      **(i)** Add energy to the electrons emitted by the photocathode under a potential difference of 20 to 40 kV between the photocathode and the output screen/anode.
      **(ii)** Focus the electrons generated in the active area of the input onto the fixed size output screen.
      **(iii)** Multi-mode IIs have a separate set of electrodes for each input field size.
      **(iv)** Concentrate all of the signal intensity produced at the input screen onto the smaller output screen.
      **(v)** Intensity gain is proportional to the ratios of the areas of the input and output screens (minification).
   **e.** **Output screen**
      **(i)** Consists of a layer of ZnCdS coated onto either a glass or fiber optic output window.
      **(ii)** Produces an image of fixed diameter irrespective of the size of the active input layer.
      **(iii)** Limiting resolution of an II is inversely proportional to the input screen's diameter.

**f. Optical distributor**

   **(i)** Couples the output phosphor image to the video camera with optical lenses or direct fiberoptics.

   **(ii)** Optical aperture adjusts the output light levels for fluoroscopy and fluorography.

   **(iii)** Images are transferred from the output screen via a digital video camera.

   **(iv)** The video image of the output screen is the same size for any FOV setting of the II.

**g.** Brightness gain = Minification gain × Electronic gain (acceleration of electrons)    [9-1]

   **(i)** The input dose level is inversely proportional to the area of the input screen.

   **(ii)** Maintaining the constant light output requires a higher x-ray flux for magnified modes.

**h. Conversion factor** is the light intensity exiting the II divided by the exposure rate at the input.

   **(i)** A measure of overall performance including brightness gain

   **(ii)** Decreases over time due to degradation of the photocathode

**2. Flat-Panel Detectors**

**a.** Replacement for the II tube, optical system, and cameras.

   **(i)** Directly converts x-rays into a digital form.

   **(ii)** Carbon fiber covers reduce x-ray attenuation and increase DQE compared to II.

**b.** Composed of arrays of detector elements (DEXELS) packaged in a square or rectangular area (Fig. 9-4).

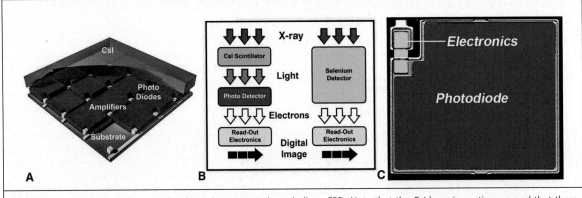

■ **FIGURE 9-4** Flat-panel detectors (FPD). **A.** Components in an indirect FPD. Note that the CsI layer is continuous and that there is space between individual dexels. The dexels in a direct x-ray system are also separated (not shown). **B.** Information flow through indirect and direct FPDs. **C.** The photodiode and some of the electronics in a single indirect dexel. ⬚ **F. 9-5**

**c. Indirect systems** have a phosphor layer that absorbs the x-rays and converts a fraction of their energy into light and a photodiode that converts the x-ray–induced light from the phosphor into a corresponding charge.

**d. Direct systems** have a semiconductor (*e.g.*, selenium) that produces x-ray–induced charge directly, which is captured by the electronics within the same dexel as the x-ray absorption event.

**e. FPD readout**

   **(i)** For fluoroscopy, after the capacitor is drained, the charge continues to be stored for the next frame.

   **(ii)** Real-time x-ray data are collected as the charge continues to be stored in a steady-state manner.

**f. Dexel arrays**

   **(i)** Reducing the FOV on spatial resolution differs for an image-intensifier and a FPD (Fig. 9-5).

   **(ii)** In an II, the FOV is reduced by electro-optically focusing a smaller portion of its input screen onto the fixed size output screen, to provide a fixed image size (image-matrix size) for the camera and image processor.

   **(iii)** In a flat-panel detector, the FOV is reduced by selecting a subarray of dexels; larger numbers of DEXELS for large FOVs and smaller numbers of DEXELS for small FOVs (Fig. 9-5; Table 9-1).

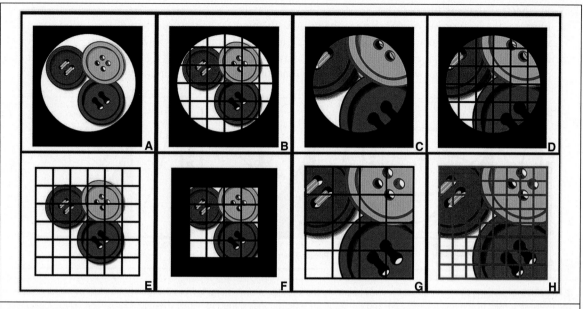

■ **FIGURE 9-5** Pixel size and magnification mode—image intensifier and flat-panel detector. **A–D.** Image intensifier—analog and digital camera outputs. The full pixel array of the digital camera captures the output of the II at any magnification mode. **E–G.** Flat-panel detector with a fixed dexel array (*e.g.,* Table 9-1 small detector). The same dexel covers the same portion of the patient irrespective of magnification mode (**E and F**). Resolution does not change when the image is digitally magnified. **H.** Flat-panel detector with unbundled dexels (*e.g.,* Table 9-1 large detector, small FOV). Resolution is improved if the FPD unbundles dexels when using a small FOV. ▭ F. 9-6

### TABLE 9-1 DEXELS, PIXELS, AND FIELD OF VIEW

| FIXED DEXEL = 0.18 | | | | | | BINNABLE DEXEL = 0.15 | | | | | |
|---|---|---|---|---|---|---|---|---|---|---|---|
| *Active Dexels* | | *Fluoro/Cine* | | *Digital Angio* | | *Active Dexels* | | *Fluoro/Cine* | | *Digital Angio* | |
| FOV | DEXELS | PIXELS 6–30 FPS | PSIZE | PIXELS >6 FPS | PSIZE | FOV | DEXELS | PIXELS 6–30 FPS | PSIZE | PIXELS >6 FPS | PSIZE |
| 26 (18) | 1,000 | 1,000 | 0.18 | 1,000 | 0.18 | 42 (30) | 2,000 | 1,000 | 0.30 | 2,000 | 0.15 |
| 20 (14) | 800 | 800 | 0.18 | 800 | 0.18 | 30 (20) | 1,400 | 700 | 0.30 | 1,400 | 0.15 |
| 13 (9) | 500 | 500 | 0.18 | 500 | 0.18 | 21 (15) | 1,000 | 1,000 | 0.15 | 1,000 | 0.15 |
| | | | | | | 15 (10) | 700 | 700 | 0.15 | 700 | 0.15 |

## 9.3 FLUOROSCOPIC X-RAY SOURCE ASSEMBLY

1. **X-ray tube**
   a. Have higher heat-storage capacity and faster cooling rates than radiographic tubes.
   b. Small focal spot is used for fluoroscopy and large for fluorography (CINE/DA/DSA).
      (i)  Spatial resolution is likely to decrease when going from fluoroscopy to fluorography.
      (ii)  Some tubes also have an additional micro-focus focal spot for geometrically magnified procedures.
   c. For all modes of operation, newer systems select the smallest focal spot that can accommodate the immediate x-ray power level and may result in spatial resolution differences for thin and thick body parts.
2. **Collimator**
   a. Dynamically adjusts the overall x-ray field size in response to a combination of inputs from both the operator and the system to confine the x-ray beam to the smallest area within the active area of the image receptor consistent with immediate clinical requirements.
   b. Wedge filters are used to equalize image receptor inputs when anatomical structures providing very different attenuation (*e.g.,* lung and mediastinum) are simultaneously in the beam.
   c. Collimation automatically limits the x-ray beam to the active FOV whenever the FOV is changed and to changes in the source to image-receptor distance (SID).

3. **X-ray spectral shaping filters**
   a. Increases the fraction of x-ray photons in the beam with energies slightly above the K absorption edge material of interest, to improve conspicuity of higher Z elements (*e.g.*, iodine at 33.2 keV).
   b. Copper filter (0.1 to 1.0 mm) and restricted x-ray tube voltage (lower kV, *e.g.*, 60) reduce the number of photons in the beam below the iodine edge and limits the number of higher energy photons (Fig. 9-6).

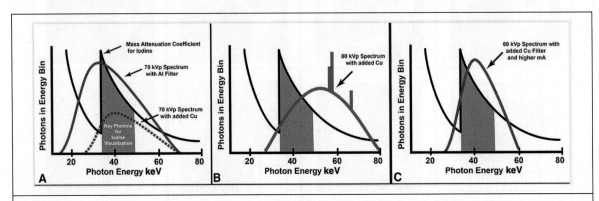

■ **FIGURE 9-6** Shaping the spectrum of the x-ray beam. **A.** The x-ray spectrum emerging from the tube is modified by a copper layer. The overall intensity of the beam is reduced, and the resultant spectrum has shifted to higher average energy. This figure shows the original spectrum, the attenuation coefficient of iodine as a function of energy, and the resultant modified spectrum with a higher fraction of photons above the iodine K edge. **B.** Increasing kV shifts the spectrum further, but most of the higher-energy photons are far from the iodine K edge and do not contribute very much to iodine visualization. Tungsten K characteristic photons are seen here as well. **C.** Reducing kV moves more of the spectrum toward the iodine K edge. There are fewer low-energy photons that would contribute to skin dose but not to the image. The photons, with energies above 60 kV, shown in **(B)** are not produced. X-ray tubes need to have high power capabilities so that they can provide adequate x-ray flux without increasing kV. ▢ **F. 9-7**

   c. Most modern systems have variable thickness copper filters in the collimator assembly.
   d. Acquisition selection (*e.g.*, low-dose rate fluoro, standard-dose rate fluoro) and automatic exposure rate control (AERC) can determine filter thickness and beam HVL (see textbook Figure 9-8, page 320 for AERC control of added filtration).
   e. Limited x-ray tube power output may require the filter thickness to decrease and the kV to increase.
   f. HVL may decrease with an increase in kV if there is a simultaneous decrease in copper thickness.

## 9.4  CONTROLS

1. **Automatic exposure rate control**
   a. Delivers constant x-ray intensity to the image receptor irrespective of tissue thickness in the beam path.
   b. Goal is reasonably constant *detector SNR* over its working range by maintaining a constant detector entrance dose rate.
   c. AERC collects detected x-ray intensity information observed by a predetermined subset of dexels.
      (i) Low average signal causes AERC to command the generator to increase x-ray output.
      (ii) High average signal causes AERC to decrease x-ray output.
   d. AERC output adjustments
      (i) Changes in FOV or frame rate adjust x-ray tube output to stabilize perceived image noise.
      (ii) X-ray factors (kV, mA, pulse width), focal spot, and beam filtration provide different balances between patient dose and image quality for various system options (Fig. 9-7).
      (iii) Image presentation to the operator is further influenced by these changes.
2. **Field of view and magnification modes**
   a. The active FOV of an *image intensifier* is established by focusing a portion of its input screen onto the full area of the output screen, with an increase in image magnification as the FOV decreases (Fig. 9-5).
   b. The active FOV of a *flat-panel detector* is reduced by accepting information from a smaller area of the image receptor, and the subsequent image is digitally resized to fill the fluoroscope's display (Fig. 9-5).
   c. The brightness gain of an II decreases as the magnification increases—the AERC compensates by boosting the x-ray exposure rate, typically by the square of the input phosphor diameter ratios.
   d. Flat-panel systems adjust dose rate when pixels are unbinned, and additional exposure rate increases are applied for all FOVs to meet perceptual requirements, usually linear with changes in active FOV area.

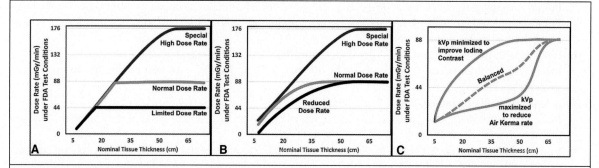

■ **FIGURE 9-7** Output dose rates as a function of patient size are a configurable property of the fluoroscopic system. **A.** System with three maximum fluoroscopic dose rate modes. In this system, the dose rate is identical for all modes until the individual mode limit is exceeded. **B.** The lower two fluoroscopic modes converge near the regulatory limit. The high-dose-rate mode is higher for all patient thicknesses and has double the usual regulatory limit. **C.** Hypothetical trajectories. Keeping the kV low for as long as possible improves iodine contrast at the expense of higher skin dose for heavy patients (highest relative dose rate for any tissue thickness). Raising the kV quickly minimizes patient dose at the expense of iodine contrast for many patients (lowest relative dose rate). Balanced curves (intermediate relative dose rate) represent a different trade-off between dose and iodine visibility. 📖 F. 9-9

## 9.5    MODES OF OPERATION

1. **Continuous fluoroscopy**
   a. An uninterrupted x-ray beam with an image stream partitioned into discrete frames by the video system.
   b. The typical frame rate is 30 frames per second (FPS).
   c. Quantum noise and anatomical motion occurring in a single frame (1/30 s) is averaged and blurred.
   d. A second stage of averaging occurs in the observer's eye due to temporal averaging.
   e. A single frame stored and viewed on a display monitor will appear nosier and sharper than the live image because observer temporal averaging no longer influences perception.

2. **Pulsed fluoroscopy and fluorography**
   a. X-ray generator produces a series of short pulses with an on-time smaller than the frame time (Fig. 9-8A).
   b. Short pulses (*e.g.*, 3 to 10 ms) reduce blurring of moving objects in individual images.
   c. Appearance of a moving object when viewed dynamically is dependent on the interactions of object motion, frame rate, processing of gap-filling display frames, and temporal filtering.
   d. An object will often appear sharper when a single image is viewed because there is no temporal averaging in either the image processor or the human visual system.
   e. The digital imaging system provides an output frame rate high enough to avoid image flicker by displaying each image multiple times when low acquisition frame rates are used (Fig. 9-8B).

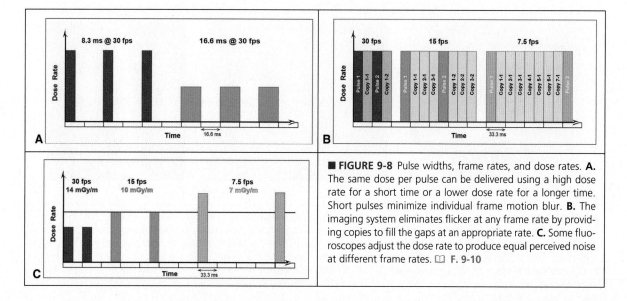

■ **FIGURE 9-8** Pulse widths, frame rates, and dose rates. **A.** The same dose per pulse can be delivered using a high dose rate for a short time or a lower dose rate for a longer time. Short pulses minimize individual frame motion blur. **B.** The imaging system eliminates flicker at any frame rate by providing copies to fill the gaps at an appropriate rate. **C.** Some fluoroscopes adjust the dose rate to produce equal perceived noise at different frame rates. 📖 F. 9-10

f. Pulsed imaging can reduce radiation because the acquisition frame rate is decoupled from the display rate.

g. Fluorographic images are intended to be viewed individually and therefore requires the same dose per pulse at any frame rate to maintain image SNR.

h. Fluoroscopic images will appear noisier if the same dose per pulse is used for all frame rates.

i. Increasing the fluoroscopy dose per pulse by about 1.4 when the FPS is halved maintains constant noise perception (Fig. 9-8C).

3. **Fluorography (unsubtracted)**

a. Fluorographic images, also known as digital angiography, DA images, or cine, should only be obtained if the intent is to store them for later review.

b. Enough dose per image is needed to reduce quantum noise to an acceptable value without relying on temporal averaging in the observer's eye.

c. A single fluorographic frame (not intended for DSA) will require about 10 times the radiation needed for a comparable fluoroscopic frame.

d. Frames intended for DSA will require 50 to 100 times as much radiation as a fluoroscopic frame (Fig. 9-9).

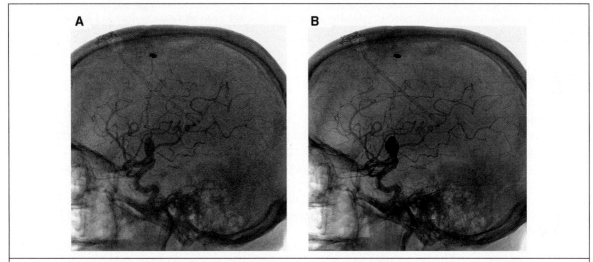

■ **FIGURE 9-9** Fluoroscopic and fluorographic images. These two images were taken a few seconds apart. The fluorographic DA image **(B)** from a DSA series required approximately 50 times the dose needed for the single fluoroscopic frame **(A)**. Note the increased quantum noise in the fluoroscopic image. 📖 **F 9-11**

4. **Fluorography (subtracted)**

a. DSA is performed by acquiring a series of DA images (*e.g.*, 1 to 6 images per second) while a contrast agent (*e.g.*, iodine or $CO_2$) is injected (Fig. 9-10).

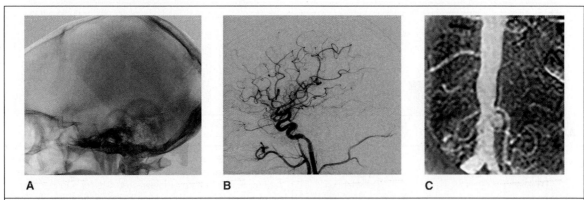

■ **FIGURE 9-10** Image subtraction. **A.** Mask image: This image will be subtracted from a later image in the series (not shown) in which iodine is present in the patient's arterial tree. **B.** Result of the subtraction: Structures common to both images have been removed. X-ray quantum noise from both images is present. The contrast of the image has been increased to improve the conspicuity of the vessels. It is necessary to use high radiation doses when acquiring the images to reduce the visibility of quantum noise. **C.** $CO_2$ subtraction image of the abdominal aorta. The $CO_2$ bubble does not fill the entire aorta at any one time. This image is reconstructed by subtracting the mask from a sequence of $CO_2$ containing images and then combining them to reconstruct the vascular tree. 📖 **F. 9-12**

**b.** The first few images contain no contrast agent, and one or an average of images is selected as the mask.

**c.** The contrast agent moves through the vessels, images contain both anatomy and contrast-enhanced vessels.

**d.** The mask image is subtracted (pixel by pixel) from the images with contrast images, resulting in the subtraction of the anatomical background.

**e.** Software tools permit automatic or manual reregistration of images to minimize motion artifacts.

**f.** DSA removes fixed information common to both the mask and live image.

**g.** Random noise adds and produces more quantum noise in the difference image than in either initial image.

**h.** Display contrast is increased to improve visibility of blood vessels or other moving structures. This increases the visibility of quantum noise in the image.

**i.** Suppressing quantum noise requires the use of more per-image radiation.

**j.** Nominally, up to 10 times the dose is needed for a single DSA frame than for a comparable unsubtracted fluorographic (DA) image.

**k.** Using low frame rates, where practicable, reduces radiation.

**5. Cine fluorography (analog and digital)**

**a.** The same digital image chain supports fluoroscopy, DSA, and cine. Imaging modes are changed by configuring fluoroscopic hardware and software.

**b.** Frame rates can be set to conform to procedure specific requirements. Reduction in cine frame rate produces a major reduction in patient dose.

**c.** Retrospectively stored fluoroscopy (if of adequate quality) can be substituted for acquisitions in the clinical image stream, saving both radiation and the volume of contrast media used in a procedure.

## 9.6  IMAGE PROCESSING

**1. Single image processing**

**a.** This section discusses blurring and unsharp masking applied uniformly across the entire image.

**b.** Newer algorithms use processing to differentially modify the visibility of objects in different parts of the same image.

**c.** Image blurring to reduce the visibility of noise (Fig. 9-11).

**d.** Unsharp masking parameters (Fig. 9-12).

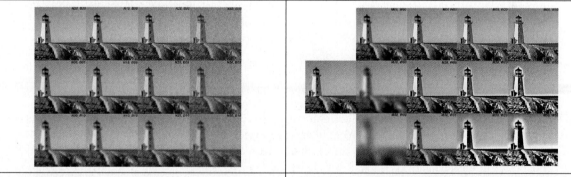

■ **FIGURE 9-11** Image blurring to reduce the visibility of noise. The original image (512 × 512 pixels, 8-bit gray scale) is in the upper left corner. **Columns:** Gaussian noise (N) added to the original image at four levels (0%, 5%, 25%, 50%). **Rows:** The resultant images were then blurred using Gaussian blurring (B) using radii of 0 (no blur), 5, and 10 pixels. ⊞ **F. 9-13**

■ **FIGURE 9-12** Unsharp masking parameters. The original (unblurred) image is on the left. **Each row** has constant Gaussian blur radius M of 5, 20, 50 pixels. **Each column** has the same weighted combination of blurred and original image weighting factors W of 0% (blur only), 50%, 200%, 500%. ⊞ **F. 9-14**

**2. Temporal image processing (multi-frame)**

**a.** Individual fluoroscopic images are relatively noisy, with noise patterns statistically changing from frame to frame.

**b.** Appropriately combining several fluoroscopic frames will improve the perceived SNR while maintaining the system's inherent spatial resolution at a potential cost of blurring moving objects.

**c.** Similar processing is seldom needed during fluorography (*e.g.*, cine) because the higher dose per frame is intended to reduce noise.

**d.** Image processors facilitate task-specific temporal blurring such as recursive filtering (Fig. 9-13).

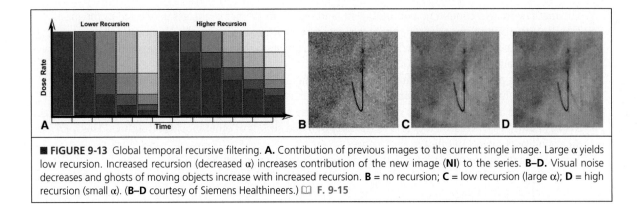

■ **FIGURE 9-13** Global temporal recursive filtering. **A.** Contribution of previous images to the current single image. Large α yields low recursion. Increased recursion (decreased α) increases contribution of the new image (**NI**) to the series. **B–D.** Visual noise decreases and ghosts of moving objects increase with increased recursion. **B** = no recursion; **C** = low recursion (large α); **D** = high recursion (small α). (**B–D** courtesy of Siemens Healthineers.) ▯ **F. 9-15**

   e. The displayed image (DI) is calculated using a fraction (α) of the just acquired new image (NI), which is added to the previously displayed image (PDI) using

$$\text{Displayed Image}\,(\text{DI}) = \alpha\,\text{NI} + (1-\alpha)\,\text{PDI} \qquad [9\text{-}1] \qquad ▯\ \text{E. }9\text{-}2$$

   f. In Equation 9-1, the parameter α ranges from 0 to 1; as α is reduced, the contribution of the current image (NI) is reduced, the contribution of the previously displayed image is enhanced, and the amount of lag is increased. As α is increased, the amount of lag is reduced, and at α = 1, no lag occurs.

3. **Display transform function (DTF)**
   a. An arbitrary look-up table to transform the image processor's output pixel levels into display brightness levels.
   b. Most fluoroscopes have several DTFs intended for different imaging tasks.

4. **Local and adaptive image processing**
   a. Faster image processing hardware now allows the use of different algorithms in different image regions.
   b. Optimizing local image processing in each region relies on a combination of a priori knowledge of the purpose of the procedure and feature extraction within an image or a sequence of images.
   c. A fluoroscopic image of a small portion of a static test object used for daily quality assurance in an interventional laboratory illustrates locally adaptive image processing (Fig. 9-14).
     (i) The image processor interpreted the lead markers as contrast-filled arteries, where the "artery" was of high contrast and might move during fluoroscopy.
     (ii) Recursive filtering was locally disabled in that region of the image, and an edge-enhancement filter was applied, resulting in sharp borders of the "artery" and increased noise in this region.
     (iii) The periphery of the image was interpreted to have nothing of clinical interest; therefore, recursive filtering was applied in this region to suppress quantum noise.

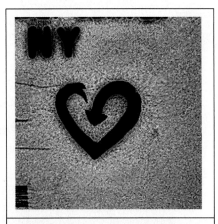

■ **FIGURE 9-14** Example of locally adaptive image processing (fluoroscopic single frame image of a small portion of an enhanced daily QA test object). The image processor interpreted the lettering, lead-wire heart, and guidewires as vessels and assumed that they might move during a fluoroscopic sequence. It reduced the amount of temporal filtering in their vicinity resulting in increased local noise visibility. Compare this region with the reduced noise seen in the temporally filtered region in the lower right corner of the image. ▯ **F. 9-16**

5. **Image displays**
   a. Viewing monitors and the human eye are the links in the imaging chain that transfer information extracted from the patient into the observer's brain (Fig. 9-15A).
     (i) For photopic vision, the eye's relative contrast sensitivity peaks around 1 minute of visual angle.
   b. An optimum viewing distance exists for different sized objects in a fixed sized radiograph (Fig. 9-15B).
   c. Practical implications of monitor size when trying to detect clinically important objects
     (i) Using a 20-inch monitor, the observer leans forward to maximize opacified vessel visibility (Fig. 9-15C).
     (ii) Using a 55-inch monitor, the observer stands back while examining similar size vessels (Fig. 9-15D).

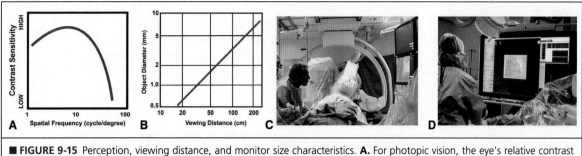

■ **FIGURE 9-15** Perception, viewing distance, and monitor size characteristics. **A.** For photopic vision, the eye's relative contrast sensitivity peaks around 1 minute of visual angle. **B.** The effect of viewing distance for full sized radiographs demonstrates that the observer should be further from a fixed size image when trying to detect large objects. **C.** Using a 20-inch display monitor, the operator leans forward to maximize the ability to see the opacified vessels. **D.** Using a 55-inch monitor while examining similar size vessels, the operator is seen standing back and away from the beam to maximize viewing. This yields two increases in operator safety: (1) Increased distance decreases the intensity of the operator's scatter field. (2) Standing upright, instead of leaning over, decreases orthopedic load and helps reduce the effects of wearing heavy personal protective equipment. 📖 **F. 9-17**

d. Large format display monitors can increase operator safety:
  **(i)** Increased distance decreases the intensity of the scatter field at the operator's working position.
  **(ii)** Standing upright, instead of leaning over, decreases orthopedic load and will help reduce the strain produced by wearing heavy radiation personal protective equipment (RPPE).
e. In-room fluoro monitors can seldom be meaningfully tested like in a manner similar to primary diagnostic monitors (*e.g.*, chest, mammo).
  **(i)** Sufficient monitor luminance is necessary to allow room lights to be on.
  **(ii)** A simple test can be used to verify visualization of 0% to 5% and 95% to 100% contrast patches in SMPTE pattern (see display monitors in Chapter 5).

## 9.7 IMAGE QUALITY IN FLUOROSCOPY

Clinically useable image quality components and considerations:

- Appropriate hardware-level image quality
- A priori information regarding the patient
- Observer's general medical knowledge
- Observer's imaging preferences

Image processing has evolved from global spatial and temporal techniques to regional processing around local features in individual images (single image processing) and across time (multiple image processing).

Image processing pipeline (Fig. 9-16) contains images in two distinct states:

- Between the image receptor hardware and the final image processor: "*For Processing*" images
- Displayed to the operator or archived when the system is in clinical mode: "*For Presentation*" images

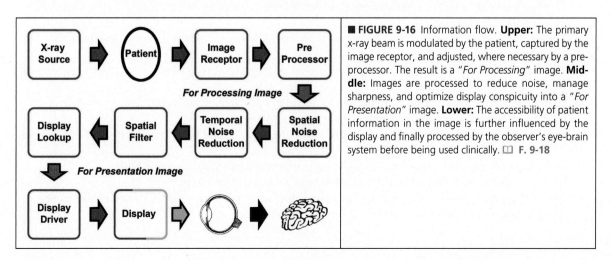

■ **FIGURE 9-16** Information flow. **Upper:** The primary x-ray beam is modulated by the patient, captured by the image receptor, and adjusted, where necessary by a pre-processor. The result is a "*For Processing*" image. **Middle:** Images are processed to reduce noise, manage sharpness, and optimize display conspicuity into a "*For Presentation*" image. **Lower:** The accessibility of patient information in the image is further influenced by the display and finally processed by the observer's eye-brain system before being used clinically. 📖 **F. 9-18**

1. **Spatial resolution**
   a. Limiting resolution of an II increases when magnification is increased (smaller FOV).
   b. Limiting resolution of an FPD is determined by the pitch of its dexels (Table 9-1).
      (i) Secondary limits are often imposed with a large active FOV and/or high frame rate.
   c. Focal spot size and geometric magnification are key contributors to overall spatial resolution (Fig. 9-17).
2. **Noise limited imaging**

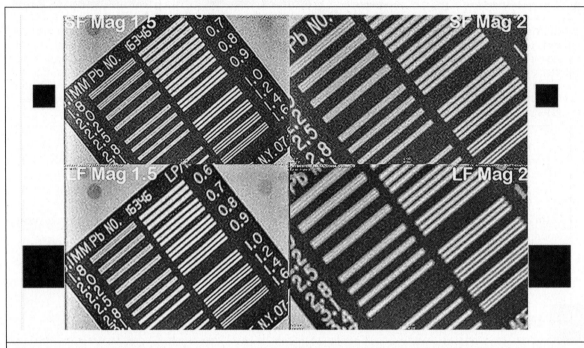

■ **FIGURE 9-17** Spatial resolution as a function of geometry and focal spot size. **Left column:** Magnification of 1.5× comparing the small focal spot (*top*) and the large focal spot (*bottom*). **Right column:** Magnification of 2.0× comparing the small focal spot (*top*) and the large focal spot (*bottom*). Spatial resolution with the small focal spot improves with magnification—System resolution is image receptor limited. Spatial resolution with the large focal spot degrades with magnification—System resolution is focal spot size limited. 📖 **F. 9-20**

   a. The perception of key clinical objects is influenced by image noise.
   b. Visual noise can be grouped into two categories
      (i) Quantum noise, produced by statistical variations in the numbers of x-ray photons converted to a signal, is dependent on the local x-ray dose level.
      (ii) System noise, the combination of all other noise sources in the imaging chain and the observer's eye-brain system, is independent of x-ray dose but may be dependent on factors such as electronic noise and illumination level.
   c. The total amount of noise in an image changes with dose only when quantum noise is dominant.
3. **Temporal resolution**
   a. The primary purpose of fluoroscopy (and associated fluorography) is to observe and document motion, requiring temporal resolution appropriate to the clinical task.
   b. Clinical temporal resolution includes the effects due to eye physiology, including:
      (i) Image averaging in the eye (approximately 200 ms)
      (ii) The eye's sensitivity to images provided at low frame rates (critical flicker frequency [CFF] of approximately 30 FPS)
   c. Eye integration does not apply when a single image is continuously displayed (Fig. 9-9).
      (i) Perceived noise is limited by the x-ray dose used to acquire that image.
      (ii) A single fluoroscopic image will appear noisier than when the same scene is viewed as a sequence.
      (iii) Fluorographic images are intended to be viewed one-by-one.

## 9.8 PATIENT RADIATION MANAGEMENT

Pragmatic radiation management points that should be known to the operator and staff are listed in Table 9-2.
**Points to consider:**

- The automatic exposure rate control (AERC) adjusts radiation output in response to changes in patient anatomy and SID.
- AERC provides the following:
  ◆ Selections such as the dose rate family associated with a specific clinical mode
  ◆ Choices between normal and low-dose-rate fluoroscopy and fluorography
- AERC program often adjusts maximum fluoroscopic dose rates to values well below regulatory limits.
- There are no regulatory limitations on dose rates or total doses for any acquisition mode (*e.g.*, cine, digital angiography, DSA).
- There are no regulatory limitations on total fluoroscopic time or fluoroscopic dose used in a procedure.
- Operational changes of x-ray equipment factors and imaging geometry will influence image quality as well as radiation dose to patients and staff (Table 9-2).

1. **Patient dose metrics**
   a. Fluoroscopic time (5-minute timer)
      (i) Intend to remind the operator about the use of radiation.
      (ii) About half of the patient's total irradiation dose in interventional procedures is attributable to fluorography.
      (iii) Fluoro-time alone supplies little useful information on potential patient tissue reactions or of stochastic risk to patients or staff.
   b. Kerma area product (KAP, DAP)
      (i) The same at any location between the x-ray tube and the patient (area of diverging beam is offset by inverse square law of output air kerma)

**TABLE 9-2 SUMMARY OF OPERATIONAL FACTORS THAT AFFECT IMAGE QUALITY AND RADIATION DOSE TO THE PATIENT AND STAFF**

| | EFFECT ON IMAGE QUALITY AND RADIATION DOSE | | |
|---|---|---|---|
| **OPERATIONAL CHANGE** | *Image Quality* | *Radiation Dose to the Patient* | *Radiation Dose to the Staff* |
| Increase in patient size | Worse (increased scatter fraction) | Higher | Higher |
| Increase in tube current (mA) with constant kV (*i.e.*, AERC off) | Better (lower image noise) | Higher | Higher |
| Increase in tube potential (kV) with AERC active | Soft tissue: Better (lower noise) | Lower | Lower |
| | Bone and contrast material: Worse: (decreased subject contrast) | | |
| Increase in tube filtration from 0.2 to 9.4 mm Cu with AERC active | Little change | Lower | Lower |
| Increase in source to skin distance | Slightly better | Lower | Little change |
| Increase in skin to image receptor distance (fixed source-skin distance) | Slightly better (less scatter) excluding x-ray tube focal spot size effects | Higher | Higher |
| Increase in image receptor magnification factor | May be better (improved spatial resolution) | Higher | Higher |
| Increase in collimator opening | Worse (increased scatter fraction) | Little change (however higher integral and effective dose) | Higher |
| Increase beam on time | No effect | Higher | Higher |
| Increase in pulsed fluoroscopy frame rate | Better (improved temporal resolution) | Higher | Higher |
| Grid is used | Better (decreased scatter fraction) | Higher | Higher |
| Image recording modes (cine, DSA, radiographic) | Better (lower noise, higher resolution) | Higher | Higher |

(ii) Does not provide a direct indicator of the possibility of skin reactions because a procedure producing the same KAP can deliver low skin dose to a large surface with large field sizes or a high skin dose to a small surface with a small field

(iii) Provides useful information for estimating stochastic risk to both patients and staff

c. Reference air kerma ($K_{a,r}$)

   (i) Provides real-time information to the operator on the total air kerma (without backscatter) delivered to a reference point on the system.

   (ii) Different reference points are defined for different types of fluoroscopic systems; the reference point on an interventional fluoroscope is on the central ray of the x-ray beam and 15 cm from isocenter toward the x-ray tube.

   (iii) On an interventional C-arm, the reference point moves with the gantry and is seldom exactly on the patient's skin (Fig. 9-18).

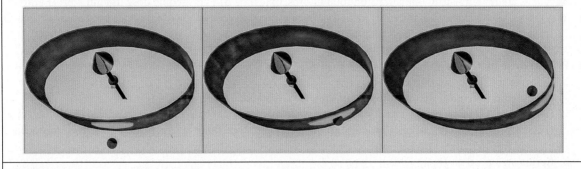

■ **FIGURE 9-18** Dose reference point (DRP) motion for an interventional C-arm fluoroscope. The reference point (indicated by the *red dot*) is outside the patient for the PA projection, on the patient's skin at 45°, and inside the patient near the lateral projection. The actual location will vary depending on patient size and table height. 📖 **F. 9-22**

d. Skin dose maps

   (i) Models the distribution of dose on the surface of a mathematical patient.

   (ii) Calculated from the $K_{a,r}$ from a single irradiation event (*e.g.*, foot-peddle actuation), a backscatter factor, collimator settings, gantry angle, and table position.

   (iii) Dose distributions add in the same area if there is no beam motion. Distributions are mapped to different regions when motion occurs.

   (iv) Radiation is additive between irradiations in regions of overlap.

   (v) The peak skin dose (PSD) is simply the highest dose on the model. It is an indicator of the highest dose on the patient's skin.

   (vi) Displays often include additional information that facilitates repositioning the beam if possible when currently-in-beam surface dose is of concern (Fig. 9-19).

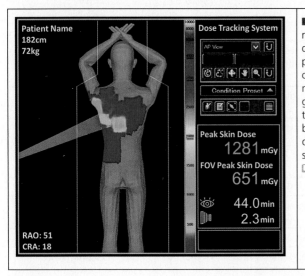

■ **FIGURE 9-19** Example of a real-time skin dose map. The fluoroscope uses its geometric and dosimetric data to "paint" the distribution of radiation on a mathematical model of the patient's skin in real time. The map shows the total distribution of radiation using a color code. The peak skin dose is indicated numerically. The current location of the x-ray beam is shown graphically. In this case, the current beam location corresponds to PSD. Operators' can use these data as part of ongoing patient benefit-risk evaluations during the procedure. Real-time skin dose maps will be provided on all new interventional fluoroscopes in the early 2020s. (Courtesy of Canon Medical Systems.) 📖 **F. 9-23**

2. **Patient radiation documentation and follow-up**
   a. Records of doses to the patient from each procedure should be kept for quality assurance.
   b. If the estimated skin doses are large enough to cause skin injury, clinical follow-up is recommended.
   c. Such large skin doses are most likely to be imparted by prolonged procedures or multiple procedures performed in the same anatomical area within a few months.

## 9.9 OPERATOR AND STAFF RADIATION SAFETY

Occupational exposures of physicians, and other personnel who routinely work in fluoroscopic suites, is often unavoidable. Table 9-2 outlines the effects of changing imaging parameters on staff irradiation. Measures that staff can take to reduce their own exposure are presented in Section 21.6.1 of the textbook.

1. **Worker dose monitoring and tracking**
   a. Scatter fields produced by fluoroscopy vary in time and space during procedures (Fig. 9-20).
   b. Modified by radioprotective devices (*e.g.*, face shields, table-mounted drapes).
   c. Staff move within these fields as they perform their duties.
   d. Because of this variability, radiation monitors should be worn by every person working in a fluoro room.

## 9.10 LOOKING AHEAD

1. **Increased image processing power** has had a substantial impact on improving conspicuity of clinically relevant objects and reducing dose in the same time interval.
2. **Algorithms** rely on a priori knowledge of the examination in progress as supplied by the operator.
3. **Collecting information** on current and historical images might improve performance in future systems.
4. **Combination modalities** such as real-time ultrasound and volumetric CT data can potentially be used to reduce the use of live fluoroscopy and fluorography through parallel image displays and image fusion.

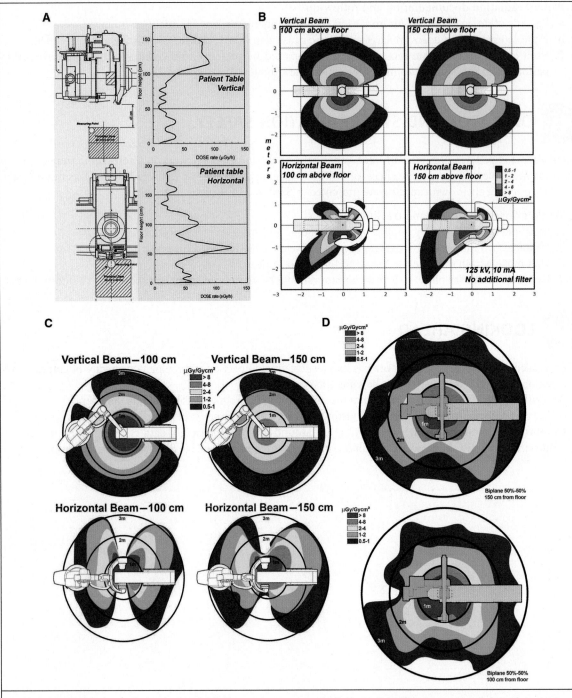

**■ FIGURE 9-20** Scatter radiation maps provided in system user manuals. **A.** Zone of significant occupancy (where the operator usually stands) for a general purpose R/F system. **B and C.** Area around two different single-plane interventional systems. Horizontal plots at 100, 150 cm above floor for horizontal and vertical beam orientations. Portions of the gantry and x-ray tube attenuate the scatter. In both **(B)** and **(C)** (lateral at 100 cm), it is seen that there is no stray radiation field behind the x-ray tube assembly. This indicates that there is minimal tube-leakage contribution to the stray field. The asymmetry in scatter from the patient can be seen in the lateral plots. In the absence of protective devices, an operator standing near the x-ray tube would be exposed to 1 to 10 mGy/h; on the image receptor side, the value is reduced by an order of magnitude. **D.** Area around a biplane interventional system. Both planes are operating simultaneously. Each plane supplies 50% of the KAP and thus contributes to the scatter field. At any point, however, the fraction of scatter supplied by each plane differs. Plots **(B–D)** are scaled in KAP; lower dose rates and better collimation will reduce operator dose. (Adapted with permission from **(A)** Canon Medical Systems, **(B)** Philips, **(C)** Siemens Healthineers, and **(D)** GE Healthcare) 📖 **F. 9-24**

# Section II Questions and Answers

1. Fluoroscopic systems are NOT intended to:
   A. observe motion of anatomical structures
   B. observe motion of introduced devices
   C. radiographically document anatomical structures
   D. radiographically document the presence of contrast media
   E. replace projection radiography

2. During a procedure, the operator's controls provide the ability to set the:
   A. configuration of the examination protocol selection button (EPSB)
   B. maximum total fluoroscopic time for the procedure
   C. maximum total patient dose for the procedure
   D. size and shape of the automatic exposure rate control (AERC) measuring field
   E. size and shape of the active image

3. All current fluoroscopic imaging chains include:
   A. analog video tubes
   B. collimators
   C. direct conversion fluoroscopic screens
   D. image documentation using photofluorographic cameras
   E. optical viewing of image intensifier outputs

4. Modern fluoroscopes no longer provide:
   A. cine fluorography
   B. digital fluorography
   C. digital subtraction fluorography
   D. pulsed fluoroscopy
   E. spot film radiographic cassettes

5. The x-ray image intensifier:
   A. contains a flat CsI input screen
   B. has a photocathode
   C. provides a direct digital image
   D. provides an output image whose physical size varies with the operator selected FOV
   E. uses the approximately 25 kV potential difference between anode and cathode as the only source of brightness gain

6. The fluoroscopic flat-panel image receptor:
   A. is surrounded by a vacuum envelope
   B. requires a slightly higher radiation dose rate than an image intensifier for fluoroscopy
   C. typically has a detective quantum efficiency (DQE) that is three times as high as an image intensifier
   D. uses a smaller electronic amplification factor for fluoroscopy than fluorography

7. A flat-panel detector:
   A. does not require an antiscatter grid
   B. does not require electron optics
   C. has significantly higher detective quantum efficiency (DQE)
   D. has significantly higher intrinsic spatial resolution
   E. requires higher dose rate increases when the active FOV is reduced

8. In comparison to a radiographic x-ray tube, an interventional fluoroscopic tube usually has a:
   A. grounded anode
   B. higher heat capacity
   C. lower cooling rate
   D. lower maximum power limits
   E. single focal spot

9. An interventional fluoroscopic collimator usually has:
   A. a 5 cm minimum distance from the focal spot to the end of the collimator
   B. a light localizer to visually indicate the x-ray beam size
   C. automatic compensation for anode heel effects
   D. sensors that automatically adjust the radiation dose rate for different body parts
   E. the ability to automatically adjust beam size as the image receptor's SID is changed

10. Beam filters used to improve the conspicuity of iodinated contrast media are made of:
    A. carbon
    B. copper
    C. iodine
    D. silver
    E. tungsten

11. The fluoroscope's automatic exposure rate control (AERC) is designed to limit:
    A. changes in image receptor dose rate
    B. patient maximum skin dose rate to 88 mGy/min for DSA
    C. patient maximum skin dose rate to 88 mGy/min for fluoroscopy
    D. patient total skin dose for DSA
    E. patient total skin dose for fluoroscopy

12. For pulsed fluoroscopy:
    A. images are always displayed to the operator at the acquisition pulse rate
    B. patient skin dose rate is always proportional to the pulse rate
    C. shorter pulses reduce potential motion unsharpness
    D. shorter pulses reduce the visibility of x-ray quantum noise
    E. the most common pulse rate is 30 pulses per second

13. A fluoroscope is equipped to perform fluoroscopy, digital angiography, and digital subtraction angiography. The ratios of the relative doses per frame (FL:DA:DSA) are approximately:
    A. 1:1:1
    B. 1:1:10
    C. 1:1:100
    D. 1:10:100
    E. 1:100:100

14. A DSA sequence:
    A. can only be produced by injecting iodinated contrast media during the sequence
    B. can only be produced if there is no patient motion during the sequence
    C. could be produced by injecting $CO_2$ during the sequence
    D. could be produced by injecting saline during the sequence

15. Digital cine fluorography:
    A. is performed at the same dose rate (mGy/min) at any frame rate
    B. is performed at the same frame rate used for film-based cine cameras
    C. must be used if the image sequences are to be saved
    D. requires separate image handling video hardware than fluoroscopy
    E. runs can be eliminated if stored fluoroscopic sequences are of adequate quality

16. The relationship between the x-ray intensity at a pixel in the image receptor and the brightness of the corresponding pixel on the display monitor is determined by:
    A. a software look-up table in the fluoroscope
    B. the composition of the x-ray conversion layer in the image receptor
    C. the display monitor's construction (*e.g.*, CRT or LED)
    D. the percentage of scatter in the image
    E. the x-ray factors used to generate the image

17. A "moving vessel" recursive-filtering protocol is selected to obtain anatomic information of a contrast-filled artery rapidly moving over a relatively homogeneous background. When temporal adaptive image processing is applied:
    A. the sharpness of the image will be decreased
    B. the sharpness of the image will be increased
    C. visible noise near the artery will be decreased
    D. visible noise near the artery will be increased

18. The fluoroscopic image perceived by the operator is usually:
    A. identical for large and small viewing monitors
    B. identical to image captured by the image receptor
    C. processed to reduce contrast range
    D. processed to reduce image noise
    E. processed to reduce spatial resolution

19. Perceived noise in a fluoroscopic image IS NOT reduced by:
    A. averaging nearby pixels in a single image
    B. averaging the same pixel in sequential images
    C. increasing the frame rate
    D. increasing the x-ray dose rate at the image receptor
    E. reducing the x-ray dose rate at the image receptor

20. The limiting spatial resolution (LSR) of an isocentric fluoroscopic system is tested using a lead bar pattern placed at isocenter and an SID of 80 cm (FOV 40 cm, no collimation). A baseline image is acquired using the small focal spot at a reference air kerma rate of 10 mGy/min. The LSR can usually be improved by:
    A. decreasing the FPD's FOV from 40 to 30 cm
    B. increasing the AK rate used to acquire the image
    C. increasing the SID to 120
    D. reducing the fluoroscopic pulse width
    E. selecting a larger focal spot

21. The low-contrast detectability (LCD) of an isocentric fluoroscopic system is tested using a contrast test tool placed at isocenter and an SID of 80 cm (FOV 40 cm, no collimation). A baseline image is acquired using the small focal spot and a reference air kerma rate of 10 mGy/min. The LCD can usually be improved by:
    A. decreasing the FPD's FOV from 40 to 30 cm
    B. increasing the AK rate used to acquire the image
    C. increasing the SID 120 cm
    D. reducing the fluoroscopic pulse width
    E. selecting a larger focal spot

22. The sharpness of an image in an isocentric fluoroscopic system is tested by moving an 0.035 guidewire placed at isocenter and an SID of 80 cm (FOV 40 cm, no collimation). A baseline image is acquired using the small focal spot and a reference air kerma rate of 10 mGy/min. The sharpness of the guidewire can usually be improved by:
    A. decreasing the FPD's FOV from 40 to 30 cm
    B. increasing the AK rate used to acquire the image
    C. increasing the SID 120 cm
    D. reducing the fluoroscopic pulse width
    E. selecting a larger focal spot

23. For a C-arm fluoroscope, the maximum normal fluoroscopic dose rate during a clinical procedure is:
    A. accurately displayed to the operator as reference AK during a procedure
    B. limited by FDA regulations to 88 mGy/min 30 cm from the focal spot
    C. limited by FDA regulations to 88 mGy/min 30 cm from the image receptor
    D. the same at any distance from the focal spot
    E. unlimited provided that the patient is an adult

24. The peak skin dose delivered by a clinical procedure is:
    A. accurately displayed to the operator as reference AK at the end of a procedure
    B. limited by FDA regulations to 2,000 mGy to prevent any possible tissue reaction
    C. limited by the Joint Commission to 5,000 mGy to prevent a severe tissue reaction
    D. no more than can be clinically justified
    E. unlimited provided that the patient is an adult

25. Which of the following dose metrics can be best used to estimate the patient's stochastic risk from a fluoroscopic procedure?
    A. Fluoroscopy time
    B. Kerma area product
    C. Peak skin dose
    D. Reference air kerma

26. In the absence of external shields (*e.g.*, lead drapes), the main source of stray radiation reaching the operator is attributable to:
    A. leakage from the x-ray tube assembly
    B. scatter from the patient
    C. scatter from the patient support
    D. secondary scatter from the walls of the procedure room
    E. transmission through the image receptor

27. The distribution of dose to a fluoroscopist's organs during a single procedure:
    A. can vary by a factor of less than 10
    B. can vary by a factor of more than 10
    C. is directly proportional to fluoroscopic time
    D. is not correlated with the fluoroscopist's height
    E. is uniform

28. The secondary radiation field produced by a monoplane isocentric fluoroscope without secondary shielding (*e.g.*, lead drapes):
    A. differs on both sides of the table at 100 cm above the floor when the beam is horizontal (direction left to right)
    B. differs on both sides of the table at 100 cm above the floor when the beam is vertical (direction floor to ceiling)
    C. enhanced behind the x-ray tube because of tube leakage
    D. increases with height above the table when the beam is vertical (direction floor to ceiling)

# Answers

1. **E**  Fluoroscopy systems provide the temporal resolution necessary for the operator to use image guidance for the placement of medical devices (*e.g.*, catheters, stents, etc.) or to observe temporal physiological phenomena. *(Pg. 309)*
Projection radiography provides static images for interpretation and archiving. Projection radiographs generally have higher spatial resolution than images acquired through a fluoroscopic system.

2. **E**  Image acquisition and display controls include x-ray generator settings including automatic exposure rate control (AERC), image-receptor FOV, image processing methods, and image display adjustments. *(Fig. 9-1)*
The EPSB selection set and accompanying AERC parameters are installed into the fluoroscope by service personnel; these settings cannot be permanently reprogrammed by an operator during a procedure. However, most configurations do provide certain adjustments to accommodate clinical requirements (*e.g.*, normal or low dose rate). Systems never limit total fluoroscopic time or patient dose.

3. **B**  All current fluoroscopic imaging chains include collimators. *(Fig. 9-2)*
Direct conversion fluoroscopic screens convert the x-ray beam into an unamplified light image. The first generation of image intensifiers relied on optical viewing. Photofluorographic cameras recorded the output of the image intensifier onto photographic film. The analog video camera directly transmitted images to an analog viewing monitor, with very limited associated image processing or recording.

4. **E**  Modern fluoroscopes no longer provide spot film radiographic cassettes. *(Pg. 311)*
The spot film changer mechanically placed a radiographic cassette between the patient and the image intensifier to obtain archival images. This facility was no longer required once the images produced through the fluoroscopic chain were of diagnostic quality.

5. **B**  The x-ray image intensifier has a photocathode. *(Fig. 9-3)*
The photocathode follows the image intensifier's curved input screen and converts the light image into electronic form. The electron optics converge this image onto a fixed size output screen while producing brightness gain by a combination of minification and electron acceleration.

6. **B**  The fluoroscopic flat-panel image receptor requires a slightly higher radiation dose rate than an image intensifier for fluoroscopy. *(Pg. 317)*
The brightness gain in an image intensifier provides more light to the electronics than the amount available in a flat panel. Thus, the FP's electronics must operate at a higher gain, resulting in higher system noise at fluoroscopy levels. Thus, a slightly higher fluoroscopic dose rate is needed to produce a clinically acceptable noise level. However, less amplification is needed at fluorographic dose levels, noise is determined by the x-ray beam, and dose rates are similar for both technologies.

7. **B**  A flat-panel detector does not require electron optics. *(Fig. 9-5)*
Scatter reaching the image receptor is the same for both technologies, grids are thus needed. The inputs to both the II and FP are CsI layers, the DQE and spatial resolution are similar. IIs have reduced brightness gain when the active FOV is reduced due to less minification gain. This is compensated by increasing the dose rate. FPs generally use fewer dexels for reduced FOVs. There is no need to compensate for lost brightness. However, noise is more visible in the images produced at small FOVs; modest increases in dose rate are applied to provide equal perceived noise at smaller FOVs.

8. **B**  In comparison to a radiographic x-ray tube, an interventional fluoroscopic tube usually has a higher heat capacity. *(Pg. 317)*

Copper spectral filters used in interventional tubes will produce reduced beam intensity relative to tubes using conventional aluminum filters. Tubes with higher heat capacity achieve the necessary beam intensity by increasing mA while limiting kV increases. Limiting kV improves iodine conspicuity.

9. **E**    An interventional fluoroscopic collimator usually has the ability to automatically adjust beam size as the image receptor's SID is changed. *(Pg. 318)*
Safety requires that the x-ray beam be confined to the active area of the image receptor. Automatic beam size adjustments are needed to meet this requirement as SID is changed. The physical of the x-ray beam emerging from the collimator is smaller at large SID.

10. **B**    Beam filters used to improve the conspicuity of iodinated contrast media are usually made of copper. *(Pg. 319)*
Copper is used because it is more efficient in removing low-energy photons than lower atomic number (Z) materials such as carbon. Prefiltering with iodine will reduce the number of photons in the energy band needed to "see" contrast media. High Z materials suppress the entire useful spectrum.

11. **A**    AERC controls limits changes in image receptor dose rate. *(Pg. 320)*
The purpose of AERC is to maintain constant signal-to-noise ratio as patient size changes. To accomplish this, radiation output is controlled to maintain a constant image receptor dose rate. The AERC does not limit total doses or dose rates for DSA. Regulations limit maximum fluoro dose rate under test conditions, not at the patient's skin.

12. **C**    For pulsed fluoroscopy, shorter pulses reduce potential motion unsharpness. *(Fig. 9-10)*
The relationship between patient skin dose rate and pulse rate is programmable. Some systems deliver the same dose per pulse irrespective of pulse rate. Others increase the dose per pulse as the pulse rate decreases to maintain constant perceived image noise.

13. **D**    The ratios of the relative doses per frame (FL:DA:DSA) are approximately 1:10:100. *(Pg. 324)*
Higher doses are required for DA than fluoro to minimize visual noise when DA frames are viewed statically. DSA consists of subtracting two DA frames and then stretching the image contrast. Subtraction does not remove quantum noise; contrast stretching increases noise visibility.

14. **C**    A DSA sequence could be produced by injecting $CO_2$. *(Pg. 324–325)*
Iodine or $CO_2$ provide the necessary attenuation in the "live" frame needed for visualization; saline does not. Patient motion can be corrected by pixel shifting the mask and "live" frames before subtraction.

15. **E**    Cine fluorography runs can be eliminated if stored fluoroscopic sequences are of adequate quality. *(Pg. 326–327)*
Digital cine is captured and stored through the same imaging channel as fluoroscopy. Fluoroscopic runs can be retrospectively saved on most fluoroscopes. There is no need to repeat runs for documentation using cine if the stored fluoro sequence meets clinical needs.

16. **A**    The relationship between the x-ray intensity at a pixel in the image receptor and the brightness of the corresponding pixel on the display monitor is determined by a software look-up table in the fluoroscope. *(Pg. 330)*
The output of the image receptor is a pixel-by-pixel array of digital numbers representing the local detected x-ray intensities. A software look-up table (LUT) transforms these values to monitor brightness in a manner intended to maximize clinical utility of the image. Some aspects of the LUT, such as brightness and contrast, are readily controllable by the operator.

17. **D**    When temporal adaptive image processing is applied, visible noise near the artery will be increased. *(Fig. 9-16)*
Adaptive image processors may locally reduce recursive filtering near an artery to reduce motion blur or ghosting. This increases noise.

18. **D**    The fluoroscopic image perceived by the operator is usually processed to reduce image noise. *(Fig. 9-15)*
The image produced by the receptor is processed before display to improve its clinical utility. Typically, contrast is increased while preserving spatial resolution. The perceived image is further influenced by the physiology of the operator's eye-brain system.

19. **E**    Perceived noise in a fluoroscopic image is not reduced by reducing the x-ray dose rate at the image receptor. *(Pg. 323)*
X-ray quantum noise in the image is the limiting factor in perceived noise. Reducing dose rate at the image receptor will always increase quantum noise.

20. **C**   The limiting spatial resolution can usually be improved by increasing the SID to 120 cm. (*Fig. 9-20*)
Spatial resolution when using the small focal spot is usually limited by the FPDs pixel matrix. In this example, the same pixel size is used for the 40 and 30 cm FOV. Geometric magnification by increasing the SID results in each pixel in the image representing a smaller area on the text pattern, thus improving spatial resolution.

21. **B**   Fluoroscopic LCD can usually be improved by increasing the AK rate used to acquire the image. (*Pg. 326*)
LCD is determined by image noise, primarily x-ray quantum noise. Increasing the AK rate increases the number of available photons in an image, thereby reducing quantum noise and increasing LCD.

22. **D**   The sharpness of a moving guidewire can usually be improved by reducing the fluoroscopic pulse width. (*Pg. 323*)
The static 0.035 wire is easily resolved. Its image is blurred by its motion during a single pulse. Reducing pulse width increases apparent sharpness.

23. **C**   The maximum normal fluoroscopic dose rate during a clinical procedure is limited by FDA regulations to 88 mGy/min 30 cm from the image receptor. (*Pg. 339*)
To meet regulatory testing requirements, this point was chosen to be near the patient's entrance skin location assuming that the image receptor is close to the patient. The reference AK displayed to the operator is 15 cm from isocenter toward the x-ray tube. These two points are seldom identical.

24. **D**   The peak skin dose (PSD) delivered by a clinical procedure is no more than can be clinically justified. (*Pg. 339*)
Appropriate total radiation use is part of the practice of medicine. The displayed AK does not include patient or gantry motion and usually does not represent PSD. Newer fluoroscopes will include real-time dose maps to provide PSD information to the operator.

25. **B**   Kerma area product (KAP) provides the best estimate of the patient's stochastic risk. (*Pg. 339*)
KAP is proportional to the total x-ray energy delivered to the patient. PSD and reference air kerma are doses delivered to a point and are relatively the same for large or small fields. Fluoroscopic time is a poor indicator of any of the other quantities and therefore a poor predictor of any kind of radiological risk.

26. **B**   The main source of stray radiation reaching the operator is attributable to scatter from the patient. (*Pg. 343*)
X-ray tube assemblies and image receptors have built-in shielding that limits leakage and transmission to well below patient scatter levels. Scatter from the patient support is small. The intensity of backscatter from the walls is less than 1% of the intensity of the scatter reaching the wall.

27. **B**   The distribution of dose to a fluoroscopist's organs during a single procedure can vary by a factor of more than 10. (*Pg. 344*)
A standard lead apron attenuates at least 90% of the beam producing a factor of 10 gradient by itself. The scatter distribution from the patient produces further gradients in operator exposure, thus increasing inhomogeneity. The eyes of a short fluoroscopist are closer to the patient than those of a taller individual; this results in differences in eye dose.

28. **A**   Differs on both sides of the table at 100 cm above the floor when the beam is horizontal (direction left to right). (*Fig. 9-24*)
Scatter is much greater on the x-ray tube side. Scatter maps are shown in Fig. 9-20 (*Fig. 9-24*)

# Section III Key Equations and Symbols

| QUANTITY | EQUATION | EQ#/PAGE/COMMENTS |
|---|---|---|
| Image intensifier brightness | Brightness gain = Minification gain × Electronic gain | Eq. 9-1/Pg. 314/Minification gain in an image intensifier is proportional to the ratios of the active area of the input and the fixed area output screen. Thus, brightness gain decreases when the FOV is reduced, this requires an increase in dose rate. |
| Image recursion | $DI = \alpha NI + (1 - \alpha)PDI$ | Eq. 9-2/Pg. 329. <br><br> DI: Displayed image <br><br> NI: Newly acquired image <br><br> PDI: Previously displayed image. |

| SYMBOL | QUANTITY | UNITS |
|---|---|---|
| *AERC* | Automatic exposure rate control | N/A |
| CFF | Critical flicker frequency | ~30 frames/second—the number of frames/s where flicker is not perceived |
| CINE | Cine fluorography | N/A |
| DA | Digital angiography | N/A |
| DEXEL | Image receptor detector element | mm × mm |
| DI | Displayed image | Image displayed to the operator after temporal averaging |
| DRP | Dose reference point | Point in space where a fluoroscope reports $K_{a,r}$ |
| DSA | Digital subtraction angiography | N/A |
| DTF | Display transfer function | Look-up table to convert digital pixel values into display brightness levels |
| FOV | Field of view | cm, inch |
| FPD | Flat-panel detector | N/A |
| HVL | Half value layer | mm of a stated material (*e.g.*, Al) |
| $K_{a,r}$ | Air kerma at reference point | mGy |
| KAP (DAP) | Kerma area product <br><br> Dose area product | Gy cm$^2$, cGy cm$^2$, mGy cm$^2$, mGy m$^2$ |
| NI | Newly acquired image | Latest single frame produced by the fluoroscope |
| PDI | Previously displayed image | Image displayed to the operator before adding the newly acquired image (NI) |
| PIXEL | Picture element (in an image) | N/A |
| PSD | Peak skin dose | mGy, Gy |
| Pulse rate | Number of pulses per second | number |
| Pulse width | Duration of a fluoro pulse | milliseconds |
| RPPE | Radiation personal protective equipment | *e.g.*, lead apron, thyroid shield, lead eyewear |
| SID | Source to image receptor distance | cm |

# CHAPTER 10

# Computed Tomography

## 10.0  INTRODUCTION

Computed tomography (CT) has experienced enormous growth in clinical use over the past three decades primarily due to significant advances in image quality and a dramatic reduction in acquisition time as the technology has advanced. Image quality has increased because of better detector sampling along the long axis ($z$-dimension) of the patient with multiple detector array systems of 40 to 160 mm beam coverage in one rotation. CT reconstruction has advanced from filtered backprojection (FBP) to generations of iterative reconstruction and deep learning (DL)-based adjuncts, providing lower noise images at lower radiation dose levels for improved spatial resolution and contrast resolution. With half-second gantry rotation (or shorter), 80 mm of patient length can be acquired in 1 second (s), and hence 400 mm of patient length can be scanned in 5 s.

CT imaging has gained widespread use across many clinical applications for abdominal, thoracic, head, musculoskeletal, CT angiography (CTA), organ-specific CT perfusion, and dual-energy CT. Thin-slice axial images, multiplanar reconstruction, and 3D volume rendering reconstruction allows segmentation of bone structures from soft tissue, accurate assessment of iodinated contrast in CT angiograms, and the ability to use volumetric data for 3D printing. Coronal and sagittal CT visualization provides important additional information to the interpreting physician, for spinal alignment, orientation of pathology, and normal anatomy including identifying feeding vessels, gastrointestinal tract topography, abdominal organ placement and orientation, trauma, and other factors.

1. **Acquisition geometry**—x-ray tube rotates in a gantry around the long axis of the body
   a. For one rotation, multiple projections are acquired and reconstructed into axial images.
   b. Two-dimensional images are comprised of pixels with equal dimensions in horizontal ($x$) and vertical ($y$) axes.
   c. The image represents a volumetric section of the patient with a thickness $\Delta z$ (Fig. 10-1).
   d. Dimensions of each voxel are on the order of 0.6 mm ($\Delta x$ and $\Delta y$) by 0.5 mm ($\Delta z$).
   e. A 75-kg person can be imaged with over 400 million voxels using CT.
2. **Volume data set and multiplanar reconstruction** from thin-slice axial images (Fig. 10-2)
   a. Routine reformatting into the coronal and sagittal planes provide intuitive anatomical display.

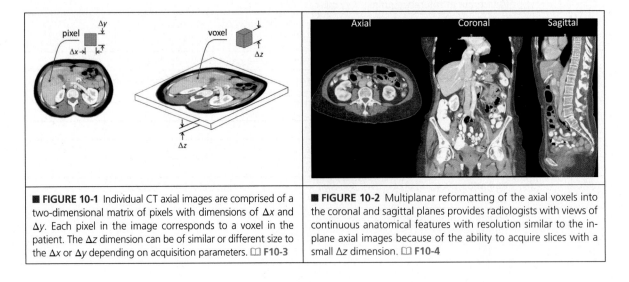

■ **FIGURE 10-1** Individual CT axial images are comprised of a two-dimensional matrix of pixels with dimensions of $\Delta x$ and $\Delta y$. Each pixel in the image corresponds to a voxel in the patient. The $\Delta z$ dimension can be of similar or different size to the $\Delta x$ or $\Delta y$ depending on acquisition parameters. 📖 **F10-3**

■ **FIGURE 10-2** Multiplanar reformatting of the axial voxels into the coronal and sagittal planes provides radiologists with views of continuous anatomical features with resolution similar to the in-plane axial images because of the ability to acquire slices with a small $\Delta z$ dimension. 📖 **F10-4**

## 10.1  BASIC CONCEPTS

1. X-ray tube potential for routine scanning—120 kV; other tube voltages also used
   a. Tube voltage is varied to optimize image quality versus radiation dose for clinical applications.
   b. Protocols and selection of voltage are based on patient size and clinical need or diagnosis.
   c. Tube voltage options (typical): 80, 100, 120, 140 kV (Fig. 10-3).
      (i)   Added filtration in beam creates a "hard" x-ray spectrum.
      (ii)  Physical properties (attenuation) of tissues are based on these spectra.
   d. Effective energy for kV spectra range from approximately 43 to approximately 70 keV (Fig. 10-4).
   e. Compton scatter is 10-fold more likely than photoelectric or Rayleigh scatter interactions for soft tissue.
   f. For bone and iodinated contrast agents, the photoelectric interaction does play an important role.
2. Attenuation coefficient for Compton interactions, Equation 10-1:

$$\mu_{Compton} \propto \rho N \frac{Z}{A}$$

[10-1]

where $N$ is Avogadro's number ($6.023 \times 10^{23}$), $Z$ is the atomic number, and $A$ is the atomic mass

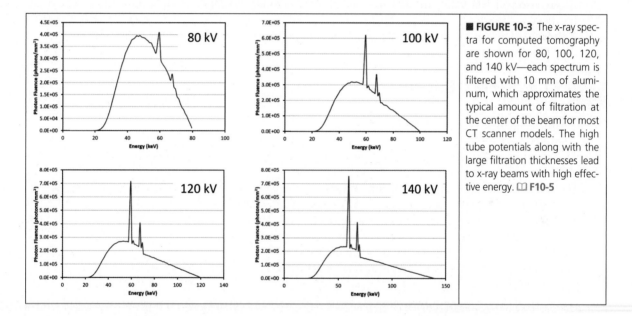

■ **FIGURE 10-3** The x-ray spectra for computed tomography are shown for 80, 100, 120, and 140 kV—each spectrum is filtered with 10 mm of aluminum, which approximates the typical amount of filtration at the center of the beam for most CT scanner models. The high tube potentials along with the large filtration thicknesses lead to x-ray beams with high effective energy. ▭ **F10-5**

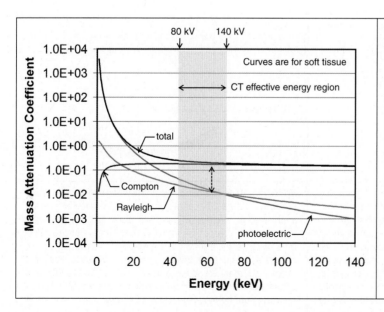

■ **FIGURE 10-4** What physical parameter does the grayscale in a CT image correspond to? The mass attenuation coefficient of soft tissue is shown as a function of x-ray energy in this graph. The curves correspond to the attenuation coefficients for the photoelectric effect, Rayleigh, and Compton scattering. The effective energy in CT is outlined by the vertical band. In this region, it is seen that the Compton cross-section is approximately 10-fold that of the Rayleigh or photoelectric cross-sections, meaning that the grayscale (Hounsfield unit) in CT for soft tissue is primarily determined by the physical dependency of Compton scattering—electron density. ▭ **F10-6**

**a.** For most elements (except *H*), *Z/A* ratio is ½; density tends to dominate when comparing adipose-rich tissues (lower density) to soft tissues in terms of attenuation at these energies.

**3.** The *Hounsfield unit* (so named after a principal developer of CT, Sir Godfrey Hounsfield)

   **a.** Preprocessing of CT acquired data applies a logarithmic function to the ratio of incident to transmitted x-ray intensity: $ln \frac{I_o}{T}$; this effectively linearizes the effective attenuation coefficient.

   **b.** Subsequent reconstruction provides grayscale encoding (Eq. 10-2), a function of the linear attenuation coefficient, called the Hounsfield unit (HU).

$$HU_K \cong 1,000 \left[ \frac{\mu_K - \mu_w}{\mu_w} \right]$$

[10-2]

   For a given voxel in the image, K, which contains average $\mu_K$, the HU is scaled to $\mu_w$, the linear attenuation coefficient of water.

   **c.** The HU is defined at water ($\mu_K = \mu_w$); $HU_{water} = 0$, and air ($\mu_K = \mu_{air}$); $HU_{air} = -1,000$.

   **d.** $\mu$ has relatively strong dependencies on x-ray beam energy as $\mu(E)$.

   **(i)** The notation for $\mu$ in Equation 10-2 represents the *effective* linear attenuation coefficient, $\mu_{eff}$.

   **(ii)** Calibration of HU is slightly different at each tube voltage, but for water HU = 0 at all tube voltages; other tissues such as liver and bone will have slightly different HU values at different tube potentials.

   **e.** Imprecision in HU values results from calibration, scattered radiation, quantum noise, and beam hardening.

   **f.** Typical HU for water is usually within ±5 HU with often larger deviations for other tissues and air.

## 10.2 CT SYSTEM DESIGNS

**1. The gantry—geometry and detector configuration**

   **a.** Clinical CT scanners have the x-ray source and detector arrays arranged in an arc (Fig. 10-5).

   **b.** Detector arrays aligned along a radius of curvature provide perpendicular incidence of the beam.

   **c.** A *fan-beam* projection incident on individual detectors.

   **(i)** For a given view (tube position and view angle), the individual x-rays (*rays*) define a line integral extending from the source to each individual detector along the detector array.

   **(ii)** The collection of all rays across the detector elements constitutes a *view* or *projection*.

   **(iii)** Raw data collected during a scan are comprised of rays and views.

   **d.** Basic geometry of a CT scanner and dimensions (Fig. 10-6).

   **(i)** Isocenter of rotation is almost always the center of the reconstructed image.

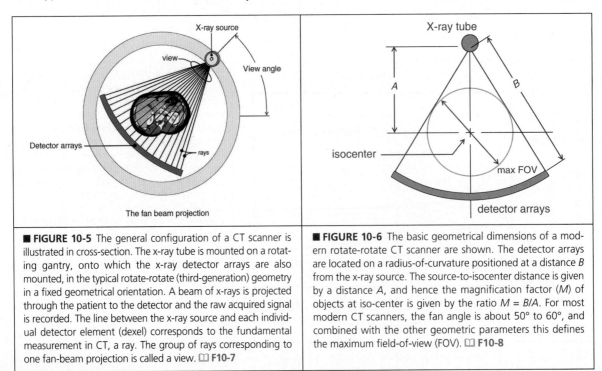

■ **FIGURE 10-5** The general configuration of a CT scanner is illustrated in cross-section. The x-ray tube is mounted on a rotating gantry, onto which the x-ray detector arrays are also mounted, in the typical rotate-rotate (third-generation) geometry in a fixed geometrical orientation. A beam of x-rays is projected through the patient to the detector and the raw acquired signal is recorded. The line between the x-ray source and each individual detector element (dexel) corresponds to the fundamental measurement in CT, a ray. The group of rays corresponding to one fan-beam projection is called a view. ☐ **F10-7**

■ **FIGURE 10-6** The basic geometrical dimensions of a modern rotate-rotate CT scanner are shown. The detector arrays are located on a radius-of-curvature positioned at a distance *B* from the x-ray source. The source-to-isocenter distance is given by a distance *A*, and hence the magnification factor (*M*) of objects at iso-center is given by the ratio *M = B/A*. For most modern CT scanners, the fan angle is about 50° to 60°, and combined with the other geometric parameters this defines the maximum field-of-view (FOV). ☐ **F10-8**

(ii) For source to isocenter distance $A$, and source to detector distance $B$, magnification $M = B/A$.
(iii) Detector width and length specified at isocenter: if $B = 95$ cm and $A = 50$ cm, $M = 1.9$ and detector width specified as 0.5 mm has an actual physical width of $1.9 \times 0.5 = 0.95$ mm.
(iv) Fan angle of the x-ray beam is approximately 50° to 60° and defines maximum scan FOV.
  e. Multidetector array CT scanner (MDCT) geometry (Fig. 10-7).
    (i) 16, 64, 256, or more detector arrays are abutted to create a larger sampling along the $z$-axis.
    (ii) Divergence of the x-ray beam in the $z$-direction results in a cone angle.
    (iii) Example: a 64 detector array of 0.625 mm width measures 40 mm along $z$, requiring a similar beam width obtained by opening the collimator slit at the x-ray tube port.
    (iv) Systems allow detectors to bin data from adjacent detector arrays to increase slice thickness.
    (v) Larger slice thickness: less image noise (both electronic and quantum), less storage required.
    (vi) Larger slice thickness: more partial volume artifact, less $z$-axis resolution.
    (vii) MDCT reconstructed slice thickness and collimated x-ray beam width are separate parameters.
    (viii) MDCT allows acquisition of faster scans (whole body in seconds for large width arrays).
    (ix) MDCT allows thinner slice acquisitions (thinnest slices are sometimes termed "raw" data).

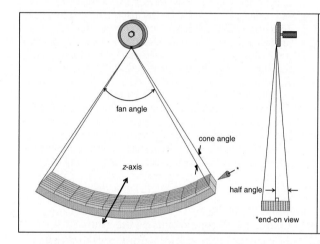

■ **FIGURE 10-7** The angles associated with a modern rotate-rotate CT scanner using multidetector arrays are shown. The fan angle is defined between the x-ray source and the extent of the detector arrays in-plane. All modern multiple detector array CT scanners (MDCT) can be considered cone-beam CT systems, with full-cone angles of 4.2° for a 40-mm detector width at isocenter, and 17.2° for a 160-mm detector width. This cone angle is fully considered in the reconstruction algorithm used to convert the raw acquired data into the final CT volume data set. ⬚ **F10-9**

## 2. Wide-beam (cone-beam) CT systems

  a. All whole-body scanners with ≥64 detector channels are technically cone-beam CT systems.
  b. True cone-beam scanners: where the half cone angle approaches 9°.
  c. Reconstruction algorithms for synthesizing data must take into account the cone angle.
  d. Challenges and benefits of wide cone-angle CT systems.
    (i) Challenges: increased x-ray scatter detection and cone-beam artifacts
    (ii) Benefits: whole organ imaging without table motion (*e.g.*, head, heart, organ perfusion; the latter with high temporal resolution)
  e. Cone-beam systems with flat-panel detectors (Fig. 10-8).
    (i) Full cone angles almost as large as the fan angle are possible.

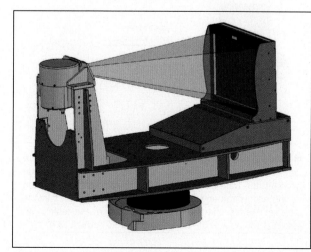

■ **FIGURE 10-8** While modern whole-body CT systems are rightly considered as (small cone angle) cone-beam systems, more traditional specialty application cone-beam CT systems typically use a flat-panel detector opposed to an x-ray source in a rotate-rotate (third-generation) cone-beam geometry, as illustrated. The system in this diagram is designed for pendant-geometry breast imaging and rotates in the horizontal plane. Flat-panel–based cone-beam CT systems enable dedicated CT applications in orthopedic, dental, breast, radiation therapy positioning, and angiographic applications and typically provide higher spatial resolution images albeit with greater artifact potential. ⬚ **F10-10**

    **(ii)** Full 2D bank of detectors and flat geometry, with different reconstruction geometry.

    **(iii)** Detector calibration includes *flat-fielding* to correct for inverse square variations and heel effect.

    **(iv)** Parallax error (nonnormal incidence to the detector at wide angles) cannot be corrected.

    **(v)** Detector readout rates limit acquisition speed; pulsed x-ray tube projections limit motion.

    **(vi)** Applications: dental CT, breast CT, orthopedic, angiographic, and radiation therapy.

**3. The slip ring**

    **a.** The CT gantry x-ray tube and detector array rotate continuously in one direction with a slip ring.

    **b.** The slip ring has a number of electrically conductive tracks and associated contactors (Fig. 10-9).

        **(i)** This maintains electrical contact with the stationary frame to the rotating gantry.

        **(ii)** The x-ray transformer is mounted on the gantry to avoid high voltage and electrical arcing.

        **(iii)** Numerous small conductive tracks with low electronic noise transfer digital signal data out.

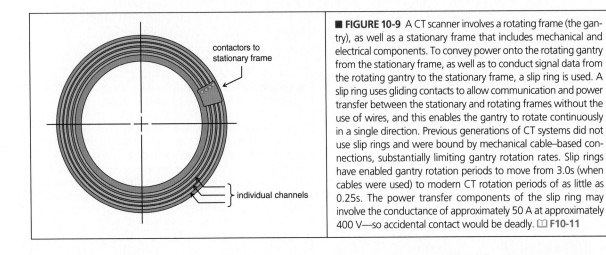

■ **FIGURE 10-9** A CT scanner involves a rotating frame (the gantry), as well as a stationary frame that includes mechanical and electrical components. To convey power onto the rotating gantry from the stationary frame, as well as to conduct signal data from the rotating gantry to the stationary frame, a slip ring is used. A slip ring uses gliding contacts to allow communication and power transfer between the stationary and rotating frames without the use of wires, and this enables the gantry to rotate continuously in a single direction. Previous generations of CT systems did not use slip rings and were bound by mechanical cable–based connections, substantially limiting gantry rotation rates. Slip rings have enabled gantry rotation periods to move from 3.0s (when cables were used) to modern CT rotation periods of as little as 0.25s. The power transfer components of the slip ring may involve the conductance of approximately 50 A at approximately 400 V—so accidental contact would be deadly. 📖 **F10-11**

*(labels in figure: contactors to stationary frame; individual channels)*

    **c.** Helical and high-speed rotations are enabled, with high centrifugal forces exceeding 20 g's.

        **(i)** Special design considerations and hardware are required for all components on the gantry.

        **(ii)** X-ray tube focal spots have flat emitter design with magnetic/electrostatic focusing coils to withstand high gyroscopic forces (see Chapter 6 for details).

**4. The patient table (couch)**

    **a.** The table is an important and highly integrated CT scanner component.

    **b.** The CT computer controls longitudinal table motion with precision motors and feedback.

        **(i)** Precise control and positioning of the table is important, particularly for helical acquisition.

        **(ii)** Accuracy of anatomic positioning is essential.

        **(iii)** Table position accuracy is evaluated during routine CT scanner testing.

    **c.** Height adjustment allows for convenient patient access and centering in the FOV (Figs. 10-10 and 10-11).

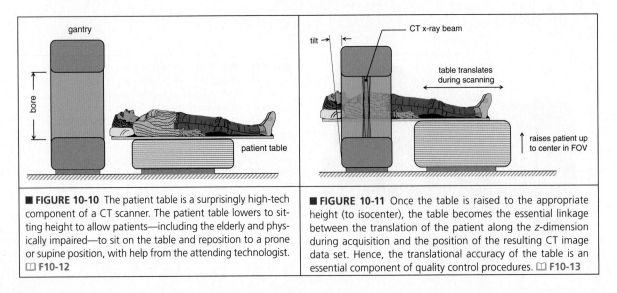

■ **FIGURE 10-10** The patient table is a surprisingly high-tech component of a CT scanner. The patient table lowers to sitting height to allow patients—including the elderly and physically impaired—to sit on the table and reposition to a prone or supine position, with help from the attending technologist. 📖 **F10-12**

■ **FIGURE 10-11** Once the table is raised to the appropriate height (to isocenter), the table becomes the essential linkage between the translation of the patient along the *z*-dimension during acquisition and the position of the resulting CT image data set. Hence, the translational accuracy of the table is an essential component of quality control procedures. 📖 **F10-13**

*(labels in figures: gantry; bore; patient table; CT x-ray beam; tilt; table translates during scanning; raises patient up to center in FOV)*

## 5. The x-ray tube and CT detector characteristics

**a.** CT x-ray tubes have the highest power loading and heat dissipation ratings.

  **(i)** MDCT acquisition geometry: better use of tube output with larger collimator and beam width.

  **(ii)** Plane of anode rotation is parallel to plane of gantry rotation to reduce gyroscopic forces.

  **(iii)** Anode-cathode axis is parallel to the $z$-axis of the scanner—so is the heel effect (Fig. 10-12).

  **(iv)** The x-ray output is limited angularly in the anode-cathode direction, but not in the fan angle (Fig. 10-13).

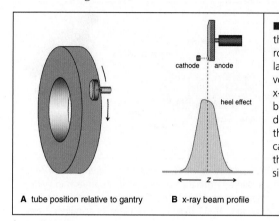

**■ FIGURE 10-12 A.** The plane of the x-ray tube anode is parallel with the rotation of the x-ray tube around the gantry, as illustrated. The high rotational velocity and the large mass of the x-ray tube anode creates large gyroscopic forces, and when considered with the high rotational velocity of the gantry, the only practical mechanical orientation of the x-ray tube is to have the rotational planes of the anode and the gantry be parallel. **B.** With the orientation of the x-ray tube and the gantry as defined in **(A)**, the anode-cathode direction is aligned with the z-axis of the CT scanner. Hence, the heel effect (always parallel to the anode-cathode axis) runs along the z-dimension of the scanner, which is also the dimension of table/patient travel corresponding to the vertical dimension of coronal and sagittal CT images. 📖 **F10-15**

**A** tube position relative to gantry     **B** x-ray beam profile

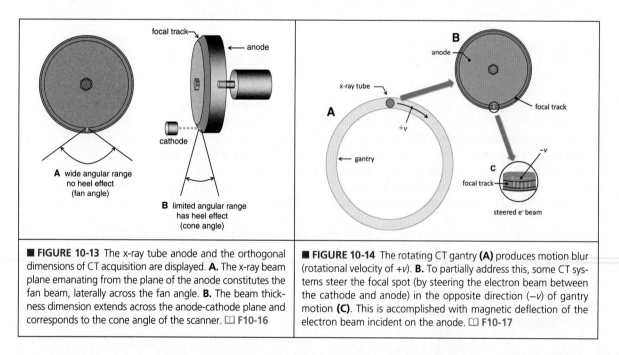

**■ FIGURE 10-13** The x-ray tube anode and the orthogonal dimensions of CT acquisition are displayed. **A.** The x-ray beam plane emanating from the plane of the anode constitutes the fan beam, laterally across the fan angle. **B.** The beam thickness dimension extends across the anode-cathode plane and corresponds to the cone angle of the scanner. 📖 **F10-16**

**■ FIGURE 10-14** The rotating CT gantry **(A)** produces motion blur (rotational velocity of +v). **B.** To partially address this, some CT systems steer the focal spot (by steering the electron beam between the cathode and anode) in the opposite direction (−v) of gantry motion **(C)**. This is accomplished with magnetic deflection of the electron beam incident on the anode. 📖 **F10-17**

**b.** Continuous x-ray output is used by most CT scanner manufacturers.

  **(i)** Detector sampling time is the acquisition time for each CT projection acquired.

  **(ii)** Sampling dwell times: approximately 0.2 to 0.5 ms.

  **(iii)** Approximately 1,000 to 3,000 projections are acquired for a 0.5 s gantry rotation over 360°.

  **(iv)** At the periphery of the FOV, the angular displacement of the focal spot during the sampling dwell time is greater than at the center, causing a relatively greater sampling distance, and resulting in blurring and loss of spatial resolution.

  **(v)** Compensation (some CT scanners) steers the focal spot in the opposite direction (Fig. 10-14).

  **(vi)** Some CT scanner manufacturers use focal spot steering to "oversample" the z-dimension to cause a shift in the source position—this effectively doubles the unique angular projection data sampling per rotation, relative to the number of detector channels.

**c.** Pulsed x-ray output by some manufacturers is used to switch x-ray voltage for dual-energy CT.

  **(i)** Every other pulse is a high (*e.g.,* 140 kV) or low (*e.g.,* 80 kV) projection (see Section 10.3.8).

**d.** Wider x-ray beam collimation with MDCT increases the detected scatter fraction.
   **(i)** 2D antiscatter grids are used to reduce scatter (Fig. 10-15).
**e.** Indirect detection (scintillator) solid-state detectors are most widely used (Fig. 10-16).
   **(i)** Scintillator materials are sintered to increase density and improve detection efficiency.
   **(ii)** Ceramic phosphors are scored to produce individual detector elements.
   **(iii)** Opaque filler between detector elements is added to reduce cross-talk.

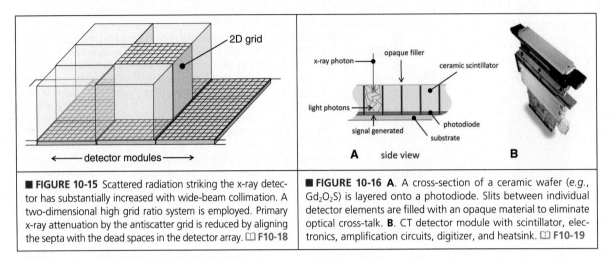

■ **FIGURE 10-15** Scattered radiation striking the x-ray detector has substantially increased with wide-beam collimation. A two-dimensional high grid ratio system is employed. Primary x-ray attenuation by the antiscatter grid is reduced by aligning the septa with the dead spaces in the detector array. 📖 **F10-18**

■ **FIGURE 10-16 A.** A cross-section of a ceramic wafer (*e.g.*, $Gd_2O_2S$) is layered onto a photodiode. Slits between individual detector elements are filled with an opaque material to eliminate optical cross-talk. **B.** CT detector module with scintillator, electronics, amplification circuits, digitizer, and heatsink. 📖 **F10-19**

   **(iv)** Each ceramic detector element has a contact photodiode to generate charge from light.
   **(v)** The detectors are designed in modules with electronics to acquire the digital data.
**f.** Emerging photon-counting detectors use solid-state detector technology.
   **(i)** Energy discrimination allows individual photons to be assigned a discrete energy bin.
   **(ii)** Multispectral imaging is possible without multiple scans at different tube potentials.
   **(iii)** Technical challenge is the bandwidth of the electronics to measure high photon flux.
**6. Over beaming and geometrical efficiency**
   **a.** Overbeaming results from the presence of penumbra due to the finite focal spot size (Fig. 10-17).
   **b.** Collimation extends *beyond* the active detector array configuration to ensure uniform beam.
      **(i)** Active detectors in the penumbra region will generate a skewed slice sensitivity profile.
      **(ii)** Manufacturers must increase the beam collimation beyond the outer active detectors.

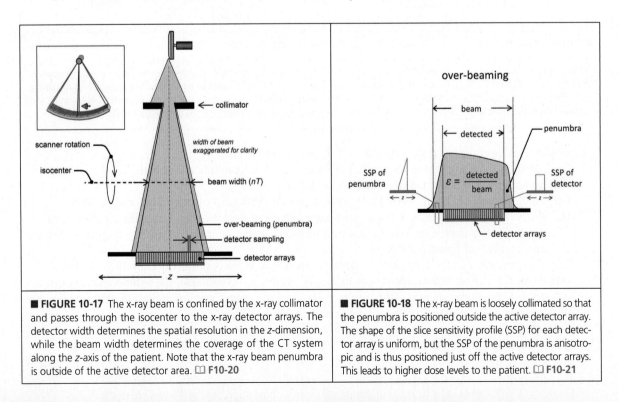

■ **FIGURE 10-17** The x-ray beam is confined by the x-ray collimator and passes through the isocenter to the x-ray detector arrays. The detector width determines the spatial resolution in the *z*-dimension, while the beam width determines the coverage of the CT system along the *z*-axis of the patient. Note that the x-ray beam penumbra is outside of the active detector area. 📖 **F10-20**

■ **FIGURE 10-18** The x-ray beam is loosely collimated so that the penumbra is positioned outside the active detector array. The shape of the slice sensitivity profile (SSP) for each detector array is uniform, but the SSP of the penumbra is anisotropic and is thus positioned just off the active detector arrays. This leads to higher dose levels to the patient. 📖 **F10-21**

    **c.** Beam geometrical efficiency is a function of the active detector width to beam width (Fig. 10-18).

        **(i)** The penumbra width remains constant, independent of beam collimation.

        **(ii)** For wider active detector arrays, efficiency is improved.

        **(iii)** Smaller active detector widths (*e.g.*, 8 channels of a 64 channel array) have poorer efficiency.

        **(iv)** Dose due to overbeaming can be a large fraction of the total dose when a small number of detector arrays are active—low-dose efficiency triggers a warning on the CT scanner.

**7. Adapting data acquisition to patient anatomy: noise propagation in CT images**

    **a.** Noise in a pixel is the consequence of all projection data intersecting the voxel representing the pixel.

    **b.** Noise variance ($\Sigma^2$) within the pixel results from the propagation of noise variance of the projections:

$$\sigma^2_{\text{CT image}} = \sigma^2_{p1} + \sigma^2_{p2} + \sigma^2_{p3} + \cdots + \sigma^2_{pN}$$

    **c.** "Noise adding in quadrature" means larger subcomponents of noise contribute more to the total noise.

        **(i)** Total noise (the standard deviation) is the square root of $\sigma^2_{\text{CT image}}$.

    **d.** Methods to reduce noise are focused on the components of the total noise that have greater impact.

        **(i)** Bowtie filters modify the incident beam to achieve a more uniform x-ray transmission from the center to the periphery of the patient.

        **(ii)** Tube current modulation varies the incident radiation as the x-ray tube rotates around the patient and adjusts current (x-ray output) on the attenuation path for each projection.

        **(iii)** These issues are discussed next and later in the guide.

**8. Beam shaping filters**

    **a.** Most body parts are circular or approximately circular in shape.

    **b.** Transmission of x-rays through the patient head or torso is greater in the periphery of the projection.

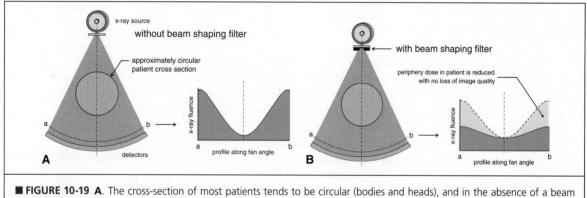

**■ FIGURE 10-19 A**. The cross-section of most patients tends to be circular (bodies and heads), and in the absence of a beam shaping filter leads to the transmitted x-ray distribution with high levels at the periphery and low levels under the center of the patient. **B**. A beam shaping filter is positioned near the x-ray source to reduce the high x-ray fluence levels at the periphery of the fan beam relative to the center. The bow tie filter reduces the imbalance of signal levels received, and in doing so provides considerable radiation dose reduction to the periphery of the patient—with no loss in image quality. 📖 **F10-22**

    **c.** The *bowtie filter* shapes the incident radiation fluence to adjust for the attenuation variability presented by the patient (Fig. 10-19).

    **d.** Reducing the beam intensity peripherally reduces dose to the patient with no appreciable loss of quality.

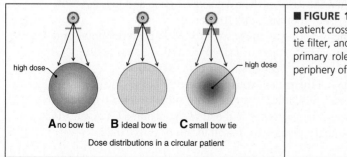

**A** no bow tie    **B** ideal bow tie    **C** small bow tie

Dose distributions in a circular patient

**■ FIGURE 10-20** The relative dose distributions in the circular patient cross-section with **(A)** no bow tie, **(B)** a well-designed bow tie filter, and **(C)** a bow tie filter that is too centrally focused. The primary role of the bow tie filter is to reduce the dose to the periphery of the patient. 📖 **F10-23**

e. In the absence of a bowtie filter, the dose to the periphery is increased (Fig. 10-20A).

f. With the wrong bowtie filter mismatched to patient anatomy, dose increases centrally (Fig. 10-20C).

9. **View sampling**

a. The data acquisition system (DAS) is intrinsic to the view sampling rate and sampling size.

b. The rotation period of the gantry about 360° occurs with continuous radiation output.

   (i) View sampling rate (frequency) over the rotation period determines sampling size (Fig. 10-21).

   (ii) A rate of 2,000 to 3,000 samples/s per detector element is necessary to maintain resolution.

c. View sampling size increases as $r\, d\theta$ (Fig. 10-21B), for angular sampling of $d\theta$.

   (i) Spatial resolution decreases from the center to the edge of the FOV.

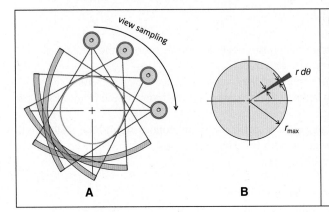

■ **FIGURE 10-21 A.** Most CT scanners operate the x-ray tube in continuously on mode during CT acquisition, that is, the x-ray source is not pulsed. View sampling is defined by the data acquisition system associated with the detector arrays, which operate with relatively high bandwidth. For example, to acquire 1,000 views over 360° rotation of the gantry in 0.35 s, each detector needs to be sampled at almost 3,000 samples per second. **B.** This figure shows that for a given view sampling width/angle, the width of the sampling sector increases from the center of the field-of-view to the periphery, as $r\, d\theta$. 📖 **F10-24**

d. Focal spot dithering (Fig. 10-14) can help mitigate the loss of peripheral detail.

10. **High-resolution CT scanners**

a. Specialty, small FOV scanners have been developed for years (small animal, specimen scanners).

   (i) "Micro-CT" can deliver voxel dimensions on the order of 10 μm (but 30 minute scan time…).

b. Cone-beam CT scanners have high resolution because of small detector elements in the flat panel.

c. Whole-body CT scanners are now available to provide high spatial resolution in humans.

   (i) One vendor provides 0.25 mm detector widths and 0.25 × 0.25 mm in-plane sampling.

   (ii) Focal spots can limit spatial resolution, so six focal spots are provided from very small to large.

   (iii) Reconstructed image matrix sizes for these scanners are 1,024 × 1,024 and 2,048 × 2,048.

d. Image noise is a challenge at high resolution—innovative reconstruction algorithms using artificial intelligence and deep learning algorithms may be a solution.

e. High-resolution CT may improve CT diagnostic accuracy across an array of clinical applications.

## 10.3 ACQUISITION MODES

1. **The CT scan radiograph**

a. X-ray tube and detector array are stationary—table moves through gantry with x-rays on.

   (i) Scanned projection radiograph localizer also known as "scout" "topogram" "scanogram" …etc.

   (ii) Technique factors use variable kV (often the same as the axial acquisitions) and low mA.

b. X-ray tube position at 0° (top), 90° (right), 180° (bottom), or 270° (left).

   (i) Depending on patient position (supine/prone), anterior/posterior (AP) or posterior/anterior (PA) projections are acquired at 0° or 180°, and lateral projections at 90° or 270°.

   (ii) Acquisition of both PA or AP and LAT localizer radiographs are common practice.

   (iii) Lateral projection identifies positioning of the patient with the isocenter of rotation (table height).

   (iv) PA acquisition is preferred to keep breast dose lower than AP acquisition for female patients.

c. The localizer defines anatomy slightly beyond the beginning and end of the planned CT acquisition.

   (i) Using CT console software, the technologist plans the CT scan locations (Fig. 10-22).

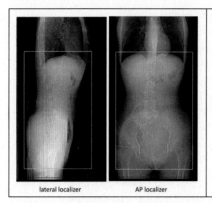

■ **FIGURE 10-22** Most CT examinations start with the acquisition of the localizer, also known as the scan projection radiograph. This figure shows both the AP and lateral localizer images, which require separate scans. These images are acquired by keeping the gantry stationary (no rotation) while translating the patient on the table through the gantry. The scan projection radiograph is used by the technologists to define the position of the CT scan with respect to the patient's anatomy, including stop and start points in z, and to adjust different regions of the scan for different acquisition parameters or post-acquisition parameters. 📖 **F10-25**

lateral localizer        AP localizer

2. **Axial (sequential) acquisition**
   a. Basic "step and shoot" where the tube and detector rotate around stationary patient/table (Fig. 10-23).
   b. X-rays turn on for 360° to acquire raw data for a number of CT slices, then turn off.
   c. Table is then moved with beam off to the next position and axial scan is repeated with stationary table.
   d. Between each acquisition, the table moves a distance $D$, equal to the sampling distance at isocenter.
      **(i)** For contiguous data acquisition $D = nT$, resulting in contiguous CT images along the $z$-direction
      **(ii)** $n$ = *number of array channels* and $T$ = *detector width*; $nT$ = *collimated beam width* + overbeaming
   e. In some protocols, $nT < D$, which provides better sampling in $z$ (e.g., for 3D volume rendering), but increases dose if the same technique factors are used.

3. **Helical (spiral) acquisition**
   a. Table moves simultaneous to tube and detector rotation, creating a helical path (Fig. 10-24).
   b. X-rays are on constantly; eliminating table start/stop—removes intertial constraints.
   c. The *pitch* describes the relative advance of the CT table per 360° rotation

$$\text{pitch} = \frac{F_{\text{table}}}{nT}$$

where $F_{\text{table}}$ is the table feed distance per 360°

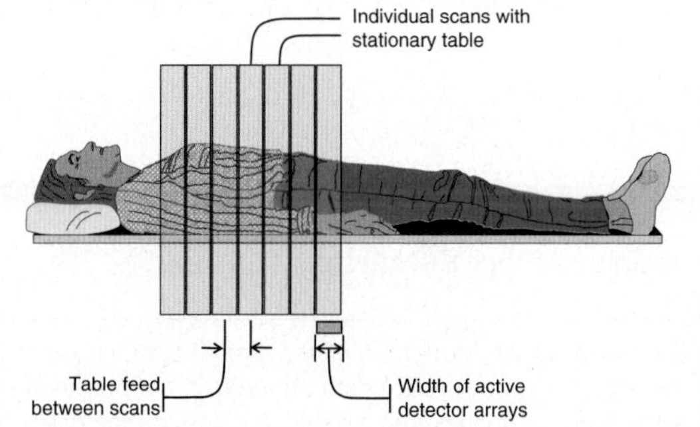

■ **FIGURE 10-23** Axial (sequential) CT acquisition. With a stationary table, one data set is acquired over one rotation with x-rays on then off. The table translates a distance equal to the width of active detector arrays for contiguous scans, and the sequence is repeated to acquire the full dataset. 📖 **F10-26**

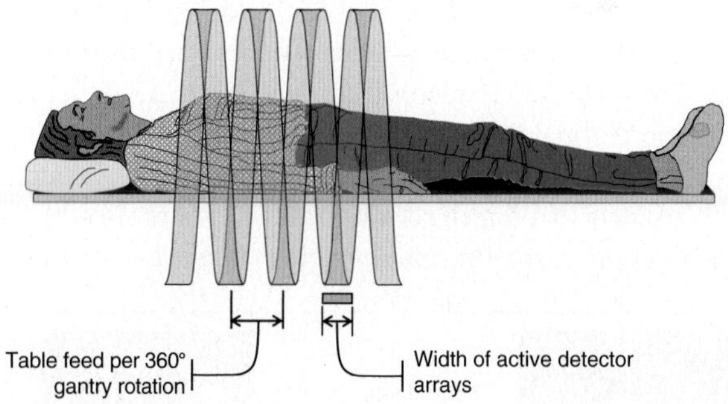

Individual scans with stationary table
Table feed between scans        Width of active detector arrays

■ **FIGURE 10-24** Helical (or spiral) CT is performed with continuous rotation of the gantry while the table is moving. Helical CT was made possible when slip rings were introduced to CT. With the gantry rotating, once the table is up to speed, helical CT scans proceed with no inertial impediment until the scan is completed. 📖 **F10-27**

Table feed per 360° gantry rotation        Width of active detector arrays

Example: 40 mm = $nT$ and 360° rotation time = 0.5 s; pitch = 1 occurs when $F_{\text{table}}$ = 80 mm/s
   d. Pitch = 1 corresponds to contiguous axial scanning in principle.
   e. Pitch >1 represents underscanning of some regions of the body.
      **(i)** Allows for faster scanning (shorter total scan time) to reduce patient motion (*e.g.*, pediatrics)
      **(ii)** For technique factors held constant (except pitch), then

$$\text{dose} \propto \frac{1}{\text{pitch}}$$

**f.** Pitch < 1 represents overscanning of the same regions of the body (and higher dose).
  **(i)** Useful for multiplanar reformatting (sagittal, coronal) and 3D volume rendering.
  **(ii)** Often, the technique factors (mAs) are reduced such that the dose is kept constant.
**g.** Comparison of axial, low pitch helical, and high pitch helical coverage (Fig. 10-25).
**h.** Acquired data at the beginning and end of scans do not have sufficient angular coverage to reconstruct artifact-free CT images (Fig. 10-26A), requiring *over*-Useful for multiplanar reformatting *ranging*.
  **(i)** Results in wasted dose when the x-ray tube is on, equal to ½ nT at beginning and ½ nT at end
**i.** Adaptive beam collimation on some CT scanners eliminates the overranging penalty (Fig. 10-26B).

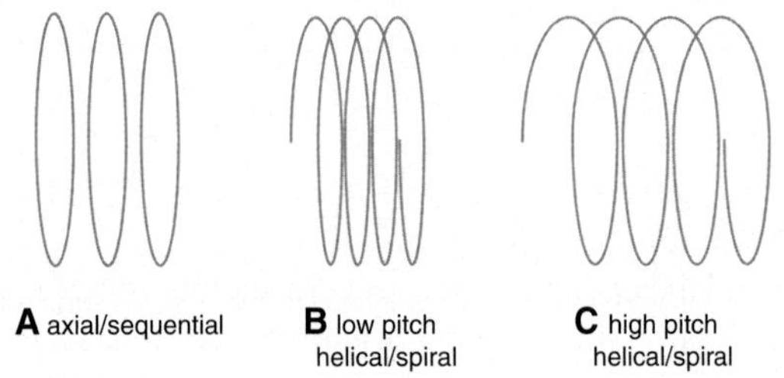

■ **FIGURE 10-25** The trajectory of the x-ray source around the patient is shown for **(A)** axial (sequential) imaging, **(B)** low pitch helical (spiral) imaging, and **(C)** high pitch helical imaging. 📖 **F10-28**

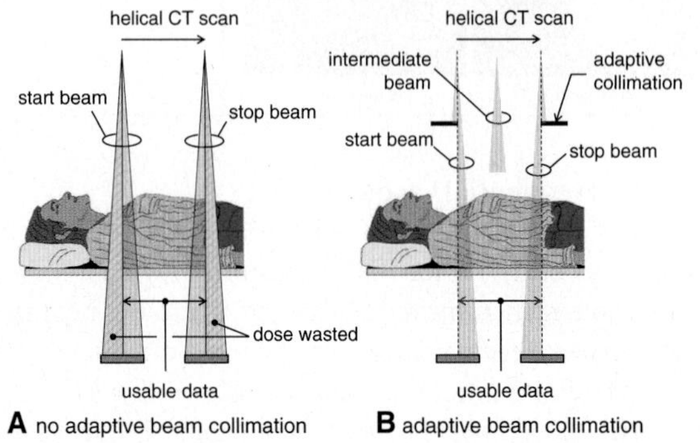

■ **FIGURE 10-26 A.** For helical CT scanning, a minimum of 180° of acquisition data is necessary to reconstruct image data, resulting in wasted irradiation. This is called overranging. **B.** Adaptive beam collimation reduces (but not completely eliminates) the overranging problem by narrowing the collimated beam width at both the beginning and the end of the helical CT scan. Overranging does not occur in axial scanning mode. 📖 **F10-29**

**4. Selection of CT slice width**
  **a.** MDCT scanners adjust the beam collimation width to the active detector channels and detector width.
  **b.** Each detector array has its own data channel, representing the smallest resolution element.
  **c.** Raw projection data are recorded for each detector element, and with this, CT image reconstructions can be produced over a range of slice thicknesses: for example, for $T = 0.625$ mm, 1.25, 2.5, and 5.0 mm thickness can be reconstructed—from the same acquisition.
  **d.** Thin-section CT reconstructions (small $\Delta z$ such as 0.625 mm) are useful as raw data for producing sagittal and coronal images, or volume-rendered images.
  **e.** Thicker slice reconstructions present with fewer images have lower quantum noise but more partial volume artifacts (for 5 mm slice versus 0.625 mm slice, there are 8× photons and $\sqrt{8}$× lower noise).
  **f.** Compromise of resolution versus noise is to reconstruct a variety of slice thicknesses (Fig. 10-27).

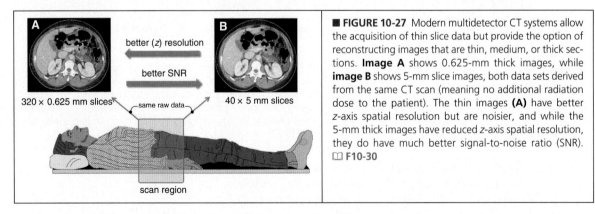

■ **FIGURE 10-27** Modern multidetector CT systems allow the acquisition of thin slice data but provide the option of reconstructing images that are thin, medium, or thick sections. **Image A** shows 0.625-mm thick images, while **image B** shows 5-mm slice images, both data sets derived from the same CT scan (meaning no additional radiation dose to the patient). The thin images **(A)** have better z-axis spatial resolution but are noisier, and while the 5-mm thick images have reduced z-axis spatial resolution, they do have much better signal-to-noise ratio (SNR). 📖 **F10-30**

**5. X-ray tube current modulation**
  **a.** Many body regions present thicknesses that vary as a function of view angle.
  **b.** For a constant x-ray beam tube current, fewer x-ray photons are detected for thicker dimension.
  **c.** Noise variance in the reconstructed image is dominated by the thicker projections with fewer photons.
  **d.** Higher detected number of photons in the projections over the thin region is essentially wasted.

e. A variable x-ray output (mA) adjusts for attenuation and equalizes noise contributions to lower dose.
  (i) In-plane adjustments occur as a function of view angle (Fig. 10-28).
  (ii) Longitudinal adjustments of mA occur as a function of table position and anatomical thickness (Fig. 10-29).

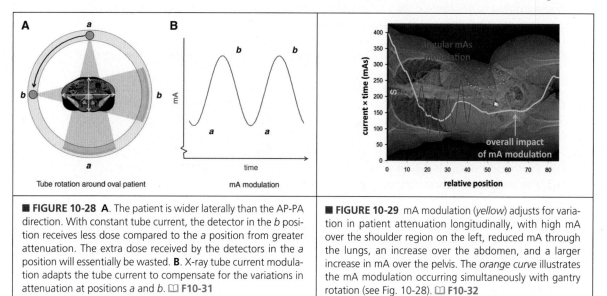

■ **FIGURE 10-28 A**. The patient is wider laterally than the AP-PA direction. With constant tube current, the detector in the *b* position receives less dose compared to the *a* position from greater attenuation. The extra dose received by the detectors in the *a* position will essentially be wasted. **B**. X-ray tube current modulation adapts the tube current to compensate for the variations in attenuation at positions *a* and *b*. 📖 **F10-31**

■ **FIGURE 10-29** mA modulation (*yellow*) adjusts for variation in patient attenuation longitudinally, with high mA over the shoulder region on the left, reduced mA through the lungs, an increase over the abdomen, and a larger increase in mA over the pelvis. The *orange curve* illustrates the mA modulation occurring simultaneously with gantry rotation (see Fig. 10-28). 📖 **F10-32**

f. Overall role of tube current modulation is analogous to *automatic exposure control* in radiography.
g. Vendors have parameters that deliver CT images with either a specified noise level or a standard effective mAs, dependent on the exam type and tolerable quantum noise in the reconstructed images.
  (i) *Noise index* is an approach to determining CT technique, based on the standard deviation of HU, where a lower noise index results in radiation doses that are overall much higher (dose $\propto 1/SD^2$).
  (ii) *Reference mAs* is another approach, which sets a nominal mAs level for a "standard" patient to use as guidance for patients of different size; a higher nominal mAs setting results in a higher dose to the patient.
6. **Acquisition modes focused on temporal aspects: CT angiography and CT perfusion**
  a. CT angiography (Fig. 10-30) image acquisition tracks iodine contrast flow through the vasculature.
  b. Blood vessel visualization provides information on vessel structure (stenosis, disease, aneurysms, etc.).
  c. Arterial, venous, and late phase imaging are used to visualize perfusion of the liver and other organs.
    (i) Multiphase imaging (*e.g.*, 4-phase liver) increases dose by a factor of 4.
  d. CT brain perfusion (Fig. 10-31) acquires data for evaluating stroke by measuring temporal uptake.

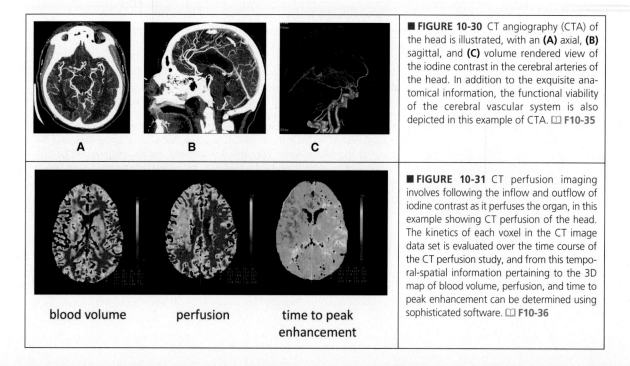

■ **FIGURE 10-30** CT angiography (CTA) of the head is illustrated, with an **(A)** axial, **(B)** sagittal, and **(C)** volume rendered view of the iodine contrast in the cerebral arteries of the head. In addition to the exquisite anatomical information, the functional viability of the cerebral vascular system is also depicted in this example of CTA. 📖 **F10-35**

■ **FIGURE 10-31** CT perfusion imaging involves following the inflow and outflow of iodine contrast as it perfuses the organ, in this example showing CT perfusion of the head. The kinetics of each voxel in the CT image data set is evaluated over the time course of the CT perfusion study, and from this temporal-spatial information pertaining to the 3D map of blood volume, perfusion, and time to peak enhancement can be determined using sophisticated software. 📖 **F10-36**

blood volume          perfusion          time to peak enhancement

   **(i)**   The same regions of the brain are scanned over 30 to 50 s, either with a "shuttle mode" for narrow collimation beams or without table motion for wide collimation beams (*e.g.*, 160 mm).
   **e.** The high Z of iodine provides an opportunity to use lower kV (80 to 100) to enhance the signal strength.
   **f.** A lower dose can be achieved with a reasonable signal to noise ratio of the iodinated signal.
7. **Acquisition modes to account for motion: cardiac CT**
   **a.** Cardiac motion is challenging for CT imaging.
      **(i)**   CT gantry rotation periods of 0.25 to 0.35 s are too long to freeze motion, where less than 100 ms is desired.
      **(ii)**  Periodic motion allows data to be sorted according to phases of the heart (*e.g.*, end-diastole).
   **b.** Cardiac gating methods acquire CT data over several cardiac cycles in conjunction with EKG trace.
   **c.** *Retrospective gating* uses a continuous acquisition throughout the heart cycles (Fig. 10-32A).
      **(i)**   Retrospective methods deliver a high dose with the tube on during the entire study.
   **d.** *Prospective gating* times the acquisition of short segments at the same phase (Fig. 10-32B).
      **(i)**   Prospective methods deliver a high, intermittent dose, with overall low-dose delivery.
      **(ii)**  For irregular heartbeats, an incomplete CT dataset may result.

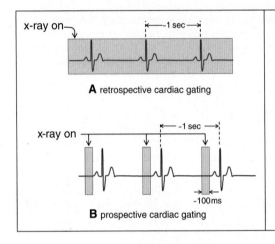

■ **FIGURE 10-32 A**. In retrospective cardiac gating, the x-ray beam is on throughout the entire cardiac cycle, over many cardiac cycles. This type of study can be used to portray the "beating heart" in three dimensions; however, the temporal information provided is not considered necessary for the valuation of coronary artery patency. The downside is the activation of the x-ray tube during the entire procedure, leading to high radiation dose levels to the heart, thorax, and breasts. **B**. Prospective cardiac gating involves the use of the ECG signal to actively pulse the x-ray tube in the CT scanner over a narrow window of the cardiac cycle at end-diastole. The acquired data set is sufficient to produce 3D volume sets of the heart to enable patency evaluation of the coronary arteries. While only one snapshot in time is available, the data set delivered is adequate enough to diagnose the most common form of cardiac disease. As illustrated, the beam is on for a much shorter period in prospective gating, making it a much lower dose technique than retrospective gating. ▢ **F10-37**

   **e.** Scanner z-axis field of view (collimation) width can impact the cardiac procedure time.
      **(i)**   Limited collimation (*e.g.*, 40 mm) requires approximately four table positions to image the heart.
      **(ii)**  Wide collimation (*e.g.*, 160 mm) does not require table repositioning.
   **f.** Dual-source cardiac CT scanner.
      **(i)**   Two x-ray tubes and detector arrays mounted at 90° within the gantry (Fig. 10-33).
      **(ii)**  Tube A has a larger array and FOV, while tube B has a smaller array and FOV.
      **(iii)** CT reconstruction requires 180° + fan angle; with orthogonal tubes, a full 180° can be acquired with 90° rotation—if full 360° rotation is 0.33 s, ¼ × 0.33 s ≈ 83 ms acquisition.

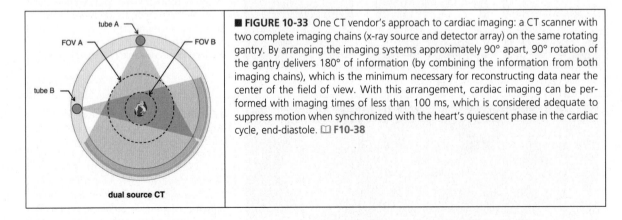

■ **FIGURE 10-33** One CT vendor's approach to cardiac imaging: a CT scanner with two complete imaging chains (x-ray source and detector array) on the same rotating gantry. By arranging the imaging systems approximately 90° apart, 90° rotation of the gantry delivers 180° of information (by combining the information from both imaging chains), which is the minimum necessary for reconstructing data near the center of the field of view. With this arrangement, cardiac imaging can be performed with imaging times of less than 100 ms, which is considered adequate to suppress motion when synchronized with the heart's quiescent phase in the cardiac cycle, end-diastole. ▢ **F10-38**

8. **Acquisition modes to acquire dual-energy CT data**
   a. Dual-energy methods can separate physical density from material elemental composition.
   b. Acquisitions at 80 and 140 kV generate energy-dependent HU values (Fig. 10-34).
   c. Methods of acquisition:
      (i) Dual-source CT operates at low and high kV for each tube.
      (ii) Single source switched kV pulses during acquisition (adjacent views are low and high kV).
      (iii) Single source single kV with two-layer detectors (top absorbs low E, bottom absorbs high E).
      (iv) Single source single kV with a beam-hardening filter covering half field for energy separation.
      (v) Single source dual kV using two passes of the anatomy at low and high kV (motion a problem).
   d. Different technologies enable various degrees of separation between low and high energy scans.
   e. Methods of reconstruction:
      (i) Raw data sets for each view subjected to logarithmic weighted subtraction—and then the subtracted dataset is used to reconstruct CT images with different x-ray energy ranges.
      (ii) Low kV and high kV image sets reconstructed with algorithmic methods applied in the CT image domain to generate the energy-weighted subtraction decomposition (more common).
   f. Example image of the foot with 3D volume rendering and dual-energy CT gout detection (Fig. 10-35).

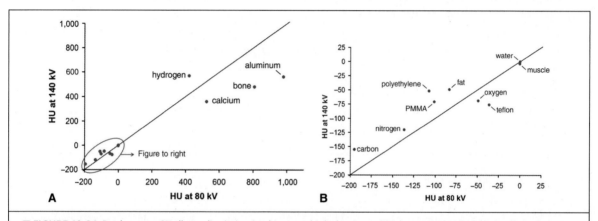

■ **FIGURE 10-34** Dual-energy CT allows discrimination between high density and high atomic number, both of which increase the numerical value of the Hounsfield unit. This plot shows the HU values at 140 kV, as a function of HU values at 80 kV. In **image A**, higher atomic number materials are below the line of identity, while lighter materials are above the line of identity. In **image B**, a blowup of the cluster of materials between −200 and 0 HU is illustrated. Dual-energy CT algorithms use tables such as that shown here to identify specific materials on a voxel-by-voxel basis. 📖 **F10-39**

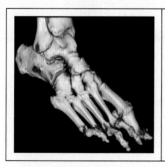

■ **FIGURE 10-35** Probably the best clinical application of dual-energy CT is the identification of gout, as illustrated in this figure. The bony foot is illustrated in this pseudo-3D rendering, with regions of uric acid crystals (the manifestation of gout) shown color-coded in *purple*. 📖 **F10-40**

## 10.4 RECONSTRUCTION

1. **CT protocols**
   a. Detailed methods for acquiring a CT exam and processing the CT exam.
   b. Acquisition parameters include type of scan (axial, helical, perfusion, etc.); kV, mA (including AEC or tube current modulation); rotation time; slice thickness; pitch; scan FOV; display FOV; scanned projection radiograph acquisition; contrast delay; voice commands.
   c. Reconstruction parameters include *algorithms* (FBP with kernel type; iterative reconstruction with type and strength of noise reduction; artificial intelligence and deep learning reconstructions); *output imaging parameters* (slice thickness; window/level settings; reconstructed FOV; multiplanar reformatting).

**d.** Access to raw data allows for reconstruction with new parameters without rescanning the patient; often the raw data are available for only a few days unless specifically protected from deletion.

**2. Preprocessing**

 **a.** "Air calibration scans" characterize bowtie filter attenuation and individual detector response.

 **b.** Dead detector compensation with interpolation of outputs from adjacent detectors.

 **c.** Scatter correction algorithms, if used, must be applied prior to projection data logarithm application.

 **d.** Data normalization and logarithmic transformation (correct for x-ray exponential attenuation).

  **(i)** Each projection is a measure of the discrete intensity, $I_j$, at each detector element $j$, with scalar constant, $k_j$ for gain values, inverse square law, bowtie filter attenuation, etc. (Fig. 10-36):

$$S_j = k_j I_0 e^{-(\mu_1 t + \mu_2 t + \mu_3 t + \cdots + \mu_n t)}$$

  **(ii)** Normalization is implemented by measuring unattenuated beam, $I_0$, with a reference detector outside of the FOV

$$S_r = k_r I_0$$

  **(iii)** Logarithmic transformation of discrete transmitted intensity measurement at detector element $j$, is the corrected projection value, $P_j$:

$$P_j = \ln\left\{\frac{\alpha S_r}{S_j}\right\} = t\left(\mu_1 + \mu_2 + \mu_3 + \ldots + \mu_n\right)$$

  where $\alpha = k_j/k_r$. The projection corresponds to linear sums of the attenuation coefficients.

 **e.** The *sinogram* is represented by $P(j,\theta)$ where $j$ corresponds to each detector, and $\theta$ to the view angle (Fig. 10-37).

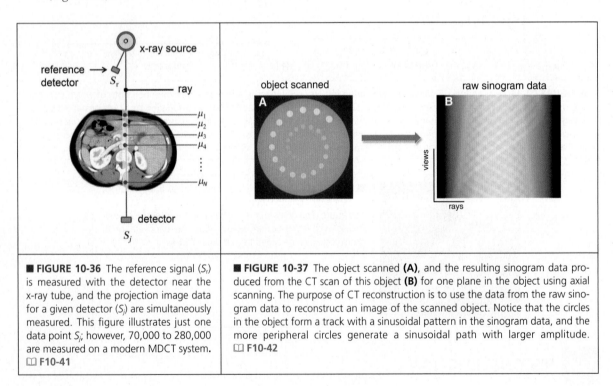

■ **FIGURE 10-36** The reference signal ($S_r$) is measured with the detector near the x-ray tube, and the projection image data for a given detector ($S_j$) are simultaneously measured. This figure illustrates just one data point $S_j$; however, 70,000 to 280,000 are measured on a modern MDCT system. 📖 **F10-41**

■ **FIGURE 10-37** The object scanned **(A)**, and the resulting sinogram data produced from the CT scan of this object **(B)** for one plane in the object using axial scanning. The purpose of CT reconstruction is to use the data from the raw sinogram data to reconstruct an image of the scanned object. Notice that the circles in the object form a track with a sinusoidal pattern in the sinogram data, and the more peripheral circles generate a sinusoidal path with larger amplitude. 📖 **F10-42**

**3. Simple backprojection**

 **a.** Computation of the CT image from the projection data with algebraic reconstruction (Fig. 10-38)

 **b.** Forward projection: creating projections from the measured data (Fig. 10-39)

  **(i)** Measured projections are backprojected into the reconstruction plane, suffering a 1/r blurring.

  **(ii)** Correction requires a mathematical convolution or FBP.

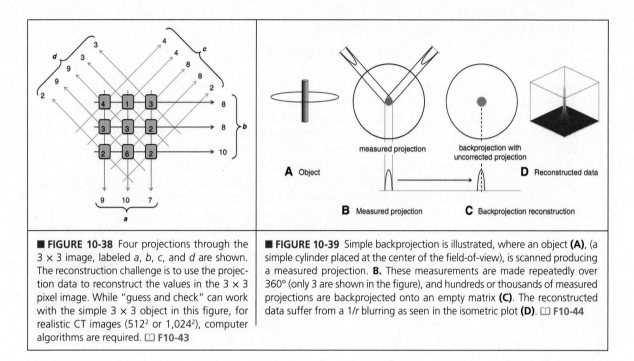

**■ FIGURE 10-38** Four projections through the 3 × 3 image, labeled *a*, *b*, *c*, and *d* are shown. The reconstruction challenge is to use the projection data to reconstruct the values in the 3 × 3 pixel image. While "guess and check" can work with the simple 3 × 3 object in this figure, for realistic CT images ($512^2$ or $1,024^2$), computer algorithms are required. 📖 **F10-43**

**■ FIGURE 10-39** Simple backprojection is illustrated, where an object **(A)**, (a simple cylinder placed at the center of the field-of-view), is scanned producing a measured projection. **B.** These measurements are made repeatedly over 360° (only 3 are shown in the figure), and hundreds or thousands of measured projections are backprojected onto an empty matrix **(C)**. The reconstructed data suffer from a 1/*r* blurring as seen in the isometric plot **(D)**. 📖 **F10-44**

## 4. Convolution backprojection

a. Undoing convolution can be implemented by deconvolution with a kernel that, in this case, adds negative weighting in the filter to create projections that when backprojected, creates the desired output

$$p'(x) = \int_{x'=-\infty}^{\infty} p(x')\, h(x-x')\mathrm{d}x' = p(x) \otimes h(x)$$

where $p(\cdot)$ is each measured projection, $h(\cdot)$ is the deconvolution kernel, and $p'(x)$ is the corrected projection (Fig. 10-40).

b. The deconvolution of the measured projections and backprojection results in a faithful representation of the object (Fig. 10-41).

c. Convolution backprojection is a specific implementation for FBP—a general "sharpening" of the resultant image.

## 5. Fourier-based filtered reconstruction

a. Convolution can be performed more efficiently in the frequency domain with the Fourier transform.

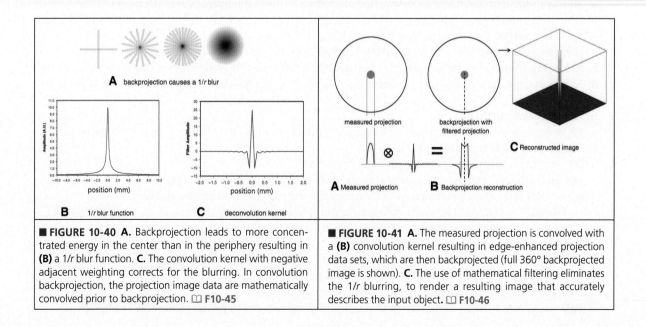

**■ FIGURE 10-40 A.** Backprojection leads to more concentrated energy in the center than in the periphery resulting in **(B)** a 1/*r* blur function. **C.** The convolution kernel with negative adjacent weighting corrects for the blurring. In convolution backprojection, the projection image data are mathematically convolved prior to backprojection. 📖 **F10-45**

**■ FIGURE 10-41 A.** The measured projection is convolved with a **(B)** convolution kernel resulting in edge-enhanced projection data sets, which are then backprojected (full 360° backprojected image is shown). **C.** The use of mathematical filtering eliminates the 1/*r* blurring, to render a resulting image that accurately describes the input object. 📖 **F10-46**

The equation expressed in Section 10.4.A becomes

$$p'(x) = FT^{-1}\left\{FT\left[p(x)\right] \times FT\left[h(x)\right]\right\}$$

where FT [·] is the Fourier transform and FT⁻¹ [·] is the inverse Fourier transform.

**b.** The Fourier transform of the deconvolution filter, FT[$h(x)$] is termed $H(f)$ and is the "ramp filter."

   **(i)** The blurring function $1/r$ in the spatial domain is $1/f$ in the frequency domain (Fig. 10-42).

   **(ii)** The $1/f$ dependency of FT[$p(x)$] thus can be corrected by the product of $|1/f| \times H(f)$.

   **(iii)** A roll-off of the ramp filter, called *apodization*, is always applied in CT because noise (where quantum noise dominates) reduction is required to make the CT images acceptable.

   **(iv)** Filter "kernels" with different bandpass cutoffs are exam specific; that is, "soft tissue," "bone," "lung," "detail," or such as H45 (head), B30 (body) giving specifics on bandpass characteristics.

**c.** Fourier filtering is applied to the raw sinogram data followed by backprojection (Fig. 10-43).

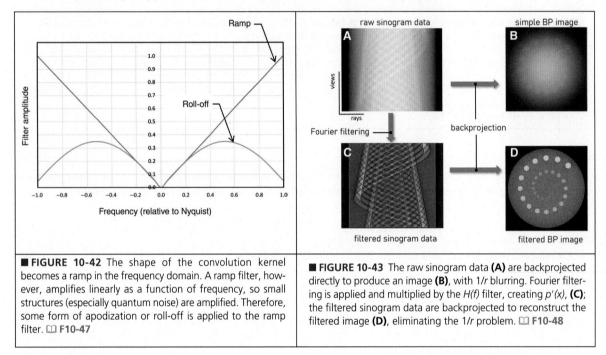

■ **FIGURE 10-42** The shape of the convolution kernel becomes a ramp in the frequency domain. A ramp filter, however, amplifies linearly as a function of frequency, so small structures (especially quantum noise) are amplified. Therefore, some form of apodization or roll-off is applied to the ramp filter. 📖 **F10-47**

■ **FIGURE 10-43** The raw sinogram data **(A)** are backprojected directly to produce an image **(B)**, with $1/r$ blurring. Fourier filtering is applied and multiplied by the $H(f)$ filter, creating $p'(x)$, **(C)**; the filtered sinogram data are backprojected to reconstruct the filtered image **(D)**, eliminating the $1/r$ problem. 📖 **F10-48**

**6. Cone-beam reconstruction**

   **a.** Similar to standard fan-beam reconstruction algorithms, with beam divergence in the $z$-axis.

   **(i)** Must consider beam divergence (the cone angle), where the projections become a function of detector fan position, $j$, view angle, $\theta$, and cone angle, $\phi$, as: $p(j,\phi,\theta)$

   **b.** Basic reconstruction algorithm is called the Feldkamp, Davis, and Kress algorithm, FDK.

   **c.** The entire volume data set (a series of CT images and thicknesses) is reconstructed simultaneously.

   **d.** Reconstruction methods violate mathematical sampling requirements leading to cone-beam artifacts (see Section 10.6.6).

**7. Iterative reconstruction**

   **a.** Iterative reconstruction techniques go through a series of iterations in the process of CT reconstruction.

   **b.** Statistical iterative reconstruction (IR):

   **(i)** Initial reconstruction begins with FBP (Fig. 10-44).

   **(ii)** Subsequent iterations use statistical methods to adaptively reduce noise (Fig. 10-45).

   **(iii)** Edges and details are preserved while large areas are smoothed for noise reduction.

   **(iv)** Going "too far" introduces overprocessing and "plastic-like" appearing images with loss of low contrast content; most manufacturers use a "blend" of FBP and statistical reconstruction.

   **c.** Model-based iterative reconstruction (MBIR):

   **(i)** Uses models of the physical parameters of the CT scanner (focal spot, x-ray spectrum, bowtie filters), properties of the detector arrays, influence of scattered radiation.

   **(ii)** MBIR images have higher SNR at the same dose or similar SNR at a lower dose than IR images.

   **(iii)** Computation and reconstruction times for MBIR are minutes to hours; clinical use is limited.

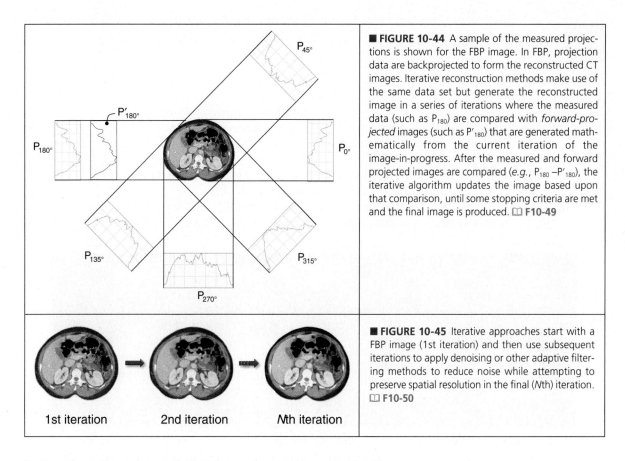

■ **FIGURE 10-44** A sample of the measured projections is shown for the FBP image. In FBP, projection data are backprojected to form the reconstructed CT images. Iterative reconstruction methods make use of the same data set but generate the reconstructed image in a series of iterations where the measured data (such as $P_{180}$) are compared with *forward-projected* images (such as $P'_{180}$) that are generated mathematically from the current iteration of the image-in-progress. After the measured and forward projected images are compared (*e.g.*, $P_{180} - P'_{180}$), the iterative algorithm updates the image based upon that comparison, until some stopping criteria are met and the final image is produced. ☐ **F10-49**

■ **FIGURE 10-45** Iterative approaches start with a FBP image (1st iteration) and then use subsequent iterations to apply denoising or other adaptive filtering methods to reduce noise while attempting to preserve spatial resolution in the final (*N*th) iteration. ☐ **F10-50**

8. **Deep learning and convolutional neural network reconstruction**
    a. Artificial intelligence and deep learning algorithms "learn" from training image sets (*e.g.*, FBP noisy image and corresponding MBIR "optimal" image) by weighting interconnections (Fig. 10-46).
    b. During training, an algorithm adjusts individual connection weights to compute the desired output.
    c. Thousands of image sets later, the weighing provides built-in intelligence for the specific task.
    d. Generalizability is limited, but the algorithms are fast and achieve superior levels of denoising.
    e. Comparison of four reconstruction methods are shown (Fig. 10-47).

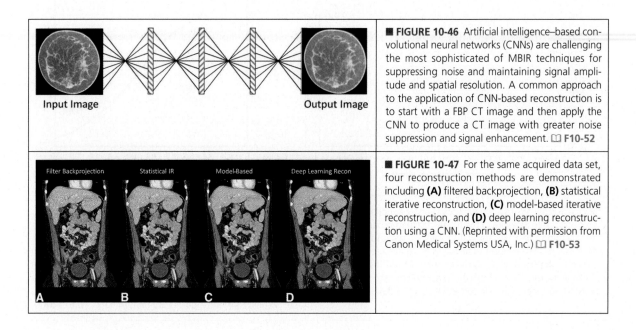

■ **FIGURE 10-46** Artificial intelligence–based convolutional neural networks (CNNs) are challenging the most sophisticated of MBIR techniques for suppressing noise and maintaining signal amplitude and spatial resolution. A common approach to the application of CNN-based reconstruction is to start with a FBP CT image and then apply the CNN to produce a CT image with greater noise suppression and signal enhancement. ☐ **F10-52**

■ **FIGURE 10-47** For the same acquired data set, four reconstruction methods are demonstrated including **(A)** filtered backprojection, **(B)** statistical iterative reconstruction, **(C)** model-based iterative reconstruction, and **(D)** deep learning reconstruction using a CNN. (Reprinted with permission from Canon Medical Systems USA, Inc.) ☐ **F10-53**

## 10.5 IMAGE QUALITY IN CT

1. **Spatial resolution**
   **a.** Spatial resolution in the reconstruction $(x,y)$ plane
   - **(i)** Factors: focal spot size/distribution; detector dimensions; magnification factor; gantry motion compensation; patient motion, scan field of view (SFOV), display field of view (DFOV); filter kernels and reconstruction algorithms; reconstructed slice thickness; matrix (512 × 512 typical)
   - **(ii)** Measurement methods: traditional line-pair phantoms (Fig. 10-48); modulation transfer function (MTF) measurements of a wire or metal foil edge to generate a line spread function (LSF) followed by Fourier transformation to calculate the MTF (Fig. 10-49)
   - **(iii)** High-resolution clinical scanners have 1,024 × 1,024 and 2,048 × 2,048 matrices, combined with selectable focal spots of small dimension (limiting factor is tube output) (Fig. 10-50)

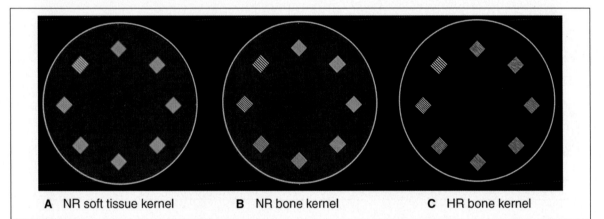

| A NR soft tissue kernel | B NR bone kernel | C HR bone kernel |

■ **FIGURE 10-48** The American College of Radiology phantom reconstructed with **(A)** a soft tissue kernel and **(B)** a bone kernel, for a normal resolution CT scanner. The higher spatial frequency characteristics of the bone kernel are apparent by observing the higher frequency line pair modules. **(C)** The same phantom is shown imaged on a high-resolution CT scanner, with all of the line pair modules resolved. ▱ **F10-54**

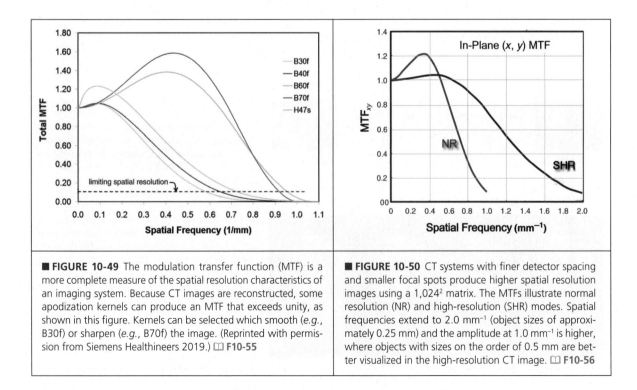

■ **FIGURE 10-49** The modulation transfer function (MTF) is a more complete measure of the spatial resolution characteristics of an imaging system. Because CT images are reconstructed, some apodization kernels can produce an MTF that exceeds unity, as shown in this figure. Kernels can be selected which smooth (*e.g.*, B30f) or sharpen (*e.g.*, B70f) the image. (Reprinted with permission from Siemens Healthineers 2019.) ▱ **F10-55**

■ **FIGURE 10-50** CT systems with finer detector spacing and smaller focal spots produce higher spatial resolution images using a 1,024² matrix. The MTFs illustrate normal resolution (NR) and high-resolution (SHR) modes. Spatial frequencies extend to 2.0 mm⁻¹ (object sizes of approximately 0.25 mm) and the amplitude at 1.0 mm⁻¹ is higher, where objects with sizes on the order of 0.5 mm are better visualized in the high-resolution CT image. ▱ **F10-56**

**b.** Spatial resolution along the *z*-axis

    **(i)** Minimum dimension is determined by the detector width backprojected to the isocenter; typical values are 0.5, 0.6, 0.625; 0.25 mm is available for high-resolution CT.

    **(ii)** Historical measurement: the slice-sensitivity profile (SSP)—a plot of system contrast from a point input in the *z*-direction—the ACR CT phantom has a series of high contrast rods spaced 0.5 mm apart at a 45° angle (Fig. 10-51).

    **(iii)** MTF measurement: using a slit or edge oriented in the *z*-dimension can provide the LSF, which is Fourier transformed to create the MTF of the SSP (Fig. 10-52).

    **(iv)** Isotropic resolution indicates similar resolution is achieved in the *z*-direction (for thin slices) when compared to resolution in the *x*-*y* plane.

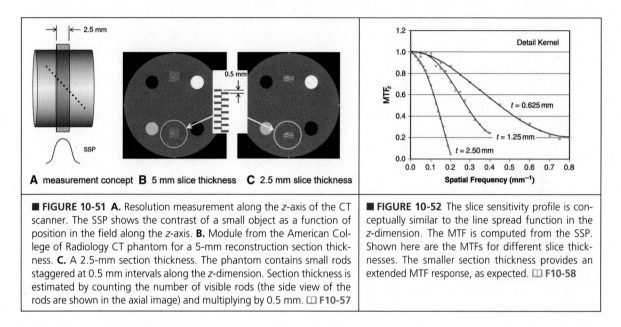

**A** measurement concept **B** 5 mm slice thickness **C** 2.5 mm slice thickness

■ **FIGURE 10-51 A.** Resolution measurement along the *z*-axis of the CT scanner. The SSP shows the contrast of a small object as a function of position in the field along the *z*-axis. **B.** Module from the American College of Radiology CT phantom for a 5-mm reconstruction section thickness. **C.** A 2.5-mm section thickness. The phantom contains small rods staggered at 0.5 mm intervals along the *z*-dimension. Section thickness is estimated by counting the number of visible rods (the side view of the rods are shown in the axial image) and multiplying by 0.5 mm. ▭ **F10-57**

■ **FIGURE 10-52** The slice sensitivity profile is conceptually similar to the line spread function in the *z*-dimension. The MTF is computed from the SSP. Shown here are the MTFs for different slice thicknesses. The smaller section thickness provides an extended MTF response, as expected. ▭ **F10-58**

**2. Noise assessment in CT**

    **a.** Contrast detectability phantom: visual assessment (Fig. 10-53)

        **(i)** Low contrast targets of large to smaller areas in known regions of the reconstructed slice.

        **(ii)** ACR CT phantom module provides a "subjective" measure of detectability as a function of noise.

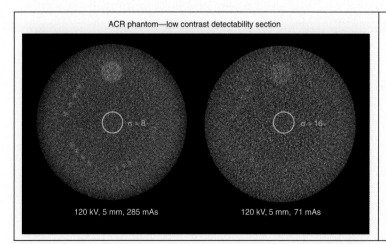

ACR phantom—low contrast detectability section

120 kV, 5 mm, 285 mAs      120 kV, 5 mm, 71 mAs

■ **FIGURE 10-53** Traditional estimation of the noise in computed tomography images make use of a low contrast phantom, comprised of a homogeneous material with cylindrical inserts of different diameters and different contrast levels. The low contrast phantom section of the American College of Radiology CT phantom is imaged at dose levels that vary by a factor of four—the high-dose image on the left shows a measured standard deviation that is about half of the low-dose image on the **right**. Furthermore, more of the objects embedded in the phantom are visible on the high-dose image **(left)** compared to the low-dose image on the right. This is a classic demonstration of contrast resolution. ▭ **F10-60**

b. Image noise in CT: the standard deviation, $\Sigma$
   (i)  Std Dev (root-mean-square) is a direct measure of the variation of Hounsfield units in a region

$$\sigma = \sqrt{\frac{\sum_{i=1}^{N}\left(HU_i - \overline{HU}\right)^2}{N-1}}$$

   (ii) Consistent with Poisson statistics (uniform area, all other factors fixed):
        noise $\propto 1/\sqrt{mAs}$—4× increase in mAs reduces noise by $1/\sqrt{4} = \frac{1}{2}$ (*e.g.*, a factor of 2)
        noise $\propto 1/\sqrt{slice\ thickness}$—4× increase in thickness (1.25 to 5.0 mm) reduces noise by ½
   (iii) Correlated noise might make these proportionalities inexact
c. Noise texture in CT: the noise power spectrum (NPS)
   (i)  The NPS is a mathematical metric describing the image noise variance ($\Sigma^2$) in the frequency domain—that is, the frequency dependence of the image noise, much like the MTF describes the transferred spatial domain image signal in the frequency domain.
   (ii) The NPS identifies noise *correlation*—where noise in one part of the image is affected by noise in the adjacent parts of the image.
   (iii) The Fourier transform of a noise patch of a 2D region of a CT image creates a 2D NPS estimate.
   (iv) The Fourier transform of a noise volume of a 3D volume of interest creates a 3D NPS estimate.
   (v)  Typically many NPS estimates are averaged together for a more accurate noise measurement.
   (vi) Estimates for kernels, dose, and reconstruction show the power of NPS analysis (Fig. 10-54).

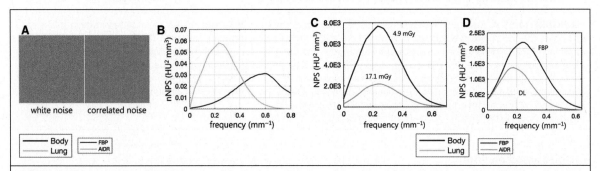

■ **FIGURE 10-54** The quantitative measurement of noise in CT includes the noise amplitude in addition to noise texture. The noise texture is demonstrated by the frequency dependence of the noise amplitude, as characterized by the noise power spectrum (NPS). **A.** Examples of white noise and correlated noise are shown. **B.** The normalized NPS for body and lung reconstruction kernels is illustrated. **C.** The NPS for different radiation dose levels (CTDI$_{vol}$ values are shown) are illustrated, demonstrating the lower dose image data have greater noise amplitude. **D.** NPS curves show the difference between standard FBP and a deep learning algorithm approach toward reconstruction for the same acquired data set. 📖 **F10-61**

## 10.6 CT IMAGE ARTIFACTS

1. **Beam hardening**
   a. Refers to the increase in effective energy of the x-ray beam as it passes through tissue (Fig. 10-55).
   b. The beam intensity decreases with tissue depth, but lower energy photons are attenuated more.
   c. Beam hardening occurs to a greater extent in tissues with higher atomic number (*e.g.*, bone).
   d. Results in lower attenuation coefficient estimate, and lowering HU values.
   e. More visible due to the backprojection process (Fig. 10-56).
   f. Only occurs in the presence of a polyenergetic x-ray spectrum.
   g. Impact of beam hardening can be lessened using "prehardened" (filtered) x-ray beams.
2. **Streak artifacts**
   a. Origins: highly attenuating objects in the patient (*e.g.*, metallic implants or dental fillings).
   b. Discontinuity in signal level challenges the linearity of the detector system.
   c. Slight motion causes the emanation of streaks (Fig. 10-57).
   d. Metal artifact reduction algorithms use mapping between voxels in the CT volume data and raw projection dataset—iteration adjusts the raw data to reduce artifacts.

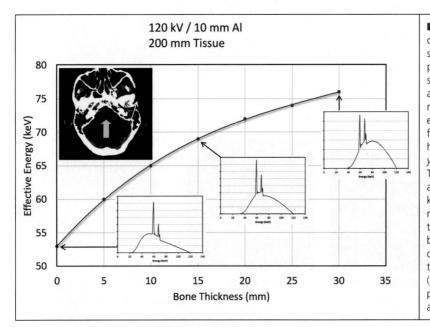

120 kV / 10 mm Al
200 mm Tissue

(y-axis) Effective Energy (keV)
(x-axis) Bone Thickness (mm)

■ **FIGURE 10-55** Beam hardening occurs as the x-ray beam traverses tissue (and especially bone) through the patient. Because CT images are reconstructed from different projection angles, and the spectral changes that result from beam hardening are different for each projection, a streaking artifact can occur between objects with high attenuation, as indicated by the *yellow arrow* on the head CT image. The plot shows the effective energy as a function of bone thickness, for a 120-kV x-ray beam (with 10 mm Al and 200 mm soft tissue filtration). The shape of the spectrum changes with increasing bone thickness, gradually being depleted of low-energy components in the spectrum at greater thicknesses (the spectra are normalized—overall photon number is considerably smaller at large thickness). 📖 **F10-62**

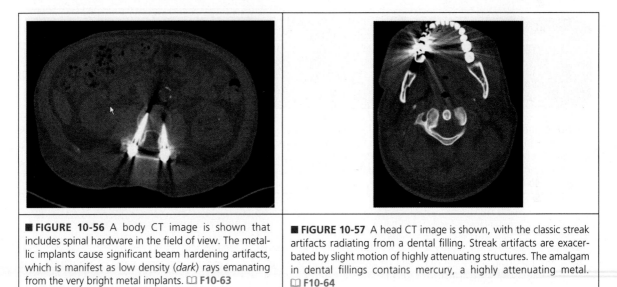

■ **FIGURE 10-56** A body CT image is shown that includes spinal hardware in the field of view. The metallic implants cause significant beam hardening artifacts, which is manifest as low density (*dark*) rays emanating from the very bright metal implants. 📖 **F10-63**

■ **FIGURE 10-57** A head CT image is shown, with the classic streak artifacts radiating from a dental filling. Streak artifacts are exacerbated by slight motion of highly attenuating structures. The amalgam in dental fillings contains mercury, a highly attenuating metal. 📖 **F10-64**

3. **View aliasing**
   a. Insufficient sampling of the *number of views* for high-frequency signals during backprojection.
   b. Artifacts project radially (Fig. 10-58).

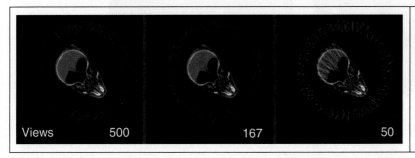

Views    500    167    50

■ **FIGURE 10-58** View aliasing is illustrated in the CT images of a mouse skull, acquired on a micro-CT scanner. No view aliasing is detected with 500 views, some view aliasing is seen for 167 views, and significant view aliasing (as well as image noise) is seen with only 50 views used in the reconstruction. 📖 **F10-65**

**4. Ring artifacts**

    **a.** Characteristic of third-generation (rotate-rotate) CT geometry.

    **b.** Detectors provide information along a given annulus of the reconstructed image.

    **c.** Malfunctioning or uncalibrated detectors cause a ring at a radius equal to the distance between the center detector in the gantry and the malfunctioning detector for an *axial scan* (Fig. 10-59).

    **d.** *Helical scan* ring artifacts occur partially in the scan plane *and* in the z-dimension (Fig. 10-60).

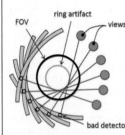
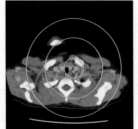
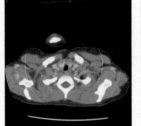

**A** description      **B** rings highlighted      **C** ring artifacts

■ **FIGURE 10-59** The cause of ring artifacts is illustrated graphically in **(A)**. In third-generation CT, a given detector contributes to an annulus in the reconstructed image; any miscalibration of the detector may result in a ring artifact. **B.** A body CT image is illustrated, and the three-ring artifacts are highlighted with the overlaid graphics. **C.** The CT image is displayed without the overlaid graphics, showing three-ring artifacts. 📖 **F10-66**

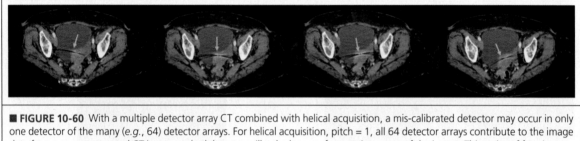

■ **FIGURE 10-60** With a multiple detector array CT combined with helical acquisition, a mis-calibrated detector may occur in only one detector of the many (*e.g.*, 64) detector arrays. For helical acquisition, pitch = 1, all 64 detector arrays contribute to the image data for every reconstructed CT image—a bad detector will only show up for certain sectors of the image. This series of four images show streak artifacts for subsequent images (along the z-axis), with the position of the artifact located at different regions in the image. 📖 **F10-67**

**5. Partial volume**

    **a.** The CT voxel is the smallest volume element with a uniform HU value.

    **b.** A combination of tissues (*e.g.*, soft tissue and calcium) results in a weighted average of the combination, and a reduction in contrast (Fig. 10-61).

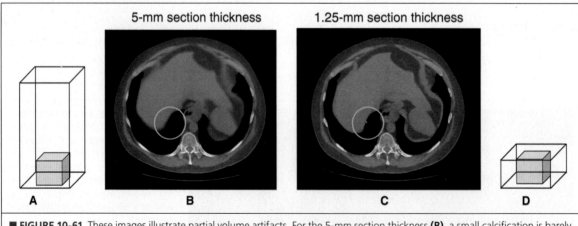

5-mm section thickness      1.25-mm section thickness

**A**      **B**      **C**      **D**

■ **FIGURE 10-61** These images illustrate partial volume artifacts. For the 5-mm section thickness **(B)**, a small calcification is barely seen because the length of the voxel is much longer than the calcification (as shown in **A**), and thus the average linear attenuation coefficient (which scales to the Hounsfield unit) is low. For the 1.25-mm section thickness **(C)**, the high attenuation of the calcification is less diluted in the volume (see graphic in **D**), resulting in a higher linear attenuation coefficient (and HU values) in the image with significantly better detectability. 📖 **F10-68**

    **c.** The volume averaging in the *z*-dimension with larger slice thickness creates a "partial volume" effect.

    **d.** Larger voxels generate larger partial volume artifacts.

**6. Cone-beam artifacts**

    **a.** Circular scan cone-beam acquisition geometry leads to undersampling in the cone-angle dimension.

    **b.** Loss of sampling occurs as the beam diverges (high cone angle).

    **c.** "Tuy's condition" is a cone-beam data insufficiency problem that states "every plane that intersects the object of interest must contain a cone-beam focal point."

    **d.** The Defrise phantom (a stack of parallel disks demonstrates the artifact (Fig. 10-62).

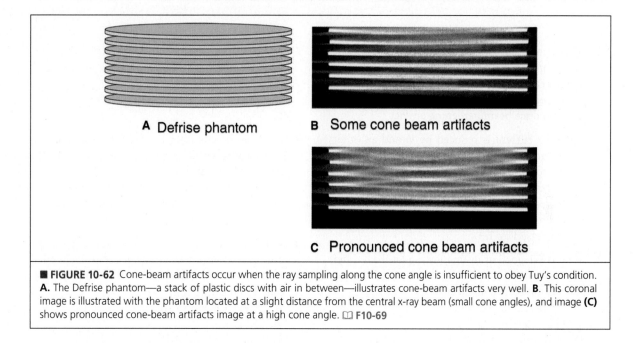

**A** Defrise phantom      **B** Some cone beam artifacts

**C** Pronounced cone beam artifacts

■ **FIGURE 10-62** Cone-beam artifacts occur when the ray sampling along the cone angle is insufficient to obey Tuy's condition. **A.** The Defrise phantom—a stack of plastic discs with air in between—illustrates cone-beam artifacts very well. **B.** This coronal image is illustrated with the phantom located at a slight distance from the central x-ray beam (small cone angles), and image **(C)** shows pronounced cone-beam artifacts image at a high cone angle. 📖 **F10-69**

# Section II Questions and Answers

1. Why is the preprocessing step LN($I_0$/$I$) performed?
   A. To linearly scale attenuation coefficients
   B. To scale CT numbers from −1,000 to +3,000
   C. To reduce the number of reconstruction steps
   D. To reduce beam hardening artifact

2. The tube current is reduced by ½ and all other factors are maintained. How much has the noise (standard deviation) in the CT image changed?
   A. Increased by 2×
   B. Increased by 1.4×
   C. Decreased by 2×
   D. Decreased by 1.4×

3. Why is CT good at distinguishing fat from other soft tissues?
   A. Vast difference in effective $Z$
   B. Decreased density of fat
   C. Photoelectric effect
   D. Hydrophobic nature of fat
   E. Increased refractive index

4. What is the definition of pitch for helical CT scanning?
   A. Sampling distance in the plane of acquisition
   B. Table travel speed in mm/s
   C. Table translation per 360° gantry rotation divided by the nominal beam width
   D. Collimated beam width divided by the table translation per 360°

5. Which one of the following tissues/materials has the lowest CT number?
   A. Water
   B. Lipoma
   C. Trabecular bone
   D. Lung
   E. Vitreous humor

6. What is the most likely x-ray interaction that occurs during CT scanning of a patient?
   A. Photoelectric absorption
   B. Compton scatter
   C. Rayleigh scatter
   D. Electron capture

7. At 120 kV, $\mu_{water} = 0.19$ cm$^{-1}$. For all else the same, what CT number will $\mu_{material} = 0.38$ cm$^{-1}$ have?
   A. −1,000
   B. −500
   C. 38
   D. 500
   E. 1,000

8. If a head bowtie filter is used for CT acquisition of a patient with a large abdomen, how will the dose be distributed?
   A. Concentrated in the center of the patient
   B. Concentrated in the periphery of the patient
   C. Homogeneous across the patient

9. A CT study uses 0.625 mm sampling in the z-direction. Reconstructions generate 1.25 and 5 mm slices. What is the SNR of the 5 mm compared to the 1.25 mm slice?
   A. $SNR_{5.0} = 4 \times SNR_{1.25}$
   B. $SNR_{5.0} = 2 \times SNR_{1.25}$
   C. $SNR_{5.0} = \sqrt{2} \times SNR_{1.25}$
   D. $SNR_{5.0} = \frac{1}{2} \times SNR_{1.25}$

10. Why is the dose efficiency of a multirow CT scanner improved with a greater width of active arrays?
    A. Detectors have better absorption efficiency
    B. X-ray tube loading is reduced
    C. The penumbra is a smaller fraction of the beam
    D. X-ray tube current is reduced

11. What is the limiting resolution in a reconstructed CT image for a 25 cm FOV and matrix of 500 pixels in *lp/cm*?
    A. 0.5
    B. 1
    C. 2
    D. 5
    E. 10

12. What does the filtering in filtered backprojection refer to?
    A. A mathematical operation
    B. Addition of copper in the beam
    C. A beam hardening correction procedure
    D. Voltage ripple reduction in the x-ray beam
    E. A process that uses only certain projections

13. What is the chief cause of beam hardening in CT?
    A. Excess scatter on the detector array
    B. Removal of the hardest x-rays in the spectrum
    C. Preferential attenuation of low energy x-rays
    D. Operating at a very low kV
    E. Characteristic x-rays that dominate the spectrum

14. Of the following relative conditions, which one will have the largest CT noise power spectrum amplitude?
    A. Low mAs, filtered backprojection
    B. High mAs, filtered backprojection
    C. Low mAs, iterative reconstruction
    D. High mAs, iterative reconstruction

15. In which direction is the x-ray tube heel effect manifested in a conventional CT scanner?
    A. In the $x$-$y$ plane
    B. In the $z$-dimension
    C. In the radial direction
    D. Heel effect is not considered for CT scanners

16. In CT, to what does the "ramp filter" refer?
    A. Shape of copper placed in the x-ray beam
    B. Shape of the kernel in the frequency domain
    C. Shape of the kernel in the spatial domain
    D. Shape of the tube current modulation kernel
    E. Shape of the bowtie thickness radius

17. How does tube current modulation reduce radiation dose and maintain CT image quality?
    A. Equalizes view-dependent projection noise
    B. Compensates for the bowtie filter attenuation
    C. Uses lower kVs to maximize subject contrast
    D. modulates the gantry rotation speed
    E. Provides focal spot switching to optimize detail

18. In CT *simple* backprojection of a uniform object, what are characteristics of the reconstruction?
    A. Adjacency aliasing throughout the image
    B. Higher signal in the center
    C. Higher signal in the periphery
    D. Signal is uniform throughout

19. What protocol below (same kV and constant mAs as indicated) delivers the lowest dose?
    A. Pitch = 1.4, mAs/rotation = 220 mAs
    B. Pitch = 1.0, mAs/rotation = 200 mAs
    C. Pitch = 0.7, mAs/rotation = 120 mAs
    D. Pitch = 0.5, mAs/rotation = 60 mAs

20. What is the major parameter determining circumferential spatial resolution in CT?
    A. Number of photons at the object's periphery
    B. Number of detector rows for a multislice system
    C. Number of rays acquired in a projection
    D. Number of views acquired in a rotation

21. In cardiac CT imaging, which parameter will have the greatest impact on lowering radiation dose?
    A. Dual-source x-ray system
    B. Low kV
    C. Prospective gating
    D. Retrospective gating
    E. Beta-blocker to slow the heart rate

22. In general, for dual-energy CT, how will the HU values scale at 80 kV compared to 140 kV for materials with HU < 0?
    A. 80 kV HU > 140 kV HU
    B. 80 kV HU < 140 kV HU
    C. 80 kV HU = 140 kV HU

# Answers

1. **A**  The natural logarithm ($LN[e^x]$) is the inverse function of $e^x$, thus, $LN[e^x] = x$. This operation linearizes the exponential attenuation of x-rays transmitted through an object along a given ray when the measured incident intensity $I_0$ is divided by the transmitted intensity $I$. *(Pg. 383–384 and Eqs. 10-6 through 10-8)*

2. **B**  The tube current and time product (mAs) is proportional to tube output per slice and thus the number of photons used in the acquisition of the image. Poisson statistics are considered for noise propagation with the standard deviation, $\sigma$, the direct measurement of noise. The measured noise is proportional to the square root of the ratio of the mAs values, $\sqrt{(mAs_1/mAs_2)}$; for $mAs_1 = 2\ mAs_2$, the noise is increased (lower number of photons) by a factor of $\sqrt{2} = 1.4\times$, or 40% *(Pg. 398–399, Eq. 10-2, and Fig. 10-60)*

3. **B**  CT numbers (HU) are chiefly dependent on the linear attenuation coefficient due to the Compton interaction, which is proportional to the density and the atomic number ($N$) to atomic number ($A$) ratio. The lower tissue density of fat ($r = 0.94\ g/cm^3$) results in a lower $\mu_{Compton}$ and thus a lower HU (negative values $-40$ to $-10$) when compared to water (HU = 0). *(Pg. 350–351, Eq. 10-1)*

4. **C**  Pitch is defined as the CT table feed distance (mm) per 360° rotation of the gantry divided by the collimated beam width (mm). *(Pg. 370–371, Eq.10-4)*

5. **D**  The CT number (HU) is determined by the weighted average of the attenuation coefficients within a voxel of the object scanned, as represented by each pixel in the reconstructed image. Lung has a significant fraction of air (HU = $-1,000$) where the effective linear attenuation coefficient will be significantly lower, thus resulting in the lowest CT number in the list of tissues. *(Pg. 350–351, Eq. 10-2)*

6. **B**  The typical range of x-ray energies produced by a tube voltage of 80 to 140 kV used in CT acquisition generates an effective energy from approximately 45 to approximately 70 keV, where the x-ray interactions are dominated by the Compton scattering interaction. *(Pg. 349–350, Fig. 10-6)*

7. **E**  The HU is based upon the attenuation coefficient of the material subtracted from the attenuation coefficient of water, and normalized by the attenuation coefficient of water and scaled by 1,000; thus 1,000 $\times$ $(0.38 - 0.19)/0.19 = 1,000$. *(Pg. 351, Eq. 10-2)*

8. **A**  The bowtie filter is constructed to modify the incident radiation fluence on the patient in accordance with the patient thickness the beam encounters so that the distribution of transmitted x-rays is uniform over the anatomy being imaged. The head bowtie filter is constructed over a smaller diameter than the abdomen of a patient, thus there will be more transmission centrally and less peripherally, resulting in dose concentrated in the center of the patient's abdomen *(Pg. 365-367, Fig. 10-23)*

9. **B**  Slice thickness represents the third dimension of the voxel and determines the relative number of x-ray photons that are detected in the volume element. A reconstruction into larger slice thickness re-bins the raw data, such that the number of photons is proportional to the volume. For a 5 mm slice, there will be *4 times* as many photons (on average) as there will be in a 1.25 mm slice. Thus, the noise will *decrease* and the signal to noise ratio will *increase* by a factor of $\sqrt{4} = 2\times$. The downside is the potential increase of partial volume artifacts and loss of detail resolution and contrast. *(Pg. 372–373, Fig. 10-30; Pg. 398–399, Eq. 10-12, Pg. 405 partial volume artifact discussion)*

10. **C**  For multichannel, multislice CT scanners, the collimated beam width can be opened to the full area of the detector array, or can likewise be reduced to cover a smaller area of active detectors. In each instance of collimation, the focal spot penumbra must be projected outside of the active detector area. Geometric efficiency is the fraction of the active detector area width divided by the collimated beam width that includes the

penumbra. This represents the relative efficiency of the radiation geometry, because the penumbra fraction irradiates the patient but is unused in the reconstruction. For a multislice scanner using a small fraction of the active detector elements (*e.g.*, using a 10 mm width active detector array), the geometric and radiation dose efficiency will be very poor, as the penumbra fraction is a substantial fraction of the detected beamwidth. On the other hand in this situation, the amount of scatter reaching the detectors is reduced, so contrast resolution is improved. (*Pg. 363–364, Fig. 10-21*)

11. **E**  Limiting resolution is chiefly determined by the sample size in the plane of the image, determined by the FOV, and the number of samples across the FOV. The Nyquist sampling theorem states that two samples per cycle are needed to avoid aliasing, thus limiting resolution = 500 samples (pixels)/(2 × 25 cm) = 10 lp/cm. Actual resolution is often limited by the reconstruction kernel or focal spot size. (*Pg. 394–395*)

12. **A**  Filtered backprojection is a mathematical operation that corrects the 1/r blurring that occurs with a simple backprojection, where the kernel is the "filter" that has specific characteristics to emphasize contrast (*e.g.*, Shepp-Logan) for soft tissue discrimination or detail (*e.g.*, "bone" or "ramp") to emphasize high contrast spatial resolution where quantum noise is less of an issue. (*Pg. 386–390*)

13. **C**  Beam hardening occurs by the preferential attenuation of the lower energy x-rays in the spectrum that affects the effective energy of the beam as it passes through greater thicknesses of tissue or higher atomic number tissues such as bone, leading to projections with many fewer photons (photon starvation) and subsequent artifacts. (*Pg. 401–403, Figs. 10-62 and 10-63*)

14. **A**  The noise power spectrum (NPS) describes the noise in terms of $HU^2$ $mm^3$ as a function of spatial frequency. Thus, the conditions that generate the highest variance (lowest number of photons) and least amount of smoothing (FBP) will have the highest amplitude NPS. (*Pg. 399–401, Fig. 10-61*)

15. **B**  The heel effect is caused by the self-attenuation of x-rays generated in the anode, causing a reduction of fluence on the anode side of the projected x-ray field. For CT scanners, this occurs in the z-dimension, which means that larger collimated beam widths and cone-beam CT scanners will have a measurable loss of fluence along the cone angle. (*Pg. 359–360, Figs. 10-15 and 10-16*)

16. **B**  The "ramp" filter refers to the frequency domain filter, $|H(f)|$ which is equal to the absolute value of $f$, multiplied by the blurring function $1/f$, to undo the blurring, followed by the inverse Fourier transform. Note that the Fourier transform of the 1/r convolution blurring is $1/f$. (*Pg. 387–389, Eq. 10-10, Fig. 10-47*)

17. **A**  Noise in the overall reconstructed image is dominated by the most highly-attenuating projections as a function of angle and plane attenuation. Tube current modulation (also known as automatic exposure control) modifies the tube current to compensate for attenuation, ensuring all projections have a similar relative noise. The thinner patient projections have reduced dose. (*Pg. 373–376, Figs. 10-31 and 10-32*)

18. **B**  Simple backprojection is a summation process that has higher density in the center of the reconstruction and, therefore, higher signal than in the periphery. (*Pg. 384–387, Fig. 10-45*)

19. **D**  The highest pitch doesn't necessary lead to the lowest dose. In this situation, [mAs/pitch] that is the lowest value determines the lowest dose [A. 157; B. 200; C. 171; D. 120]. (*Pg. 370–371, Eq. 10-5*)

20. **D**  Circumferential spatial resolution is determined by the number of views obtained during a rotation about the object. View aliasing is an associated artifact due to undersampling. (*Pg. 366–367, Fig. 10-24; 402–403, Fig. 10-65*)

21. **C**  Prospective gating uses the EKG trace to time the acquisition of views during the quiescent (diastolic) phase of the heart, thus significantly limiting the x-ray beam "on" time. (*Pg. 377–380, Fig. 10-37*)

22. **B**  At 80 kV, since the attenuation values (and thus HU) are usually higher than at 140 kV, for materials with HU < 0 (*e.g.*, fat), the numbers, in general, will be more negative than at 140 kV, and the reverse will be true for materials with HU > 0. It is the energy-dependent variations in attenuation and HU values that provide an ability to generate energy-selective tissue decomposition. (*Pg. 380–382, Figs. 10-39 and 10-40*)

# Section III Key Equations and Symbols

| QUANTITY | EQUATION | EQ NO./PAGE/COMMENTS |
|---|---|---|
| Attenuation coefficient for Compton interaction | $\mu_{\text{Compton}} = \rho N \dfrac{Z}{A}$ | Eq. 10-1/Pg. 351/Where $r$ is mass density, $N$ is Avogadro's number, $Z$ is atomic number, $A$ is atomic mass. |
| Hounsfield unit, HU | $HU_K \equiv 1{,}000 \left[ \dfrac{\mu_K - \mu_w}{\mu_w - \mu_{\text{air}}} \right] \cong 1{,}000 \left[ \dfrac{\mu_K - \mu_w}{\mu_w} \right]$ | Eq. 10-2/Pg. 351/For a given voxel $K$ in the image, linear attenuation coefficients $\mu_K$, $\mu_w$, and $\mu_{\text{air}}$ for material $K$, water, and air; second equality is a simplification. |
| Overbeaming and radiation efficiency | Radiation efficiency = detected width/beam width | Figure 10-21/Pg. 364/For multidetector arrays, the penumbra is a fixed fraction of the collimated beam; efficiency is increased for larger detected width. |
| Propagation of noise | $\sigma^2_{\text{CT image}} = \sigma^2_{p1} + \sigma^2_{p2} + \sigma^2_{p3} + \cdots + \sigma^2_{pN}$ | Eq. 10-3/Pg. 365/The total noise in CT adds in quadrature for each projection $pN$; larger contributions dominate overall noise. |
| Pitch | $\text{pitch} = \dfrac{F_{\text{table}}}{nT}$ | Eq. 10-4/Pg. 370/$F_{\text{table}}$ is the table feed distance per 360°; $n = $ *number of array channels, and* $T = $ *detector width.* |
| Dose and pitch relationship | $\text{dose} \propto \dfrac{1}{\text{pitch}}$ | Eq. 10-5/Pg. 371/Holds only when all other factors are held constant. |
| Measurement of the "ray" at position $j$ along the projection | $S_j = k_j I_0 e^{-(\mu_1 t + \mu_2 t + \mu_3 t + \cdots + \mu_n t)}$ | Eq. 10-6/Pg. 383/Each projection, $S_j$, is a measure of the discrete intensity, $I_j$, at each detector element $j$, with scalar constant, $k_j$ for each attenuation coefficient along the ray path for incident $I_0$. |
| Normalization with reference detector measurement | $S_r = k_r I_0$ | Eq. 10-7/Pg. 383/Measurement of unattenuated beam $I_0$, with $k_r$ scalar constant. |
| Reference corrected projection measurement | $P_j = \ln\left\{ \dfrac{\alpha S_r}{S_j} \right\} = t(\mu_1 + \mu_2 + \mu_3 + \ldots + \mu_n)$ | Eq. 10-8/Pg. 384/$\alpha = k_j/k_r$ and the projection $P_j$ corresponds to the linear sum of the attenuation coefficients. |
| Sinogram representation | $P(j, \theta)$ | Pg. 384/where $j$ corresponds to each detector position, and $\theta$ to the view angle (Fig. 10-42B, Pg. 385). |
| Convolution backprojection | $p'(x) = \int_{x'=-\infty}^{\infty} p(x')\, h(x - x')dx' = p(x) \otimes h(x)$ | Eq. 10-9/Pg. 386/$p(\cdot)$ is each measured projection, $h(\cdot)$ is the deconvolution kernel, and $p'(x)$ is the corrected projection. |
| Fourier-based filtered reconstruction | $p'(x) = FT^{-1}\{FT[p(x)] \times FT[h(x)]\}$ | Eq. 10-10/Pg. 387/Where FT is the Fourier transform and $FT^{-1}$ is the inverse Fourier transform. |
| Frequency domain filter for $1/f$ degradation | $|H(f)| = \alpha \times f$ | Eq. 10-11/Pg. 389/Where $\alpha$ is a scaling factor. This is the "ramp" filter. |

| QUANTITY | EQUATION | EQ NO./PAGE/COMMENTS |
|---|---|---|
| Image noise in CT | $$\sigma = \sqrt{\dfrac{\sum_{i=1}^{N}\left(HU_i - \overline{HU}\right)^2}{N-1}}$$ | Eq; 10-12/Pg. 398/$\sigma$ is the standard deviation within a region of interest. |

| SYMBOL | QUANTITY | UNITS |
|---|---|---|
| Voxel | Volume element | mm³ |
| HU | Hounsfield unit | Unitless (normalized to water) |
| Ray | X-ray photon trajectory | Unitless |
| View | Collection of rays at one angle | Unitless |
| View angle | Angle of x-ray tube about 360° | Degrees |
| Fan angle | X-ray beam in the *x-y* plane | Degrees |
| Cone angle | X-ray beam in the *z* plane | Degrees |
| Geometric efficiency | The ratio of active detector width to collimated beam width | Unitless |
| SSP | Slice sensitivity profile | mm |
| Kernel | Mathematical reconstruction filter | Description of filter |

# X-Ray Dosimetry in Projection Imaging and Computed Tomography

## 11.0 INTRODUCTION

Radiation dosimetry encompasses the measurement and calculation of ionizing radiation energy deposition into matter—this chapter addresses the application of dosimetry to x-ray projection imaging and x-ray computed tomography.

## 11.1 X-RAY TRANSMISSION

1. **X-ray energy spectrum incident on a patient**
   a. Typical spectrum at 100 kV is shown with 3 mm inherent aluminum filtration (Fig. 11-1).
   b. Interactions within tissues have energy dependencies that are considered for accurate dosimetry.

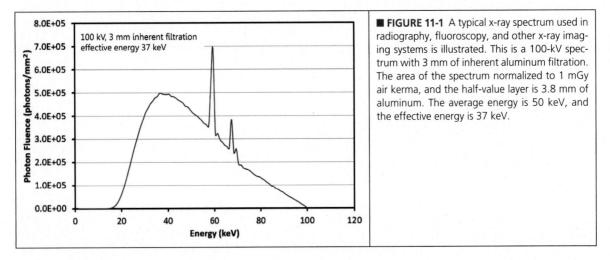

■ **FIGURE 11-1** A typical x-ray spectrum used in radiography, fluoroscopy, and other x-ray imaging systems is illustrated. This is a 100-kV spectrum with 3 mm of inherent aluminum filtration. The area of the spectrum normalized to 1 mGy air kerma, and the half-value layer is 3.8 mm of aluminum. The average energy is 50 keV, and the effective energy is 37 keV.

2. **Dose, D, deposited by *primary photons*** at a specific depth $x$ is given by (Eq. 11-1):

$$D(x) = \int_{E_{min}}^{E_{max}} \left\{ \frac{\mu_{en}(E)}{\rho} \right\} E\phi(E)e^{-\mu(E)x} \, dE \qquad [11\text{-}1]$$

where the photon fluence is $\phi(E)$ in #photons/cm², the mass-energy absorption coefficient is $\mu_{en}(E)/\rho$ for photons of energy $E$, $\rho$ is the density of the material, and $\mu(E)$ is the linear attenuation coefficient for photons of energy $E$.

   a. The *transmitted x-ray* fluence for *primary photons* (Eq. 11-2) is reduced by attenuation (Fig. 11-2) as

$$D(x) = D_o e^{-\mu_{eff} x} \qquad [11\text{-}2]$$

where $\mu_{eff}$ is the "match" of the *effective* attenuation of the 100 kV spectrum in Figure 11-1.

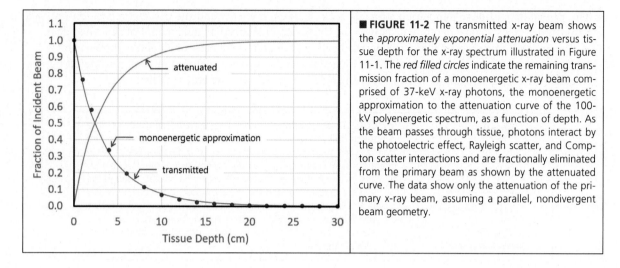

■ **FIGURE 11-2** The transmitted x-ray beam shows the *approximately exponential attenuation* versus tissue depth for the x-ray spectrum illustrated in Figure 11-1. The *red filled circles* indicate the remaining transmission fraction of a monoenergetic x-ray beam comprised of 37-keV x-ray photons, the monoenergetic approximation to the attenuation curve of the 100-kV polyenergetic spectrum, as a function of depth. As the beam passes through tissue, photons interact by the photoelectric effect, Rayleigh scatter, and Compton scatter interactions and are fractionally eliminated from the primary beam as shown by the attenuated curve. The data show only the attenuation of the primary x-ray beam, assuming a parallel, nondivergent beam geometry.

    **b.** The intensity of the beam is reduced independent of attenuation by the *inverse square law*, as x-rays are emitted from a point source (the focal spot) with a diverging beam (Fig. 11-3)

**3. Generation of x-ray scatter**: the complex geometry of x-ray scatter and other factors requires the use of computer-based Monte Carlo techniques to track the passage of primary and scatter photons.

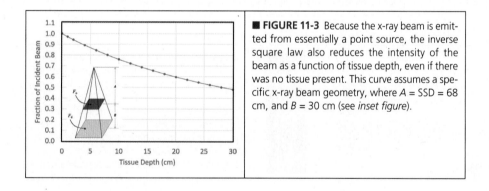

■ **FIGURE 11-3** Because the x-ray beam is emitted from essentially a point source, the inverse square law also reduces the intensity of the beam as a function of tissue depth, even if there was no tissue present. This curve assumes a specific x-ray beam geometry, where *A* = SSD = 68 cm, and *B* = 30 cm (see *inset figure*).

## 11.2  MONTE CARLO SIMULATION

All modern x-ray dosimetry relies extensively on Monte Carlo simulation. Sophisticated computer programs and algorithms track simulated x-ray photons as they are incident on the patient and in the tissue, photon by photon. Photons that do not interact with the patient, the primary photons, are those used to form the image. The vast majority of photons that do interact with the tissue (greater than 90% of the total) deposit dose through the photoelectric effect and Compton scattering. The statistical probabilities of the interactions and noninteractions followed for billions of photons derived from a polyenergetic spectrum provide a way to determine the dose to the skin and various organs in the body as explained in this section.

**1. Computing the random walk of each x-ray photon**
    **a.** Each incident x-ray from a bremsstrahlung spectrum is followed through stochastic processes and random number generators (Fig. 11-4).
    **b.** Included are attenuation and geometry-dependent inverse square law processes described in **Section 11.1**, as well as photoelectric absorption and Compton scatter probabilities for each x-ray photon history.
    **c.** The simulation loops over the energies (*e.g.*, in 1 keV steps) in the filtered bremsstrahlung spectrum.
**2. The quantity absorbed dose** (Eq. 11-3) is the energy deposited (d*E*) by ionizing radiation per unit mass (d*m*):

$$D_{absorbed} = \frac{dE}{dm}$$

[11-3]

3. **The probability of dose deposition** depends on x-ray photon energy and the tissue composition (fat, soft tissue, bone) at a specified depth to determine the likelihood of interaction and amount of deposited dose.
   a. The photoelectric absorption interaction results in local deposition of most or all of the photon energy.
   b. The Compton scatter interaction deposits a fraction of the incident photon dose, and a scattered photon continues on the random walk, emitted at an angle dependent on its energy and the tissue.

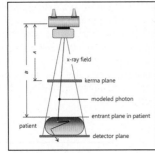

■ **FIGURE 11-4** A typical design for Monte Carlo simulation of dose deposition is illustrated. The simulated (virtual) x-ray beam is emitted from a point source and is collimated onto a detector plane. X-ray interactions are computed in a virtual patient, where the dose deposition and its distribution are tallied. The air kerma passing through the kerma plane is recorded, and the radiation dose in the patient is also tallied. This geometry can then be used to define a coefficient, which is the ratio of patient dose to incident air kerma. More specific anatomical geometry can also tally dose to specific organs and other interaction sites of interest.

4. **Normalization point for entrance air kerma**
   a. Radiography and fluoroscopy: air kerma at the surface of the patient
   b. Computed tomography: air kerma at the center of rotation (the isocenter)
5. **Mathematical phantoms**
   a. Simple geometrical phantoms to detailed anatomical models (Fig. 11-5) are used to simulate the body.
   b. Anatomical models are segmented into relatively large (2 × 2 × 2 mm voxels) for use in simulations.

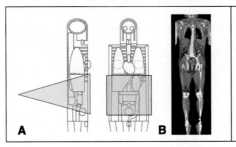

■ **FIGURE 11-5 A.** Historically, Monte Carlo studies made use of anatomical models defined by simple geometrical shapes; here, the Medical Internal Radiation Dose (MIRD) phantom is illustrated. **B.** The power of modern computers combined with the availability of high-resolution anatomical data from CT scans have allowed Monte Carlo simulations to be performed with very detailed anatomical models.

## 11.3 THE PHYSICS OF X-RAY DOSE DEPOSITION

1. **X-ray interactions with electrons deposit dose to tissue**
   a. Photoelectric effect and Compton scatter ionize atoms/molecules at the site of interaction
   b. An ejected electron further interacts with tissue in a very small local volume.
   c. Electron collision with other electrons (called secondary electrons or "delta rays") imparts energy.
   d. Energy deposition can cause chemical changes (*e.g.*, creation of hydroxyl radicals) that can damage DNA.
2. **Kerma**
   a. Kerma—"**K**inetic **e**nergy **r**eleased in **ma**tter."
   b. *Air kerma* is a special case of the energy released in air (Fig. 11-6).
   c. X-ray interactions transfer energy to electrons—the absorbed energy is the difference of the energy transferred ($E_{tr}$) and the energy radiated ($E_r$) out of the volume (Fig. 11-7) as given by Equation 11-4.

$$E_{en} = E_{tr} - E_r$$

[11-4]

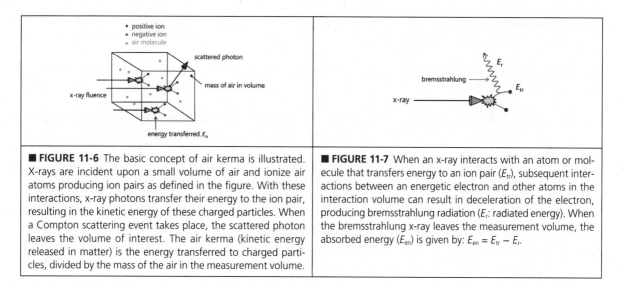

**FIGURE 11-6** The basic concept of air kerma is illustrated. X-rays are incident upon a small volume of air and ionize air atoms producing ion pairs as defined in the figure. With these interactions, x-ray photons transfer their energy to the ion pair, resulting in the kinetic energy of these charged particles. When a Compton scattering event takes place, the scattered photon leaves the volume of interest. The air kerma (kinetic energy released in matter) is the energy transferred to charged particles, divided by the mass of the air in the measurement volume.

**FIGURE 11-7** When an x-ray interacts with an atom or molecule that transfers energy to an ion pair ($E_{tr}$), subsequent interactions between an energetic electron and other atoms in the interaction volume can result in deceleration of the electron, producing bremsstrahlung radiation ($E_r$: radiated energy). When the bremsstrahlung x-ray leaves the measurement volume, the absorbed energy ($E_{en}$) is given by: $E_{en} = E_{tr} - E_r$.

### 3. Absorbed dose in a medium (Fig. 11-8)

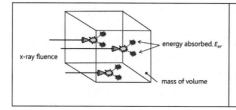

**FIGURE 11-8** When x-ray photons are incident upon the measurement volume (x-ray fluence density), energy is initially transferred ($E_{tr}$), and some energy may be radiated away (as shown in Fig. 11-7). The energy remaining, $E_{en}$, divided by the mass of the volume represents the absorbed dose. The volume of interest in this figure could be filled with air, and hence, the dose would be the air dose; however, this can also be a small volume of tissue, corresponding to the absorbed dose in tissue.

## 11.4  DOSE METRICS

There are a number of metrics that describe dose in different ways

1. **Entrance skin air kerma (ESAK)**
   a. The amount of radiation incident on the surface of the patient (formerly entrance skin exposure [ESE]).
   b. ESAK is an appropriate metric for radiographic, mammographic, and fluoroscopic procedures.
   c. The ESAK value is estimated and derived from known output characteristics and geometry at the skin surface and is equal to the air kerma, $K_{air}$, at that point.
      (i)   Value is "free-in-air"—meaning that there is no influence of scatter from any medium in proximity.
   d. For diagnostic radiology energies, the air kerma, $K_{air}$, approximates the dose to air, $D_{air}$: $K_{air} \approx D_{air}$
2. **Entrance skin dose**
   a. Radiation dose imparted to the initial layers of skin.
   b. The entrance skin dose includes (i) the dose in air, $D_{air}$ (without backscatter); (ii) dose deposited to the skin by photons backscattered from the tissue volume; and (iii) the ratio of the tissue to air mass-energy attenuation coefficients relating the dose to tissue, $D_{tissue}$, to that measured in air, $D_{air}$.
   (i)   The ESAK is equivalent to the dose in air, $D_{air}$, without backscattered radiation.
   (ii)  *Backscattered radiation* contributes to the dose at the entrance surface—the backscatter factor is variable, dependent on tissue thickness and field size irradiated, ranging from approximately 1.1 to approximately 1.5.
   (iii) The ratio of the tissue to air mass-energy attenuation coefficients for a small irradiated area accounts for an increase to the dose in tissue, where $D_{tissue} \cong 1.09\, D_{air}$ (Eq. 11-5).

$$D_{tissue} = D_{air} \times \frac{\left\{\dfrac{\mu_{en}}{\rho}\right\}_{tissue}}{\left\{\dfrac{\mu_{en}}{\rho}\right\}_{air}}$$

[11-5]

3. **Absorbed dose**
   a. Considered to be the fundamental concept of radiation dose.
   b. Absorbed dose is the energy absorbed per unit mass (Eq. 11-3).
   c. With energy expressed in joules and mass expressed in kilograms, the unit is the gray (Gy); 1 Gy = 1 J/kg.
   d. Absorbed dose is specified at a specific point—the dose nearly always varies with position in the patient.
   e. Dose is often misinterpreted as a metric directly related to "risk" as described below:
      (i) Specification of the total mass of tissue that receives a given absorbed dose can have widely different impacts in terms of risk: for example, 10 Gy to a 20-mg finger versus average dose of 10 mGy to a 20-kg abdomen.
      (ii) In the example, the finger and the abdomen receive the same absorbed dose, but the same risk?
      (iii) Deposition of dose into organs or tissues affects the risk (see *effective dose* description, part 6 below).
   f. Absorbed dose or just "dose" is the gold standard measurement describing one or more radiation exposure events.
4. **Mean glandular dose (also known as average glandular dose)**
   a. The mean glandular dose (MGD) is the dose metric for describing dose to the breast tissue, composed of fibroglandular, adipose (fat), and skin tissues—methods to determine MGD are explained in Chapter 8.
   b. Radiosensitivity of glandular tissue is far greater than skin or adipose tissue.
   c. MGD is the standard metric for computing dose in the breast.
5. **Organ dose**
   a. Metrics
      (i) Average (mean) dose delivered to the specific organ of interest
      (ii) For paired organs (*e.g.*, kidneys or breasts), if a targeted examination deposits dose in only one (*e.g.*, 0.2 mGy to the left kidney), the average dose to both kidneys for the procedure would be 0.1 mGy.
      (iii) Implicit assumption is that the stochastic risk is the same whether one half of the organ receives all of the radiation or if the radiation dose was evenly distributed throughout the entire organ.
   b. Anthropomorphic phantoms
      (i) Organ doses from x-ray exposures in anthropomorphic phantoms can be estimated with Monte Carlo techniques (for further details, see Fig. 11-5, and textbook Pg. 418, Fig. 11-9)
      (ii) A balance between accuracy and simulation efficiency for organ dose comes in the form of "hybrid modeling," which combines analytical and Monte Carlo simulation methods on stylized or computational human phantoms ranging from the newborn to (male and female) adults
   c. No one dose metric can do it all.
      (i) A tally of organ doses represents the comprehensive assessment of radiation dose from imaging.
      (ii) There is no *single* metric that can quantify "dose" and the corresponding radiosensitivity of an organ.
      (iii) Different radiation types (x-rays, gamma rays, electrons, protons, alpha particles) can deposit dose quite differently in tissues, and increase the probability of stochastic effects like cancer for the same absorbed dose; the dose metric called *equivalent dose* accounts for differences in the type of radiation.
6. **Equivalent dose**
   a. Accounts for the biological damage to tissues based upon the consequence of linear energy transfer (LET) deposition of different radiation types through the use of weighting factors, $w_R$ (Eq. 11-6).
   b. Sparsely ionizing low LET radiations (*e.g.*, x-rays, γ-rays, electrons) are assigned $w_R = 1$.
   c. Densely ionizing high LET radiations (*e.g.*, protons, alpha particles) are assigned $w_R$ greater than 1; for example, $w_R = 20$ for alpha particles (*See Chapter 3, Pg. 65–66, and Table 3-4 in the textbook*).
   d. The quantity *equivalent dose, H,* is

   $$H = D \times w_R \qquad [11\text{-}6]$$

   e. Note: for x-rays, the *equivalent dose* is numerically equal to the absorbed dose, but they are different quantities—unit of equivalent dose is the sievert (Sv), and unit of absorbed dose is the gray (Gy).
7. **Effective dose, E**
   a. Like H, E is a *calculated value* that is not really a dose in the physical sense. E is a radiation protection term that provides a *single value metric* for the cumulative long-term potential for harm (detriment) to a population for exposures to different areas of the body.
   b. Originally proposed for assessment of environmental and industrial exposure to radiation workers.
   c. Organs that do not receive dose do not contribute to *E*.
   d. Incorporates an approximation of organ sensitivities and assigns a *tissue weighting factor, $w_T$*.
      (i) For *uniform whole-body irradiation*, the total tissue weighting is 1.0—thus, the individual organ $w_T$ sum to 1.0.

(ii)  A proportion of the total is the $w_T$ of the organs, assigned according to organ-tissue sensitivity, (mostly radiogenic cancer).

(iii) $w_T$ ranges from 0.01 for radioresistant tissues to 0.12 for sensitive tissues (Table 11-1).

  e. Quantifying effective dose, $E$, is a two-step process.
  (i)  Organ absorbed dose, $D$ (Gy), is converted to organ equivalent dose, $H_T$ (Sv), using Equation 11-6.
  (ii) The effective dose $E$ (units of Sv) is calculated using Equation 11-7 for all organs irradiated $T$, as the sum over $T$ of the product of $w_T$ and the corresponding organ equivalent dose $H_T$ as:

$$E(Sv) = \sum_T \left[ w_T \times H_T(Sv) \right]$$

[11-7]

### TABLE 11-1  TISSUE WEIGHTING FACTORS ($W_T$) FOR VARIOUS TISSUES AND ORGANS (ICRP 103)

| TISSUE | $W_T$ |
|---|---|
| Bone marrow, breast, colon, lung, stomach, remainder | 0.12 |
| Gonads | 0.08 |
| Bladder, esophagus, liver, thyroid | 0.04 |
| Brain, bone surface, salivary glands, skin | 0.01 |

  f. Strengths of effective dose, $E$
  (i)   $E$ takes into consideration partial body exposure.
  (ii)  $E$ provides a method to include doses from radiopharmaceuticals (see Chapter 16).
  (iii) $E$ provides a *single value metric* for the long-term potential for harm (detriment) to a population for multiple exposures to different areas of the body.
  (iv)  $E$ can be used to make numerical comparisons to radiation doses associated with medical imaging procedures in a more understandable context for patients and healthcare workers—for example, comparison of annual background radiation of 3.1 mSv at sea level to a head CT effective dose of 2.5 mSv.
  g. Weaknesses of effective dose
  (i)  As defined by the ICRP, $E$ was never meant and should not be used as a risk-related metric for a specific person or population that differs from the population used to define the weighting factors. Unfortunately, all too often, $E$ has been popularized as a quantitative measure of individual future cancer risk, a use for which it was never intended.
  (ii) As a risk metric, $E$ does not take into consideration patient-specific factors such as health status, clinical indication, patient sex, patient age—all factors that must be considered when evaluating potential risks against the benefits of a particular imaging procedure,
  h. $E$ is useful in comparing imaging modality doses (*e.g.*, CT versus radiography) to the same patient population.

## 11.5  RADIATION DOSE IN PROJECTION RADIOGRAPHY

1. **X-ray system radiation output levels**
  a. Measurable normalized values of radiation output (Fig. 11-9).
  b. Information is typically provided by annual testing of radiographic equipment.
  c. Air kerma (mGy) per 100 mAs at 100 cm as a function of x-ray tube kV (and any added filtration).
2. **Computing the patient ESAK**—(Eqs. 11-8 to 11-10)
  a. Distance: source to skin distance (SSD) and source to image distance (SID) (Fig. 11-10)
  b. Inverse square law: relates measured x-ray tube output air kerma at 100 cm to $x$ SSD (cm)

$$C_1 = \left[ \frac{100\,cm}{SSD} \right]^2$$

[11-8]

  c. Tube current-time product (mAs): relates mAs used for the examination, $x$, to 100 mAs measured output

$$C_2 = \frac{x\,mAs}{100\,mAs}$$

[11-9]

  d. Determine air kerma from output curve graph (Fig. 11-9) for the kV used in the examination, AK (kV)
  e. Calculate the ESAK as the product of $C_1$, $C_2$, and AK (kV)

$$ESAK = C_1 C_2 AK\,(kV)$$

[11-10]

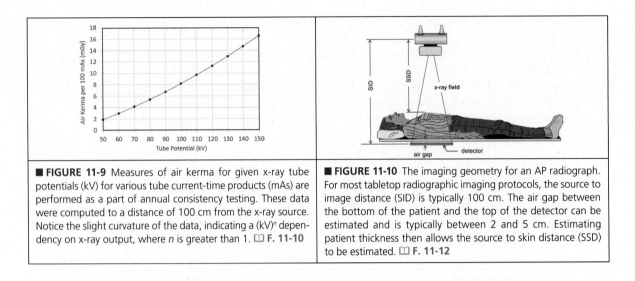

**■ FIGURE 11-9** Measures of air kerma for given x-ray tube potentials (kV) for various tube current-time products (mAs) are performed as a part of annual consistency testing. These data were computed to a distance of 100 cm from the x-ray source. Notice the slight curvature of the data, indicating a $(kV)^n$ dependency on x-ray output, where $n$ is greater than 1. 📖 **F. 11-10**

**■ FIGURE 11-10** The imaging geometry for an AP radiograph. For most tabletop radiographic imaging protocols, the source to image distance (SID) is typically 100 cm. The air gap between the bottom of the patient and the top of the detector can be estimated and is typically between 2 and 5 cm. Estimating patient thickness then allows the source to skin distance (SSD) to be estimated. 📖 **F. 11-12**

3. **Estimating effective dose**
   a. Tabular data are available for computing organ doses and effective doses from ESAK for specific examinations.
      (i) See textbook, Page 425, Table 11-3: Effective dose per entrance surface dose (mSv/mGy) conversion factors for various kV, filters, and radiographic projections
   b. Digital radiography systems provide kerma area product (KAP) measurements directly; this metric is often called dose area product (DAP)
      (i) The KAP, sometimes indicated as $P_{KA}$, is equal to the product of the cross-sectional area of the x-ray beam and air kerma exiting collimator and provides a dose metric that is constant with distance.
      (ii) Air kerma at a specific distance can be determined by indicated KAP divided by the beam area projected at that distance (*e.g.*, onto the patient at the SSD).
      (iii) Total energy imparted to the patient is proportional to KAP and also to effective dose.
      (iv) Monte Carlo routines for projection radiography can be used to estimate effective dose for specific projections by knowing the acquisition technique factors (kV, mAs, tube filtration/half-value layer, field area projected onto the anthropomorphic phantom).
      (v) A graphic relationship of KAP to effective dose conversion factor can be determined as the slope of the linear regression fit of data points for different patients (Fig. 11-11).

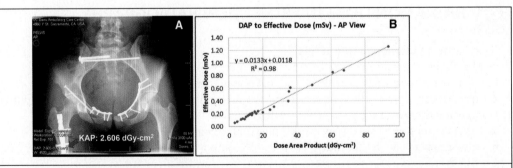

**■ FIGURE 11-11** The kerma area product (KAP), also referred to as the dose area product (DAP) in the DICOM header, is a metric available on modern digital radiography systems. **A.** An anterior-posterior (AP) projection of the pelvis in a thin patient, with a measured KAP of 2.61 dGy-cm². (Note, dGy-cm² is the standard DICOM unit for KAP, not the more commonly used, but equivalent unit of mGy-cm².) **B.** Plot of the calculated effective dose versus indicated KAP for a range of patient sizes using x-ray acquisitions with automatic exposure control. The linear regression fit gives the slope (mSv/dGy-cm²) and offset, which is used to estimate effective dose directly from the KAP for any similar examination. For the patient radiograph shown in (**A**), the effective dose is estimated to be 0.046 mSv (0.0118 + 0.0133 × 2.606). 📖 **F. 11-13**

**RADIATION DOSE IN FLUOROSCOPY**

1. **Considerations relative to radiography**
   a. Acquisitions vary over an extended time, with variations in tube current.
   b. Geometrically, fluoroscopy changes with interactive movements for patient repositioning.
   c. Several magnification modes can be selected that change air kerma rate and FOV.
   d. The operator can change the beam projection angle throughout the procedure.
   e. SID often changes throughout the procedure with table height and detector adjustments.
   f. FOV collimation can be circular, square, or rectangular.
   g. kV and filtration are interactive, dependent on fluoro mode used (*e.g.*, low, medium, high dose).
2. **Automatic exposure (air kerma) rate control (AERC)**
   a. AERC adjusts the kV and mA to achieve an acceptable image as needed by the examination.
   b. Adjustments include selection of low dose, medium dose, or high contrast as required.
   c. Measurements in the field with various attenuator thicknesses can validate operation (Fig. 11-12).

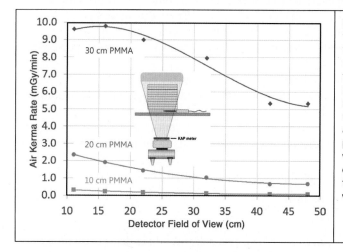

■ **FIGURE 11-12** Virtually all modern fluoroscopic systems work in automatic exposure rate control mode, and therefore, characterization of the output of the system needs to embrace this. The air kerma rate is shown as a function of the detector field of view, for three thicknesses of polymethyl methacrylate (PMMA), a tissue surrogate. For calculation of patient dose in fluoroscopy using the data shown in the figure, the medical physicist also needs to know (for each touch of the fluoroscopic pedal) the patient thickness and the detector field of view. For patient thicknesses that are substantially different from the three shown (10, 20, and 30 cm) exponential, interpolation can be used at each detector field of view setting. □ F. 11-14

3. **Estimates of radiation dose in fluoroscopy**
   a. Integrated air kerma at the *reference point*, $K_{a,r}$, and kerma-area product (KAP or $P_{KA}$) are required.
      (i) For interventional systems, $K_{a,r}$ is 15 cm closer to the x-ray tube from the isocenter of rotation.
      (ii) For mobile C-arm fluoroscopy units, $K_{a,r}$ is determined 30 cm from the detector entrance surface.
   b. DICOM Radiation Dose Structured Report (RDSR) provides a recording of each irradiation event with all x-ray output parameters, collimation, geometric orientation, and operation mode.
   c. The cumulative $K_{a,r}$ is a surrogate for estimating *peak skin dose* for possible tissue reactions and injuries.
      (i) Dose to the skin can be estimated from $K_{a,r}$ and distance, $d$, to the reference point from the focal spot to the skin, SSD, by inverse square correction, the backscatter factor (*BSF*) that ranges from 1.1 to 1.5 dependent on field size and patient thickness, and tissue-to-air ratio of approximately 1.09 in Equation 11-5 above.
      (ii) Estimates of peak skin dose (PSD) or $D_{skin}$ use $K_{a,r}$ data and beam geometry/orientation from the RDSR data and *BSF* (Eq. 11-11), as well as attenuation of the table/pad as described in Chapter 9

$$D_{skin} = K_{a,r} \left( \frac{d_{ref\,point}}{SSD} \right)^2 \times BSF \times \frac{(\mu_{en}/\rho)_{tissue}}{(\mu_{en}/\rho)_{air}}$$  [11-11]

   (iii) A *sentinel event* as defined by The Joint Commission is an acute PSD of 15,000 mGy (15 Gy) or consecutive studies that exceed 15,000 mGy when summed over a 6-month period.
   (iv) "Procedural pause" occurs when $K_{a,r}$ reaches predetermined limits (*e.g.*, 5,000 mGy, 7,000 mGy, etc.) to identify next steps and as a reminder to spread dose over a large area of the body.
   d. The KAP ($P_{KA}$) allows the determination of energy imparted to the patient and can be used with conversion factors to estimate effective dose (and thereby an estimate of risk) for the fluoro examination
      (i) Methods are similar to those described above in Section 11.5.3.b.
      (ii) Conversion factors with units of mSv/mGy-cm² for various procedures are available in the literature.

## 11.7 RADIATION DOSE IN COMPUTED TOMOGRAPHY

The computed tomography dose index (CTDI) is a metric that considers the unique characteristics of CT, including no well-defined entrant surface, rotation about an isocenter, spatial dependence of beam-shaping filters, and acquisition parameters that impact the delivered dose to the patient. CTDI *is not patient dose* and does not consider the size of the patient. It does, however, represent a measure of the radiation output of the CT scanner.

1. Computed Tomography Dose Index, $CTDI_{100}$
   a. $CTDI_{100}$ uses a 100-mm-long "pencil" ionization chamber of approximately 9 mm diameter and approximately 3 cm$^3$ volume with a uniform radiation response along its length.
   b. A cylindrical polymethyl methacrylate (PMMA) phantom of 15 cm length is used for measurements.
      (i) 16-cm phantom: output measurements to represent adult and pediatric head scans
      (ii) 32-cm phantom: output measurements to represent the adult body and a *majority of* pediatric body scans
      (iii) 16-cm phantom: to represent small diameter pediatric body studies by some CT scanner vendors, although many vendors use the large 32-cm-diameter phantom for *all* pediatric body studies
   c. Each phantom has several parallel holes for insertion of the pencil ionization chamber (Fig. 11-13).
      (i) One central position and peripheral position holes at 12, 3, 6, and 9 o'clock are used for measurement.
      (ii) During measurements, all open holes are filled with PMMA rod "plugs."
   d. Table height is adjusted to match the center of the phantom with the isocenter of rotation, and longitudinal/lateral table position is adjusted to position the beam central axis in the geometric center.
   e. For narrow collimation (up to approximately 40 mm beam width), the 100-mm chamber measures the primary and a significant fraction of the scattered radiation, $K_{measured}$ (kerma), along the length of the ionization chamber as shown in Figure 11-14.
      (i) Partial irradiation of the chamber by the nominal primary beam width, $B$, requires correction, as:

$$K_{corrected} = \frac{100\,mm}{B\,mm} \times K_{measured} \qquad [11\text{-}12]$$

      (ii) In Equation 11-12, $B$ is the product of the number of data channels, $n$, and the detector width for each channel, $T$; for example, 64 channels with 0.625 mm detector width has 40 mm beam width (at the isocenter).
      (iii) A single scan (1 rotation) estimates the average dose of a multiple, contiguous scan at each measurement location as determined from primary and scattered radiation detection.
   f. For wider beams, the 100-mm ionization chamber and measurement methodology fails (Fig. 11-15), chiefly due to the inability to capture the scattered radiation.
      (i) An alternate, preferred measurement uses a small thimble chamber (0.6 cm$^3$).
      (ii) The *total* scan is required for each measurement, and partial volume correction is not needed because the entire length of the probe is irradiated.
      (iii) This methodology is required for wide collimation (≥80 mm) and cone-beam scanners.

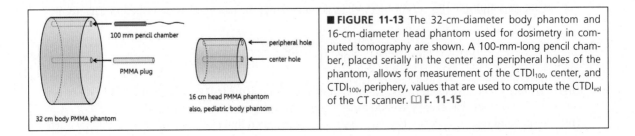

**■ FIGURE 11-13** The 32-cm-diameter body phantom and 16-cm-diameter head phantom used for dosimetry in computed tomography are shown. A 100-mm-long pencil chamber, placed serially in the center and peripheral holes of the phantom, allows for measurement of the $CTDI_{100}$, center, and $CTDI_{100}$, periphery, values that are used to compute the $CTDI_{vol}$ of the CT scanner. ▢ F. 11-15

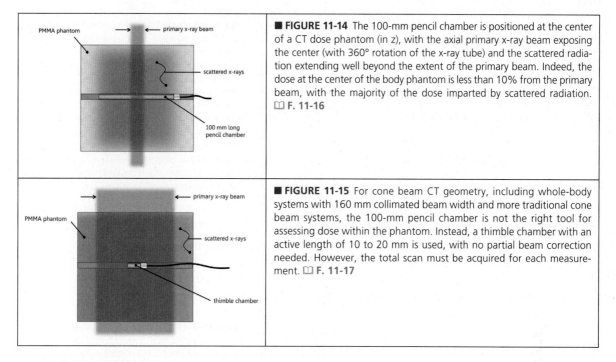

■ **FIGURE 11-14** The 100-mm pencil chamber is positioned at the center of a CT dose phantom (in z), with the axial primary x-ray beam exposing the center (with 360° rotation of the x-ray tube) and the scattered radiation extending well beyond the extent of the primary beam. Indeed, the dose at the center of the body phantom is less than 10% from the primary beam, with the majority of the dose imparted by scattered radiation. 📖 F. 11-16

■ **FIGURE 11-15** For cone beam CT geometry, including whole-body systems with 160 mm collimated beam width and more traditional cone beam systems, the 100-mm pencil chamber is not the right tool for assessing dose within the phantom. Instead, a thimble chamber with an active length of 10 to 20 mm is used, with no partial beam correction needed. However, the total scan must be acquired for each measurement. 📖 F. 11-17

## 2. Weighted CTDI (CTDI_w), volume CTDI (CTDI_vol), and DLP

**a.** The $CTDI_{100}$ is an integral of a dose distribution, $D(z)$, from a single rotation of the scanner having a nominal beam width of $nT$ (Eq. 11-13)

$$CTDI_{100} = \frac{1}{nT} \int_{L=-50\ mm}^{+50\ mm} D(z)dz$$  [11-13]

**b.** Measurements are made in the center ($CTDI_{100,\ center}$) and in the periphery ($CTDI_{100,\ periphery}$).
   **(i)** Multiple measurements (typically 3) at each location are averaged.
**c.** $CTDI_w$ (Eq. 11-14) combines the center and peripheral measurements to estimate the average dose to the phantom.

$$CTDI_w = \frac{1}{3} CTDI_{100,center} + \frac{2}{3} CTDI_{100,periphery}$$  [11-14]

**d.** For helical (spiral) scanning, the pitch is defined as the table translation distance (mm) for a full gantry rotation divided by the nominal beam width, $nT$ (mm), and the dose is inversely proportional to pitch (Eq. 11-15) when all other factors (kV, mAs) are constant:

$$dose \propto \frac{1}{pitch}$$  [11-15]

**e.** Dependency of dose on pitch adjusts the $CTDI_w$ (Eq. 11-16), resulting in the volume CTDI ($CTDI_{vol}$)

$$CTDI_{vol} = \frac{CTDI_w}{pitch}$$  [11-16]

**f.** Estimated $CTDI_{vol}$ is displayed prior to a scan, based on parameters (kV, mAs, pitch, collimation width), and the CTDI phantom used (16 or 32 cm diameter); actual $CTDI_{vol}$ is indicated after the scan.
**g.** The dose length product (DLP) is the product of the $CTDI_{vol}$ and the scan length, L, along the z-axis over which the table travels during the scan, Equation 11-17:

$$DLP = CTDI_{vol} \times L$$  [11-17]

   **(i)** Since *dose = energy/mass*, rearranging gives: *energy = dose × mass*; as mass scales linearly with length, *DLP is proportional to the energy imparted to the patient and is thus proportional to effective dose* (see Effective dose estimates in CT 11.7.5)
   **(ii)** DLP is reported with the phantom diameter (head, 16 cm, or body, 32 cm) in which it was measured.
**h.** For constant mAs (tube current × rotation time), $CTDI_{vol}$ increases with kV (Fig. 11-16).
   **(i)** The CTDI head phantom (16 cm diameter) is larger than the CTDI body phantom (32 cm diameter).

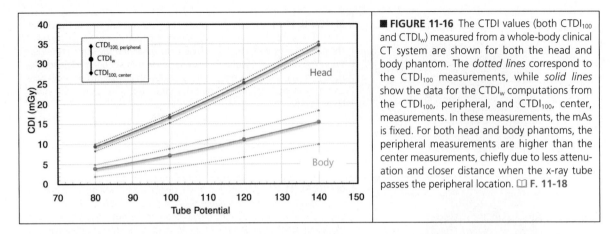

■ **FIGURE 11-16** The CTDI values (both CTDI$_{100}$ and CTDI$_w$) measured from a whole-body clinical CT system are shown for both the head and body phantom. The *dotted lines* correspond to the CTDI$_{100}$ measurements, while *solid lines* show the data for the CTDI$_w$ computations from the CTDI$_{100}$, peripheral, and CTDI$_{100}$, center, measurements. In these measurements, the mAs is fixed. For both head and body phantoms, the peripheral measurements are higher than the center measurements, chiefly due to less attenuation and closer distance when the x-ray tube passes the peripheral location. ⌷ **F. 11-18**

    **(ii)** The peripheral measurement of CTDI$_{100}$ is greater than the center measurement.
  **i.** A very large fraction of the measured CTDI comes from scatter and is of long range (Fig. 11-17).
    **(i)** The 100-mm pencil chamber captures the most proximal scatter dose (± 50 mm).
    **(ii)** A large fraction of scatter is consequently not recorded with the PMMA phantom.

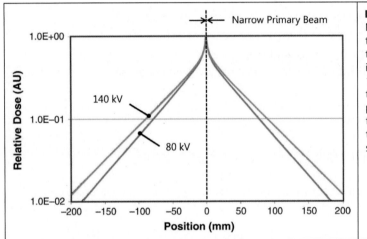

■ **FIGURE 11-17** These data are derived from Monte Carlo studies and demonstrate the longitudinal spread of scattered radiation from a very thin (0.1 mm) primary CT beam. The vertical axis is logarithmic, with a linear horizontal axis. For 140 kV, more than 2% of the dose from scattered radiation is deposited 200 mm from the primary beam (more than 1% on each side). Due to the lower energy of the scattered radiation, the longitudinal spread of the 80 kV beam is slightly less. ⌷ **F. 11-19**

**3. CT dose consideration for different scan lengths**
  **a.** Because of scatter, the dose to the center of the patient increases as the scan length increases (Fig. 11-18).
  **b.** A "rise to equilibrium" dose (graph insert in Fig. 11-18) with increased scan length indicates the influence of scattered radiation.
  **c.** Relative dose profiles demonstrate the long-range and additive contribution of scattered radiation to dose as shown in Figure 11-19 for a position centrally located in the scan length.

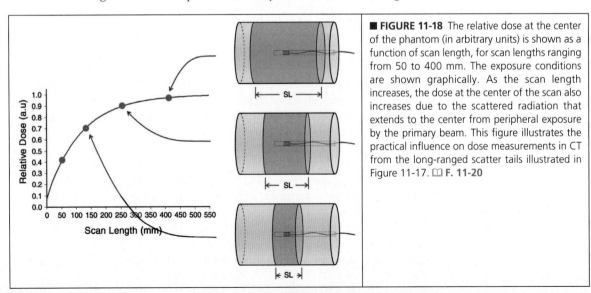

■ **FIGURE 11-18** The relative dose at the center of the phantom (in arbitrary units) is shown as a function of scan length, for scan lengths ranging from 50 to 400 mm. The exposure conditions are shown graphically. As the scan length increases, the dose at the center of the scan also increases due to the scattered radiation that extends to the center from peripheral exposure by the primary beam. This figure illustrates the practical influence on dose measurements in CT from the long-ranged scatter tails illustrated in Figure 11-17. ⌷ **F. 11-20**

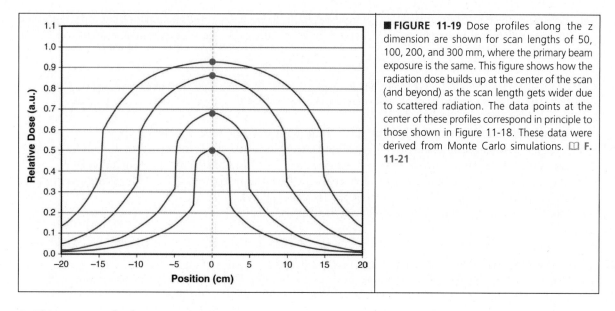

■ **FIGURE 11-19** Dose profiles along the z dimension are shown for scan lengths of 50, 100, 200, and 300 mm, where the primary beam exposure is the same. This figure shows how the radiation dose builds up at the center of the scan (and beyond) as the scan length gets wider due to scattered radiation. The data points at the center of these profiles correspond in principle to those shown in Figure 11-18. These data were derived from Monte Carlo simulations. ◻ **F. 11-21**

4. **The size-specific dose estimate, SSDE**
   a. $CTDI_{vol}$ is a dose metric that indicates the average dose to a plastic phantom, not to a specific patient.
      (i) $CTDI_{vol}$ underestimates dose when the patient size is smaller than the phantom diameter (this is for most patients).
      (ii) The higher density of PMMA (1.19 g/cm³) makes the phantom attenuation appear as approximately 38 cm diameter of tissue.
   b. The *SSDE* (a method developed by the American Association of Physicists in Medicine, Task Group 204 report) uses the $CTDI_{vol}$ and corrects for the mismatch between the phantom and patient size.
      (i) Water equivalent diameter, $D_w$, is the diameter of a circular cross section of water that has the same attenuation properties of the cross section of a patient and is calculated from the CT slice using Equation 11-18:

$$A = \sum_x \sum_y \Delta \left[ \frac{HU(x,y)+1000}{1000} \right]; \quad D_w = 2\sqrt{\frac{A}{\pi}} \qquad [11\text{-}18]$$

where $A$ is the area of the tissue (excluding air in and around the object), $\Delta$ is the area of a single pixel, $HU(x,y)$ is the CT number at position $x,y$ in the image, and $D_w$ is the water equivalent diameter.
      (ii) Higher-density tissues (higher HU) are weighted more (*e.g.*, bone), and lower-density/diameter tissues (lower HU) less (*e.g.*, lung)—the result is the approximation of the water-equivalent diameter, $D_w$.
      (iii) In order to be accurate, the complete patient's anatomy must be visible on the CT image with no cutoff by the reconstructed field of view.
      (iv) The localizer scan raw data and vendor-specific determination of $D_w$ are used as an alternate method.
   c. Dose values for 32-cm and 16-cm-diameter CTDI phantoms are normalized for various water equivalent diameters (Fig. 11-20) and computer fit to the exponential equation in Equation 11-19:

$$f = ae^{-bD_w} \qquad [11\text{-}19]$$

where $f$ is the normalized dose coefficient, and the fitting coefficients $a$ and $b$ are: for the body—$a = 3.7043$ and $b = 0.03672$ cm⁻¹; and for the head—$a = 1.9852$ and $b = 0.0486$ cm⁻¹.

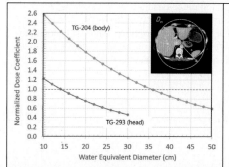

■ **FIGURE 11-20** The normalized dose coefficients as a function of water equivalent diameter are shown for both the head and body phantoms. These coefficients are used to estimate the size-specific dose estimate (SSDE), where the results are described in AAPM Report 204 (body) and Report 293 (head). The computer fits from a comprehensive mix of measured data (both physical measurements and Monte Carlo simulation data) from several groups are shown. ◻ **F. 11-22**

    **d.** The size-corrected absorbed dose ($D_{abs}^{z=0}$) from the indicated CTDI$_{vol}$ of the examination for a patient water equivalent diameter at the center ($z = 0$) of the scan length along the z-axis is determined in Equation 11-20:

$$D_{abs}^{z=0} = f \times CTDI_{vol}$$ [11-20]

    **(i)** The CTDI$_{vol}$ *for a given CT acquisition technique* will be the same regardless of patient size.

    **(ii)** The SSDE is a function of $D_w$ and therefore a better estimate of absorbed dose to the patient.

**5. Effective dose estimates in CT**

    **a.** Monte Carlo calculations provide organ doses for given scan areas and examination types.

    **b.** Since the dose length product (DLP) is linear with energy imparted in CT, for several studies, the organ dose data are used for estimating effective dose (see Section 11.4.6) and related to the examination DLP.

    **c.** The relationship is fit with linear regression techniques to yield the slope term, $k$, of the resulting curve (Fig. 11-11 shows a similar methodology developed for radiography).

    **d.** Effective dose, $E$, can thus be estimated from the DLP as

$$E = k \times DLP$$ [11-21]

    where $E$ has units of mSv, DLP has units of mGy-cm, and $k$ has units of mSv/mGy-cm.

    **e.** Table 11-2 lists $k$ for several CT examination types (for adult patients—pediatric values not indicated).

**TABLE 11-2 CONVERSION FACTORS ("$K$ FACTORS") FOR ESTIMATION OF EFFECTIVE DOSE (mSv) FROM DOSE LENGTH PRODUCT (mGy-cm), FOR VARIOUS CT EXAMINATION TYPES (FROM AAPM REPORT 96)**

| CT EXAMINATION TYPE | $K$ FACTOR (mSv/[mGy-cm]) |
| --- | --- |
| Head | 0.0021 |
| Chest | 0.017 |
| Abdomen | 0.015 |
| Abdomen-pelvis | 0.015 |
| Pelvis | 0.015 |

📖 T. 11-4

## 11.8 DOSE REPORTING SOFTWARE AND DOSE REGISTRIES

1. In the 2008–2010 time frame, there were several radiation dose accidents using CT in the United States that prompted scrutiny by the FDA, The Joint Commission, and several states, including California.
2. Radiation Dose Management Systems were developed subsequently to record radiation dose metrics in CT.
3. Automatic recording of the dose metrics from the DICOM images and Radiation Dose Structured Report (RDSR) has led to a better understanding of the relative dose metrics across CT examinations (Fig. 11-21).
4. The ACR has implemented a nationwide Dose Index Registry (DIR) to allow comparisons of dose metrics for several types of institutions (academic, large regional, small rural hospitals) and regions across the United States.
5. The automatic assessment of dose metrics has led to the use of Diagnostic Reference Levels (next section).

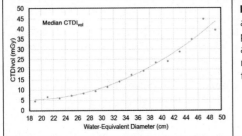

■ **FIGURE 11-21** Dose reporting in CT has spread across the United States and has led to the development of databases that can now be used for comprehensive protocol assessment for CT scanners at the same institution and across the country. The data in this figure show the median CTDI$_{vol}$ for abdomen CT scans as a function of water equivalent diameter, for a CT scanner that routinely uses x-ray tube current modulation. 📖 F. 11-23

## 11.9 DIAGNOSTIC REFERENCE LEVELS AND ACHIEVABLE DOSES

1. A **DRL** represents the 75th percentile of the dose distribution for an imaging study or acquisition protocol across a cohort of similar examinations.
2. An **achievable dose** is the 50th percentile (median) of the dose distribution and is a potential target for those facilities in the top quartile above the DRL.
   a. Radiology practices above the DRL should consider revising acquisition protocols to reduce dose.
   b. The achievable dose is a reasonable target for imaging practices in the top quartile.
3. *Examples:* in a recent study, the reported **DRL** for abdomen CT was 20 mGy CTDI$_{vol}$/1,004 mGy-cm DLP, and the **Achievable Dose** was 13 mGy CTDI$_{vol}$/657 mGy-cm DLP over the all-size category; for head CT, the **DRL** was 57 mGy/1,011 mGy-cm, and the **Achievable Dose** was 49 mGy/1,011 mGy-cm.
4. The use of DRLs and achievable doses for radiation protection are discussed in Chapter 21.

## 11.10 SUMMARY—TYPICAL EFFECTIVE DOSES FOR RADIOGRAPHIC PROCEDURES (TABLE 11-3)

**TABLE 11-3 TYPICAL EFFECTIVE DOSES FOR VARIOUS RADIOGRAPHIC PROCEDURES**

| PROCEDURE | AVERAGE EFFECTIVE DOSE (mSv) |
|---|---|
| **Radiographic Procedures** | |
| Skull | 0.14 |
| Cervical spine | 0.36 |
| Thoracic spine | 1.0 |
| Lumbar spine | 1.4 |
| PA and lateral chest | 0.10 |
| Mammography | 0.36 |
| Abdomen | 0.6 |
| Pelvis | 0.6 |
| Hip | 0.4 |
| Shoulder | 0.006 |
| Knee | 0.003 |
| Upper GI series[a] | 6.0 |
| Barium enema[a] | 6.0 |
| **CT Procedures** | |
| Head | 1.6 |
| Calcium scouring | 1.7 |
| Chest | 6.2 |
| Abdomen and pelvis | 7.7 |
| Three-phase liver | 15 |
| Spine | 8.8 |
| CT colonography | 10 |

[a]Includes dose from fluoroscopy.

Adapted with permission from National Council on Radiation Protection and Measurements (NCRP). *Report No. 184 Medical Radiation Exposure of Patients in the United States;* 2019. http://NCRPonline.org. 📖 T. 11-5

# Section II Questions and Answers

1. The SI unit of *absorbed dose* is the:
   A. curie
   B. gray
   C. roentgen
   D. rad
   E. sievert

2. One milligray is equal to how many joules per kilogram?
   A. $10^{-6}$
   B. $5 \times 10^{-5}$
   C. $10^{-4}$
   D. 0.001
   E. 0.01

3. The SI unit for air kerma is:
   A. curie
   B. gray
   C. roentgen
   D. rad
   E. sievert

4. A typical *effective dose*, *E*, for an adult noncontrast brain CT is approximately:
   A. 2 mSv
   B. 8 mSv
   C. 20 mSv
   D. 60 mSv
   E. 100 mSv

5. A typical *effective dose* for an abdominal CT of an average size adult patient is approximately:
   A. 3 mSv
   B. 10 mSv
   C. 30 mSv
   D. 60 mSv
   E. 100 mSv

6. Why is the DLP used for estimating the effective dose of patient CT scan instead of $CTDI_{vol}$?
   A. DLP is independent of $CTDI_{vol}$.
   B. DLP is proportional to the energy imparted.
   C. DLP is less affected by tube current modulation.
   D. DLP includes compensation for patient size.

7. What is the detriment to the patient that effective dose takes into account?
   A. Cataracts
   B. Acute radiation syndrome
   C. Cancer and severe hereditary effects
   D. Deterministic effects
   E. Deterministic and stochastic effects

8. The $CTDI_{vol}$ (32-cm-diameter phantom) for a large patient of 40 cm effective diameter is 25 mGy. How will the SSDE value compare to the $CTDI_{vol}$?
   A. Smaller
   B. Larger
   C. The same

9. For a kerma area product of 1,500 mGy-cm², an SID of 100 cm, and collimated square field size of 10 × 10 cm at the patient surface, what is the air kerma?
   A. 1.5 mGy
   B. 15 mGy
   C. 150 mGy
   D. 1,500 mGy
   E. 15,000 mGy

10. The DLP for a chest CT scan is 600 mGy-cm. What is the estimated effective dose for the examination?
    A. 5 mSv
    B. 10 mSv
    C. 15 mSv
    D. 20 mSv
    E. 25 mSv

11. At what percentile of a dose distribution is the Diagnostic Reference Level (DRL) determined?
    A. 5th
    B. 25th
    C. 50th
    D. 75th
    E. 95th

12. What is the rationale for using the 100-mm CT ionization chamber for determining CTDI?
    A. Measure scatter and primary radiation in 1 scan
    B. Get a better measurement for cone beam CT
    C. Use with collimated beam widths greater than 100 mm
    D. Provide accurate measurements for helical scans

13. When the magnification mode is used in digital fluoroscopy with AERC, what happens to the entrance skin air kerma rate?
    A. Increases
    B. Decreases
    C. Remains the same

14. A helical CT scan technique uses 150 mAs, pitch = 1.0. What is the relative dose when using 75 mAs, pitch = 0.5 with all other acquisition parameters the same?
    - **A.** 2.0 ×
    - **B.** 1.5 ×
    - **C.** 1.0 ×
    - **D.** 0.5 ×

15. The reference point air kerma, $K_{a,r}$, utilized in interventional fluoroscopy approximates:
    - **A.** HVL
    - **B.** effective mA
    - **C.** effective kV
    - **D.** entrance dose
    - **E.** effective dose

16. A sentinel event as described by The Joint Commission for peak skin dose in interventional radiology is greater than which of the following, in units of mGy?
    - **A.** 1,500
    - **B.** 5,000
    - **C.** 15,000
    - **D.** 50,000

17. Calculation of $CTDI_w$ requires central and peripheral measurements of $CTDI_{100}$ in the phantom. What are the weights of the measurements?
    - **A.** 1/4 central + 3/4 peripheral
    - **B.** 1/3 central + 2/3 peripheral
    - **C.** 1/2 central + 1/2 peripheral
    - **D.** 2/3 central + 1/3 peripheral
    - **E.** 3/4 central + 1/4 peripheral

18. Which one of the following dose metrics *directly* takes into account linear energy transfer of radiation types?
    - **A.** Absorbed dose
    - **B.** Effective dose
    - **C.** Equivalent dose
    - **D.** Mean glandular dose
    - **E.** Entrance skin dose

19. For an interventional fluoroscopy system, where is the location of the reference point, $K_{a,r}$?
    - **A.** 30 cm from the detector surface
    - **B.** 15 cm from the isocenter closer to the detector
    - **C.** 15 cm from the isocenter closer to the x-ray tube
    - **D.** 30 cm from the x-ray tube focal spot

20. The *achievable dose* represents what fraction of the population dose distribution for a procedure?
    - **A.** 0.05
    - **B.** 0.25
    - **C.** 0.50
    - **D.** 0.75
    - **E.** 0.95

21. A 4-year-old pediatric patient has an abdominal CT examination on a unit that uses the 32-cm CTDI phantom. How does the SSDE compare with the CTDIvol?
    - **A.** SSDE is higher.
    - **B.** SSDE is lower.
    - **C.** SSDE is the same.

22. In *radiography*, which one of the following radiation dose metrics can directly be used to estimate the risk of an examination with a conversion factor?
    - **A.** ESAK
    - **B.** KAP
    - **C.** DLP
    - **D.** MGD

23. For the organs listed below, which one has the *highest* tissue weighting factor?
    - **A.** Gonads
    - **B.** Thyroid
    - **C.** Brain
    - **D.** Lung
    - **E.** Skin

24. For the following properly exposed radiographic examinations, which has the lowest radiation risk?
    - **A.** Cranial-caudal mammogram
    - **B.** PA chest
    - **C.** Lateral skull
    - **D.** PA and LAT knee
    - **E.** AP hip

25. When using a 100-mm pencil ionization chamber for measuring CTDI, the correction factor necessary to produce an accurate dose estimate to the phantom is which one of the following?
    - **A.** Nominal beam width
    - **B.** CT gantry rotation speed
    - **C.** Helical pitch value
    - **D.** Focal spot penumbra width
    - **E.** Tube current modulation fraction

26. The reference point air kerma, $P_{KA}$, is a method to identify a potentially high peak skin dose. Which two parameters are necessary to determine the PSD from $P_{KA}$? (*Select two*—note, credit only given for the two correct choices—no partial credit)
    - **A.** Backscatter factor
    - **B.** Kerma area product
    - **C.** Half-value layer
    - **D.** Source to patient surface distance
    - **E.** X-ray beam quality

# Answers

1. **B** By definition, the SI unit for dose is the gray; the old definition is the rad. (*Pg. 416*)

2. **D** 1 gray = 1 J/kg, thus 1 milligray = 0.001 J/kg. (*Pg. 416*)

3. **B** Air kerma has units of Gy (typically mGy used for diagnostic imaging). (*Pg. 415*)

4. **A** The *typical* effective dose for a single acquisition brain CT scan is about 2 mSv. (*Pg. 440, Table 11-5*)

5. **B** The CTDI$_{vol}$ for a single acquisition abdominal scan of a normal adult size will likely range from 15 to 25 mGy, a DLP (assuming 30 cm acquisition) of 450 to 750 mGy-cm and a corresponding effective dose (using a k factor of 0.015): 450 × 0.015 to 750 × 0.015 = 6.75 to 11.25 mSv, closest to 10 mSv. (*Pg. 437, 440, Table 11-5*)

6. **B** DLP, Dose Length Product, is the product of the average CTDI$_{vol}$ and the table travel for a given examination. As such, it is an estimate of the total energy imparted to the patient, and for a specific area of the body, it can be used with "k" factors to generate an estimate of the effective dose for the head (k = 0.0021 mSv/mGy-cm), chest (k = 0.017 mSv/mGy-cm), abdomen (k = 0.015 mSv/mGy-cm) Note: k values do vary depending upon the reference; these are estimates for an adult from the references in the textbook. (*Pg. 433, 437, Table 11-4*)

7. **C** Effective dose provides a single-value metric that is used to represent the long-term detriment (primarily an increase in cancer risk) to a generic population incorporating committee-selected weighting factors for radiation quality and organ sensitivity. These weighting factors are averaged across all ages and both genders and thus do not apply to any specific individual or radiosensitive subpopulations such as children. (*Pg. 419–421*)

8. **A** The CTDIvol is determined for an adult body examination with the 32-cm-diameter CTDI phantom. As the patient is larger (40 cm diameter) and the patient mass is larger, then the actual dose (energy deposited/mass) as estimated by the SSDE paradigm is smaller than the estimated CTDIvol. Therefore, the SSDE results in a smaller (and closer) estimate of the dose compared to the actual dose to the patient. (*Pg. 435–436, Fig. 11-22*)

9. **B** The kerma area product is a value independent of the distance for a diverging point source with a fixed collimated beam. Therefore, a 10 × 10 cm field has an area of 100 cm$^2$ and for a 1,500 mGy-cm$^2$ KAP, the kerma at that distance is calculated as 1,500 mGy-cm$^2$/100 cm$^2$ = 15 mGy. (*Pg. 424–425, Fig. 11-13*)

10. **B** To determine effective dose from DLP, the conversion factor *k* must be known. For a chest CT examination, the *k* factor is 0.017 mSv/mGy-cm. *E* is 0.017 mSv/mGy-cm × 600 mGy-cm = 10.2 mSv. (*Pg. 437, Table 11-4*)

11. **D** The DRL is determined at the 75th percentile of a specific dose distribution. (*Pg. 439*)

12. **A** The 100-mm pencil ion chamber was implemented with legacy CT scanners and smaller collimated widths to measure both primary and scatter distributions for a single scan that could provide an estimate of the multiple scan average dose (MSAD) instead of acquiring a whole scan. (*Pg. 428–431, Fig. 11-16*)

13. **A** Magnification mode for digital detectors that do not use pixel binning results in a smaller collimated field of view expanded over a larger image area on the display, which provides improved sampling and better visible detail and object resolution for the fluoroscopist. Because quantum noise will also be more visible, the system adjusts (increases) the input dose to the patient approximately inversely linear to the magnification factor. Note, for pixel binning digital fluoroscopy detectors and image intensifier/TV systems, the input dose is increased inversely quadratic to the magnification factor. (*Pg. 425–428, Fig. 11-14*)

14. **C** For a given CT technique (kV and mAs), the dose is proportional to the mAs and to the inverse of the pitch. For the indicated technique factors, the doses as estimated by CTDIvol (150 mAs/1 and 75 mAs/0.5) are equivalent. This demonstrates an important point that dose depends on pitch *and* mAs; in many instances, particularly for 3D reconstructions, a pitch less than 1 is used with lower mAs to improve the sampling of the anatomy for better rendering without increasing dose, of course as long as the patient remains still. (*Pg. 432*)

15. **D**    The reference point air kerma location for an interventional fluoroscopy system is located at a point 15 cm below the isocenter of rotation closer to the x-ray tube as an estimate of the patient surface location and thus *entrance dose* when the table is centered. For conventional fluoroscopy (RF) systems and C-arm fluoroscopes, the reference point air kerma location is set 30 cm from the detector surface. *(Pg. 428, 341, Chapter 9)*

16. **C**    A sentinel dose event in interventional fluoroscopy occurs when a peak skin dose (PSD) exceeds a value of 15 Gy (15,000 mGy) to a specific area of skin on a patient undergoing a procedure. For multiple procedures, the PSD should be tracked over a time period of 6 months. *(Pg. 428, Section11.6.3.c.iii above)*

17. **B**    Weighted CTDI, CTDIw, is a combination of $CTDI_{100}$ measurements in the center and the periphery of the CTDI phantom with a weighted average of 1/3 central and 2/3 peripheral. *(Pg. 432, Eq. 11-14)*

18. **C**    Linear energy transfer (LET), discussed in Chapter 3, accounts for differences in the degree of biological damage produced by different types of radiation for the same total energy deposited in tissues. To take account of the differences in LET, the absorbed dose, D, is transformed to a radiation protection quantity called *equivalent dose*, H (in units of Sv), by using radiation weighting factors ($w_R$) assigned to the type of ionizing radiation as a function of its LET, as $H = D \times w_R$. For x-rays, $w_R = 1$, while for particulate radiation such as alpha particles, $w_R = 20$. *(Pg.415–421, specifically Pg. 419; also Chapter 3, Pg. 65–66)*

19. **C**    The interventional reference point, $K_{a,r}$, also known as the reference point air kerma, is located 15 cm from the geometric isocenter of rotation closer to the x-ray tube in order to get an estimate of the skin dose to the patient. *(Pg. 427–428, and Question 15 above)*

20. **C**    The *achievable dose* is determined from a distribution of reported radiation dose metrics for a specific examination or acquisition protocol using the 50th percentile (median) value of the distribution. *(Pg. 439)*

21. **A**    For pediatric CT examinations of the body, some manufacturers always use the 32-cm-diameter CTDI phantom, while some manufacturers use the 16-cm-diameter phantom, particularly for smaller and younger pediatric patients. Using the 32-cm-diameter phantom will typically result in an underestimate by the CTDIvol dose metric compared to the actual dose as estimated by SSDE. This is because the effective diameter of a pediatric patient will almost always be smaller, and for a given acquisition technique, the actual dose to the patient will be higher, often by a factor of 2 or more. *(Pg. 435–537, Fig. 11-22)*

22. **B**    The risk of an examination due to radiation dose is proportional to the energy imparted to the patient, and the age and sex specific risk coefficients of the organs irradiated. In the case of radiography (and fluoroscopy), the energy imparted to the patient is given by the KAP—kerma area product (or dose area product). With known (published) conversion factors, the effective dose can be estimated from the KAP. The other acronyms are ESAK, entrance surface air kerma; DLP, dose length product; MGD, mean glandular dose. *(Pg. 424–426, Fig. 11-13)*

23. **D**    The tissue weighting factor is a value assigned by the International Commission on Radiation Protection and Measurements (ICRP), whose most recent publication, ICRP-103, lists the organs and their respective weighting factors based primarily on epidemiological evidence on the impact of radiation dose and biological detriment. For the organs listed, the lung has the highest tissue weighting factor, $w_R$. *(Pg. 419–421, Table 11-1)*

24. **D**    Radiation risk depends on the absorbed dose and the organs receiving the dose. Patient extremity examinations (*e.g.*, hands, wrist, elbows, knees, shoulders) have few radiosensitive tissues and typically require a lower incident radiation dose to achieve an acceptable radiograph, thus resulting in a very low detriment and effective dose estimate. Thus, the knee radiograph will have the lowest risk. *(Pg. 439–440, Table 11-5)*

25. **A**    The primary x-ray beam width relative to the 100 mm length of the ionization chamber is necessary to correct for the partial volume exposure since an ionization chamber can only produce an accurate dose estimate if the entire sensitive volume is irradiated by the x-ray beam. Note that the beam width for CT is the product of the z-axis collimation, T (*the active detector width for an active channel*), and the number of channels, n: *for T = 0.625 mm and n = 64*, the beam width is 40 mm and the corrected ion chamber reading (in mGy) is the measured reading (mGy) × 100/40 mm. *(Pg 430–431, Fig 11-16, Eq. 11-12)*

26. **A and D**    The reference point air kerma is a "free-in-air" estimate of the incident radiation at the reference point, which for an interventional fluoro unit, is 15 cm closer to the x-ray tube from the isocenter. This value does not include radiation scatter; when the patient intercepts the beam at the skin surface, a significant fraction of the radiation absorbed dose is due to backscatter and this *backscatter factor, BSF*, accounts for 20% to 50% of the skin dose (i.e., BSF=1.2 to 1.5). Another necessary correction is for any deviation in the source to surface [skin] distance relative to the geometrical location of the reference point, which requires an inverse square correction factor. *(Pg. 428, Eq. 11-11)*

# Section III Key Equations and Symbols

| QUANTITY | EQUATION | EQ. NO./PAGE/COMMENTS |
|---|---|---|
| Dose deposited by *primary photons* in a medium at a depth $x$ | $D(x) = \int_{E_{min}}^{E_{max}} \left\{ \dfrac{\mu_{en}(E)}{\rho} \right\} E\phi(E) e^{-\mu(E)x} dE$ | Eq. 11-1/Pg. 407/mass energy absorption coefficient in brackets, for photons of energy $E$; f($E$) is fluence (photons/cm²); $r$ is material density. and m($E$) is linear attenuation coefficient for photons of energy $E$ |
| Monoenergetic approximation of a polyenergetic spectrum | $D(x) = D_o e^{-\mu_{eff}x}$ | Eq. 11-2/Pg. 408/m$_{eff}$ is the effective linear attenuation coefficient for a 37-keV photon emulating a 100 kV x-ray spectrum for a known beam filtration |
| Absorbed dose: defined as energy deposited by ionizing radiation per unit mass | $D_{absorbed} = \dfrac{dE}{dm}$ | Eq. 11-3/Pg. 411/$E$ is energy and $m$ is mass |
| Energy absorbed in a volume of air resulting from energy transferred and energy released | $E_{en} = E_{tr} - E_r$ | Eq. 11-4/Pg. 414/Absorbed energy $E_{en}$; transferred energy $E_{tr}$; radiated energy $E_r$ |
| Dose to tissue is equal to the dose in air times the ratio of mass-energy attenuation coefficients: tissue to air | $D_{tissue} = D_{air} \times \dfrac{\left\{ \dfrac{\mu_{en}}{\rho} \right\}_{tissue}}{\left\{ \dfrac{\mu_{en}}{\rho} \right\}_{air}}$ | Eq. 11-5/Pg. 416/Value is ~1.09 (except for higher-density tissues such as bone) |
| Equivalent dose | $H = D \times w_R$ | Eq. 11-6/Pg. 419/Weighting factor $w_R$ dependent on LET; $H$ in Sv |
| Effective dose | $E(Sv) = \sum_T \left[ w_T \times H_T(Sv) \right]$ | Eq. 11-7/Pg. 420/$E$ is a product of tissue weighting factor $w_T$ and equivalent dose $H$ summed over T |
| Inverse square law | $C_1 = \left[ \dfrac{100 \text{ cm}}{SSD} \right]^2$ | Eq. 11-8/Pg. 423/$C_1$ is a correction term for the inverse square law for 100 cm SID for a source to skin distance, SSD |
| Radiation output mAs linearity | $C_2 = \dfrac{x \text{ mAs}}{100 \text{ mAs}}$ | Eq. 11-9/Pg. 423/$C_2$ is a correction term for relating output of x-ray tube normalized to 100 mAs |
| Entrance surface (skin) air kerma | $ESAK = C_1 C_2 K_{air}(kV)$ | Eq. 11-10/Pg. 423/ESAK estimated from the inverse square and mAs for air kerma as a function of kV (Fig. 11-10 Pg. 422) |
| Dose to skin (fluoroscopy) | $D_{skin} = K_{a,r} \left( \dfrac{d_{ref\,point}}{SSD} \right)^2 \times BSF \times \dfrac{(\mu_{en}/\rho)_{tissue}}{(\mu_{en}/\rho)_{air}}$ | Eq. 11-11/Pg. 428/$K_{a,r}$ is the reference point air kerma; BSF is the backscatter factor |

**(Continued)**

| QUANTITY | EQUATION | EQ. NO./PAGE/COMMENTS |
|---|---|---|
| Corrected exposure for partial exposure to 100-mm pencil ionization chamber | $K_{corrected} = \dfrac{100 \text{ mm}}{B \text{ mm}} \times K_{measured}$ | Eq. 11-12/Pg. 431/CT dose using 100-mm pencil chamber: correction for nominal collimated beam width B |
| Computed tomography dose index for 100-mm pencil chamber measurement | $CTDI_{100} = \dfrac{1}{nT} \displaystyle\int_{L=-50\text{ mm}}^{+50\text{mm}} D(z)\,dz$ | Eq. 11-13/Pg. 432/$CTDI_{100}$ is the integral of the dose distribution (primary + scatter) over a 100 mm distance along the z-axis; $nT$ is the beam width B (above)—$n$ = #channels; $T$ = detector width projected to isocenter |
| Weighted CTDI ($CTDI_w$) | $CTDI_w = \dfrac{1}{3}\,CTDI_{100,center} + \dfrac{2}{3}CTDI_{100,periphery}$ | Eq. 11-14/Pg. 432/$CTDI_{100}$ is measured at the center and periphery (12 o'clock position) of the CTDI phantom |
| Dose corrected for pitch | $\text{dose} \propto \dfrac{1}{\text{pitch}}$ | Eq. 11-15/Pg. 432/Pitch is the table travel per rotation divided by the collimated beam width, $B$, for a helical scan. **This is for all other acquisition parameters (kV, mA, time) fixed** |
| Volume computed tomography dose index | $CTDI_{vol} = \dfrac{CTDI_w}{\text{pitch}}$ | Eq. 11-16/Pg. 432/The weighted CTDI for a scan is adjusted for pitch |
| Dose length product | $DLP = CTDI_{vol} \times L$ | Eq. 11-17/Pg. 433/L is the scan length of the acquisition; DLP is proportional to the effective dose |
| Water equivalent diameter | $A = \displaystyle\sum_x \sum_y \Delta\left[\dfrac{HU(x,y)+1000}{1000}\right];\quad D_w = 2\sqrt{\dfrac{A}{\pi}}$ | Eq. 11-18/Pg. 436/$A$ is the area of the tissue, $D$ is the area of a pixel, HU is the CT number in the image at position $x,y$; the expression in the bracket corrects for the fractional water equivalence at position $x,y$ |
| Conversion factor $f$: value to convert $CTDI_{vol}$ to size-specific dose estimate | $f = ae^{-bD_w}$ | Eq. 11-19/Pg. 436/Least-squares fit of $D_w$ to measured and Monte Carlo dose estimates that are normalized to 32- and 16-cm-diameter phantoms (see Fig. 11-22 in text, Pg. 437); $a$ and $b$ are the fitting parameters |
| Size-specific dose estimate (estimated absorbed dose, $D_{abs}$ at center slice) | $D_{abs}^{z=0} = f \times CTDI_{vol}$ | Eq. 11-20/Pg. 436/The SSDE at the center slice is determined from the measured $D_w$ for a specific patient and the corresponding $f$ factor using the appropriate fit parameters for 16- or 32-cm CTDI phantom diameter |
| Effective dose (determined from DLP) | $E = k \times DLP$ | Eq. 11-21/Pg. 437/Conversion factor $k$, in mSv/mGy-cm, is determined for various CT examinations; values are shown in Table 11-4, Pg. 437 |

| SYMBOL | QUANTITY | UNITS |
|---|---|---|
| $D$ | Dose | Gy |
| $\mu$ | Linear attenuation coefficient | $cm^{-1}$ |
| $\mu_{en}$ | Absorbed energy linear attenuation coefficient | $cm^{-1}$ |
| $\mu/\rho$ | Mass attenuation coefficient | $cm^2/gm$ |
| $\mu_{en}/\rho$ | Mass energy attenuation coefficient | $cm^2/gm$ |
| $w_R$ | Radiation weighting factor for type of radiation | unitless |
| LET | Linear energy transfer | unitless |

*(Continued)*

*(Continued)*

| QUANTITY | EQUATION | EQ. NO./PAGE/COMMENTS |
|---|---|---|
| $H$ | Equivalent dose | Sv |
| $w_T$ | Tissue weighting factor for various organs | unitless |
| $E$ | Effective dose | Sv |
| ESAK | Entrance surface air kerma | Gy |
| SSD | Source to surface (Skin) distance | cm |
| KAP or $P_{KA}$/DAP | Kerma area product/dose area product | Gy-cm$^2$ |
| AERC | Automatic exposure (air kerma) rate control | unitless |
| $K_{a,r}$ | Air kerma at the reference point | Gy |
| BSF | Backscatter fraction (factor) | unitless |
| PSD | Peak skin dose | Gy |
| CTDI | Computed tomography dose index | Gy |
| CTDI$_{100}$ | CTDI measured with 100-mm ion chamber | Gy |
| CTDI$_w$ | Weighted CTDI | Gy |
| CTDI$_{vol}$ | Volume CTDI | Gy |
| DLP | Dose length product | Gy-cm |
| $D_w$ | Water equivalent diameter | cm |
| SSDE | Size-specific dose estimate | Gy |
| DRL | Diagnostic reference level | mGy, mGy-cm, mGy-cm$^2$ |

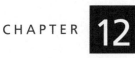

# CHAPTER 12

# Magnetic Resonance Basics: Magnetic Fields, Nuclear Magnetic Characteristics, Tissue Contrast, Image Acquisition

The protons and neutrons of the nucleus have a *magnetic* field associated with their nuclear spin and charge distribution. *Resonance* is an energy coupling that causes the individual nuclei to absorb and release energy unique to those nuclei and their surrounding environment. This chapter reviews the basic properties of magnetism, concepts of resonance, tissue magnetization and relaxation events, generation of image contrast, and basic methods of acquiring image data.

## 12.1 MAGNETISM, MAGNETIC FIELDS, AND MAGNETIC PROPERTIES OF MATERIALS

**1. Magnetism**
A fundamental property of matter generated by moving charges, usually electrons. Magnetic properties of materials result from the organization and motion of the electron.

**2. Magnetic fields**
  **a.** Magnetic fields exist as dipoles and can be induced by a moving electric charge in a wire (Fig. 12-1).
  **b.** Units of magnetic fields are tesla (T) and gauss (G): **1 T = 10,000 G**.
  **c.** The earth's magnetic field is 0.5 G or 5 mT; A 1.5 T MRI scanner has 30,000 times stronger field.

**3. Magnetic properties of materials**
  **Magnetic susceptibility** describes the extent to which a material becomes magnetized in a magnetic field.
  **a.** Diamagnetic materials have negative susceptibility and oppose the magnetic field (Fig. 12-2, left).
    **(i)** Examples of diamagnetic materials are calcium, water, and most organic materials.
  **b.** Paramagnetic materials have positive susceptibility and enhance the magnetic field (Fig. 12-2, right).
    **(i)** That is, molecular oxygen ($O_2$), deoxyhemoglobin, methemoglobin, and gadolinium-based agents
  **c.** Ferromagnetic materials are "superparamagnetic" and augment the magnetic field substantially.

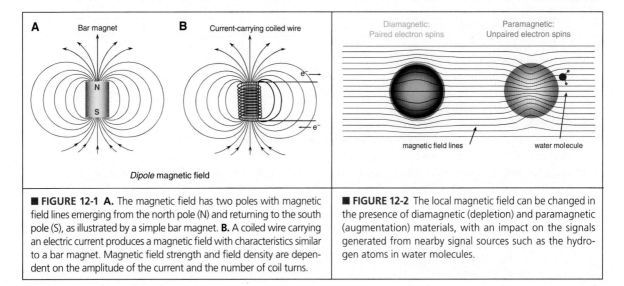

■ **FIGURE 12-1 A.** The magnetic field has two poles with magnetic field lines emerging from the north pole (N) and returning to the south pole (S), as illustrated by a simple bar magnet. **B.** A coiled wire carrying an electric current produces a magnetic field with characteristics similar to a bar magnet. Magnetic field strength and field density are dependent on the amplitude of the current and the number of coil turns.

■ **FIGURE 12-2** The local magnetic field can be changed in the presence of diamagnetic (depletion) and paramagnetic (augmentation) materials, with an impact on the signals generated from nearby signal sources such as the hydrogen atoms in water molecules.

4. **Magnetic characteristics of the nucleus**
   a. The nucleus exhibits magnetic characteristics of the constituent protons and neutrons (Table 12-1).
   b. Magnetic properties are influenced by spin and charge distributions intrinsic to the proton and neutron.
   c. A magnetic dipole is created for the proton and the neutron resulting from associated nuclear spin.
      (i) Dipoles are in opposite direction and approximately the same strength.
   d. The nuclear magnetic moment is represented as a dipole vector indicating magnitude and direction.
      (i) The nuclear magnetic moment is determined through the pairing of protons and neutrons.
      (ii) For the sum of constituent protons (P) and neutrons (N) even, magnetic moment is zero.
      (iii) For N even and P odd, or N odd and P even, the nuclear magnetic moment is non-zero.

### TABLE 12-1 PROPERTIES OF THE NEUTRON AND PROTON

| CHARACTERISTIC | NEUTRON | PROTON |
|---|---|---|
| Mass (kg) | $1.674 \times 10^{-27}$ | $1.672 \times 10^{-27}$ |
| Charge (coulomb) | 0 | $1.602 \times 10^{-19}$ |
| Spin quantum number | ½ | ½ |
| Magnetic moment (J/T) | $-9.66 \times 10^{-27}$ | $1.41 \times 10^{-26}$ |
| Magnetic moment (nuclear magneton) | $-1.91$ | 2.79 |

5. **Nuclear magnetic characteristics of the elements**
   a. Biologically relevant elements for producing MR signals are listed (Table 12-2).
   b. Hydrogen, with largest magnetic moment and greatest abundance, is best element for clinical utility.
   c. Other elements are orders of magnitude less sensitive—$^{23}$Na and $^{31}$P have been used for imaging.

### TABLE 12-2 MAGNETIC RESONANCE PROPERTIES OF MEDICALLY USEFUL NUCLEI

| NUCLEUS | SPIN QUANTUM NUMBER | % ISOTOPIC ABUNDANCE | MAGNETIC MOMENT[a] | % RELATIVE ELEMENTAL ABUNDANCE[b] | RELATIVE SENSITIVITY | GYROMAGNETIC RATIO, $\gamma/2\pi$ (MHZ/T) |
|---|---|---|---|---|---|---|
| $^1$H | ½ | 99.98 | 2.79 | 10 | 1 | 42.58 |
| $^3$He | ½ | 0.00014 | $-2.13$ | 0 | – | 32.43 |
| $^{13}$C | $-$½ | 0.011 | 0.70 | 18 | – | 10.71 |
| $^{17}$O | ⁵⁄₂ | 0.04 | $-1.89$ | 65 | $9 \times 10^{-6}$ | 5.77 |
| $^{19}$F | ½ | 100 | 2.63 | <0.01 | $3 \times 10^{-8}$ | 40.05 |
| $^{23}$Na | ³⁄₂ | 100 | 2.22 | 0.1 | $1 \times 10^{-4}$ | 11.26 |
| $^{31}$P | ½ | 100 | 1.13 | 1.2 | $6 \times 10^{-5}$ | 17.24 |

[a]Moment in nuclear magneton units = $5.05 \times 10^{-27}$ J/T.

[b]*Note*: By mass in the human body (all isotopes).

6. **Magnetic characteristics of the proton**
   a. Unbound protons have randomized directions of the nuclear dipoles (Fig. 12-3A).
   b. In the presence of external magnetic field, $B_0$, magnetic forces cause the nuclei to tend to realign with the applied field in parallel and antiparallel directions (Fig. 12-3B).
   c. An excess of a few protons per million are oriented parallel to the $B_0$ field.
   d. Sum of nuclear magnetic moments, **net magnetization**, is along the $B_0$ direction.
   e. Magnetic moment of spins rotates around the static magnetic field as a *precession*.
   f. The angular frequency of precession, $\omega_0$, is proportional to the magnetic field strength $B_0$ (Fig. 12-4).
      (i) The Larmor equation describes dependence between $B_0$ and $\omega_0$:

$$\omega_0 = \gamma B_0,$$

      (ii) The $\gamma$ is the **gyromagnetic ratio** unique to each element—for protons, $\gamma = 42.58$ MHz/T, which yields 63.87 MHz resonance frequency at 1.5 T and 127.74 MHz at 3.0 T

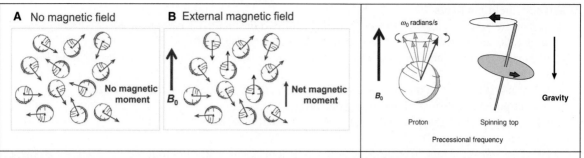

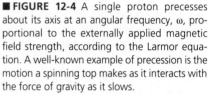

■ **FIGURE 12-3** Simplified distributions of "free" protons without and with an external magnetic field are shown. **A.** Without an external magnetic field, a group of protons assumes a random orientation of magnetic moments, producing an overall magnetic moment of zero. **B.** Under the influence of an applied external magnetic field, $B_0$, a few per million protons aligns in two possible orientations: parallel and antiparallel to the applied magnetic field. A slightly greater number of protons exist in the parallel direction, resulting in a measurable *net magnetic moment* in the direction of $B_0$.

■ **FIGURE 12-4** A single proton precesses about its axis at an angular frequency, ω, proportional to the externally applied magnetic field strength, according to the Larmor equation. A well-known example of precession is the motion a spinning top makes as it interacts with the force of gravity as it slows.

## 12.2 MR SYSTEM

The MR system is composed of several components.

1. **Magnet**
   **a.** Air core magnets: wire-wrapped cylinders produce magnetic field by an electric current in the wires
      **(i)** The magnetic field produced is parallel to the long axis of the cylinder (Fig. 12-5A).
   **b.** Solid core magnets: permanent magnets, a wire-wrapped iron core "electromagnet," or a hybrid
      **(i)** The magnetic field runs between the poles of the magnet, most often vertically (Fig. 12-5B).
   **c.** *Superconductivity*: a characteristic of certain metals that exhibit no resistance to electric current
      **(i)** Superconductive wires require extremely low temperatures (liquid helium; less than 4°K).
      **(ii)** A superconductive magnet with field strength of 1.5 or 3 T is common for clinical systems.

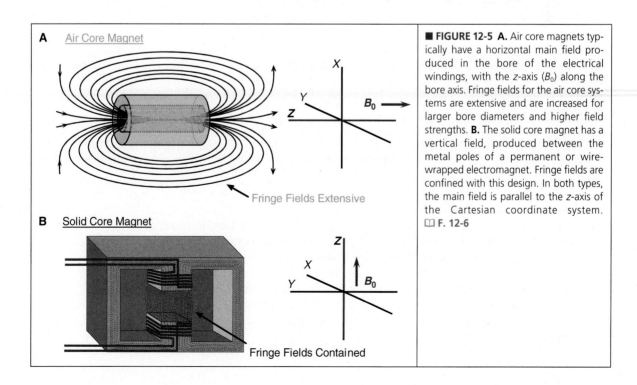

■ **FIGURE 12-5 A.** Air core magnets typically have a horizontal main field produced in the bore of the electrical windings, with the $z$-axis ($B_0$) along the bore axis. Fringe fields for the air core systems are extensive and are increased for larger bore diameters and higher field strengths. **B.** The solid core magnet has a vertical field, produced between the metal poles of a permanent or wire-wrapped electromagnet. Fringe fields are confined with this design. In both types, the main field is parallel to the $z$-axis of the Cartesian coordinate system. 📖 F. 12-6

## 2. Magnetic field gradients

a. Generated by superimposing the magnetic fields of two or more coils carrying a direct current of specific amplitude and direction with a precisely defined geometry (Fig. 12-6).

b. Inside the magnet bore, three sets of gradients reside along the logical coordinate axes in three directions, *x*, *y*, and *z*.

c. Linear magnetic field gradients selectively excite or spatially localize MR signals (Fig. 12-7).

d. Two important properties of magnetic gradients:

  (i) *Gradient field strength*: determined by its peak amplitude and slope (change over distance)—typically ranges from 1 to 50 mT/m.

  (ii) *Slew rate* is the time to achieve the peak gradient magnetic field amplitude—typical slew rates of gradient fields are from 5 to 250 mT/m/ms.

e. Protons maintain precessional frequencies corresponding to local magnetic field strength.

  (i) Middle of the gradient is called the gradient isocenter—no change in the field strength or precessional frequency.

  (ii) A linear gradient increases and decreases magnetic field strength linearly.

  (iii) The gradient field adds/subtracts to the static magnetic field as does the precessional frequency.

  (iv) The angular precessional frequency at a location within a linear gradient, $\omega$, is:

$$\omega = \gamma(B_0 + G_{net} \cdot d)$$

where $G_{net}$ is the net gradient and $d$ is the distance from the gradient isocenter.

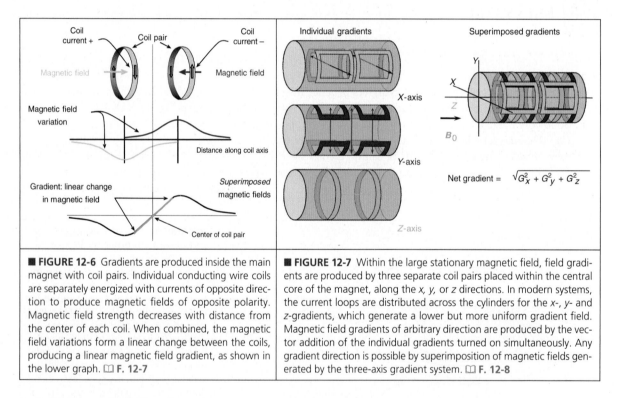

■ **FIGURE 12-6** Gradients are produced inside the main magnet with coil pairs. Individual conducting wire coils are separately energized with currents of opposite direction to produce magnetic fields of opposite polarity. Magnetic field strength decreases with distance from the center of each coil. When combined, the magnetic field variations form a linear change between the coils, producing a linear magnetic field gradient, as shown in the lower graph. 📖 **F. 12-7**

■ **FIGURE 12-7** Within the large stationary magnetic field, field gradients are produced by three separate coil pairs placed within the central core of the magnet, along the *x*, *y*, or *z* directions. In modern systems, the current loops are distributed across the cylinders for the *x*-, *y*- and *z*-gradients, which generate a lower but more uniform gradient field. Magnetic field gradients of arbitrary direction are produced by the vector addition of the individual gradients turned on simultaneously. Any gradient direction is possible by superimposition of magnetic fields generated by the three-axis gradient system. 📖 **F. 12-8**

## 3. Radiofrequency (RF) coils

a. *Transmit coils* use an electromagnetic RF energy pulse tuned to the Larmor frequency.

  (i) Resonance of the magnetization within the sample is called *excitation*.

  (ii) The created secondary field is $\boldsymbol{B}_1$ and is arranged at right angles to the main magnetic field.

  (iii) Tissue magnetization within the sample returns to equilibrium conditions over time.

  (iv) Detectable RF energy at the same frequency, in phase coherence, is released.

b. *Receive coils* are highly sensitive antennas that generate signals from the rotating magnetization vector.

c. *Volume coils* encompass the total area of the anatomy of interest and yield uniform excitation and SNR over the entire imaging volume.

d. *Phased array coils*, consisting of multiple coils and receivers, are made of several overlapping loops, which extend the imaging FOV in one direction.

e. *Surface coils* are used to image anatomy near the surface of the patient.

   **(i)** Coils are usually small and shaped for a specific imaging examination and for patient comfort.

   **(ii)** Typically receive-only designs, these coils achieve high SNR and high resolution. (Pictures of RF coils are shown in textbook F. 12-9).

**4. MR system subcomponents**

a. Control interfaces, RF source, detector, amplifier, computer system, gradient power supplies, image display (textbook F. 12-5)

b. Internal magnet components: shim coils, RF coils, gradient coils, superconducting coils, liquid helium vessel (textbook F. 12-10)

## 12.3 MAGNETIC RESONANCE SIGNAL

Application of RF energy synchronized to the precessional frequency of the protons causes absorption of energy and displacement of the sample magnetic moment from equilibrium conditions. The return to equilibrium results in the emission of energy proportional to the number of excited protons in the volume.

**1. Orientation, frame of reference, and magnetization vectors**

a. The *laboratory frame* (Fig. 12-8A) is a stationary reference frame from the observer's point of view, where the sample magnetic moment vector precesses about the $z$-axis in a circular geometry about $x$-$y$.

b. The *rotating frame* (Fig. 12-8B) is a *spinning* axis system, whereby the $x'$-$y'$ axes rotate at an angular frequency equal to the Larmor frequency—in this frame, the sample magnetic moment vector appears to be stationary when rotating at the resonance frequency.

c. The net magnetization vector of the sample, $M$, is described by three components.

   **(i)** *Longitudinal magnetization*, $M_z$, along the $z$ direction, is the component of the magnetic moment parallel to the applied magnetic field, $B_0$.

   **(ii)** *Equilibrium magnetization*, $M_0$, is the maximum longitudinal magnetization in the direction of $B_0$.

   **(iii)** *Transverse magnetization*, $M_{xy}$, is the component of the magnetic moment perpendicular to $B_0$ in the $x$-$y$ plane, and at equilibrium, $M_{xy}$ is zero.

d. When protons in the magnetized sample absorb energy, phase coherence of the spins generates a rotating vector in the transverse plane, $M_{xy}$, generating the all-important MR signal (Fig. 12-9).

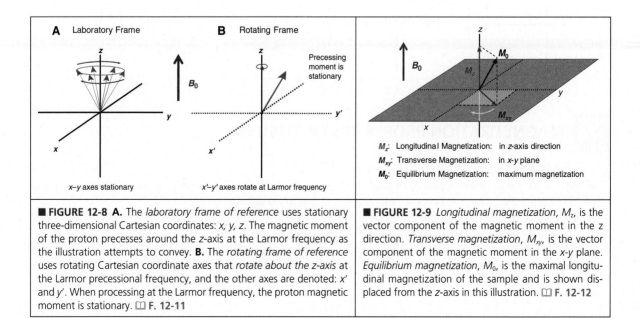

■ **FIGURE 12-8 A.** The *laboratory frame of reference* uses stationary three-dimensional Cartesian coordinates: *x, y, z*. The magnetic moment of the proton precesses around the *z*-axis at the Larmor frequency as the illustration attempts to convey. **B.** The *rotating frame of reference* uses rotating Cartesian coordinate axes that *rotate about the z-axis* at the Larmor precessional frequency, and the other axes are denoted: *x'* and *y'*. When processing at the Larmor frequency, the proton magnetic moment is stationary. ☐ **F. 12-11**

■ **FIGURE 12-9** *Longitudinal magnetization*, $M_z$, is the vector component of the magnetic moment in the z direction. *Transverse magnetization*, $M_{xy}$, is the vector component of the magnetic moment in the x-y plane. *Equilibrium magnetization*, $M_0$, is the maximal longitudinal magnetization of the sample and is shown displaced from the z-axis in this illustration. ☐ **F. 12-12**

## 2. Resonance and excitation (Fig. 12-10)

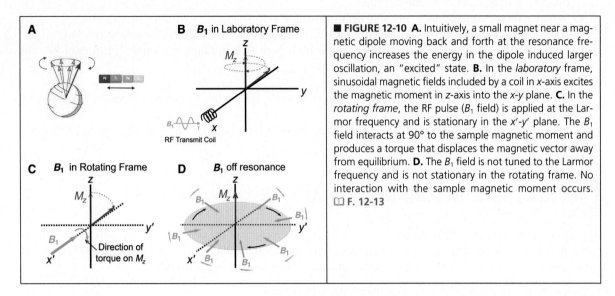

**FIGURE 12-10 A.** Intuitively, a small magnet near a magnetic dipole moving back and forth at the resonance frequency increases the energy in the dipole induced larger oscillation, an "excited" state. **B.** In the *laboratory* frame, sinusoidal magnetic fields included by a coil in x-axis excites the magnetic moment in z-axis into the x-y plane. **C.** In the *rotating frame*, the RF pulse ($B_1$ field) is applied at the Larmor frequency and is stationary in the x'-y' plane. The $B_1$ field interacts at 90° to the sample magnetic moment and produces a torque that displaces the magnetic vector away from equilibrium. **D.** The $B_1$ field is not tuned to the Larmor frequency and is not stationary in the rotating frame. No interaction with the sample magnetic moment occurs. 🔲 **F. 12-13**

## 3. Flip angles
*Flip angles* represent the degree of $M_z$ rotation by the $B_1$ field as it is applied normal to $M_z$ (Fig. 12-11)

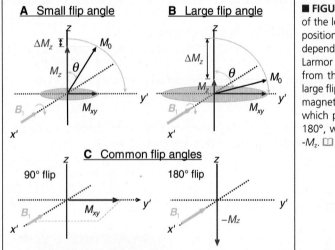

**FIGURE 12-11** Flip angles describe the angular displacement of the longitudinal magnetization vector from the equilibrium position. The rotation angle of the magnetic moment vector is dependent on the duration and amplitude of the $B_1$ field at the Larmor frequency. Flip angles describe the rotation of $M_z$ away from the z-axis. **A.** Small flip angles (less than 45°) and **(B)** large flip angles (75° to 90°) produce small and large transverse magnetization, respectively. **C.** Common flip angles are 90°, which produce the maximum transverse magnetization, and 180°, which invert the existing longitudinal magnetization to $-M_z$. 🔲 **F. 12-14**

## 12.4  MAGNETIZATION PROPERTIES OF TISSUES

## 1. Free induction decay: T2 and T2* relaxation
  a. After a 90° RF pulse is applied to a magnetized sample at the Larmor frequency, an initial phase coherence of the individual protons is established, and maximum $M_{xy}$ is achieved.
  b. Rotating at the Larmor frequency, the transverse magnetic field of the excited sample induces a damped sinusoidal electronic signal, known as the *free induction decay* (FID) (Fig. 12-12).
  c. The FID amplitude decay is caused by an exponential loss of $M_{xy}$ phase coherence.
  d. Elapsed time between the peak transverse signal and 37% of the peak level (1/e) is the *T2 relaxation time* (Fig. 12-13A), expressed as

$$M_{xy}(t) = M_0 e^{-t/\text{T2}}$$

where $M_{xy}(t)$ is the transverse magnetic moment at time $t$ for a sample that has $M_0$ transverse magnetization at $t = 0$.

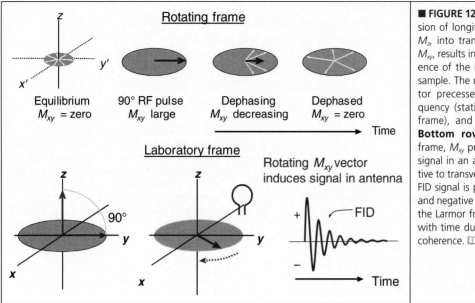

■ **FIGURE 12-12 Top row.** Conversion of longitudinal magnetization, $M_z$, into transverse magnetization, $M_{xy}$, results in an initial phase coherence of the individual spins of the sample. The magnetic moment vector precesses at the Larmor frequency (stationary in the rotating frame), and dephases with time. **Bottom row.** In the laboratory frame, $M_{xy}$ precesses and induces a signal in an antenna receiver sensitive to transverse magnetization. An FID signal is produced with positive and negative variations oscillating at the Larmor frequency and decaying with time due to the loss of phase coherence. ⌨ **F. 12-15**

**e.** Characteristics of T2 decay values depend on tissue structure and molecular size.

   **(i)** *Amorphous structures* (*e.g.*, cerebral spinal fluid [CSF] or highly edematous tissues) contain mobile molecules with fast and rapid molecular motion—without structural constraint (*e.g.*, lack of a hydration layer), these tissues do not support intrinsic magnetic field inhomogeneities and thus exhibit **longer T2**.

   **(ii)** *Increasing molecular size* results in constrained molecular motion and often the presence of an hydration layer that produces magnetic field domains within the structure, which causes increased spin dephasing and more rapid decay of the FID with **shorter T2**.

   **(iii)** *Large, nonmoving structures* such as bone maintain stationary magnetic inhomogeneities that result in a **very short T2**.

   **(iv)** *Extrinsic magnetic inhomogeneities*, such as the imperfect main magnetic field, $B_0$, or susceptibility agents in the tissues (*e.g.*, MR contrast materials, paramagnetic or ferromagnetic objects), add to the loss of phase coherence from intrinsic inhomogeneities and further reduce the decay constant, known as **T2\*** under these conditions (Fig. 12-13B).

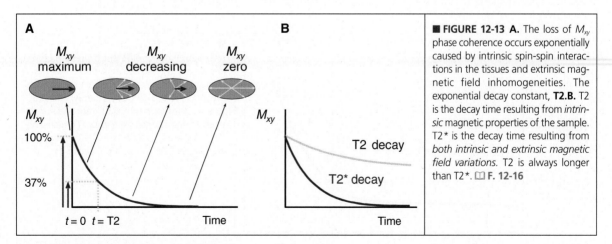

■ **FIGURE 12-13 A.** The loss of $M_{xy}$ phase coherence occurs exponentially caused by intrinsic spin-spin interactions in the tissues and extrinsic magnetic field inhomogeneities. The exponential decay constant, **T2.B.** T2 is the decay time resulting from *intrinsic* magnetic properties of the sample. T2\* is the decay time resulting from *both intrinsic and extrinsic magnetic field variations.* T2 is always longer than T2\*. ⌨ **F. 12-16**

## 2. Return to equilibrium: T1 relaxation

   **a.** *Longitudinal magnetization recovery* occurs immediately after the $B_1$ excitation pulse, simultaneous with transverse decay, but over a longer period.

   **b.** *Spin-lattice relaxation* describes the release of energy back to the lattice (the molecular structure) and the regrowth of $M_z$ that occurs exponentially as

$$M_z(t) = M_0(1 - e^{-t/T1})$$

where $M_z(t)$ is the longitudinal magnetization at time $t$ and T1 is the time needed for the recovery of 63% of $M_z$ after a 90° pulse (Fig. 12-14).

**c.** Characteristics of T1 relaxation recovery:
   **(i)** Rate of energy dissipation into the surrounding molecular lattice and hydration layer.
   **(ii)** T1 varies substantially for different tissue structures and pathologies.
   **(iii)** Molecular lattice tumbling frequency provides "conduit" of energy release at Larmor frequency.
   **(iv)** Amount of overlap with molecular frequency is inversely proportional to T1.
   **(v)** Gadolinium chelated with complex macromolecules is effective in decreasing T1 relaxation time of local tissues by creating a hydration layer that forms a spin-lattice energy sink.

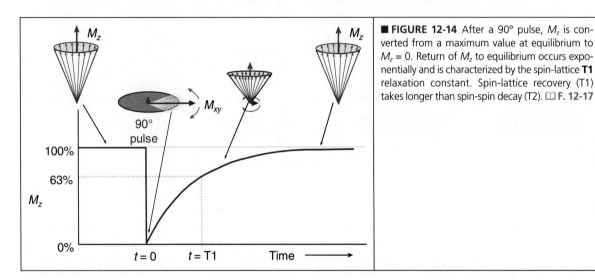

■ **FIGURE 12-14** After a 90° pulse, $M_z$ is converted from a maximum value at equilibrium to $M_z = 0$. Return of $M_z$ to equilibrium occurs exponentially and is characterized by the spin-lattice **T1** relaxation constant. Spin-lattice recovery (T1) takes longer than spin-spin decay (T2). 📖 **F. 12-17**

3. **Comparison of T1 and T2**
   **a.** T1 is on the order of 5 to 10 times longer than T2.
      **(i)** Molecular motion, size, and interactions influence T1 and T2 relaxation (Fig. 12-15).
      **(ii)** Tissues of interest for clinical MR applications are intermediate to small-sized molecules; most tissues with a longer T1 have a longer T2, with a shorter T1 have a shorter T2.
      **(iii)** Comparison of T1 and T2 values for various tissues (Table 12-3).
   **b.** Agents that disrupt the local magnetic field environment: paramagnetic blood degradation products, elements with unpaired electron spins (*e.g.*, gadolinium), cause a significant decrease in T2*.
   **c.** Macromolecules that bind water in hydration layer significantly decreases T1.

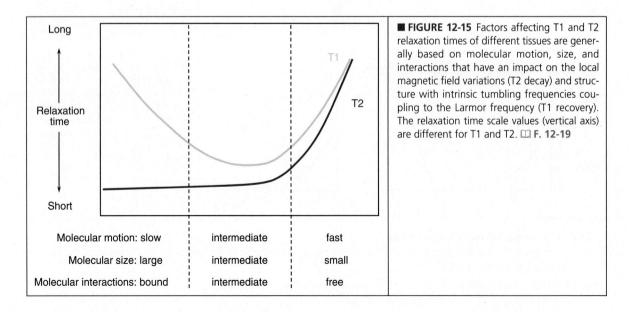

■ **FIGURE 12-15** Factors affecting T1 and T2 relaxation times of different tissues are generally based on molecular motion, size, and interactions that have an impact on the local magnetic field variations (T2 decay) and structure with intrinsic tumbling frequencies coupling to the Larmor frequency (T1 recovery). The relaxation time scale values (vertical axis) are different for T1 and T2. 📖 **F. 12-19**

**TABLE 12-3 T1 AND T2 RELAXATION CONSTANTS FOR SEVERAL TISSUES**[a]

| TISSUE | T1, 0.5 T (ms) | T1, 1.5 T (ms) | T2 (ms) |
|---|---|---|---|
| Fat | 210 | 260 | 80 |
| Liver | 350 | 500 | 40 |
| Muscle | 550 | 870 | 45 |
| White matter | 500 | 780 | 90 |
| Gray matter | 650 | 900 | 100 |
| Cerebrospinal fluid | 1,800 | 2,400 | 160 |

[a]Estimates only, as reported values for T1 and T2 span a wide range.

## 12.5   BASIC ACQUISITION PARAMETERS

The differences of T1 and T2, relaxation time constants, and proton density of the tissues are the key to the exquisite contrast sensitivity of MR images.

1. **Time of repetition (TR)**
   a. The period between $B_1$ excitation pulses.
   b. During the TR interval, T2 decay and T1 recovery occur in the tissues.
2. **Time of echo (TE)**
   a. The time between the excitation pulse and the appearance of the peak amplitude of an induced echo
   b. For a spin echo sequence, a 180° RF inversion pulse (a.k.a refocusing pulse) at TE/2
   c. For a gradient echo sequence, gradient polarity reversal at TE/2
3. **Time of inversion (TI)**
   a. The time between an initial inversion (180°) RF pulse that produces negative maximum magnetization and a 90° excitation pulse.
   b. During the TI, $M_z$ recovery occurs.
4. **Partial saturation**
   a. Saturation is a state of tissue magnetization less than equilibrium conditions.
   b. When TR is not long enough for $M_z$ to be fully recovered (TR < 5 T1) and multiple excitations occur, $M_z$ recovery is incomplete, and consequently, a "steady-state" equilibrium of $M_z$ is reached (Fig. 12-16).

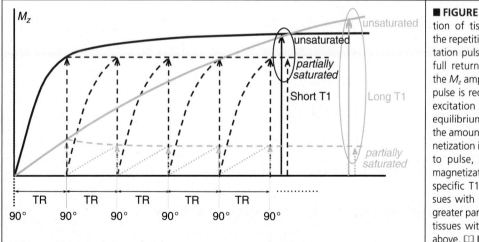

■ **FIGURE 12-16** Partial saturation of tissues occurs because the repetition time between excitation pulses does not allow for full return to equilibrium, and the $M_z$ amplitude for the next RF pulse is reduced. After the third excitation pulse, a steady-state equilibrium is reached, where the amount of longitudinal magnetization is the same from pulse to pulse, as is the transverse magnetization for a tissue with a specific T1 decay constant. Tissues with long T1 experience a greater partial saturation than do tissues with short T1 as shown above. 📖 **F. 12-20**

## 12.6  BASIC PULSE SEQUENCES

Three major pulse sequences performed for imaging: spin echo (SE), inversion recovery (IR), and gradient echo (GRE). When used in conjunction with spatial localization, "contrast-weighted" images are obtained.

1. **Spin echo (SE)**
   a. *SE* describes the excitation of the magnetized protons in a sample with a 90° RF pulse and production of an FID, followed by a refocusing 180° RF pulse to produce an echo (Fig. 12-17).
   b. Subsequent 180° RF pulses during the TR interval (Fig. 12-18) produce corresponding echoes with peak amplitudes that are reduced by intrinsic T2 decay of the tissues and are immune from extrinsic inhomogeneities.

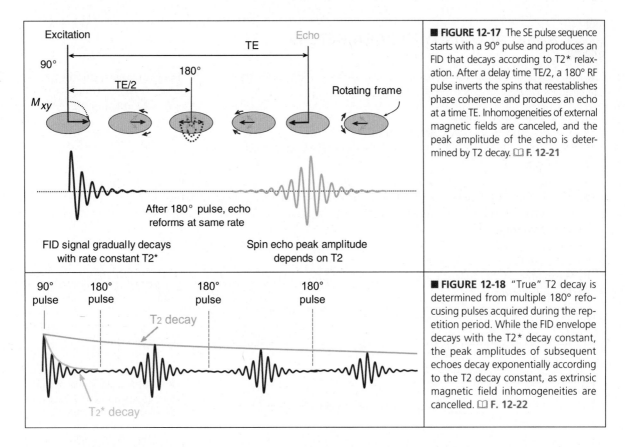

**■ FIGURE 12-17** The SE pulse sequence starts with a 90° pulse and produces an FID that decays according to T2* relaxation. After a delay time TE/2, a 180° RF pulse inverts the spins that reestablishes phase coherence and produces an echo at a time TE. Inhomogeneities of external magnetic fields are canceled, and the peak amplitude of the echo is determined by T2 decay. 📖 **F. 12-21**

**■ FIGURE 12-18** "True" T2 decay is determined from multiple 180° refocusing pulses acquired during the repetition period. While the FID envelope decays with the T2* decay constant, the peak amplitudes of subsequent echoes decay exponentially according to the T2 decay constant, as extrinsic magnetic field inhomogeneities are cancelled. 📖 **F. 12-22**

c. Spin echo contrast weighting: the signal intensity produced using a SE sequence is

$$S \propto \rho_{\mathrm{H}}\left[1-e^{-\mathrm{TR/T1}}\right]e^{-\mathrm{TE/T2}}$$

where $\rho_{\mathrm{H}}$ is the proton density, T1 and T2 are physical properties of tissue, and TR and TE are pulse sequence timing parameters—by changing the pulse sequence parameters TR and TE, the contrast dependence can be weighted toward T1, proton density, or T2 characteristics of the tissues (Table 12-4).

### TABLE 12-4  SE PULSE SEQUENCE CONTRAST WEIGHTING PARAMETERS

| PARAMETER | T1 CONTRAST | PROTON DENSITY CONTRAST[a] | T2 CONTRAST |
|---|---|---|---|
| TR (ms) | 400–600 | 2,000–4,000 | 2,000–4,000 |
| TE (ms) | 5–30 | 5–30 | 60–150 |

[a]Strictly speaking, SE images with TR less than 3,000 ms are not proton density with respect to the CSF; because of its long T1, only 70% of the CSF magnetization recovery will have occurred and will not appear as bright as for a true PD image. True PD image intensities can be obtained with fast spin echo methods (Chapter 13) with longer TR (*e.g.*, 8,000 ms).

TE, time of echo; TR, time of repetition.

**d. Proton density weighting**: Proton density contrast weighting relies mainly on differences in the number of magnetized protons per unit volume of tissue.
   **(i)**   Achieved by reducing the contributions of T1 recovery and T2 decay.
   **(ii)**  T1 differences are reduced by selecting a **long TR** value to allow substantial recovery of $M_z$.
   **(iii)** T2 differences of the tissues are reduced by selecting a **short TE** value (Figs. 12-19 and 12-20).

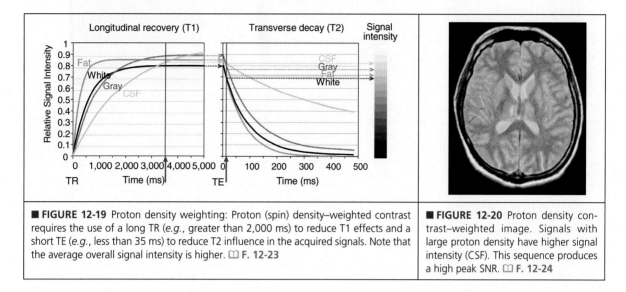

■ **FIGURE 12-19** Proton density weighting: Proton (spin) density–weighted contrast requires the use of a long TR (*e.g.*, greater than 2,000 ms) to reduce T1 effects and a short TE (*e.g.*, less than 35 ms) to reduce T2 influence in the acquired signals. Note that the average overall signal intensity is higher. ▢ **F. 12-23**

■ **FIGURE 12-20** Proton density contrast–weighted image. Signals with large proton density have higher signal intensity (CSF). This sequence produces a high peak SNR. ▢ **F. 12-24**

**e. T2 weighting** reduces T1 differences in tissues with a **long TR** and emphasizes T2 differences with a long TE (Figs. 12-21 and 12-22).

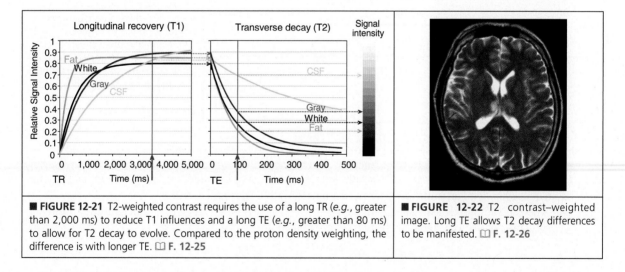

■ **FIGURE 12-21** T2-weighted contrast requires the use of a long TR (*e.g.*, greater than 2,000 ms) to reduce T1 influences and a long TE (*e.g.*, greater than 80 ms) to allow for T2 decay to evolve. Compared to the proton density weighting, the difference is with longer TE. ▢ **F. 12-25**

■ **FIGURE 12-22** T2 contrast–weighted image. Long TE allows T2 decay differences to be manifested. ▢ **F. 12-26**

**f. T1 weighting** is achieved by using a relatively short TR to maximize the differences in longitudinal magnetization recovery during the return to equilibrium and a short TE to minimize T2 decay during signal acquisition (Figs. 12-23 and 12-24).

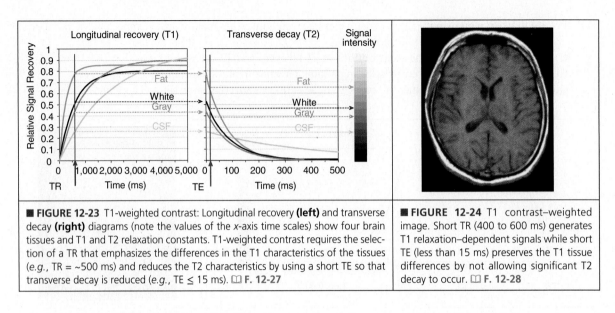

**■ FIGURE 12-23** T1-weighted contrast: Longitudinal recovery **(left)** and transverse decay **(right)** diagrams (note the values of the *x*-axis time scales) show four brain tissues and T1 and T2 relaxation constants. T1-weighted contrast requires the selection of a TR that emphasizes the differences in the T1 characteristics of the tissues (*e.g.*, TR = ~500 ms) and reduces the T2 characteristics by using a short TE so that transverse decay is reduced (*e.g.*, TE ≤ 15 ms). 🕮 **F. 12-27**

**■ FIGURE 12-24** T1 contrast–weighted image. Short TR (400 to 600 ms) generates T1 relaxation–dependent signals while short TE (less than 15 ms) preserves the T1 tissue differences by not allowing significant T2 decay to occur. 🕮 **F. 12-28**

**g.** Both proton density and T2-weighted contrast signals can be acquired during a single TR by acquiring two echoes with a short TE and a long TE (Fig. 12-25).

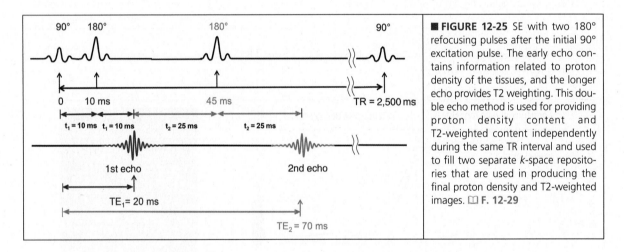

**■ FIGURE 12-25** SE with two 180° refocusing pulses after the initial 90° excitation pulse. The early echo contains information related to proton density of the tissues, and the longer echo provides T2 weighting. This double echo method is used for providing proton density content and T2-weighted content independently during the same TR interval and used to fill two separate *k*-space repositories that are used in producing the final proton density and T2-weighted images. 🕮 **F. 12-29**

**h. Inversion recovery:** emphasizes T1 relaxation times of the tissues by extending the amplitude of the longitudinal recovery with an initial 180° RF pulse: inverts $M_z$ to $-M_z$ (Fig. 12-26).

**(i)** The echo amplitude associated with a given tissue depends on TI, TE, TR, and magnitude (positive or negative) of $M_z$. The signal intensity is approximated as:

$$S \propto \rho_H (1 - 2e^{-\text{TI/T1}})(1 - e^{-(\text{TR} - \text{TI})/\text{T1}})(e^{-\text{TE/T2}})$$

Where $\rho_H$ is the proton density, and the factor of 2 in the first part of the equation arises from the longitudinal magnetization recovery from $-M_z$ to $M_z$ during TI and turned into the transverse magnetization right after the 90° RF pulse; the second term is the recovery of the longitudinal magnetization from the 90° RF pulse to the next inversion RF pulse, and the last term is T2 decay during TE.

**(ii)** For TI to control tissue contrast (mainly T1 contrast), TR must be relatively long and TE short (Fig. 12-27).

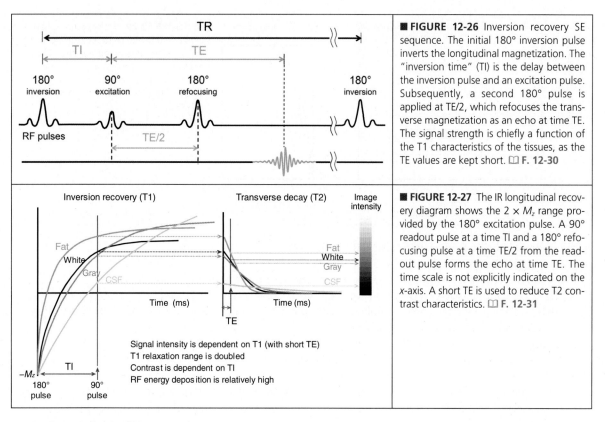

■ **FIGURE 12-26** Inversion recovery SE sequence. The initial 180° inversion pulse inverts the longitudinal magnetization. The "inversion time" (TI) is the delay between the inversion pulse and an excitation pulse. Subsequently, a second 180° pulse is applied at TE/2, which refocuses the transverse magnetization as an echo at time TE. The signal strength is chiefly a function of the T1 characteristics of the tissues, as the TE values are kept short. 📖 **F. 12-30**

■ **FIGURE 12-27** The IR longitudinal recovery diagram shows the $2 \times M_z$ range provided by the 180° excitation pulse. A 90° readout pulse at a time TI and a 180° refocusing pulse at a time TE/2 from the readout pulse forms the echo at time TE. The time scale is not explicitly indicated on the x-axis. A short TE is used to reduce T2 contrast characteristics. 📖 **F. 12-31**

Signal intensity is dependent on T1 (with short TE)
T1 relaxation range is doubled
Contrast is dependent on TI
RF energy deposition is relatively high

## 2. Gradient echo (GRE)

**a.** The *GRE* technique uses a magnetic field gradient applied in one direction and then reversed to induce the formation of an echo, instead of the 180° inversion pulse.

   **(i)** The induced GRE signal is acquired just before and after the peak amplitude (Fig. 12-28).

   **(ii)** Magnetic field ($B_0$) inhomogeneities and tissue susceptibilities caused by paramagnetic or diamagnetic tissues or contrast agents are emphasized in GRE imaging.

   **(iii)** Significant sensitivity to field nonuniformity and magnetic susceptibility agents occurs, as $M_{xy}$ decay is a strong function of T2*, which is much shorter than the "true" T2 achieved in SE sequences.

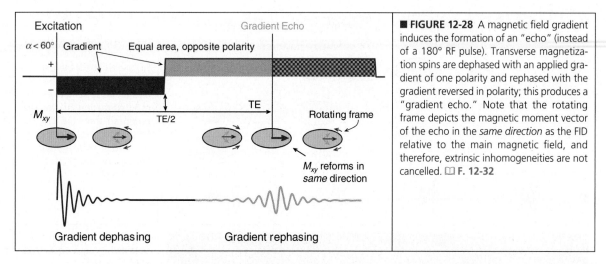

■ **FIGURE 12-28** A magnetic field gradient induces the formation of an "echo" (instead of a 180° RF pulse). Transverse magnetization spins are dephased with an applied gradient of one polarity and rephased with the gradient reversed in polarity; this produces a "gradient echo." Note that the rotating frame depicts the magnetic moment vector of the echo in the *same direction* as the FID relative to the main magnetic field, and therefore, extrinsic inhomogeneities are not cancelled. 📖 **F. 12-32**

   **(iv)** Tissue contrast in GRE pulse sequences depends on TR, TE, and flip angle along with specialized manipulation of the acquisition sequence.

   **(v)** A plot of $M_{xy}$ signal amplitude versus TR as a function of flip angle (Fig. 12-29) shows that smaller flip angles may produce more $M_{xy}$ signal than larger flip angles.

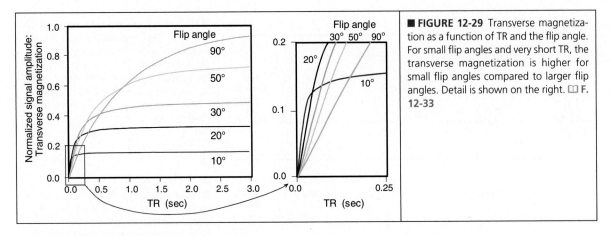

■ **FIGURE 12-29** Transverse magnetization as a function of TR and the flip angle. For small flip angles and very short TR, the transverse magnetization is higher for small flip angles compared to larger flip angles. Detail is shown on the right. 📖 **F. 12-33**

**b. Gradient echo sequences with long TR (>200 ms)**
  **(i)** TR is longer than tissue T2*—Transverse magnetization produced by an RF pulse is diminished prior to the next pulse with little or no coherent echo signals evolved by multiple RF pulses.
  **(ii)** T1 weighting is achieved with a short TE (5 to 10 ms).
  **(iii)** A relatively long TE tends to emphasize T2* contrast, useful for perfusion imaging with a contrast injection and blood oxygen level–dependent (BOLD) imaging (see Chapter 13).
**c. Gradient echo sequences with short TR (<50 ms)**
  **(i)** Residual T2* component exists from the previous TR.
  **(ii)** Persistent transverse magnetization produces two signals: (1) the FID produced from the RF pulse just applied and (2) the stimulated echo from the residual transverse magnetization (Fig. 12-30).
  **(iii)** Selective collection of signals yields different contrast and classifies different GRE sequences.
**d. Coherent GRE:** A "balanced" SSFP (bSSFP) sequence generates and utilizes accumulated gradient echo (FID) and stimulated echo signals with the use of symmetrical gradients in three spatial directions.
  **(i)** Because of its high speed, it is particularly useful for cardiac imaging or dynamic imaging.
  **(ii)** Common acronyms of this technique are TrueFISP and FIESTA (Fig. 12-31).

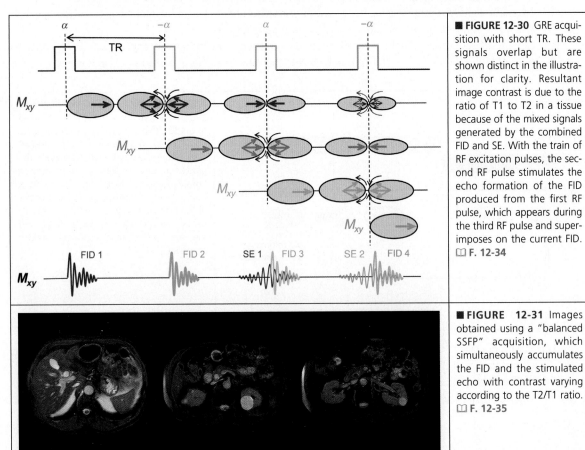

■ **FIGURE 12-30** GRE acquisition with short TR. These signals overlap but are shown distinct in the illustration for clarity. Resultant image contrast is due to the ratio of T1 to T2 in a tissue because of the mixed signals generated by the combined FID and SE. With the train of RF excitation pulses, the second RF pulse stimulates the echo formation of the FID produced from the first RF pulse, which appears during the third RF pulse and superimposes on the current FID. 📖 **F. 12-34**

■ **FIGURE 12-31** Images obtained using a "balanced SSFP" acquisition, which simultaneously accumulates the FID and the stimulated echo with contrast varying according to the T2/T1 ratio. 📖 **F. 12-35**

e. **Gradient spoiling:** The signal variations of bSSFP can be avoided using a spoiling gradient.
   (i)   Spoiler gradient spreads spin phases within a voxel and removes the transverse magnetization.
   (ii)  Gradient can be applied in any gradient direction or in a combination.
   (iii) Location of a spoiling gradient can select either the FID or SE (Fig. 12-32).
   (iv)  MR angiography images are shown with a gradient recalled echo sequence (Fig. 12-33).

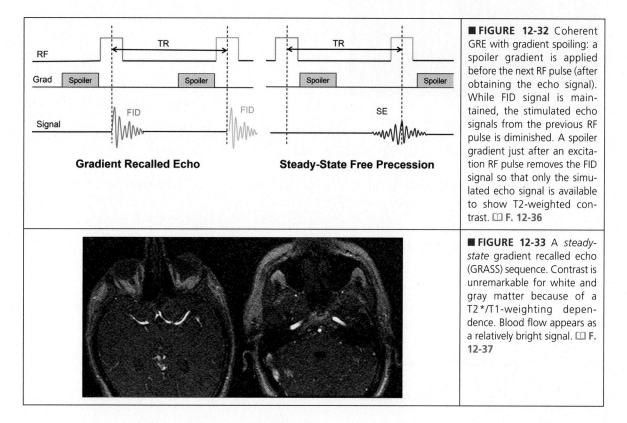

■ **FIGURE 12-32** Coherent GRE with gradient spoiling: a spoiler gradient is applied before the next RF pulse (after obtaining the echo signal). While FID signal is maintained, the stimulated echo signals from the previous RF pulse is diminished. A spoiler gradient just after an excitation RF pulse removes the FID signal so that only the simulated echo signal is available to show T2-weighted contrast. 📖 **F. 12-36**

■ **FIGURE 12-33** A *steady-state* gradient recalled echo (GRASS) sequence. Contrast is unremarkable for white and gray matter because of a T2*/T1-weighting dependence. Blood flow appears as a relatively bright signal. 📖 **F. 12-37**

f. **Incoherent, "spoiled" gradient echo techniques**
   (i)   T1 weighting with short TR: The T2* influence can be reduced by "spoiling" the steady-state transverse magnetization by introducing *incoherent* phase differences from pulse to pulse.
   (ii)  A phase shift is added to successive RF pulses during the excitation of protons, called "*RF spoiling*" (Fig. 12-34).
   (iii) The common acronyms of this technique include SPGR (spoiled gradient recall) and FLASH (fast low-angle shot)
   (iv)  T1-weighted SPGR demonstrates bright blood (Fig. 12-35).

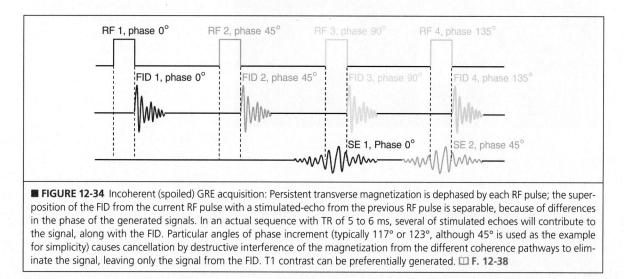

■ **FIGURE 12-34** Incoherent (spoiled) GRE acquisition: Persistent transverse magnetization is dephased by each RF pulse; the superposition of the FID from the current RF pulse with a stimulated-echo from the previous RF pulse is separable, because of differences in the phase of the generated signals. In an actual sequence with TR of 5 to 6 ms, several of stimulated echoes will contribute to the signal, along with the FID. Particular angles of phase increment (typically 117° or 123°, although 45° is used as the example for simplicity) causes cancellation by destructive interference of the magnetization from the different coherence pathways to eliminate the signal, leaving only the signal from the FID. T1 contrast can be preferentially generated. 📖 **F. 12-38**

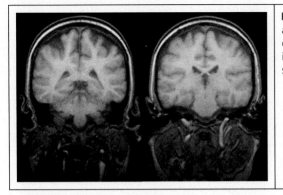

■ **FIGURE 12-35** Incoherent (spoiled) GRE images. The ability to achieve T1 contrast weighting is extremely useful for rapid three-dimensional volume imaging. Bright blood (lower portion of each image) and magnetic susceptibility artifacts are characteristic of this sequence. TR = 8 ms, TE = 1.9 ms, flip angle = 20°. ▭ **F. 12-39**

## 3. Tissue suppression techniques

One of the advantages of MRI is a capability of selectively suppressing unwanted signals (fat or CSF) in the anatomy, achieved by using T1 relaxation or chemical shift.

**a.** *Short tau inversion recovery* (STIR)

    **(i)** An inversion RF pulse applied at the *tissue null* of fat, where TI at 1.5 T is 180 ms (Fig. 12-36).

    **(ii)** STIR is immune to off-resonance fields (Fig. 12-37).

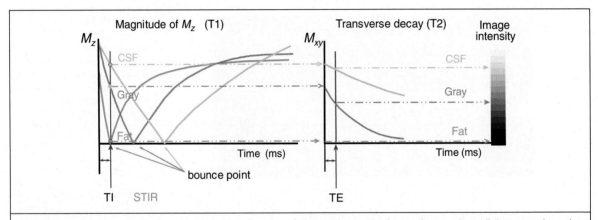

■ **FIGURE 12-36** IR longitudinal magnetization as a function of time, with magnitude signal processing. All tissues go through a null (the bounce point) at a time dependent on T1. The inversion time (TI) is adjusted to select a time to null a certain tissue type. Shown above is the STIR (short tau IR) used for suppressing the signal due to fat tissues, achieved with TI = approximately 150 ms (0.693 × 260 ms, the T1 value for fat). ▭ **F. 12-40**

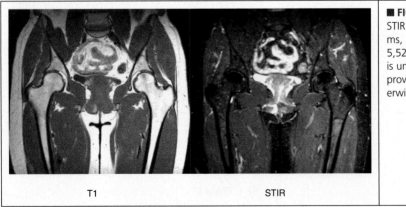

■ **FIGURE 12-37** SE T1 weighting versus STIR technique. **Left.** T1 W with TR = 750 ms, TE = 13 ms. **Right.** STIR with TR = 5,520 ms, TI = 150 ms, TE = 8 ms. The fat is uniformly suppressed in the STIR image, providing details of nonfat structures otherwise difficult to discern. ▭ **F. 12-41**

**b.** *Fat saturation RF pulse*

    **(i)** Suppresses fat signals using the chemical shift of fat of 3.5 ppm (Fig. 12-38).

    **(ii)** Compared to the STIR technique, this technique maintains full water signal, and higher SNR can be achieved.

    **(iii)** Method is sensitive to off-resonance fields, leading to imperfect suppression.

    **(iv)** Referred to as Chem Sat (chemical saturation) or CHESS (chemical shift selective)

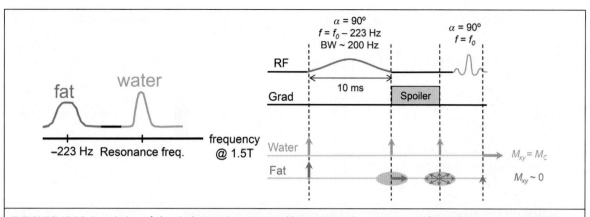

■ **FIGURE 12-38** Description of chemical saturation: Fat signal has a 223 Hz lower resonance frequency than water signal at 1.5 T because of chemical shift. A fat saturation RF pulse at the fat resonance frequency excites only fat signal and a spoiling gradient after the fat saturation RF pulse completely saturates the transverse magnetization of fat before a water excitation RF pulse. 📖 **F. 12-42**

c. *Fat separation*
   (i) Fat or water signals can be selectively imaged using the chemical shift (Fig. 12-39).
   (ii) Multiple images are acquired at different echo times: in and out of phase.
   (iii) Water- or fat-*only* images are generated after linear operation (Fig. 12-40).

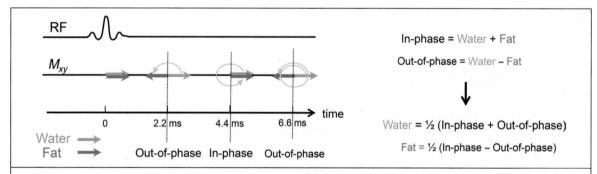

■ **FIGURE 12-39** Description of a fat/water separation technique (Dixon method): Due to the chemical shift of fat, the fat and the water spins are out of phase at 2.2, 6.6 ms, and so on while in phase at 0, 4.4 ms, and so on right after the excitation RF pulse is applied. From the images collected while fat and water spins are in-phase and out-of-phase, the amount of fat and water can be estimated by the linear operation. The method produces four different images: in-phase, out-of-phase, water, and fat images. 📖 **F. 12-43**

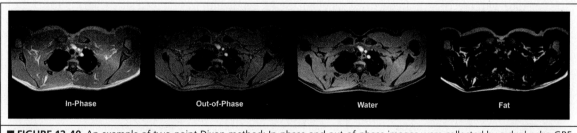

■ **FIGURE 12-40** An example of two-point Dixon method: In-phase and out-of-phase images were collected by a dual-echo GRE sequence with a TE of 2.6 and 1.4 ms, respectively, at 3 T. 📖 **F. 12-44**

d. *Fluid-attenuated inversion recovery (FLAIR)*
   (i) Reduces CSF signal and other water-bound anatomy by using a T1 selected at or near the bounce point of CSF, 1,700 ms at 1.5 T (Fig. 12-41).
   (ii) A comparison of T1, T2, and FLAIR sequences demonstrates the contrast differences achievable by reducing signals of one tissue to be able to visualize another (Fig. 12-42).

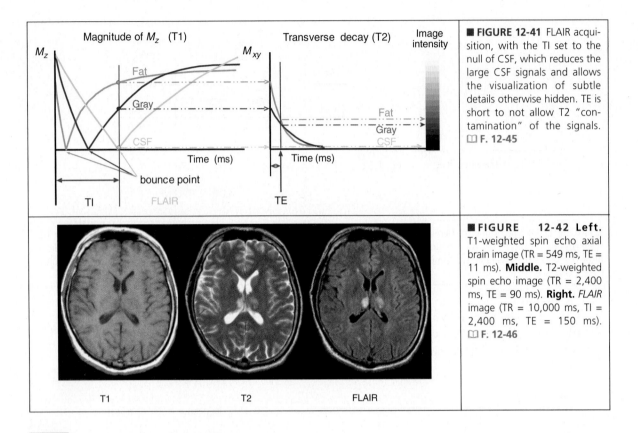

■ **FIGURE 12-41** FLAIR acquisition, with the TI set to the null of CSF, which reduces the large CSF signals and allows the visualization of subtle details otherwise hidden. TE is short to not allow T2 "contamination" of the signals. 📖 **F. 12-45**

■ **FIGURE 12-42 Left.** T1-weighted spin echo axial brain image (TR = 549 ms, TE = 11 ms). **Middle.** T2-weighted spin echo image (TR = 2,400 ms, TE = 90 ms). **Right.** *FLAIR* image (TR = 10,000 ms, TI = 2,400 ms, TE = 150 ms). 📖 **F. 12-46**

## 12.7 MR SIGNAL LOCALIZATION

Spatial localization of MR signal is achieved by superimposing linear magnetic field variations on the $B_0$ field to generate corresponding position-dependent variations in precessional frequency of the protons.

1. **Slice selection:**
   a. RF transmitters determine the slice location of the protons in the tissues that absorb energy.
   (i) Slice-select gradient (SSG) incrementally increases or decreases proton precessional frequency dependent on their distance from the gradient isocenter.
   (ii) Frequency and bandwidth of the RF pulse simultaneous to the SSG determines the slice location of the tissues that absorb energy.
   (iii) A selective, narrow band RF frequency pulse of known duration and amplitude excites only those protons with precessional frequencies matching the RF bandwidth in a defined slice (Fig. 12-43).

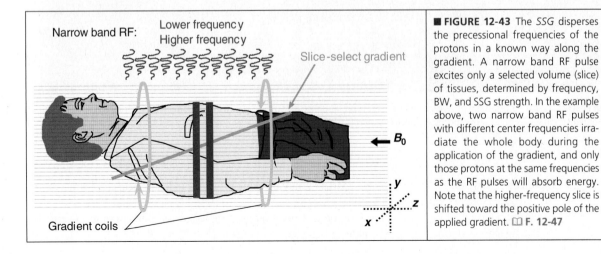

■ **FIGURE 12-43** The *SSG* disperses the precessional frequencies of the protons in a known way along the gradient. A narrow band RF pulse excites only a selected volume (slice) of tissues, determined by frequency, BW, and SSG strength. In the example above, two narrow band RF pulses with different center frequencies irradiate the whole body during the application of the gradient, and only those protons at the same frequencies as the RF pulses will absorb energy. Note that the higher-frequency slice is shifted toward the positive pole of the applied gradient. 📖 **F. 12-47**

**b.** Slice thickness is chiefly determined by the frequency BW of the RF pulse and the gradient strength across the slice (Fig. 12-44).

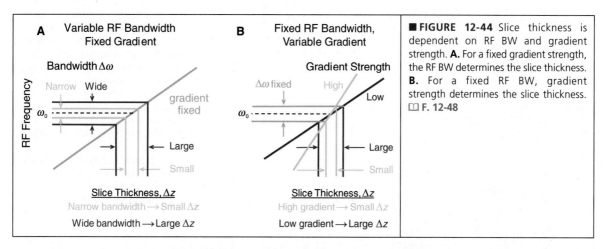

**A** Variable RF Bandwidth Fixed Gradient

Bandwidth $\Delta\omega$

Narrow  Wide

$\omega_0$

gradient fixed

Large

Small

Slice Thickness, $\Delta z$

Narrow bandwidth → Small $\Delta z$

Wide bandwidth → Large $\Delta z$

**B** Fixed RF Bandwidth, Variable Gradient

Gradient Strength

$\Delta\omega$ fixed   High

Low

$\omega_0$

Large

Small

Slice Thickness, $\Delta z$

High gradient → Small $\Delta z$

Low gradient → Large $\Delta z$

■ **FIGURE 12-44** Slice thickness is dependent on RF BW and gradient strength. **A.** For a fixed gradient strength, the RF BW determines the slice thickness. **B.** For a fixed RF BW, gradient strength determines the slice thickness. 📖 **F. 12-48**

**c.** The strength and duration of the RF pulse determines the effective flip angle.
**d.** After the SSG is turned off, a rephasing gradient is required to maintain phase coherence across the slice (Fig. 12-45)

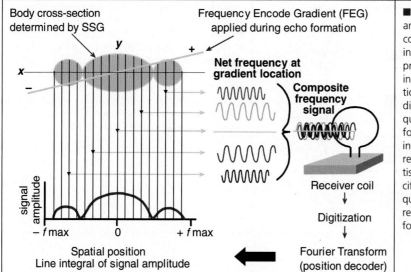

RF pulse

SSG

Rephasing Gradient

Equal area

out of phase

in phase       in phase

Relative phase

■ **FIGURE 12-45** SSG rephasing. At the peak of the RF pulse, all protons in the slice are in phase, but the SSG causes the spins to become dephased after the gradient is turned off. To reestablish phase coherence, a reverse polarity gradient is applied equal to one half the area of the original SSG. At the next pulse, the relative phase will be identical. 📖 **F. 12-49**

**2. Frequency encoding:**
   **a.** When the frequency-encoding gradient (FEG) is applied along the logical *x*-axis, net changes in precessional frequencies are distributed symmetrically from 0 at the gradient isocenter to $+f_{max}$ and $-f_{max}$ at the edges of the FOV (Fig. 12-46).
   **b.** The composite signal is processed by the Fourier transform to convert frequency into spatial position (Fig. 12-47).

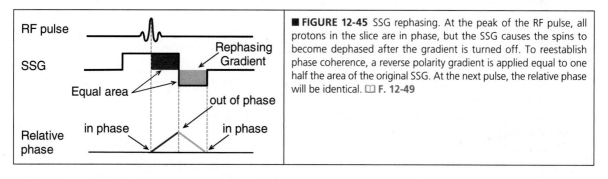

Body cross-section determined by SSG

$y$

$x$

Frequency Encode Gradient (FEG) applied during echo formation

Net frequency at gradient location

Composite frequency signal

Receiver coil

↓

Digitization

↓

Fourier Transform (position decoder)

signal amplitude

$-f$max    0    $+f$max

Spatial position

Line integral of signal amplitude

■ **FIGURE 12-46** The *FEG* is applied in an orthogonal direction to the SSG and confers *a spatially dependent variation* in the precessional frequencies of the protons. Acting only on those protons in a slice determined by the SSG excitation, the composite signal is acquired, digitized, demodulated (Larmor frequency removed), and Fourier transformed into frequency and amplitude information. A one-dimensional array represents a *projection* of the slice of tissue (amplitude and position) at a specific angle. (Demodulation into net frequencies occurs *after* detection by the receiver coil; this is shown in the figure for clarity only.) 📖 **F. 12-50**

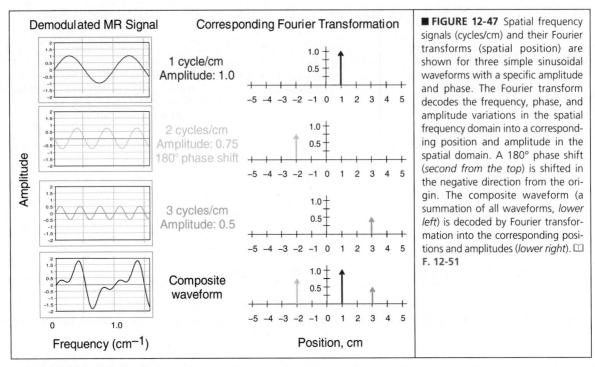

**■ FIGURE 12-47** Spatial frequency signals (cycles/cm) and their Fourier transforms (spatial position) are shown for three simple sinusoidal waveforms with a specific amplitude and phase. The Fourier transform decodes the frequency, phase, and amplitude variations in the spatial frequency domain into a corresponding position and amplitude in the spatial domain. A 180° phase shift (*second from the top*) is shifted in the negative direction from the origin. The composite waveform (a summation of all waveforms, *lower left*) is decoded by Fourier transformation into the corresponding positions and amplitudes (*lower right*). 📖 **F. 12-51**

    **c.** The strength of FEG determines the bandwidth across FOV. SNR is inversely proportional to the receiver BW:

$$\text{SNR} \propto \frac{1}{\sqrt{\text{BW}}} \; ; \text{therefore, narrow BW and low gradient strength are preferred.}$$

    **d.** Artifacts due to *chemical shift* is more pronounced with narrow BW (see Chapter 13, Section 13.5, Chemical Shift Artifacts).

    **e.** Trade-offs in image quality must be considered when determining the optimal RF bandwidth.

**3. Phase encoding**

    **a.** Position of the protons in the logical *y*-axis is determined with a phase-encoding gradient (PEG).

    **b.** Specific known phase changes are a function of position across the FOV for each TR.

    **c.** Each location along *y*-axis is spatially encoded by the amount of phase shifts experienced by the protons (Fig. 12-48).

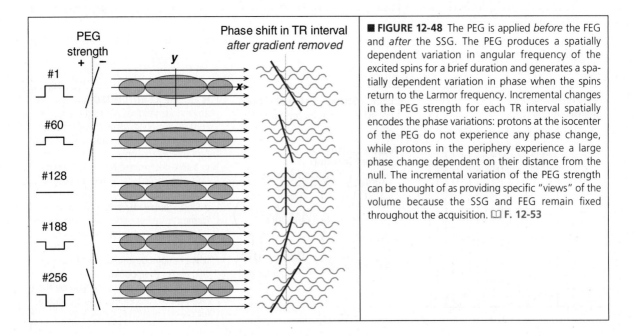

**■ FIGURE 12-48** The PEG is applied *before* the FEG and *after* the SSG. The PEG produces a spatially dependent variation in angular frequency of the excited spins for a brief duration and generates a spatially dependent variation in phase when the spins return to the Larmor frequency. Incremental changes in the PEG strength for each TR interval spatially encodes the phase variations: protons at the isocenter of the PEG do not experience any phase change, while protons in the periphery experience a large phase change dependent on their distance from the null. The incremental variation of the PEG strength can be thought of as providing specific "views" of the volume because the SSG and FEG remain fixed throughout the acquisition. 📖 **F. 12-53**

### 4. Gradient sequencing

Acquisition of a *spin echo* pulse sequence including all three gradients (Fig. 12-49)

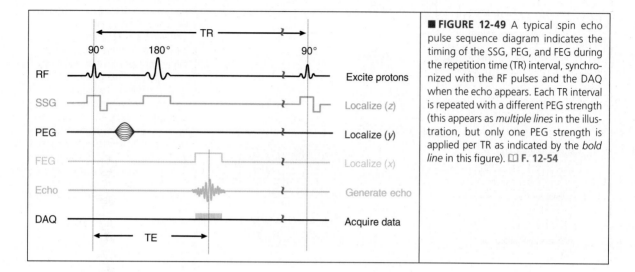

■ **FIGURE 12-49** A typical spin echo pulse sequence diagram indicates the timing of the SSG, PEG, and FEG during the repetition time (TR) interval, synchronized with the RF pulses and the DAQ when the echo appears. Each TR interval is repeated with a different PEG strength (this appears as *multiple lines* in the illustration, but only one PEG strength is applied per TR as indicated by the *bold line* in this figure). 📖 **F. 12-54**

## 12.8  *"K-SPACE"* DATA ACQUISITION AND IMAGE RECONSTRUCTION

MR data are initially stored in the *k*-space matrix, the "frequency domain" repository (Fig. 12-50).

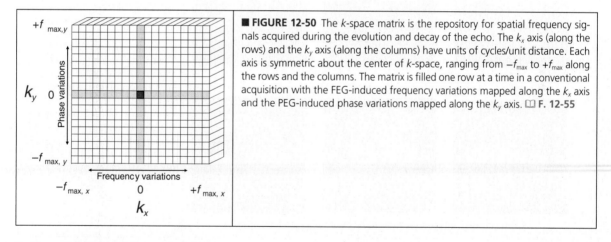

■ **FIGURE 12-50** The *k*-space matrix is the repository for spatial frequency signals acquired during the evolution and decay of the echo. The $k_x$ axis (along the rows) and the $k_y$ axis (along the columns) have units of cycles/unit distance. Each axis is symmetric about the center of *k*-space, ranging from $-f_{max}$ to $+f_{max}$ along the rows and the columns. The matrix is filled one row at a time in a conventional acquisition with the FEG-induced frequency variations mapped along the $k_x$ axis and the PEG-induced phase variations mapped along the $k_y$ axis. 📖 **F. 12-55**

### 1. Two-dimensional data acquisition

   **a.** A *k*-space matrix is filled to produce the desired variations across the frequency- and phase-encoding directions (Fig. 12-51).

   **b.** The bulk of image information representing the lower spatial frequencies is contained in the center of k-space, whereas the higher spatial frequencies are contained in the periphery, as shown in Figure 12-52.

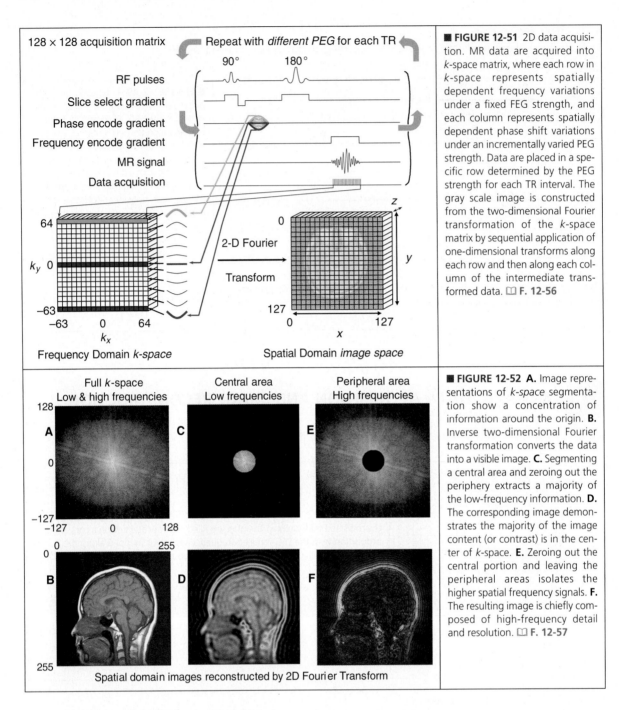

**FIGURE 12-51** 2D data acquisition. MR data are acquired into *k*-space matrix, where each row in *k*-space represents spatially dependent frequency variations under a fixed FEG strength, and each column represents spatially dependent phase shift variations under an incrementally varied PEG strength. Data are placed in a specific row determined by the PEG strength for each TR interval. The gray scale image is constructed from the two-dimensional Fourier transformation of the *k*-space matrix by sequential application of one-dimensional transforms along each row and then along each column of the intermediate transformed data. 📖 **F. 12-56**

**FIGURE 12-52 A.** Image representations of *k-space* segmentation show a concentration of information around the origin. **B.** Inverse two-dimensional Fourier transformation converts the data into a visible image. **C.** Segmenting a central area and zeroing out the periphery extracts a majority of the low-frequency information. **D.** The corresponding image demonstrates the majority of the image content (or contrast) is in the center of *k*-space. **E.** Zeroing out the central portion and leaving the peripheral areas isolates the higher spatial frequency signals. **F.** The resulting image is chiefly composed of high-frequency detail and resolution. 📖 **F. 12-57**

## 2. Two-dimensional multiplanar acquisition

Direct axial, coronal, sagittal, or oblique planes can be obtained by selecting (or switching) the appropriate gradient coils during the image acquisition (Fig. 12-53).

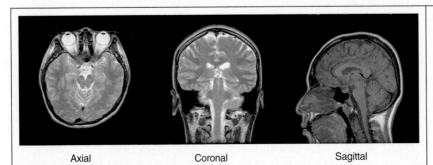

Axial    Coronal    Sagittal

**FIGURE 12-53** Direct acquisitions of axial, coronal, and sagittal tomographic images are possible by electronically energizing the magnetic field gradients in a different order without moving the patient. Oblique planes can also be obtained. 📖 **F. 12-58**

### 3. Three-dimensional image acquisition

  **a.** A *slab-selective* RF pulse excites a large volume of protons, and two-phase gradients are discretely applied in the slice encode and phase encode directions (Fig. 12-54).

  **b.** A 3D Fourier transform is applied to generate 3D volumetric images.

  **c.** 3D imaging allows reconstruction of very thin slices with good detail and high SNR but a downside is the increased probability of motion artifacts.

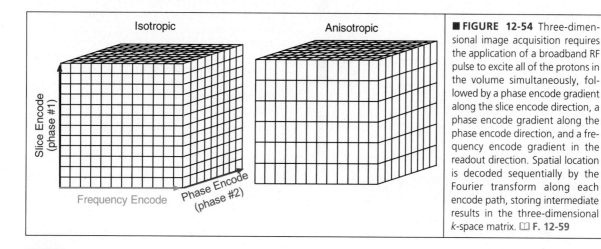

■**FIGURE 12-54** Three-dimensional image acquisition requires the application of a broadband RF pulse to excite all of the protons in the volume simultaneously, followed by a phase encode gradient along the slice encode direction, a phase encode gradient along the phase encode direction, and a frequency encode gradient in the readout direction. Spatial location is decoded sequentially by the Fourier transform along each encode path, storing intermediate results in the three-dimensional *k*-space matrix. ▢ **F. 12-59**

## 12.9  MR IMAGE CHARACTERISTICS

### 1. Spatial resolution and contrast sensitivity

  **a.** Spatial resolution is dependent on the FOV and the matrix size

  **b.** Higher field strength magnets can improve spatial resolution due to a larger SNR.

  **c.** Contrast sensitivity is dependent upon a pulse sequence and its timing parameters.

  **d.** MR contrast materials disrupt the local magnetic field to enhance T2 decay and shorten T1 recovery.

### 2. Signal-to-noise ratio, SNR, dependencies (covered in Sections 12.3 to 12.8)

  **a.** The MR image SNR is dependent on many imaging parameters.

  **b.** In general, SNR is proportional to the **intrinsic signal intensity** based on pulse sequence.

  **c.** The **voxel volume** determines the signal strength collected.

  **d.** The **square root of time** spent on the collection of *k*-space data, including number of **signal averages** ($\sqrt{\text{NEX}}$) and **receiver bandwidth** ($1/\sqrt{\text{BW}}$).

### 3. Voxel volume

  **a.** The voxel volume is equal to

$$\text{Volume} = \frac{\text{FOV}_x}{\text{No. of pixels}, x} \times \frac{\text{FOV}_y}{\text{No. of pixels}, y} \times \text{Slice thickness}, z$$

  **b.** SNR is linearly proportional to the voxel volume.

### 4. Signal averages

  **a.** Known as number of excitations, NEX, is achieved by averaging sets of data acquired using an identical pulse sequence (same PEG strength).

  **b.** The SNR is proportional to the square root of the number of signal averages: $\text{SNR} \propto \sqrt{\text{NEX}}$.

### 5. RF bandwidth

  **a.** The receiver bandwidth defines the range of frequencies to which the detector is tuned during the application of the readout gradient.

  **b.** A narrow bandwidth (a narrow spread of frequencies around the center frequency) provides a higher SNR, proportional to $1/\sqrt{\text{BW}}$.

  **c.** White noise, which is relatively constant across the bandwidth, does not change, while the signal distribution changes with bandwidth (Fig. 12-55).

   **d.** Any decrease in RF bandwidth might be unacceptable if chemical shift artifacts are of concern (see Artifacts, Chapter 13).

   **e.** Narrower bandwidths also require a longer time for sampling and therefore affect the minimum TE time that is possible for an imaging sequence.

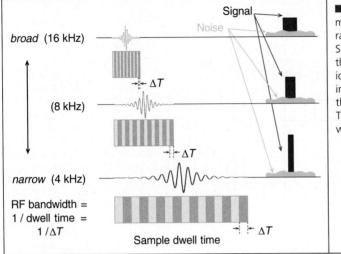

■ **FIGURE 12-55** RF, receiver bandwidth, is determined by the FEG strength, the FOV, and sampling rate. This figure illustrates the spatial domain view of SNR and corresponding sample dwell time. Evolution of the echo in the broad bandwidth situation occurs rapidly with minimal dwell time, which might be needed in situations where very short TE is required, even though the SNR is reduced. On the other hand, in T2-weighted images requiring a long TE, narrow bandwidth can improve SNR. ▢ **F. 12-60**

6. **RF coil quality factor**
      **a.** The coil quality factor is an indication of RF coil sensitivity to induced currents in response to signals emanating from the patient.
      **b.** Quadrature coils increase the SNR as two coils are used in the reception of the signal.
      **c.** Phased array coils increase the SNR even more when the data from several coils are added together.
      **d.** Body receiver coils positioned in the bore of the magnet provides lower SNR than other coils while the signal is relatively uniform across the FOV.
      **e.** Surface coils offers superb SNR when positioned proximal to the anatomy of interest while limiting the useful imaging depth and resulting in nonuniform brightness across the image.

7. **Magnetic field strength**
      **a.** Magnetic field strength influences the SNR of the image by a factor of $B^{1.0}$ to $B^{1.5}$.
      **b.** Other considerations mitigate the SNR improvement in the clinical environment, including longer T1 and greater RF absorption.

8. **Cross-excitation**
      **a.** Cross-excitation occurs from the nonrectangular RF excitation profiles in the spatial domain and the resultant overlap of adjacent slices in multislice image acquisition sequences.
      **b.** This saturates the protons and reduces contrast and the contrast-to-noise ratio.
      **c.** To avoid cross-excitation, *interslice gaps* or *interleaving procedures* are necessary.

9. **Image acquisition and reconstruction algorithms**
      **a.** Image acquisition and reconstruction algorithms have a profound effect on SNR.
      **b.** The volume of tissue that is excited is the major factor to improving the SNR and image quality.
      **c.** Reconstruction filters and image processing algorithms will also affect the SNR.
         **(i)** High-pass filtration methods that increase edge definition will generally decrease the SNR.
         **(ii)** Low-pass filtration methods smooth the image data and generally increase the SNR at the cost of reduced resolution.

# Section II Questions and Answers

1. What magnetic material decreases the local magnetic field surrounding the material because of negative magnetic susceptibility?
   A. Diamagnetic
   B. Paramagnetic
   C. Ferromagnetic
   D. Superparamagnetic

2. Which element below has magnetic moment close to zero and is not observable in MR system?
   A. $^1H$
   B. $^4He$
   C. $^{23}Na$
   D. $^{31}P$

3. If a superconducting magnet developed a leak from the bore of the magnet, what fluid/gas would be most likely to be encountered?
   A. Hydrogen
   B. Helium
   C. Oxygen
   D. Fluorine
   E. Water

4. What elemental magnetic property of calcium causes a cancellation of the $T_2$ shortening effects of the blood degradation products in an acute hemorrhage?
   A. Diamagnetic
   B. Hyperpolarization
   C. Magnetization transfer
   D. Paramagnetic
   E. Superparamagnetic

5. Of the following precessional frequencies, which one represents the closest for protons (hydrogen nuclei) in a 1.5 T magnetic field?
   A. 1.5 MHz
   B. 15 MHz
   C. 43 MHz
   D. 64 MHz
   E. 92 MHz

6. Which of the following substances often encountered in blood hemorrhage exhibits paramagnetic characteristics?
   A. Methemoglobin
   B. Hemosiderin

C. Calcium
D. Oxygen
E. Water

7. What type of receiver coils is mostly suitable to obtain uniform intensity in the image volume without using an intensity correction algorithm?
   A. Surface coils
   B. Phase array coils
   C. Volume coils

8. Which magnetization component of the tissue sample after an RF excitation is described by the T1 time constant?
   A. Transverse
   B. Spin density
   C. Longitudinal
   D. Equilibrium

9. In terms of the MR spin-lattice relaxation time, what does the lattice refer to?
   A. The $x, y, z$ coordinate system
   B. The tissue structure
   C. The magnetic field
   D. The digital image matrix
   E. The gyromagnetic ratio constant

10. Which characteristic proton tissue parameter increases as the magnetic field strength increases?
    A. T1
    B. T2
    C. T2/T1
    D. T2*

11. Which of following represents relationships among magnetic relaxation times correctly?
    A. T1 > T2 > T2*
    B. T1 < T2 < T2*
    C. T1 > T2 < T2*
    D. T1 > T2* > T2

12. In a contrast-weighted spin echo sequence with TR = 5,000 ms and TE = 5 ms, which of the following tissues will have the largest signal?
    A. White matter
    B. Gray matter
    C. Fat
    D. CSF

**13.** In a T1-weighted imaging sequence, which of the following tissues will have the LEAST signal assuming a fat suppression technique is not applied?
  A. White matter
  B. Gray matter
  C. Fat
  D. CSF

**14.** Which of the following pulse sequences will have the largest signal-to-noise ratio? (Consider similar slice thickness, image volume, and number of excitations.)
  A. T1-weighted SE
  B. Proton density–weighted SE
  C. T2-weighted SE
  D. T1-weighed spoiled GRE
  E. T2-weighted FSE

**15.** In coherent gradient echo imaging acquisitions with TR less than 15 ms, what is the chief cause of poor tissue contrast in the acquired image?
  A. Longitudinal magnetization recovery
  B. Magnetic field inhomogeneity
  C. Persistent transverse magnetization
  D. Patient motion
  E. Susceptibility effects

**16.** Which of the following gradient echo sequences produces T1 weighting?
  A. Balanced SSFP (or FIESTA)
  B. Gradient Recalled Echo
  C. Steady-state free precession
  D. Spoiled gradient echo (or FLASH)

**17.** Of the four MRI sequences illustrated, identify the STIR sequence:

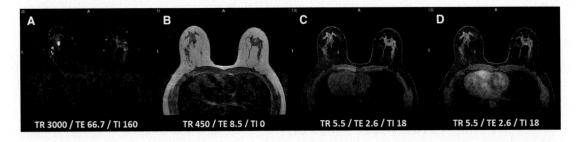

TR 3000 / TE 66.7 / TI 160     TR 450 / TE 8.5 / TI 0     TR 5.5 / TE 2.6 / TI 18     TR 5.5 / TE 2.6 / TI 18

**18.** Which of the following MRI techniques is not intended to suppress fat signals in the image?
  A. Chemical saturation
  B. Short tau (or T1) inversion recovery
  C. Gradient moment nulling
  D. Two-point Dixon

**19.** At 1.5 T, fat and water signals are in-phase every 4.4 ms. Which of the following echo times should be selected to get out-of-phase images in Dixon technique?
  A. Approximately 0 ms
  B. 4.4 ms
  C. 6.6 ms
  D. 8.8 ms

**20.** Which one of the following acquisition sequences does the diagram on the right most closely describe for generated tissue contrast?
  A. STIR
  B. FLAIR
  C. Gradient moment nulling
  D. Propeller
  E. Magnetization transfer

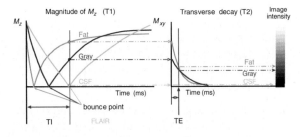

**21.** For the axial brain images shown, identify the image obtained with a T1-weighted sequence.

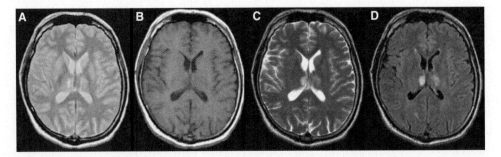

22. For the axial brain images below, identify the image obtained with a FLAIR sequence.

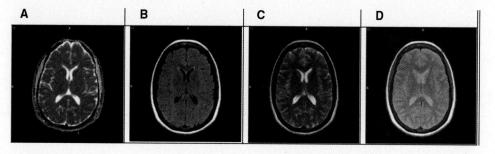

23. Which of the following pulse sequences is particularly useful for improved visualization of white matter lesions in the brain?
    A. STIR
    B. STEAM
    C. GRASS
    D. FISP
    E. FLAIR

24. What is the purpose of gradient coils during an MRI acquisition?
    A. Acquire the FID signal as it is produced in the transverse plane.
    B. Excite the protons in the body through absorption of RF.
    C. Improve the homogeneity of the magnet field.
    D. Limit the RF power deposition into the patient.
    E. Spatially vary the precessional frequency of the protons.

25. In MR imaging, what is the gradient *slew rate*?
    A. Time to invert the applied gradient field
    B. Time to achieve the peak amplitude of the gradient field
    C. Time to induce eddy currents in the gradient coil
    D. Time to superimpose the gradient fields from different coils
    E. Time to overcome patient attenuation of the gradient field

26. To acquire an *axial image* in an air-core superconducting magnet, which of the following gradients is energized during the initial RF excitation pulse?
    A. $G_X$
    B. $G_Y$
    C. $G_Z$
    D. $G_{XY}$
    E. $G_{YZ}$

27. To obtain images in the sagittal plane directly, which one of the following gradients are activated for slice selection?
    A. $G_X$
    B. $G_Y$
    C. $G_Z$
    D. $G_{XY}$
    E. $G_{YZ}$

28. When changing from a 256 × 256 matrix ($SNR_1$) with 2 NEX to a 256 × 128 matrix ($SNR_2$) with 1 NEX and the phase encoding along the 128 matrix dimension (with everything else fixed), what are the relationships between $SNR_1$ and $SNR_2$?
    A. $SNR_1 = \frac{1}{4} SNR_2$
    B. $SNR_1 = \frac{1}{2} SNR_2$
    C. $SNR_1 = SNR_2$
    D. $SNR_1 = 2 SNR_2$
    E. $SNR_1 = 4 SNR_2$

29. While maintaining all other MRI scan parameters, FOV is increased by 20% in frequency- and phase-encoding directions. How SNR will be changed?
    A. Increased by 20%
    B. Decreased by 20%
    C. Increased by 44%
    D. Decreased by 44%

30. What is the functional relationship between signal-to-noise ratio (SNR) of the *receiver RF signal* and bandwidth (BW)?
    A. $BW^{0.5}$
    B. $BW^{-0.5}$
    C. $BW^{1.0}$
    D. $BW^{-1.0}$

# Answers

1. **A** Diamagnetic elements and materials have slightly negative susceptibility and oppose the applied magnetic field, because of paired electrons in the surrounding electron orbitals. Examples of diamagnetic materials are calcium, water, and most organic materials (chiefly owing to the diamagnetic characteristics of carbon and hydrogen molecules). *(Pg. 444, Fig. 12-2)*

2. **B** To make MR signal observable, mass number of an element (the sum of the number of protons [P] and number of neutrons [N]) should be odd, resulting noninteger nuclear spin to generate a nuclear magnetic moment. Hyperpolarized $^3$He gas is used to image gas distribution throughout the lungs. *(Pg. 445, Table 12-2)*

3. **B** Superconducting magnets require temperatures close to absolute zero (0°K) to maintain current without resistance. This is achieved with liquid helium; in some older magnet systems, a second Dewar "jacket" of liquid nitrogen (not a choice in this question) could also leak. The liquid helium would immediately convert to the gas phase outside of the Dewar, however. *(Pg. 448–449)*

4. **A.** Calcium, because of its paired nuclear spins, exhibits a *diamagnetic* property that has the effect of diminishing the local magnetic field. *Paramagnetic* agents, such as methemoglobin, augment the local magnetic field. In certain situations, these properties offset (paramagnetic + diamagnetic), and the image does not exhibit the expected appearance of a hemorrhage. *(Pg. 444, Ch 13 - Pg. 527)*

5. **D** The *LARMOR FREQUENCY* equation is $\omega = \gamma B_0$; $\gamma = 42.58$ MHz/T$\omega = 1.5 \times 42.58 \approx 64$ MHz. *(Pg. 447–448, see example on Pg. 448)*

6. **A** Methemoglobin is a blood degradation product that has unpaired electron spins and exhibits paramagnetic properties, and thus, susceptibility changes allow the characterization of the age of the hemorrhage; in this case, methemoglobin represents the acute stage of evolution. *(Pg. 444)*

7. **C** Volume coils encompass the total area of the anatomy of interest and yield uniform excitation and SNR over the entire imaging volume. *(Pg. 452)*

8. **C** T1 is the spin-lattice relaxation constant for a given tissue, and it expresses the time required to reestablish 67% of the longitudinal magnetization recovery when placed in a magnetic field. *(Pg. 458–459, Fig. 12–17)*

9. **B** The lattice is the tissue environment (structure) in which the spins (protons) exist. *(Pg. 459–460)*

10. **A** Increasing the magnetic field strength increases the Larmor frequency and lengthens the T1 relaxation time, there is a loss of T1 contrast compared to the same acquisition protocols on an optimally tuned magnet of lower field strength, even though SNR is higher with larger magnetic field strength. *(Pg. 460–461, Table 12-3)*

11. **A** T1 is on the order of 5 to 10 times longer than T2. Regarding other answers, extrinsic magnetic inhomogeneities add to the loss of phase coherence reduce the decay constant, known as T2*. Therefore, T2 > T2*, but T2 itself is not affected by a change in magnetic field strength. *(Pg. 461)*

12. **D** For the spin echo sequence, a long TR and short TE are used. This is proton density weighted. At equilibrium, CSF demonstrates the largest proton density, although fat also has a large number of protons per unit mass. *(Pg. 463–467, Table 12-4)*

13. **D** CSF has the longest T1, which takes the longest time to recover back to the equilibrium. Therefore, CSF has the least amount of signal in a T1-weighted imaging sequence. *(Pg. 465–467)*

14. **B**  Proton (spin) density weighting produces the largest SNR. A long TR is required, allowing for $M_z$ recovery and associated large signal. Also, a short TE is required, thus reducing the amount of signal decay occurring for echo formation, maintaining the high signal strength. *(Pg. 464)*

15. **C**  With gradient recalled echo (GRE) acquisitions, the short TR does not allow sufficient time for transverse magnetization decay (in addition to longitudinal decay). The persistent transverse magnetization hinders the ability to develop any significant anatomical contrast; typically, any differences in the anatomy are due to a ratio of T2* to T1 relaxation times. This is advantageous with MR angiography sequences because the desire is to separate the unsaturated bright blood signal from the surrounding anatomy, which a GRASS or FISP GRE sequence does quite nicely; in combination with a maximum intensity projection (MIP) algorithm, 2D angiogram projections can be created from the volume in a time-of-flight (TOF) acquisition sequence. T1 contrast can be achieved by "spoiling" the persistent transverse magnetization by introducing successive phase shifts in the subsequent RF excitation pulses to "destroy" the persistent transverse magnetization. *(Pg. 473–474)*

16. **D**  In SPGR, The T2* influence can be reduced by spoiling the steady-state transverse magnetization by introducing incoherent phase differences from pulse to pulse. T1-weighted contrast is obtained. *(Pg. 473–474, Fig. 12-39)*

17. **A**  The STIR sequence is one that eliminates fat and uses an extended TR (3,000 ms) and an inversion time, TI (160 ms) to capture the signals at the "bounce point" of fat to be effectively nulled. Image B is a T1-weighted image demonstrating the large signal due to fatty tissues, surrounding the glandular tissues. Images C and D are 3D GRE image acquisitions pre- and postcontrast, respectively, as demonstrated by the signal intensity in the heart in Image D. These pre- and postcontrast images are used for generating quantitative flow studies of the wash in and wash out of suspected breast lesions. *(Pg. 475–477)*

18. **C**  Gradient moment nulling is a technique reducing motion ghosting caused by CSF or blood flow. This approach is also referred to as flow compensation. *(Pg. 479–481, Fig. 12-49)*

19. **C**  The chemical shift between fat and water yields the resonance frequency difference of 223 Hz at 1.5 T, which is interpreted as being in-phase every 4.4 ms. The fat and the water spins are *out of phase* at 2.2, 6.6 ms, and so on while *in phase* at 0, 4.4 ms, and so on right after the excitation RF pulse is applied. *(Pg. 475–478, Fig. 12-44)*

20. **B**  This is a typical fluid-attenuated inversion recovery (FLAIR) signal evolution. Note the "bounce point" equal to the inversion time (TI) readout pulse. *(Pg. 477–479, Fig. 12-45)*

21. **B**  T1-weighted image shows the opposite contrasts of tissue T1 values, which are fat > white matter > gray matter > CSF. *(Pg. 463–467, Fig. 12-28)*

22. **B**  The FLAIR image is characterized by dark CSF resulting from the selection of the CSF bounce point (TI = ~2,400 ms, TR = 10,000 ms) in the inversion recovery pulse sequence. Note that a T1W image will also have dark CSF due to a long T1 of CSF (not provided as a choice). Image A is an image acquired to calculate an apparent diffusion coefficient (ADC) image; Image C is T2 weighted; Image D is proton density weighted. *(Pg. 477–479, Figs. 12-45 and 12-46)*

23. **E**  FLAIR is an acronym for fluid-attenuated inversion recovery, which sets the TI (inversion time) at a point where the signals for CSF go through zero during the longitudinal magnetization recovery time, which is on the order of 2,500 ms. Reducing the very bright signal from CSF assists in visualizing adjacent white matter lesions. *(Pg. 477–479, Figs. 12-45 and 12-46)*

24. **E**  Gradient coils encode the spatial location of the protons within the patient volume as a function of variations in precessional frequency and phase changes. *(Pg. 450–451)*

25. **B**  This is the definition of gradient slew rate. Limitations of high gradient slew rates are caused by eddy currents generated by magnetic field inductions (changing magnetic field), which can be reduced by using actively shielded coils. *(Pg. 450)*

26. **C**  The orientation of the main magnetic field in a superconducting air core magnet is along the long axis of the body. By convention, the z-axis is parallel to the main magnetic field, which is parallel to the long axis of the body. Therefore, the $G_z$ coil is activated. Note that in a solid core magnet with the main magnetic field vertical, this would not be the correct answer. More information would have to be given to determine which gradient (or gradients) would have to be turned on. *(Pg. 479–480)*

27. **A**   In the sagittal plane, the slice direction is right/left (or in physical $x$) direction. Therefore, $x$ gradient should be turned on during slice selection. (*Pg. 479–481*)

28. **C**   The voxel volume is doubled, therefore related to volume differences, $SNR_2 = 2\ SNR_1$ (SNR is directly proportional to voxel volume). However, the *total* time spent is *decreased* by a factor of 4 (from 2 NEX to 1 NEX is 2X, and 256 excitations to 128 excitations [phase encoding] is 2x); therefore, related to the #excitations, $SNR_2 = 1/2\ SNR_1$ (the SNR is directly proportional to the square root of the number of excitations). The overall relative SNR of the images is therefore equal because of offsetting variables. (*Pg. 489*)

29. **C**   SNR is linearly proportional to the voxel volume. Voxel volume is increased by 44% (this is the product of the increased FOV of 20% in both the FEG and PEG directions = 1.2 x 1.2 = 1.44, an increase of 44%). Therefore, SNR is also increased by 44%. (*Pg. 489–490*)

30. **B**   $SNR \propto 1/\sqrt{BW}$. The SNR is improved by narrowing the bandwidth (BW) because the evolution of the echo occurs over a longer period, and a more accurate sampling can occur simultaneous to noise averaging within the $1/\Delta T$ period. (*Pg. 490–491, Fig. 12-60*)

# Section III Key Equations, Symbols, Quantities, and Units

| QUANTITY | EQUATION | PAGE/COMMENTS |
|---|---|---|
| Angular precessional frequency | $\omega_0 = \gamma B_0$ | Pg. 447/$\gamma$ is the gyromagnetic ratio in radians/s/T, $\omega_0$ is radians/s for field strength $B_0$ (T) |
| Precessional frequency | $f_0 = \dfrac{\gamma}{2\pi} B_0$ | Pg. 447/$f_0$ is the linear frequency in cycles/s; $\gamma/2\pi$ is the gyromagnetic ratio in MHz/T (42.58 MHz/T) |
| Angular precessional frequency at a location within a linear gradient | $\omega = \gamma(B_0 + G_{net} \cdot d)$ | Pg. 451/$\omega$ is the angular precessional frequency at a location within the linear gradient $G_{net}$ at distance $d$ from null |
| Transverse magnetization with T2 relaxation after 90° excitation at $t = 0$ | $M_{xy}(t) = M_0 e^{-t/T2}$ | Pg. 458/$M_{xy}$ is the transverse magnetization, and $M_0$ is equilibrium magnetization |
| Longitudinal magnetization with T1 recovery after 180° inversion at $t = 0$ | $M_z(t) = M_0(1 - e^{-t/T1})$ | Pg. 459/$M_z$ is the longitudinal magnetization |
| Signal intensity produced by an SE sequence | $S \propto \rho_H [1 - e^{-TR/T1}] e^{-TE/T2}$ | Pg. 463/$\rho_H$ is proton density; equation is a function of TR, time of repetition, and TE, time of echo |
| Signal intensity produced by an IR SE sequence | $S \propto \rho_H (1 - 2e^{-T1/T1})(1 - e^{-(TR-T1)/T1})(e^{-TE/T2})$ | Pg. 468/TI is inversion time |
| Time to bounce point for magnitude $M_z = 0$ recovery for inversion time, TI | $TI = \ln(2) \times T1 = 0.693 \times T1$ | Pg. 475/T1 is the longitudinal recovery time for the tissue of interest |
| SNR of a 2D image acquisition | $SNR \propto I \times voxel_{x,y,z} \times \dfrac{\sqrt{NEX}}{\sqrt{BW}} \times f(QF) \times f(B)$ $\times f(\text{slice gap})$ $\times f(\text{reconstruction})$ | Pg. 489/SNR is signal-to-noise ratio; $I$ is the intrinsic signal intensity based on the pulse sequence; voxel is the volume element; NEX is number of excitations; BW is receive bandwidth; $f(-)$ is a function of coils, magnetic field strength, slice gap, and reconstruction parameters |
| Voxel volume in a 2D image acquisition | $Volume = \dfrac{FOV_x}{\text{No. of pixels, } x} \times \dfrac{FOV_y}{\text{No. of pixels, } y}$ $\times \text{Slice thickness, } z$ | Pg. 489/The volume element, voxel, is a product of the incremental $x$-, $y$-, and $z$-dimensions of the MR acquisition |

| SYMBOL | QUANTITY | UNITS |
|---|---|---|
| $B_0$ | Static magnetic field | Tesla (T) |
| $T$ | Magnetic field strength | Tesla |
| $G$ | Magnetic field strength | Gauss; 10,000 G = 1 T |
| $\omega_0$ | Angular precessional frequency | Radian/s |
| $f_0$ | Precessional (or resonance) frequency | 1/s or Hz |
| $\gamma$ | Gyromagnetic ratio | Radian·Hz/tesla or Hz/tesla |
| $G_x, G_y, G_z$ | Gradient field strength in $x, y, z$ | Tesla/m |
| $G_{net}$ | Net gradient field strength | Tesla/m |

(Continued)

*(Continued)*

| SYMBOL | QUANTITY | UNITS |
|---|---|---|
| $d$ | Distance from the gradient isocenter | cm |
| $B_1$ | *Excitation magnetic field* | Gauss (G) or millitesla (mT) |
| $M_0$ | *Equilibrium magnetization* | NA |
| $M_z$ | *Longitudinal magnetization* | NA |
| $M_{xy}$ | *Transverse magnetization* | NA |
| $\theta$ | Flip angle | degrees |
| T1 | Longitudinal relaxation time | seconds (s) |
| T2 | Transverse relaxation time | seconds (s) |
| T2* | Transverse relaxation time including extrinsic magnetic inhomogeneities | seconds (s) |
| TR | Time of repetition | seconds (s) |
| TE | Time of echo | seconds (s) |
| TI | Time of inversion | seconds (s) |
| $\rho_H$ | Proton density | – |
| BW | Receiver bandwidth | Hz |
| $FOV_x$, $FOV_y$ | Field of view in *x, y* | centimeters (cm) |

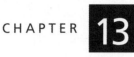

# CHAPTER 13

# Magnetic Resonance Imaging: Advanced Image Acquisition Methods, Artifacts, Spectroscopy, Quality Control, Siting, Bioeffects, and Safety

## 13.0 INTRODUCTION

Advanced pulse sequences and fast image acquisition methods; methods for perfusion, diffusion, and angiography imaging; spectroscopy; image quality metrics; common artifacts; MR siting; and MR safety issues are described and discussed with respect to the underlying physics.

## 13.1 IMAGE ACQUISITION TIME

1. Acquisition time, 2D acquisition
   a. **Time = TR × #PEG × NEX**—where TR is the repetition time, #PEG is the number of phase-encode gradient applications, and NEX is the number of excitations (averages).
   b. Matrix size defining *k*-space is often not square—typically, the smaller dimension is assigned to PEG.
   c. Tradeoff of time and SNR are considered.
2. Multislice data acquisition
   a. During the TR, cycling gradients and tuning RF excitation frequency images the volume (Fig. 13-1).
   b. Tradeoff is cross excitation of adjacent tissues and loss of contrast from nonsquare excitation pulses.
   c. **Total number of slices = TR/(TE + C)**, where C is a constant dependent on MR equipment capabilities.
   d. Longer TR (*e.g.*, *T*2-weighted SE) can have more slices acquired in the acquisition.

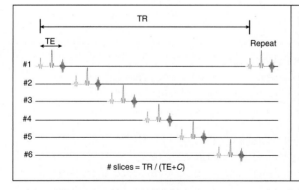

■ **FIGURE 13-1** Multislice two-dimensional image acquisition is accomplished by discretely exciting different slabs of tissue during the TR period; appropriate changes of the RF excitation bandwidth, SSG, PEG, and FEG parameters are necessary. Because of diffuse excitation profiles, RF irradiation of adjacent slices leads to partial saturation and loss of contrast. The number of slices (volume) that can be obtained is a function of the TR, TE, and C, the latter representing the capabilities of the MR system and type of pulse sequence.

3. Acquisition time, 3D acquisition
   a. The 3D acquisition is initiated with a *slice encode* excitation in addition to a phase-encode excitation.
   b. **Time (3D) = TR × # phase-encode steps (Z-axis) × phase-encode steps (X-axis) × NEX.**

## 13.2 FAST IMAGING TECHNIQUES

1. **Fast pulse sequences**
   a. Fast spin echo (FSE) uses multiple PEG steps with multiple 180° refocusing pulses per TR.
      (i) Multiple lines in *k*-space are filled per TR resulting in an echo train length (ETL) (Fig. 13-2).
      (ii) Speed increase is acquisition time × 1/ETL.
      (iii) Characteristics: high SAR, good immunity from inhomogeneities (with 180° excitations).

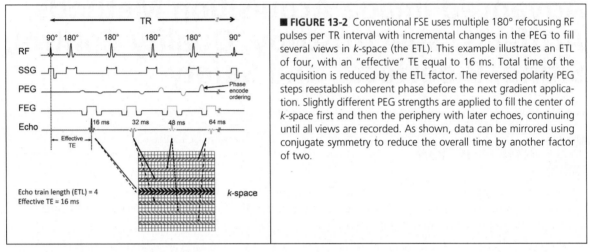

■ **FIGURE 13-2** Conventional FSE uses multiple 180° refocusing RF pulses per TR interval with incremental changes in the PEG to fill several views in *k*-space (the ETL). This example illustrates an ETL of four, with an "effective" TE equal to 16 ms. Total time of the acquisition is reduced by the ETL factor. The reversed polarity PEG steps reestablish coherent phase before the next gradient application. Slightly different PEG strengths are applied to fill the center of *k*-space first and then the periphery with later echoes, continuing until all views are recorded. As shown, data can be mirrored using conjugate symmetry to reduce the overall time by another factor of two.

   b. Echo planar image (EPI) acquisition uses oscillating readout gradient and phase-encode gradient "blips."
      (i) Can be initiated with spin echo or gradient echo (**spin echo EPI**—Fig. 13-3)
      (ii) Offers "snapshot" capability: down to 50 ms acquisition
      (iii) Characteristics: low resolution, artifacts (ghosting and geometric distortion due to susceptibility)

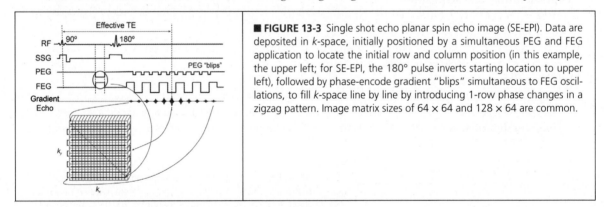

■ **FIGURE 13-3** Single shot echo planar spin echo image (SE-EPI). Data are deposited in *k*-space, initially positioned by a simultaneous PEG and FEG application to locate the initial row and column position (in this example, the upper left; for SE-EPI, the 180° pulse inverts starting location to upper left), followed by phase-encode gradient "blips" simultaneous to FEG oscillations, to fill *k*-space line by line by introducing 1-row phase changes in a zigzag pattern. Image matrix sizes of 64 × 64 and 128 × 64 are common.

   c. GRASE (gradient and spin echo) sequence combines FSE and EPI.
      (i) A series of GREs between inversion RF pulses is repeated over multiple fast spin echoes.
      (ii) Achieves benefits of GRE (speed) and SE (RF refocusing to compensate for T2* effects).
      (iii) For details, see textbook Page 499, Figure 13-4.
2. **k-Space filling**
   a. Nonsequential filling of *k*-space data to obtain optimal contrast (Fig. 13-4).
   b. *Centric k-space filling* for SNR advantage when echoes have their highest amplitude.
   c. *Keyhole filling* collects central lines later for important events such as contrast-enhanced angiography.

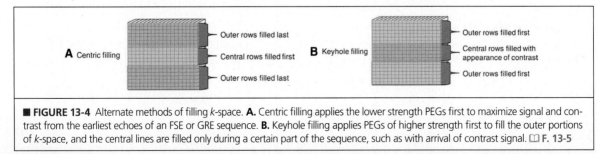

■ **FIGURE 13-4** Alternate methods of filling *k*-space. **A.** Centric filling applies the lower strength PEGs first to maximize signal and contrast from the earliest echoes of an FSE or GRE sequence. **B.** Keyhole filling applies PEGs of higher strength first to fill the outer portions of *k*-space, and the central lines are filled only during a certain part of the sequence, such as with arrival of contrast signal. 📖 **F. 13-5**

3. **Noncartesian _k_-space acquisition** (nonrectilinear filling—Fig. 13-5)
   **a.** _Radial imaging_—generates radial spokes passing through the center of _k_-space in 2D and 3D space
       **(i)**   Yields higher sampling density at the center than the periphery
       **(ii)**  Benefits applications of dynamic imaging requiring high temporal resolution (_e.g._, contrast-enhanced angiography, cardiac imaging; see text book, Fig. 13-7 for details)

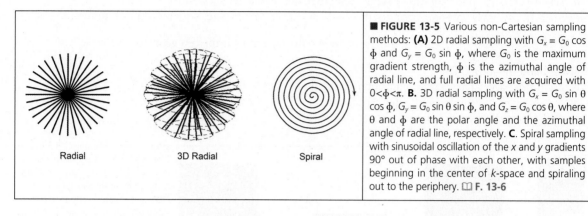

■ **FIGURE 13-5** Various non-Cartesian sampling methods: **(A)** 2D radial sampling with $G_x = G_0 \cos \phi$ and $G_y = G_0 \sin \phi$, where $G_0$ is the maximum gradient strength, $\phi$ is the azimuthal angle of radial line, and full radial lines are acquired with $0 < \phi < \pi$. **B.** 3D radial sampling with $G_x = G_0 \sin \theta \cos \phi$, $G_y = G_0 \sin \theta \sin \phi$, and $G_z = G_0 \cos \theta$, where $\theta$ and $\phi$ are the polar angle and the azimuthal angle of radial line, respectively. **C.** Spiral sampling with sinusoidal oscillation of the _x_ and _y_ gradients 90° out of phase with each other, with samples beginning in the center of _k_-space and spiraling out to the periphery. ▭ **F. 13-6**

   **b.** _Spiral imaging_—an alternate method of EPI, involving oscillation of equivalent encoding gradients
   **c.** _Propeller_—acquisition technique that mitigates motion artifacts
       **(i)**   Rectangular block of data ("a blade") is acquired and rotated about center of _k_-space.
       **(ii)**  Redundant information is used to identify and correct motion artifacts (see textbook Pg. 502–503, Fig. 13-8 for details).
4. **Data synthesis**—takes advantage of the symmetry and redundancy of _k_-space frequency domain signals
   **a.** Fractional NEX: in phase-encode direction, the number of excitations are reduced (Fig. 13-6, **left**).
   **b.** Fractional echo: in frequency-encode direction, a fraction of echo reduces TE, and more slices can be acquired in one TR period (Fig. 13-6, **right**).
   **c.** Tradeoff for both methods: loss of SNR due to fewer excitations per voxel in the volume.

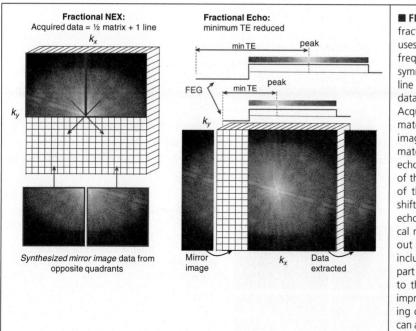

■ **FIGURE 13-6** Fractional NEX and fractional echo. **Left.** Fractional NEX uses data synthesis characteristics of the frequency domain. Phase conjugate symmetry allows ½ of the PEG + 1 extra line with the complex conjugate of the data reflected in symmetric quadrants. Acquisition time is reduced by approximately 2x (approximately 50%), but image noise is increased by approximately $\sqrt{2}$ (40%). **Right.** Fractional echo acquisition is performed with part of the echo read during the application of the FEG. The peak of the echo is shifted by the readout gradient, and the echo signals prior to the peak are identical mirror images after the peak to fill out _k_-space. The sampling window includes the peak and the dephasing part of the echo. The echo peak is closer to the RF excitation pulse, which can improve T1 and proton density weighting contrast. A larger number of slices can also be obtained with a shorter TE in a multislice acquisition. ▭ **F. 13-9**

5. **Parallel imaging**
   a. Response of multiple-receive RF coils overcome aliasing artifacts due to undersampling.
   b. SENSitivity Encoding (SENSE) uses the sensitivity profile of each coil element.
   c. A *k*-space–based approach synthesizes skipped lines directly (see textbook, Pg. 505, Fig. 13-10).
      (i) Method: GeneRalized Autocalibrating Partially Parallel Acquisition (GRAPPA)
   d. Scan time reduction factor can be higher than two, but SNR is reduced.
   e. SNR is inversely proportional to the coil geometry factor and square root of reduction factor:
   $$\text{SNR}_{\text{PI}} = \frac{\text{SNR}_{\text{Fully Sampled}}}{\sqrt{R} \cdot g},$$ where $R$ is the scan time reduction and $g$ is the coil geometry factor.

6. **Multi-band imaging (MB)**
   a. MB further accelerates image acquisition by exciting multiple slices simultaneously (Fig. 13-7).
   b. No SNR penalty from scan time reduction is incurred as multiple excitation pulses are acquired.
   c. Coil *g*-factor in slice direction reduces SNR slightly.

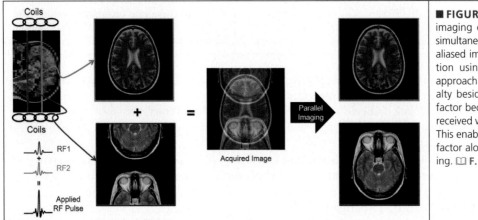

■ **FIGURE 13-7** Multiband imaging excites multiple slices simultaneously and unwraps the aliased image in the slice direction using a parallel imaging approach. There is no SNR penalty besides the coil geometry factor because a larger signal is received with multiple 2D slices. This enables a high acceleration factor along with parallel imaging. 📖 **F. 13-11**

## 13.3  SIGNAL FROM FLOW

1. **Flow-related enhancement**
   a. A process causing increased signal enhancement of moving tissue (blood, CSF).
   b. High intensity is caused by wash-in of unsaturated protons into a partially saturated volume.
   c. Elimination of bright signals can be achieved with saturation pulses outside of the imaging volume.
2. **MR angiography**—exploitation of blood flow enhancement
   a. Time-of-flight angiography
      (i) Relies on flow enhancement of "tagged" or "unsaturated" protons into the imaging volume.
      (ii) Longitudinal magnetization differences of moving blood results in differential vessel contrast.
      (iii) Use of poor anatomic contrast imaging (e.g., GRASS-FISP sequence) allows use of maximum intensity projections to generate angle-specific views of the vasculature (Fig. 13-8).

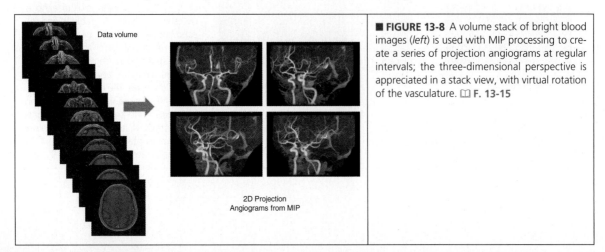

■ **FIGURE 13-8** A volume stack of bright blood images (*left*) is used with MIP processing to create a series of projection angiograms at regular intervals; the three-dimensional perspective is appreciated in a stack view, with virtual rotation of the vasculature. 📖 **F. 13-15**

**b.** Phase-contrast angiography
  **(i)**  Relies on the phase change occurring in moving protons (Fig. 13-9).
  **(ii)** The phase change is dependent on bipolar gradients in two excitations with opposite polarity.
  **(iii)** Time, $\Delta T$, between bipolar gradients is the velocity encoding (VENC) time to ensure optimal phase shift for measurements without aliasing and for gray scale encoding of velocity.
  **(iv)** Measurements are quantitative for velocity *and* direction (Fig. 13-10).

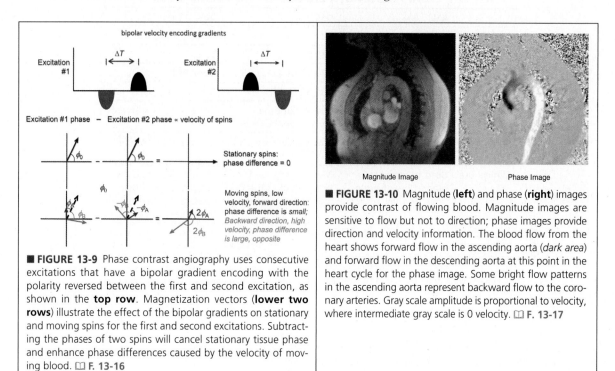

**■ FIGURE 13-9** Phase contrast angiography uses consecutive excitations that have a bipolar gradient encoding with the polarity reversed between the first and second excitation, as shown in the **top row**. Magnetization vectors (**lower two rows**) illustrate the effect of the bipolar gradients on stationary and moving spins for the first and second excitations. Subtracting the phases of two spins will cancel stationary tissue phase and enhance phase differences caused by the velocity of moving blood. 📖 **F. 13-16**

**■ FIGURE 13-10** Magnitude (**left**) and phase (**right**) images provide contrast of flowing blood. Magnitude images are sensitive to flow but not to direction; phase images provide direction and velocity information. The blood flow from the heart shows forward flow in the ascending aorta (*dark area*) and forward flow in the descending aorta at this point in the heart cycle for the phase image. Some bright flow patterns in the ascending aorta represent backward flow to the coronary arteries. Gray scale amplitude is proportional to velocity, where intermediate gray scale is 0 velocity. 📖 **F. 13-17**

**3. Gradient moment nulling** (for flow compensation)
  **a.** Flowing blood often causes flow artifacts due to the phase dispersion of moving spins (Fig. 13-11).
  **b.** Additional gradients set the phase evolution of stationary and moving spins to 0 prior to data collection.

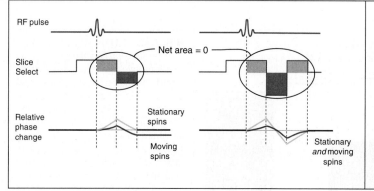

**■ FIGURE 13-11 Left.** Phase dispersion of stationary and moving spins under the influence of an applied gradient (no flow compensation) as the gradient is inverted is shown. The stationary spins return to the original phase state, whereas the moving spins do not. **Right.** Gradient moment nulling of first-order linear velocity (flow compensation) requires a doubling of the negative gradient amplitude followed by a positive gradient such that the total summed area is equal to zero. This will return both the stationary spins and the moving spins to their original phase state. 📖 **F. 13-18**

## 13.4 PERFUSION AND DIFFUSION CONTRAST IMAGING

Perfusion is the delivery of blood to a capillary bed in tissue and permits the delivery of oxygen and nutrients to the cells and removal of waste (*e.g.*, $CO_2$) from the cells—methods include ASL, DSC, DCE (Table 13-1).

**TABLE 13-1 COMPARISON OF PERFUSION MRI TECHNIQUES**

|  | ASL | DSC | DCE |
|---|---|---|---|
| GBCA | X | O | O |
| Contrast | Blood T1 | T2/T2* | T1 |
| Sequence | PASL or PCASL | T2w SE or T2*w GRE | T1w SPGR |
| Parameters | CBF | CBF, CBV, MTT | $K^{trans}$, $k_{ep}$, $V_p$, $V_e$ |
| Pros | Repeatable<br>Ease of quantification | Short scan time<br>Large signal change | Evaluation of leakage |
| Cons | Transit delay effect<br>Low spatial resolution | Low spatial resolution<br>Susceptibility artifact | Complexity of model |
| Clinical use | Used to measure blood flow of brain, heart, kidney, muscle | Most widely used for brain (strokes/tumors) and heart (ischemia) | Most widely used for evaluating tumors/ response to therapy in brain, breast, pelvis |

ASL, arterial spin labeling; DSC, dynamic susceptibility contrast; DCE, dynamic contrast enhanced; PASL, pulsed ASL; PCASL: pseudo-continuous ASL; CBF, cerebral blood flow; CBV, cerebral blood volume; MTT, mean transit time; $K^{trans}$, the rate constant from intravascular space to extravascular space; $k_{ep}$, the rate constant for efflux back into plasma; $V_p$, the volume fraction of plasma; $V_e$, the volume fraction of extravascular extracellular space. GBCA: Gadolinium-Based Contrast Agent.

1. **Arterial spin labeling (ASL)**
   a. ASL uses blood magnetization and measures blood flow (Fig. 13-12).
   b. Pulsed ASL tags blood with inversion or saturation pulse.
      **(i)** Tagged blood moves into region of interest with imaging initiated.
      **(ii)** After waiting time (1 to 2 s), another image set without inversion is acquired in same region.
      **(iii)** Subtraction of the images removes the signals from static tissues.
   c. Continuous ASL uses a long RF pulse applied in a plane while the blood signal is inverted.
      **(i)** After "post-labeling delay" images in the target area are acquired.
      **(ii)** Another acquisition of noninverted spins and subtraction yields the signals from the blood.
   d. Method suffers from low SNR, requiring multiple signal averages (20 to 60).
   e. Most important is choice of waiting time—a tradeoff of measuring vascular signals versus tissue perfusion and the T1 decay of blood signals.

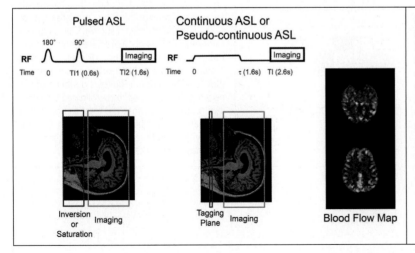

■ **FIGURE 13-12** Description of arterial spin labeling techniques: In-flowing blood spins are inverted by a single spatial inversion pulse (for pulsed ASL) or a long RF train at the tagging plane (for continuous ASL). Control and tag images are collected, and perfusion-weighted images are generated by subtraction of two. Blood flow is estimated using a kinetic model with an assumption that the entire labeled signal is delivered to the tissues because the water in the blood is freely diffusible into the tissues. 📖 **F. 13-19**

### 2. Dynamic susceptibility contrast (DSC)

**a.** Use of contrast material tagged with susceptibility agents such as gadolinium (Gd).

**b.** T2 and T2* parameters generate large signal differences in the vasculature—Gd concentrations can be tracked as a function of time in arteries and tissues (Fig. 13-13).

**c.** Blood flow can be estimated by deconvolution of the tissue residue function (Fig. 13-14).

**(i)** Mean transit time (MTT) is estimated with ratio of cerebral blood volume (CBV) and cerebral blood flow (CBF) or an integral of blood flow.

**d.** Concern with DSC is contrast agent leakage to extravascular or extracellular space, as the conventional DSC model is based on no leakage.

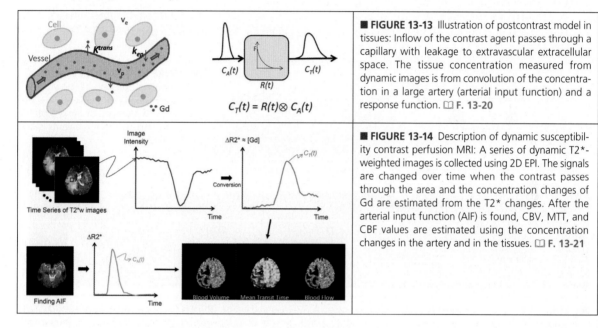

■ **FIGURE 13-13** Illustration of postcontrast model in tissues: Inflow of the contrast agent passes through a capillary with leakage to extravascular extracellular space. The tissue concentration measured from dynamic images is from convolution of the concentration in a large artery (arterial input function) and a response function. 📖 **F. 13-20**

■ **FIGURE 13-14** Description of dynamic susceptibility contrast perfusion MRI: A series of dynamic T2*-weighted images is collected using 2D EPI. The signals are changed over time when the contrast passes through the area and the concentration changes of Gd are estimated from the T2* changes. After the arterial input function (AIF) is found, CBV, MTT, and CBF values are estimated using the concentration changes in the artery and in the tissues. 📖 **F. 13-21**

### 3. Dynamic contrast enhanced (DCE)

**a.** Purpose is the measure the amount of leakage into tissues.

**b.** "Tofts" and "Extended Tofts" models are used (see textbook Pg. 515–516 for details).

**c.** Dynamic T1-weighted sequence such as SPGR is used.

**d.** Mapping of T1 signal change when Gd contrast agent is injected (Fig. 13-15).

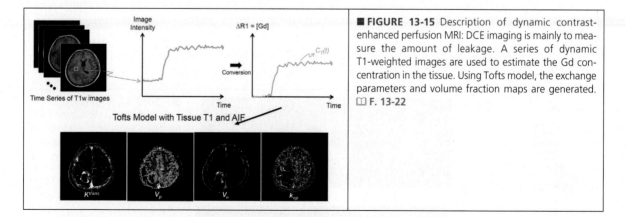

■ **FIGURE 13-15** Description of dynamic contrast-enhanced perfusion MRI: DCE imaging is mainly to measure the amount of leakage. A series of dynamic T1-weighted images are used to estimate the Gd concentration in the tissue. Using Tofts model, the exchange parameters and volume fraction maps are generated. 📖 **F. 13-22**

### 4. Diffusion MRI

Molecular diffusion is the stochastic translational motion of molecules also known as Brownian motion. Diffusion MRI sequences use strong MR gradients applied symmetrically about the refocusing pulse to produce signal differences based on the *mobility and directionality* of water diffusion.

**a.** Diffusion-weighted imaging (DWI)
   **(i)** Symmetrical gradients of amplitude G and duration δ placed before/after the 180° pulse (Fig. 13-16).
   **(ii)** Tissues with more mobility are dephased by the gradients and have a smaller signal than those with restricted diffusion (*e.g.*, ischemic injury).
   **(iii)** A T2-weighted image without diffusivity weighting is compared to a weighted image (*b* value).
   **(iv)** A *b* value (s/mm²) is a diffusion sensitivity factor, and the diffusivity *D* is the diffusion rate (mm²/s).

$$M_{xy}\left(b,\mathrm{TE}\right) = M_0 e^{-\mathrm{TE/T2}} e^{-bD}$$

   **(v)** The *b* values are typically in the range of 200 to 2,000.
   **(vi)** A higher *b* value (*e.g.*, *b* = 1,000) generates more sensitive but noisier diffusion-weighted images.
   **(vii)** Apparent diffusion coefficient (ADC) images are generated from the image pair (Fig. 13-17).

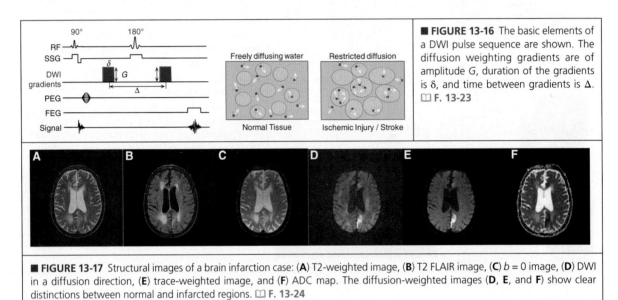

■ **FIGURE 13-16** The basic elements of a DWI pulse sequence are shown. The diffusion weighting gradients are of amplitude *G*, duration of the gradients is δ, and time between gradients is Δ. ☐ **F. 13-23**

■ **FIGURE 13-17** Structural images of a brain infarction case: (**A**) T2-weighted image, (**B**) T2 FLAIR image, (**C**) *b* = 0 image, (**D**) DWI in a diffusion direction, (**E**) trace-weighted image, and (**F**) ADC map. The diffusion-weighted images (**D**, **E**, and **F**) show clear distinctions between normal and infarcted regions. ☐ **F. 13-24**

**b.** Diffusion tensor imaging
   **(i)** Advanced form of diffusion imaging that uses encoding directionality to indicate the anisotropy of white matter by measuring the diffusion restriction and providing structure of surrounding tissues.
   **(ii)** A diffusion tensor provides quantitative diffusion metrics (diffusivity and fractional anisotropy).
   **(iii)** A minimum of six diffusion-encoding directions are required to generate the tensor; many more are actually used to improve the SNR.
   **(iv)** DTI images are color encoded to illustrate directions of diffusion (Fig. 13-18).

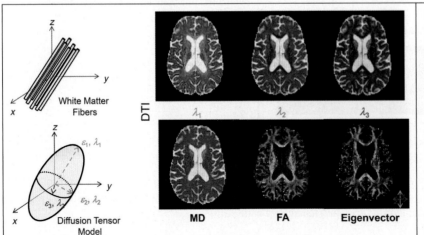

■ **FIGURE 13-18** Diffusion tensor model associated with white matter fibers represents eigenvalues and eigenvectors characterizing water diffusion and molecular structure within a voxel (*left*). From a DTI with a 1,000 *b* value in 30 diffusion directions, three orthogonal eigenvalues (*top right row*) are estimated and mean diffusivity (MD), fractional anisotropy (FA), and eigenvector color map (*bottom right row*) are calculated showing the direction of the primary eigenvectors (*blue*: S/I, *red*: R/L, and *green*: A/P directions). ☐ **F. 13-25**

## 13.5 OTHER ADVANCED TECHNIQUES

1. **Functional MRI**
   a. Technique of mapping neuronal activities in the brain and relying on a local reduction of deoxyhemoglobin, which is paramagnetic, while the neurons in the region become active
   b. Blood oxygen level–dependent (BOLD) acquisition
      (i) A series of dynamic T2*-weighted images using fast EPI GRE sequences map the brain's active regions through correlation of signals with a *repetitive task* (*e.g.*, physical, sensory, or cognitive).
      (ii) Resultant areas are color mapped onto the gray scale images (see textbook, Pg. 521, Fig. 13-26).
   c. Combination diffusion MRI and fMRI can help visualize structure and function (*e.g.*, identify areas prior to resection of a brain tumor) (see textbook, Pg. 521, Fig. 13-27).
2. **Susceptibility-weighted imaging**
   a. Based on T2*-weighted magnitude and phase images obtained with a 3D GRE sequence.
   b. Images are sensitive to local susceptibility differences from deoxyhemoglobin in venous blood, methemoglobin in blood hemorrhage, and iron deposition.
   c. Technique utilizes small and local phase differences and magnitude change with image processing to remove phase changes due to field inhomogeneities.
   d. SWI images are generated from a multiplication of phase masks with the magnitude images to emphasize small phase deviations caused by the susceptibility agents (Fig. 13-19).
   e. Improved visualization is obtained with minimum intensity projection (mIP) of the SWI image stack.

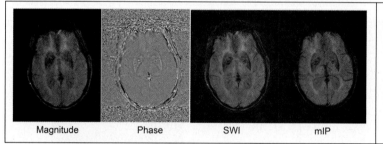

Magnitude    Phase    SWI    mIP

■ **FIGURE 13-19** Susceptibility-weighted imaging: Magnitude and phase images are obtained with 3D T2*-weighted GRE sequence. In SWI, the small phase deviations hardly detectable in normal T2*-weighted images are emphasized by multiplying the magnitude images with the phase masks multiple times. mIP (minimum intensity projection) is created by choosing the minimum value in multiple slices. 📖 **F. 13-28**

3. **MR elastography**
   a. Technique evaluates the stiffness of tissues with the use of an external mechanical wave generator.
   b. GRE imaging with motion-encoding gradients (similar to phase-contrast MRA) are used for acquisition.
      (i) 4 to 8 dynamic images are acquired of magnitude and phase during mechanical vibration.
      (ii) Displacement information is extracted from the dynamic phase information at the applied frequency.
      (iii) Submicrometer motion in the direction of mechanical wave is inversely proportional to the wave speed, from which the stiffness is determined, as stiffer tissues have faster wave speed.
   c. Typical use is assessment of tissue stiffness in the liver (Fig. 13-20).

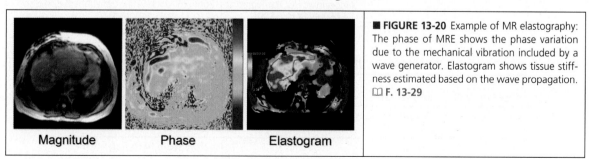

Magnitude    Phase    Elastogram

■ **FIGURE 13-20** Example of MR elastography: The phase of MRE shows the phase variation due to the mechanical vibration included by a wave generator. Elastogram shows tissue stiffness estimated based on the wave propagation. 📖 **F. 13-29**

4. **Magnetization transfer contrast**
   a. The interaction between protons in free water molecules and protons hydrated to the macromolecules of a protein provides a conduit for partial saturation with off-resonance pulse.
   b. Magnetization exchange occurs between the two proton groups.

c. *Selective saturation of the protons in the hydration layer* occurs separately from the bulk water by using narrow-band RF pulses tuned to the hydration layer with an off-resonance peak of approximately 5 kHz.

d. Transfer of the magnetization partially saturates the adjacent protons in bulk water.

e. Saturation of these spins reduces anatomic contrast and is often used in conjunction with MRA time-of-flight methods and other examinations where selective reduction of high signal assists in diagnosis, such as knee cartilage (see textbook, Pg. 522–523, Fig. 13-30).

5. **Magnetic resonance spectroscopy (MRS)**

a. A method to evaluate tissue chemistry by recording and measuring signals from metabolites.

b. MRS metabolic peaks are separable by frequency shifts relative to the frequency of water proton.

c. Metabolite precessional frequencies are bounded by that of water and fat requiring selective saturation pulses to allow the quantitative evaluation of the very weak metabolite signals (Fig. 13-21).

   (i) CHESS (Chemical Shift-Selective) or STIR (Chapter 12) signal suppression methods are used.

d. MRS signals are derived from proton metabolites in targeted tissues (Fig. 13-22, **left**, and Table 13-2).

   (i) Chemical shifts occur due to electron cloud shielding—the amount of shift identifies the metabolite.

e. Localization of the target volume is achieved with single voxel or multivoxel techniques.

   (i) Single voxel sampling areas are about 1 cm³—a STEAM (STimulated Echo Acquisition Mode) or a PRESS (Point REsolved SpectroScopy) sequence are employed to identify the volume.

   (ii) Multivoxel MRS uses a CSI (chemical shift imaging) technique to delineate multiple voxels of approximately 1 cm³ in 1, 2, or 3 planes over a block of several centimeters of tissue.

f. Magnetic resonance spectroscopic imaging (MRSI) generates the signal intensity of a single metabolite in each voxel and color encodes the values (*e.g.*, the choline/creatine ratio), which are superimposed as a map on the anatomical MR image (Fig. 13-22, **right**) indicating normal/abnormal tissues (Table 13-3).

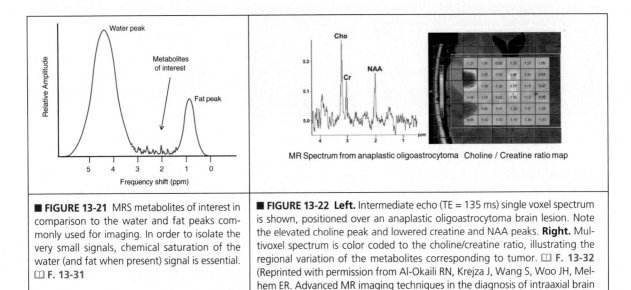

MR Spectrum from anaplastic oligoastrocytoma   Choline / Creatine ratio map

■ **FIGURE 13-21** MRS metabolites of interest in comparison to the water and fat peaks commonly used for imaging. In order to isolate the very small signals, chemical saturation of the water (and fat when present) signal is essential. ▭ **F. 13-31**

■ **FIGURE 13-22 Left.** Intermediate echo (TE = 135 ms) single voxel spectrum is shown, positioned over an anaplastic oligoastrocytoma brain lesion. Note the elevated choline peak and lowered creatine and NAA peaks. **Right.** Multivoxel spectrum is color coded to the choline/creatine ratio, illustrating the regional variation of the metabolites corresponding to tumor. ▭ **F. 13-32** (Reprinted with permission from Al-Okaili RN, Krejza J, Wang S, Woo JH, Melhem ER. Advanced MR imaging techniques in the diagnosis of intraaxial brain tumors in adults. *Radiographics.* 2006;26:S173–S189. Copyright © Radiological Society of North America. doi: 10.1148/rg.26si065513.)

### TABLE 13-2 METABOLITES IN MRS AT 1.5 T

| ABBREVIATION | METABOLITE | SHIFT (ppm) | PROPERTIES/SIGNIFICANCE IN THE BRAIN |
|---|---|---|---|
| Cho | Phosphocholine | 3.22 | Membrane turnover, cell proliferation |
| Cr | Creatine | 3.02 and 3.93 | Temporary store for energy-rich phosphates |
| NAA | *N*-acetyl-*L*-aspartate | 2.01 | Presence of intact glioneuronal structures |
| Lactate | | 1.33 (inverted) | Anaerobic glycolysis |
| Lipids | Free fatty acids | 1.2–1.4 | Necrosis |

**TABLE 13-3 RATIOS OF METABOLITE PEAKS IN MRS INDICATING "NORMAL" AND "ABNORMAL" STATUS**

| METABOLITE RATIO | NORMAL | ABNORMAL |
|---|---|---|
| NAA/Cr | 2.0 | <1.6 |
| NAA/Cho | 1.6 | <1.2 |
| Cho/Cr | 1.2 | >1.5 |

## 13.6 MR ARTIFACTS

Artifacts manifest as positive or negative signal intensities that do not accurately represent the imaged anatomy, classified in three broad areas based on the machine, the patient, and on signal processing.

1. **Magnetic field inhomogeneities**
   a. Global or focal field perturbations that lead to the mismapping of tissues
   b. Causes: ferromagnetic objects in or on the patient (makeup, implants, surgical clips, dentures)
   c. Distortion and/or mismapping of anatomy with more rapid T2* decay
   d. Reduction of inhomogeneities
      (i)   Proper site planning, self-shielded magnets, automatic shimming, preventive maintenance
      (ii)  Spin echo pulse sequence with a 180° refocusing RF pulse
2. **Susceptibility artifacts**
   a. Susceptibility is the ratio of the induced internal tissue magnetization to the external magnetic field
   b. Large changes in susceptibility distorts the local magnetic field
      (i)   Common susceptibility changes occur at tissue-air interfaces (*e.g.*, lungs and sinuses).
      (ii)  Signal loss due to rapid dephasing (T2*) is evident in gradient echo imaging (Fig. 13-23).
      (iii) In certain situations, susceptibility is useful, for example, staging of a hemorrhage with changes in the tissue characteristics of methemoglobin and hemosiderin based on imaging appearance.

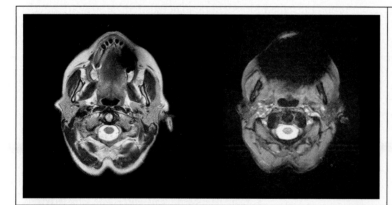

■ **FIGURE 13-23** Susceptibility artifacts due to dental fillings are shown in the same axial image slice. **Left.** Axial T2-weighted fast spin echo image illustrates significant suppression of susceptibility artifacts with 180° refocusing pulse. **Right.** Axial T2*-weighted gradient echo image illustrates significant image void exacerbated by the gradient echo, where external inhomogeneities are not canceled in the reformed echo. 📖 **F. 13-33**

3. **Gradient field artifacts**
   a. Magnetic field gradients spatially encode the location of the signals emanating from excited protons.
   b. Gradient strength has a tendency to fall off at the periphery of a large FOV.
   c. Gradient nonlinearity may cause inaccuracy of geometry (Fig. 13-24).
   d. Proper adjustment and calibration is part of a preventive maintenance routine for MRI scanners.

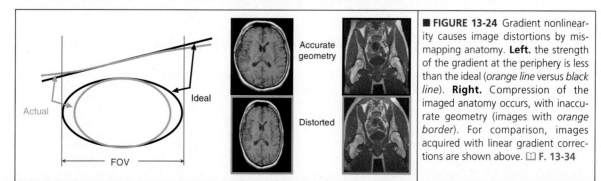

■ **FIGURE 13-24** Gradient nonlinearity causes image distortions by mismapping anatomy. **Left.** the strength of the gradient at the periphery is less than the ideal (*orange line* versus *black line*). **Right.** Compression of the imaged anatomy occurs, with inaccurate geometry (images with *orange border*). For comparison, images acquired with linear gradient corrections are shown above. 📖 **F. 13-34**

4. **RF coil artifacts**
   a. Surface coils produce variations in uniformity across the image caused by RF excitation variability, attenuation, mismatching, and sensitivity falloff with distance.
   b. Proximal to the surface coil, receive signals are intense, and with distance, signal intensity is attenuated.
   c. Gray scale shading and loss of brightness in the image occurs without calibration (Fig. 13-25).
   d. Magnetic field shimming helps reduce the disturbance of the main magnetic field by the patient.
   e. For RF quadrature coils with two amplifiers that are imbalanced, a *center point artifact* can appear that arises at "0" frequency DC offset.

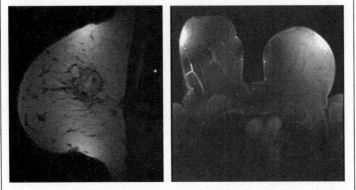

Coil close to skin    Inadequate shimming for fat saturation

■ **FIGURE 13-25** Signal intensity variations occur when surface RF receive coils are too close to the skin, as exemplified by the MR breast image on the **left**. With inadequate shimming calibration, saturation pulses for adipose tissue in the breast are uneven, causing a significant variation in the uniformity of the reconstructed image on the **right**. ▢ F. 13-35 (**Left**, reprinted by permission from Springer Nature. Hendrick RE. *Breast MRI: Fundamentals and Technical Aspects*. Copyright © 2008, Springer Science Business Media, LLC. **Right**, courtesy of R. Edward Hendrick, PhD.)

5. **RF artifacts**
   a. Precessional frequencies of MRI occupy the same frequencies of common electronic devices.
   b. A leaking Faraday cage results in a "zipper" pattern, a narrow band of black/white alternating noise.
   c. Broadband RF noise disrupts the image over a large area of the reconstructed image with diffuse, contrast-reducing "herringbone" artifacts.
   d. Appropriate site planning and the use of properly installed RF shielding materials reduce stray RF interference to an acceptably low level.
   e. Short RF pulse profiles have a wide spatial profile, causing *cross-excitation* with reductions in SNR and CNR that can be reduced by including interslice gaps or interleaving (Fig. 13-26).

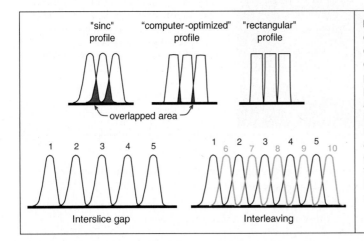

"sinc" profile    "computer-optimized" profile    "rectangular" profile

overlapped area

Interslice gap    Interleaving

■ **FIGURE 13-26 Top.** Poor pulse profiles are caused by truncated RF pulses, and resulting profile overlap causes unwanted partial saturation in adjacent slices, with a loss of SNR and CNR. Optimized pulses are produced by considering the trade-off of pulse duration versus excitation profile. **Bottom.** *Left*—Reduction of cross-excitation is achieved with interslice gaps, but anatomy at the gap location might be missed. *Right*—An interleaving technique acquires the first half of the images with an interslice gap, and the second half of the images are positioned in the gaps of the first images. The separation in time reduces the amount of contrast reducing saturation of the adjacent slices. ▢ **F. 13-36**

6. ***k*-Space errors**
   a. Each individual pixel value in *k*-space contributes to all pixel values in image space as a frequency harmonic with a signal amplitude.
   b. Errors in *k*-space encoding affect *all areas* of the reconstructed image and cause the artifactual superimposition of wave patterns across the FOV (Fig. 13-27).

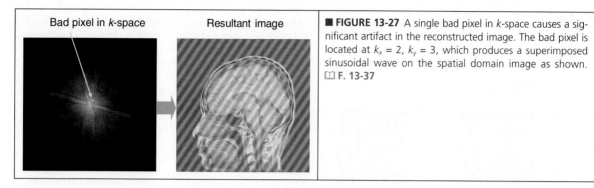

Bad pixel in *k*-space       Resultant image

■ **FIGURE 13-27** A single bad pixel in *k*-space causes a significant artifact in the reconstructed image. The bad pixel is located at $k_x = 2$, $k_y = 3$, which produces a superimposed sinusoidal wave on the spatial domain image as shown. 📖 **F. 13-37**

7. **Motion artifacts**
   a. Motion artifacts arise from voluntary and involuntary movement and flow (blood, CSF).
   b. Long acquisition times increase the probability of motion.
   c. Most occur along the phase-encode direction, as adjacent phase-encoding measurements in *k*-space are separated by a TR interval that can last 3,000 ms or longer.
   d. Slight changes in movement cause changes in phase to create ghost patterns across the FOV (Fig. 13-28).

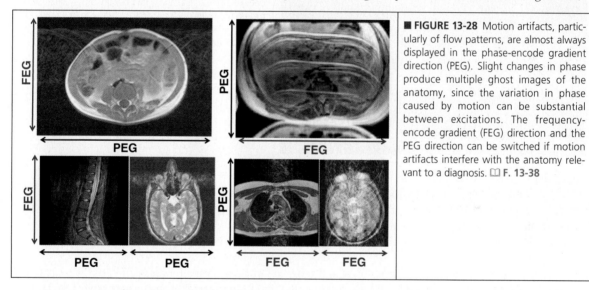

■ **FIGURE 13-28** Motion artifacts, particularly of flow patterns, are almost always displayed in the phase-encode gradient direction (PEG). Slight changes in phase produce multiple ghost images of the anatomy, since the variation in phase caused by motion can be substantial between excitations. The frequency-encode gradient (FEG) direction and the PEG direction can be switched if motion artifacts interfere with the anatomy relevant to a diagnosis. 📖 **F. 13-38**

   e. Compensation for motion-related artifacts
   (i) Switch the PEG and FEG directions to displace the artifacts out of the way (might have impact on examination time or a loss of spatial resolution or SNR).
   (ii) Use cardiac or respiratory gating (will increase acquisition time).
   (iii) Signal averaging to reduce artifacts by random motion (will increase acquisition time).
   (iv) Use short TE SE sequences, fractional echo GRE sequences (Note: T2W more susceptible to motion).
   (v) Gradient moment nulling can rephase spins that are dephased due to motion.
   (vi) Presaturation pulses to reduce signals from patient motion occurring adjacent to the imaged volume.
   (vii) Multiple redundant sampling in the center of *k*-space (*e.g.*, Propeller, radial sampling) to identify pulse sequence contributions contributing to motion and correcting the motion effects.

8. **Chemical shift artifacts of the first kind**
   a. The protons in fat resonate at a slightly lower frequency than the corresponding protons in water.
   (i) Specification in "parts per million" (PPM) is with respect to the resonance frequency of water.
   (ii) Fat has a shift of approximately 3.5 PPM and silicone approximately 5 PPM.
   (iii) At 1.5 T, the protons in fat process at a rate of $63.8 \times 10^6 \times 3.5 \times 10^{-6}$ Hz = 223 Hz *less* than water.
   b. Data acquisition methods cannot directly discriminate a frequency shift due to the application of a frequency encode gradient or a chemical shift, which results in fat-water displacement.
   (i) Displacement occurs in the applied FEG direction (Fig. 13-29).
   c. Applied gradient strength determines the frequency bandwidth across a pixel and amount of chemical shift manifested in the image (Fig. 13-30).
   (i) Low gradient strength has a narrow bandwidth, and a greater propensity for chemical shift.
   (ii) High gradient strength has a broad bandwidth, allowing the shift to be contained within the pixel.

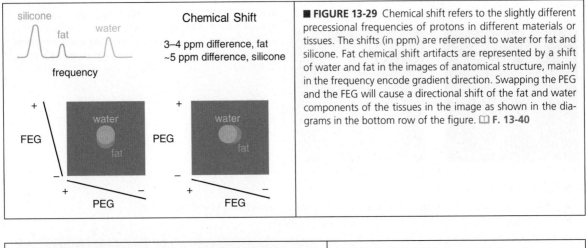

■ **FIGURE 13-29** Chemical shift refers to the slightly different precessional frequencies of protons in different materials or tissues. The shifts (in ppm) are referenced to water for fat and silicone. Fat chemical shift artifacts are represented by a shift of water and fat in the images of anatomical structure, mainly in the frequency encode gradient direction. Swapping the PEG and the FEG will cause a directional shift of the fat and water components of the tissues in the image as shown in the diagrams in the bottom row of the figure. ▭ **F. 13-40**

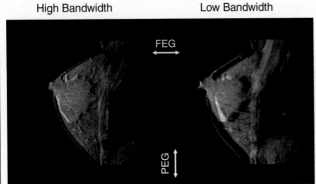

■ **FIGURE 13-30** MR images of the breast, containing glandular and adipose tissue, are acquired under a high bandwidth (32 kHz) and a low bandwidth (4 kHz), illustrating the more severe chemical shift with low read-out gradient strength and bandwidth. (Courtesy of R. Edward Hendrick, PhD.) ▭ **F. 13-41**

    d. Reducing chemical shift artifacts
       (i)   High gradient strength (reduced SNR due to broad bandwidth—SNR $\propto 1/\sqrt{BW}$)
       (ii)  Chemical presaturation ("FatSat") or STIR techniques (Chapter 12) to eliminate fat in the image

**9. Chemical shift artifacts of the second kind**
    a. For GRE imaging, the rephasing and dephasing of the echo occurs in the same direction relative to the main magnetic field.
    b. At 1.5 T, the precessional frequencies of fat and water are in phase every 4.4 ms (0, 4.4, 8.8, 12.2 ms) and maximally out of phase shifted by 2.2 ms (2.2, 6.6, 8.8 ms) for transverse magnetization (Fig. 13-31).
    c. Signal appearance of fat and water are thus dependent on the selection of TE (Fig. 13-32).
       (i)   When in phase, a typical chemical shift is manifested.
       (ii)  When out of phase, a dark rim around heterogeneous fat/water tissue occurs "India-ink artifact."

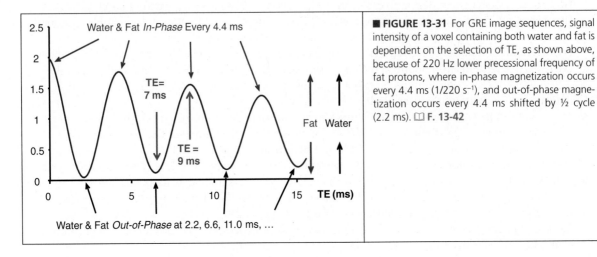

■ **FIGURE 13-31** For GRE image sequences, signal intensity of a voxel containing both water and fat is dependent on the selection of TE, as shown above, because of 220 Hz lower precessional frequency of fat protons, where in-phase magnetization occurs every 4.4 ms (1/220 s⁻¹), and out-of-phase magnetization occurs every 4.4 ms shifted by ½ cycle (2.2 ms). ▭ **F. 13-42**

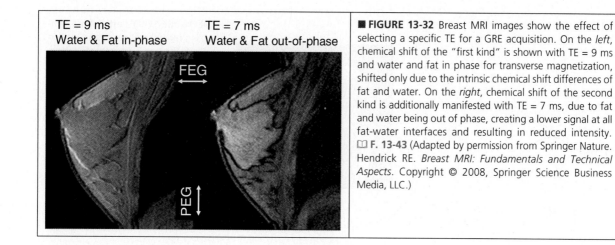

TE = 9 ms
Water & Fat in-phase

TE = 7 ms
Water & Fat out-of-phase

■ **FIGURE 13-32** Breast MRI images show the effect of selecting a specific TE for a GRE acquisition. On the *left*, chemical shift of the "first kind" is shown with TE = 9 ms and water and fat in phase for transverse magnetization, shifted only due to the intrinsic chemical shift differences of fat and water. On the *right*, chemical shift of the second kind is additionally manifested with TE = 7 ms, due to fat and water being out of phase, creating a lower signal at all fat-water interfaces and resulting in reduced intensity. 📖 **F. 13-43** (Adapted by permission from Springer Nature. Hendrick RE. *Breast MRI: Fundamentals and Technical Aspects.* Copyright © 2008, Springer Science Business Media, LLC.)

## 10. Ringing artifacts

a. Occurs near sharp boundaries and high-contrast transitions in the image.

b. Insufficient sampling of high frequencies results in bright/dark oscillations at sharp discontinuities.

c. The *k*-space matrix size determines the number of frequency harmonics—smaller matrix size results in fewer harmonics, which increases the ringing, a consequence of high-frequency aliasing (Fig. 13-33).

d. Example image shows observable ringing with 128 harmonics versus 256 harmonics (Fig. 13-34).

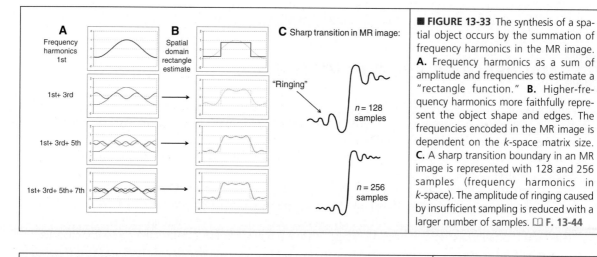

■ **FIGURE 13-33** The synthesis of a spatial object occurs by the summation of frequency harmonics in the MR image. **A.** Frequency harmonics as a sum of amplitude and frequencies to estimate a "rectangle function." **B.** Higher-frequency harmonics more faithfully represent the object shape and edges. The frequencies encoded in the MR image is dependent on the *k*-space matrix size. **C.** A sharp transition boundary in an MR image is represented with 128 and 256 samples (frequency harmonics in *k*-space). The amplitude of ringing caused by insufficient sampling is reduced with a larger number of samples. 📖 **F. 13-44**

256 (vertical) × 128 (horizontal)          256 × 256

■ **FIGURE 13-34** Example of ringing artifacts caused by a sharp signal transition at the skull in a brain image for a 256 × 128 matrix (*left*) along the horizontal axis, and the elimination of the artifact in a 256 × 256 matrix (*right*). The horizontal axis defines the PEG direction. 📖 **F. 13-45**

## 11. Wrap-around artifacts

a. Mismapping of anatomy that lies outside of the FOV but within the slice volume.

b. Insufficient sampling beyond the Nyquist frequency results in aliasing that reverses phase and masquerades as a lower frequency, causing a displacement of anatomy to the opposite side (Fig. 13-35).

c. Reducing the effects of wrap-around artifact on the acquired image.

    (i) Increase the FOV (reduces resolution)

    (ii) Use a low-pass filter in the FEG direction to eliminate higher frequencies (reduces resolution)

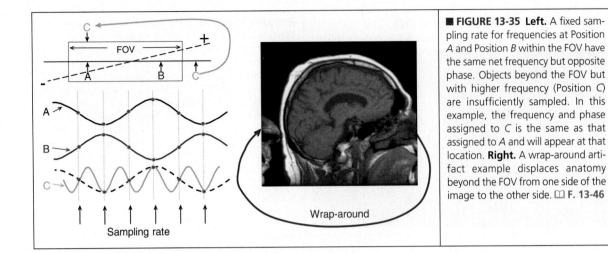

■ **FIGURE 13-35 Left.** A fixed sampling rate for frequencies at Position *A* and Position *B* within the FOV have the same net frequency but opposite phase. Objects beyond the FOV but with higher frequency (Position *C*) are insufficiently sampled. In this example, the frequency and phase assigned to *C* is the same as that assigned to *A* and will appear at that location. **Right.** A wrap-around artifact example displaces anatomy beyond the FOV from one side of the image to the other side. 📖 **F. 13-46**

    **(iii)** Increase the number of PEG steps to increase sampling (increases acquisition time)

    **(iv)** Use an "anti-aliasing" saturation pulse just beyond the periphery of the FOV (increases SAR)

    **(v)** Move the region of anatomic interest to the center of the FOV

**12. Partial volume artifacts**

    **a.** Partial volume artifacts arise from the finite size of the voxel over which the signal is averaged.

    **b.** Loss of detail and spatial resolution occurs with larger slice thickness and larger pixel dimensions.

    **c.** Minimizing partial volume requires acquisition protocols that result in smaller voxel dimensions.

    **d.** Tradeoffs include noisier images (smaller voxels) or increased imaging time (greater NEX).

## 13.7 MAGNET SITING AND QUALITY CONTROL

**1. Magnet siting**

    **a.** Two requirements must be considered for MR system siting: protect the local environment from the magnet system and protect the magnet system from the local environment.

    **b.** Superconductive magnets produce extensive magnetic *fringe fields* and create potentially hazardous conditions in adjacent areas.

      **(i)** *Passive* (thick metal walls close to the magnet) and *active* (electromagnet systems strategically placed in the magnet housing) shielding limits the extent of magnetic fringe fields (Fig. 13-36).

      **(ii)** Disruption of fringe fields can disrupt the homogeneity of the active imaging volume.

      **(iii)** Administrative control for magnetic fringe fields is 0.5 mT, requiring controlled access for areas exceeding this level.

      **(iv)** Sensitive electronic equipment (*e.g.*, image intensifiers, gamma cameras) requires less than 0.3 mT fields.

    **c.** Environmental RF noise

      **(i)** Precessional frequencies in MR overlap those common to commercial FM broadcasts.

      **(ii)** A *Faraday Cage*—an internal enclosure surrounding the magnet, consists of copper sheet and copper wire mesh to attenuate external RF signals, with special attention to the door (Fig. 13-37).

**2. Field uniformity**

    **a.** Expressed in parts per million (ppm) of the precessional frequency over a given volume

      **(i)** For 1.5 T (63.8 MHz), a 2 ppm homogeneity specification results in $63.8 \times 10^6 \times 2 \times 10^{-6} = 128$ Hz variation over the volume.

      **(ii)** Typical homogeneities: less than 10 ppm (150 mm FOV) to greater than 10 ppm (400 mm FOV).

    **b.** Achieved by manipulating the main field peripherally with passive and active "shim" coils

      **(i)** Shim coils interact with the fringe fields and adjust the variation of the central magnetic field.

**3. Quality control**

    **a.** The American College of Radiology MRI accreditation program specifies requirements for system operation, QC, and the training requirements of involved technologists, radiologists, and physicists.

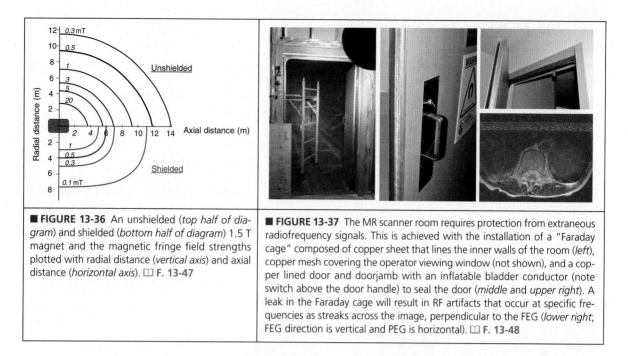

**■ FIGURE 13-36** An unshielded (*top half of diagram*) and shielded (*bottom half of diagram*) 1.5 T magnet and the magnetic fringe field strengths plotted with radial distance (*vertical axis*) and axial distance (*horizontal axis*). 🕮 **F. 13-47**

**■ FIGURE 13-37** The MR scanner room requires protection from extraneous radiofrequency signals. This is achieved with the installation of a "Faraday cage" composed of copper sheet that lines the inner walls of the room (*left*), copper mesh covering the operator viewing window (not shown), and a copper lined door and doorjamb with an inflatable bladder conductor (note switch above the door handle) to seal the door (*middle* and *upper right*). A leak in the Faraday cage will result in RF artifacts that occur at specific frequencies as streaks across the image, perpendicular to the FEG (*lower right*; FEG direction is vertical and PEG is horizontal). 🕮 **F. 13-48**

**b.** Qualifications of personnel, equipment performance, effectiveness of QC procedures, and quality of clinical images are evaluated on a periodic basis (typically every 3 years).

**c.** Quality control tests include high-contrast spatial resolution, slice thickness accuracy, slice position accuracy, RF center frequency tuning, geometric accuracy and spatial uniformity, signal uniformity, low-contrast detectability, artifact evaluation, operational controls, and review of system log book.

**d.** MRI accreditation phantom is used for acquisition of images and evaluation of QC program metrics.

   **(i)** The phantom contains many modules surrounded by a liquid filler with defined relaxation times.

   **(ii)** Seven quantitative tests are performed by scanning the phantom with specific acquisition protocols.

   **(iii)** Examples of phantom images show some of the tests (Fig. 13-38).

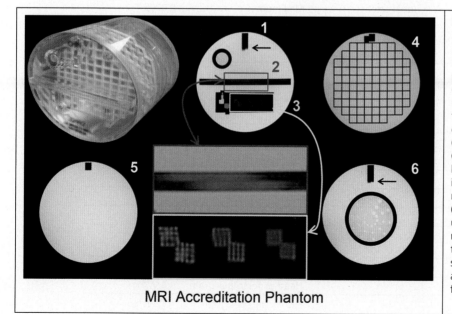

**MRI Accreditation Phantom**

**■ FIGURE 13-38** The ACR MRI accreditation phantom (*upper left*) and selected MRI axial images from the phantom are shown. (*1*) First phantom slab containing slice position accuracy ramp (*black arrow*); (*2*) slice thickness ramp (magnified and enhanced image—*red* outline); (*3*) spatial resolution module (magnified image—*yellow* outline). Other phantom slabs include (*4*) geometric distortion module; (*5*) uniformity module; (*6*) low-contrast resolution module and slice position accuracy ramp at the other end of phantom. Not all images are shown; see the ACR large phantom MRI accreditation documentation for further information. 🕮 **F. 13-49**

## 13.8 MR BIOEFFECTS AND SAFETY

Preliminary remarks (1): There are very many important bioeffects and safety issues to be considered for MR—first and foremost, for a superconducting system, **THE MAGNET IS ALWAYS ON**.

**a.** To turn off the magnet, a *quench* is necessary (removing current from the superconducting coils).

    **(i)** A controlled quench provides a level of safety but can be expensive.

    **(ii)** An uncontrolled quench can be extremely dangerous by damaging equipment, threatening life, and extremely expensive—often requiring the replacement of the system.

Preliminary remarks (2): Another important issue is the *labeling of materials* brought into the MR scanner area.

**a.** Signage exists in three categories to help identify MR conditional and MR unsafe materials

**b.** "MR safe" is put on materials and objects that are wholly nonmetallic; " MR unsafe" is placed on all ferromagnetic and many conducting metals; "MR conditional" signage is placed on objects that may be safe under specific conditions, for example cardiac implantable devices (Fig. 13-39).

MR is considered "safe" when used within the regulatory guidelines specified in Table 13-4.

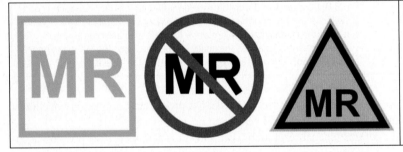

■ **FIGURE 13-39** MR labeling for materials includes (*left* to *right*) *MR safe* (items do not interact with the strong MR field or disrupt operation); *MR unsafe* (**do not** bring items past Zone 2) (see later discussion); *MR conditional* (item safety depends on conditions specified for use before scanning). 📖 **F. 13-50**

### TABLE 13-4 **MRI SAFETY GUIDELINES**

| ISSUE | PARAMETER | VARIABLES | SPECIFIED VALUE |
|---|---|---|---|
| Static magnetic field | Magnetic field ($B_0$) | Maximum strength | 3.0 T[a] |
| | Inadvertent exposure | Maximum | 0.0005 T |
| Changing magnetic field ($dB/dt$) | Axial gradients | $\tau > 120\ \mu s$ | <20 T/s |
| | | $12\ \mu s < \tau < 120\ \mu s$ | <2,400/$\tau$ ($\mu s$) T/s |
| | | $\tau < 12\ \mu s$ | <200 T/s |
| | Transverse gradients System | | <3× axial gradients |
| | | | <6 T/s |
| RF power deposition | Temperature | Core of body | <18°C |
| | | Maximum head | <38°C |
| | | Maximum trunk | <39°C |
| | | Maximum extremities | <40°C |
| | Specific absorption rate (SAR)[b] | Whole body (average) | <4 W/kg |
| | | Head (average) | <3.2 W/kg |
| | | Head or torso per gram | <8 W/kg |
| | | Extremities per gram | <12 W/kg |
| Acoustic noise levels | | Peak pressure | 200 pascals |
| | | Average pressure | 105 dBA |

$\tau$: rise time of gradients. 📖 T. 13-5
[a]In some clinical applications, higher field strengths (*e.g.*, 7.0 T) are allowed.
[b]"Normal" mode (suitable for all patients) is half the limit (2 W/kg); "first level" mode (shown) is with medical.

1. **Static magnetic fields**
   a. At lower magnetic field strengths, there have not been any reports of deleterious or nonreversible acute or chronic biologic effects.
   b. At very high field strength magnets (*e.g.*, 4 T or higher), anecdotal evidence suggests dizziness and disorientation of personnel and patients as they move through the field.
   c. Maximum field strength allowed is 3 T, except in special cases where up to 7 T is allowed (Table 13-4).

2. **Spatial field gradient**
   a. Although the static magnetic fields are stable over time, the distribution of the field is spatially varying and stronger with closer distance and at magnet bore edges as shown by the gradient map (Fig. 13-40).

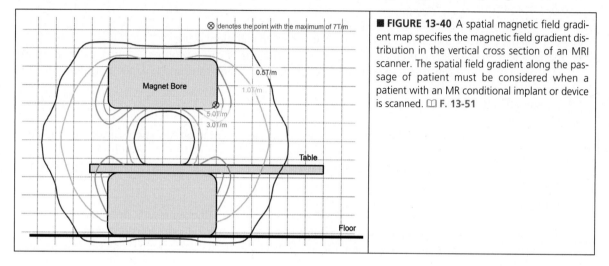

■ **FIGURE 13-40** A spatial magnetic field gradient map specifies the magnetic field gradient distribution in the vertical cross section of an MRI scanner. The spatial field gradient along the passage of patient must be considered when a patient with an MR conditional implant or device is scanned. ⏎ **F. 13-51**

   b. As a patient slides in the magnetic field, Lenz law predicts induced currents from the "effective" magnetic field changes with motion—it is important to move patients slowly in the magnet to avoid the creation of opposing magnetic fields where the patient can experience high mechanical and magnetic forces.
   c. MR conditional devices have specific requirements such as maximum field strength to ensure safety.

3. **Varying magnetic field effects**
   a. The time-varying magnetic fields encountered in the MRI system are due to the gradient switching used for localization of the protons.
   b. Magnetic fields that vary their strength with time are generally of greater concern than static fields because oscillating magnetic fields can induce electrical current flow in conductors.
      (i) Changing magnetic field gradients ($dB/dt$) are limited to less than 20 T/s for axial gradients and less than 6 T/s for transverse gradients (Table 13-4).
   c. Patients can experience burns when they inadvertently create a conductive loop with parts of their body, such as touching their fingers directly on their torso, resulting in induced current that concentrates at the fingertips.

4. **Specific absorption rate (SAR)**
   a. A measure of the energy absorption rate when the human body is exposed to RF fields.
   b. SAR in an MR examination is a function of the TR, flip angle, number of excitations per TR, field strength.
      (i) Inversion recovery spin echo and fast spin echo sequences with high ETL can deliver a high SAR.
      (ii) Short TR sequences in general have a higher SAR than long TR sequences.
   c. FDA limits SAR to an average less than 4 W/kg for the whole body and less than 3.2 W/kg for the head (Table 13-4).
      (i) "Normal" operating mode limits pulse sequences to ½ the FDA SAR limit.
      (ii) "First level" operating mode limits pulse sequences to the FDA SAR limit.
   d. MR conditional devices specify a maximum allowable SAR for an examination, types of coils (receive or transmit/receive) and regions of imaging; most restrictive are neurostimulators and associated wires.

5. **RF exposure, acoustic noise limits**
   a. RF exposure causes heating of tissues; for high SAR or extended scanning, the body accumulates heat faster than it can be removed.
      (i) Temperatures are limited to 38°C for the core of the body and for the head.
      (ii) Maximum trunk and extremity heating is limited to less than 39°C and less than 40°C, respectively.

**(iii)** RF coil safety requires periodic inspection to ensure wires and connectors are in good condition.

   **b.** Gradient coils are responsible for the banging noise one hears during imaging.

     **(i)** Flexing is caused by the torque experienced by the gradient coil from the changing magnetic field.

     **(ii)** Allowable noise levels are limited to peak pressure of 200 pascals and average pressure of 120 dBA.

     **(iii)** Hearing protection must always be available to the patient.

**6. Pregnancy-related issues and pediatric patient concerns**

   **a.** Current data have not yielded any deleterious effects on the developing fetus with common MR examinations.

   **b.** No special considerations are warranted, as long as the benefit-risk ratio of doing the study is that for any other typical patient.

   **c.** Administration of contrast should not be routinely provided.

   **d.** For pediatric patients, the more complex issues are sedation and monitoring.

   **e.** Special attention to sedation protocols, adherence to standards of care regarding sedation guidelines, and monitoring patients during the scan with MR safe temperature monitoring and isolation transport units are crucial to maintaining patient safety.

**7. MR personnel and MR safety zones**

   **a.** MR personnel.

   **b.** *Level 1 MR personnel* have passed minimal safety and education training on MR safety issues and can work in Zone 3 and Zone 4 areas.

   **c.** *Level 2 MR personnel* are more extensively trained in the broader aspects of MR safety issues and are *the gatekeepers* of access into Zone 4.

   **d.** MR safety zones (Fig. 13-41):

     **(i)** Zone 1 is freely accessible to the general public, outside of the MR magnet area and building.

     **(ii)** Zone 2 represents the interface between Zone 1 and Zone 3—typically the reception area.

     **(iii)** Zone 3 is a restricted area composed of the MR control and computer room that only specific personnel can access.

     **(iv)** Zone 4 represents the MR magnet room and is always located within the confines of Zone 3.

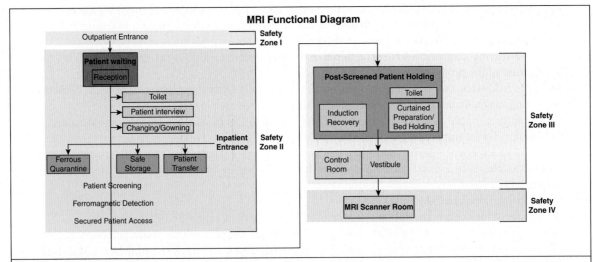

■ **FIGURE 13-41** Zoning concept for describing areas in an MR system environment include Zone 1, unrestricted access; Zone 2, interface between unrestricted and restricted areas; Zone 3, restricted area only allowed for MR personnel and screened individuals; Zone 4, the area of the scanner and high magnetic field strength. ▢ **F. 13-52** (Obtained from and modified with the permission of the Department of Veterans Affairs Office of Construction & Facilities Management, Strategic Management Office; reprinted from Kanal E, Barkovich AJ, Bell C, et al. ACR guidance document on MR safe practices: 2013. *J Magn Reson Imaging.* 2013;37:501–530. doi:10.1002/jmri.24011)

# Section II Questions and Answers

1. Which of the following descriptors most accurately indicates how fast spin echo (FSE) pulse sequences decrease imaging time?
   A. Using multiple PEG steps per TR interval
   B. Decreasing TR and TE
   C. Increasing the gradient field strength
   D. Acquiring the signal in three dimensions
   E. Applying a broadband RF pulse

2. Which of the following acquisition methods are most often used for functional imaging?
   A. Echo planar
   B. Fast spin echo
   C. FLAIR
   D. Steady-state free precession
   E. STIR

3. Propeller is an acquisition method that can reduce which kind of MR artifact?
   A. Zipper
   B. Motion
   C. Chemical shift
   D. Wrap-around
   E. Susceptibility

4. For time-of-flight MR angiography, what acquisition contrast weighting can best produce bright blood and reduced background anatomical signals in a volume acquisition?
   A. T2-weighted fast spin echo
   B. T2*/T1-weighted coherent gradient echo
   C. T1-weighted spoiled gradient echo
   D. T1-weighted spin echo
   E. T1-weighted echo planar

5. Apparent diffusion coefficient (ADC) computed from diffusion MRI signals is most likely related to:
   A. proton density
   B. tissue cellularity
   C. cerebral blood flow
   D. tissue oxygenation level

6. Which MRI technique is NOT used to map blood perfusion in the body?
   A. Dynamic susceptibility contrast MRI
   B. Dynamic contrast-enhanced MRI
   C. Arterial spin labeling MRI
   D. Magnetic resonance angiography

7. Which MRI perfusion or angiography technique utilizes blood as an endogenous contrast agent?
   A. Dynamic susceptibility contrast MRI
   B. Dynamic contrast-enhanced MRI
   C. Arterial spin labeling MRI
   D. Contrast-enhanced MR angiography

8. Which MRI technique is best used to assess tissue permeability?
   A. Dynamic susceptibility contrast MRI
   B. Dynamic contrast-enhanced MRI
   C. Arterial spin labeling MRI
   D. Magnetic resonance angiography

9. Which description below is NOT directly associated with functional brain MR?
   A. Oxyhemoglobin to deoxyhemoglobin
   B. BOLD imaging
   C. Echo planar acquisition
   D. High spatial resolution
   E. Periodic stimulus and response

10. Which artifact deteriorates image quality most often in the phase-encode direction of the MR image?
    A. Wrap-around
    B. RF zipper
    C. Motion
    D. Chemical shift
    E. Aliasing

11. What is the likely cause for the distortion of the acquired MR brain image pictured on the right?

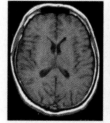 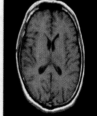

Ideal image          Distorted image

    A. Cross excitation from adjacent slices
    B. Improper shimming adjustment
    C. Main magnetic field fluctuation
    D. Nonlinear gradient field
    E. RF resonance tuning error

12. What is the most dominant source that caused the artifacts in the image shown below?

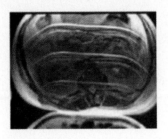

    A. Patient motion
    B. Blood flow
    C. Chemical shift
    D. RF leakage through the door

13. Which encoding gradient manifests the chemical shift artifact?
    A. Frequency encode
    B. Phase encode
    C. Slice select
    D. Slice encode

14. With an increased main magnetic field strength, how are chemical shift artifacts more likely manifested in the image?
    A. Increased
    B. Decreased
    C. Unchanged

15. Chemical shift of the second kind with GRE imaging is caused by which of the following?
    A. Shifts in the localization of protons along the phase-encode gradient
    B. Shifts in the localization of protons along the frequency-encode gradient
    C. In-phase and out-of-phase alignment of water and fat moments at various TE
    D. In-phase and out-of-phase alignment of water and fat moments at various TR

16. Which of the following is the most likely cause for a "wrap-around" artifact?
    A. Involuntary patient motion
    B. Gradient nonuniformities
    C. Small FOV for large object
    D. Inversion recovery pulsing
    E. Magnetization transfer

17. Which one of the breast MR images below demonstrates chemical shift artifact of the second kind?

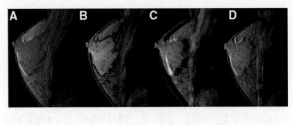

    A. A.                C. C.
    B. B.                D. D.

18. What action can be taken to eliminate the artifact shown in the image below?

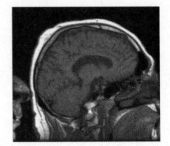

    A. Decrease the TE
    B. Decrease the slice thickness
    C. Increase the TR
    D. Increase the field of view

19. If a patient "codes" during an MRI procedure (1.5 T superconducting magnet), what is the most appropriate action to be taken?
    A. Quench the magnet and allow the code team immediate access to Zone 4.
    B. Complete the scan and then deliver patient to Zone 2 holding area.
    C. Stop the procedure and immediately move patient to Zone 3.
    D. Ensure that the code team has only magnetically compatible instruments.

20. Referring to the figure, which demarcated zone can a patient enter and be unescorted prior to an MR examination?
    A. Zone 1
    B. Zone 2
    C. Zone 3
    D. Zone 4

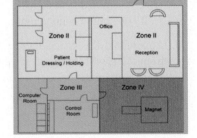

# Answers

1. **A**  FSE (fast spin echo) relies on multiple phase-encode gradient steps during each TR interval. Of importance is the technique of "phase reordering" adjusting the strength of the PEG to fill the center of $k$-space with the early echoes (higher SNR) and the periphery of $k$-space with the later echoes (less important). *(Pg. 496–497, Fig. 13-2)*

2. **A**  Functional imaging requires very fast, repeated imaging in conjunction with a stimulus to map metabolic volumes in the brain. Echo planar imaging is the fast acquisition method (50 to 100 ms/image) that provides this capability. *(Pg. 520–521, Fig. 13-26)*

3. **B**  Propeller is an acronym for *Periodically Rotating Overlapping Parallel Lines with Enhanced Reconstruction*, where the center of $k$-space is oversampled, and projections that contain motion are corrected to reduce the impact of phase changes on the reconstructed image. *(Pg. 501–503, Fig. 13-8)*

4. **B**  Time-of-flight angiography depends on "bright blood" and otherwise poor anatomical contrast, which is provided by GRASS/FISP coherent gradient echo (GRE) acquisition sequences. Poor background SNR reduces the contributions of nonvessel components with maximum intensity projection (MIP) processing. *(Pg. 508–510, Figs. 13-13 and 13-14)*

5. **B**  Apparent Diffusion Coefficient is related to the amount of water diffusion within tissue and represent tissue cellularity. *(Pg. 516–518, Figs. 13-23 and 13-24)*

6. **D**  Note the negative stem. A, B, and C are methods to map perfusion. Angiography is an imaging technique to map blood vessel structure. *(Pg. 513–517, Table 13-1 for perfusion, Pg. 508–510 for angiography)*

7. **C**  Arterial spin labeling is using blood as an endogenous contrast agent while other techniques need an injection of gadolinium-based contrast agent. *(Pg. 513–514, Fig. 13-19)*

8. **B**  Dynamic contrast-enhanced MRI is tracking the changes of T1 caused by the contrast agent staying in the extravascular extracellular space, which is the outcome of blood-brain barrier (BBB) breakdown or permeability changes. *(Pg. 515–516, Fig. 13-22)*

9. **D**  You need to look for the false answer (negative stem). In the case of functional imaging, speed of data acquisition with ability to associate stimulus and response that allows for intensive image processing and placing a premium on signal-to-noise ratio to detect very subtle signals from the background requires a tradeoff of spatial resolution (the false answer) for speed and high SNR by data averaging. The other distractors are part of the functional imaging procedure. *(Pg. 520–521)*

10. **C**  Motion artifacts most often occur in the phase-encode direction, due to even slight anatomical movement causing changes in the phase of the individual phase-encode gradient (PEG) application, which is sampled incrementally over the image sequence time. This displaces the location of the sampled anatomy, causing multiple "ghost images" to be rendered along the PEG. The second-best answer could be wrap-around, as the number of samples in the PEG direction are often reduced across the FOV, resulting in insufficient sampling with the consequence of anatomy wrapping to the opposite side of the FOV. *(Pg. 531–533, Fig. 13-38)*

11. **D**  The gradient magnetic field is assumed to be linear, or corrected to a linear response. If the gradient field falls off at the periphery, the precessional frequency of the protons will experience a similar fall off, causing the image to be distorted. This is usually manifested as a narrowing of the anatomy. *(Pg. 528–529, Fig. 13-34)*

12. **A**  The ghosting artifact is caused by patient breathing motion in the phase-encoding direction. The image also shows wrap-around artifacts as well. *(Pg. 531–533, motion; Pg. 536–538, wrap-around)*

13. **A**   The chemical shift artifact occurs due to the lower precessional frequency of protons in a lipid environment relative to a hydrated environment. The MR signal acquisition during the frequency-encode gradient application cannot distinguish between protons resonating at a given frequency due to the gradient versus those resonating at a slightly slower frequency due to chemical shift. The lipid part of the material shifts toward the weaker polarity of the applied gradient. *(Pg. 533–534, Fig. 13-40)*

14. **A**   Chemical shift occurs as a result of the magnetic shielding of protons in fat or fatty tissues, causing a reduction of the precessional frequency compared to unbound protons in water or nonfatty soft tissues. The precessional frequency difference is about 3.5 ppm, or in terms of absolute difference is a product of $3 \times 10^{-6}$ × Larmor precessional frequency; as $B_0$ increases, the amount of discrepancy between fat and tissue frequencies increase. However, as the gradient strength increases, for a given slice field of view, the frequency range across each pixel is expanded, and the displacement of fat signals is less. Be careful to note whether the main magnetic field or gradient field strength is increased. *(Pg. 533–534)*

15. **C**   Chemical shift of the second kind represents the in-phase and out-of-phase orientation of the magnetization vectors of fat and water with GRE pulse sequences. Since the chemical shift is on the order of 3.5 ppm, then at 1.5 T, the difference in the precessional frequency of fat versus water is $3.5 \times 10^{-6}$ × 42.58 MHz/T × 1.5 T = 223 cycles/second, which means that at every 1/253 s = 4.5 ms, water and fat will be in phase, and every 2.25 ms (180° or ½ rotation), water and fat will be out of phase. If the selected TE is a multiple of 4.5 ms, the water/fat will be in phase, and if the TE is a multiple of 2.25 ms, water/fat will be out of phase in all directions (independent of the FEG and PEG and SSG directions) creating a black rim around organ boundaries that have a fat and water mixture. *(Pg. 534–535, Fig. 13-42)*

16. **C**   Wrap-around is the misposition of anatomy from one side of the field of view to the other; this is caused by signals outside of the FOV producing frequencies, which exceed the "Nyquist" sampling requirement (two samples per cycle), and the computer identifies the signals as lower frequency and opposite phase. Insufficient sampling causes the signals to "alias" and be mispositioned in the output image, typically on opposite sides. Increasing the FOV can eliminate aliasing, at the cost of reduced spatial resolution. *(Pg. 536–538, Fig. 13-46)*

17. **B**   Chemical shift of the second kind is a phenomenon that affects GE images of specific TE times. Since fat and water resonate at about 220 Hz difference at 1.5 T, the protons in fat and water will be in phase every 4.4 ms and out of phase every 4.4 ms shifted by ½ cycle, or 2.2 ms. Image B is a GE image acquired at TE = 7 ms, and the out-of-phase fat signal is manifested as a dark rim around anatomical structures; Image A is the same GE sequence but acquired at 9 ms, demonstrating chemical shift of the first kind. Image C is a chemical shift image of the first kind but acquired with a lower bandwidth and lower gradient strength, illustrating the greater amount of chemical shift in the resultant image (compare to Image D acquired at a higher, typical bandwidth). This is also known as an "India Ink" artifact. *(Pg. 533–535, Figs. 13-42 and 13-43)*

18. **D**   Shown in the image is the wrap-around artifact, caused by anatomy outside of the display FOV but within the scan FOV. Protons outside of the FOV with frequencies or phase beyond the Nyquist sampling frequency will be aliased to the opposite side of the FOV. Thus, by increasing the acquisition FOV, this can be eliminated, but at the cost of spatial resolution. Alternatively, saturation pulses adjacent to the FOV boundaries can eliminate the signals. *(Pg. 536–538, Fig. 13-46)*

19. **C**   Zone 4, the scanner room, must be protected from all personnel except MR-trained personnel and those patients and/or support staff that have been screened. During a code, the procedure must be stopped and the patient must be removed from the magnet room (Zone 4) to at least Zone 3. Except under extremely dire circumstances, the magnet should not be quenched (a way to turn off a superconducting magnet in a controlled way) because of potential harm to the system, nearby personnel, and high costs to restart the system. *(Pg. 541–542)*

20. **B**   Zone 1 is the totally unrestricted zone for the general public. Upon freely entering Zone 2, there are several evaluation steps that MR personnel ask the patient and any other non-MR personnel before allowing admittance to Zone 3. That, of course, makes Zone 4 (only accessible through Zone 3) off limits as well. *(Pg. 546–547, Fig. 13-52)*

# Section III Key Equations and Symbols

| QUANTITY | EQUATION | EQ NO./PAGE/COMMENTS |
|---|---|---|
| Acquisition time for 2D SE and GRE imaging | Acquisition time = TR × # PEG Steps × NEX | Eq. 13-1/Pg. 495/TR is time of repetition; PEG is phase-encode gradient; NEX is number of excitations |
| Total number of slices during a TR for multislice acquisition | Total Number of Slices = TR/(TE + C) | Eq. 13-2/Pg. 495/C is a machine-dependent term |
| Acquisition time for 3D imaging | Acquistion time = TR × # Phase Encode Steps (Z - axis) × # Phase Encode Steps (Y - axis) × # NEX | Eq. 13-3/Pg. 496/Use of *slice encode* excitation for the Z-axis |
| SNR of parallel imaging ($SNR_{PI}$) | $SNR_{PI} = \dfrac{SNR_{\text{Fully Sampled}}}{\sqrt{R} \cdot g}$ | Eq. 13-4/Pg. 506/R: scan time reduction factor; g: coil geometry factor |
| Tofts model for DCE | $C_T(t) = R(t) \otimes C_A(t), \quad CBV \approx 0$ <br> $R(t) = K^{trans}e^{-k_{ep}t} \quad \text{or} \quad K^{trans}e^{-\frac{K^{trans}}{V_e}t}$ | Eq. 13-5/Pg. 515–516/R(t) is the response function and $C_A(t)$ is the arterial input function. $K^{trans}$, $v_e$, and $k_{ep}$ are the transfer constant from intravascular to extravascular space, volume fraction of extracellular space, and rate constant for efflux back to plasma, respectively |
| Extended Tofts model for DCE | $C_T(t) = R(t) \otimes C_A(t) + v_p C_A(t)$ <br> $R(t) = K^{trans}e^{-k_{ep}t} \quad \text{or} \quad K^{trans}e^{-\frac{K^{trans}}{V_e}t}$ | Eq. 13-6/Pg. 515–516/Inclusion of $v_p$, the plasma volume is added to the Tofts model for refining the calculation |
| Transverse magnetization of DWI | $M_{xy}(b, TE) = M_0 e^{-TE/T2}e^{-bD}$ | Eq. 13-7/Pg. 517/The b value is the diffusion sensitivity factor in s/mm²; D is the diffusivity of the molecules in mm²/s |

| SYMBOL | QUANTITY | UNITS |
|---|---|---|
| TR | Time of repetition | Seconds (s) |
| TE | Time of echo | Seconds (s) |
| NEX | Number of excitations or averages | NA |
| FSE | Fast spin echo | NA |
| ETL | Echo train length | NA |
| EPI | Echo planar imaging | NA |
| SE-EPI, GRE-EPI, GRASE | Spin echo, gradient echo, and gradient and spin echo EPI acquisitions | NA |
| SNR | Signal-to-noise ratio | NA |
| R | Scan time reduction factor | NA |
| g | Coil geometry factor | NA |
| T1 | Longitudinal relaxation time | Seconds (s) |
| T2 | Transverse relaxation time | Seconds (s) |

*(Continued)*

*(Continued)*

| SYMBOL | QUANTITY | UNITS |
|---|---|---|
| $T2^*$ | Transverse relaxation time including extrinsic magnetic inhomogeneities | Seconds (s) |
| $R1$ | Longitudinal relaxivity (1/T1) | 1/Seconds (1/s) |
| $R2^*$ | Transverse relaxivity (1/T2*) | 1/Seconds (1/s) |
| MRA | Magnetic resonance angiography | NA |
| ASL | Arterial spin labeling | NA |
| DSC | Dynamic susceptibility contrast | NA |
| DCE | Dynamic contrast enhanced | NA |
| MTT | Mean transit time | Seconds (s) |
| CBF | Cerebral blood flow | $cm^3/s$ |
| CBV | Cerebral blood volume | $cm^3$ |
| $K^{trans}$ | Transfer constant from intravascular space to extravascular space | 1/minutes (1/min) |
| $V_e$ | Volume fraction of extravascular extracellular space | NA |
| $k_{ep}$ | Rate constant for efflux back into plasma | 1/minutes (1/min) |
| $C_T(t)$ | Tissue concentration | NA |
| $R(t)$ | Response function | NA |
| $C_A(t)$ | Arterial input function | NA |
| $v_p$ | Plasma volume fraction | NA |
| $b$ | Diffusion sensitivity factor | $s/mm^2$ |
| D | Diffusivity | $mm^2/s$ |
| DWI | Diffusion-weighted imaging | NA |
| DTI | Diffusion tensor imaging | NA |
| DSI | Diffusion spectrum imaging | NA |
| HARDI | High angular resolution diffusion imaging | NA |
| NODDI | Neurite orientation dispersion and density | NA |
| fMRI | Functional MRI | NA |
| BOLD | Blood oxygen level dependent | NA |
| MRE | Magnetic resonance elastography | NA |
| MTC | Magnetization transfer contrast | NA |
| MRS | Magnetic resonance spectroscopy | NA |
| STEAM | Stimulated echo acquisition mode | NA |
| PRESS | Point resolved spectroscopy | NA |
| CSI | Chemical shift imaging | NA |
| SAR | Specific absorption rate | W/kg |

# Ultrasound

## 14.0 INTRODUCTION

The characteristics, properties, and production of ultrasound for clinical applications are described. Ultrasound interaction with tissues, instrumentation, equipment, image acquisition, processing, and display demonstrate how useful acoustic properties can be obtained, including tissue stiffness and blood velocity determinations. Common artifacts, bioeffects, and safety aspects are also considered.

## 14.1 CHARACTERISTICS OF SOUND

Sound is mechanical energy that propagates through a continuous medium by the compression (high pressure) and rarefaction (low pressure) of particles that comprise it. For ultrasound, the mechanical force is a transducer, composed of an expanding and contracting group of crystal elements creating local periodic compressions and rarefactions in the tissue medium. Mechanical energy travels at the speed of sound into the patient and "particles" of the tissue transfer energy much like a compressible spring, traveling as a longitudinal wave (Fig. 14-1).

1. **Wavelength, Frequency, Speed**
   a. *Wavelength* ($\lambda$): distance between two repeating points in a periodic wave (*i.e.*, a cycle), (*e.g.*, mm).
   b. *Frequency* (*f*) is the cycle repetition per second (s), in Hertz (Hz), where 1 Hz = 1 cycle/s.
      (i) Less than 15 Hz is infrasound; 15 to 20 kHz is audible sound; greater than 20 kHz is ultrasound Medical ultrasound: 1 to 20 MHz, up to 50 MHz and beyond for specialized applications
   c. *Period*: time duration of one wave (cycle) and is equal to 1/*f*
   d. *Speed of sound*, c: distance traveled per unit time is equal to the product of wavelength and frequency

$$c = \lambda f$$

[14-1]

   (i) Speed of sound units: m/s (meters/second), cm/s, mm/μs.
   (ii) c varies in a medium, based on compressibility, stiffness, and density characteristics; tissues with high compressibility = slow speed (e.g., air); greater stiffness = high speed (e.g., bone) (Table 14-1).
   e. Using c = 1.54 mm/μs, the wavelength in mm of soft tissue = 1.54 mm/*f* (MHz), thus the wavelength of a 10-MHz beam is easily calculated, as 1.54/10 = 0.154 mm and for a 2-MHz beam as 1.54/2 = 0.77 mm (Fig. 14-2).
   f. Higher frequencies provide better resolution, but higher attenuation and limited depth penetration.
2. **Pressure and Intensity**
   a. Pressure (*P*), expressed as Newton per square meter ($N/m^2$) with SI unit of pascal (*Pa*); "pressure amplitude" refers to the magnitude of change in pressure: note—earth's atmospheric pressure = 100,000 *Pa* and ultrasound imaging peak pressure is 1,000,000 *Pa* or 1 *MPa*—the peak US intensity is about 10 times higher than earth atmospheric pressure.
   b. Intensity, *I*, is a measure of average power per unit area and is proportional to the square of the pressure amplitude, $I \propto P^2$; medical diagnostic ultrasound intensity levels are milliwatts/cm$^2$.
   c. Relative pressure and intensity levels are scaled using the *decibel* (*dB*), a unitless value.

$$\text{Relative pressure (dB)} = 20 \log \frac{P_1}{P_2}$$

[14-2]

$$\text{Relative intensity (dB)} = 10 \log \frac{I_1}{I_2}$$

[14-3]

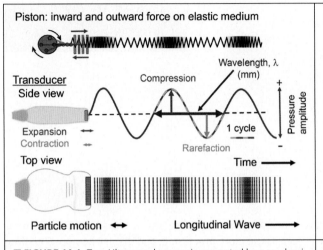

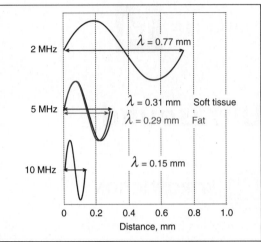

■ **FIGURE 14-1** *Top*: Ultrasound energy is generated by a mechanical displacement of a elastic medium, modeled as a compressible spring. An inward and outward force of a piston coupled to the medium creates increased pressure (compression) and decreased pressure (rarefaction) in a cyclical manner. *Mid*: Side view of transducer with crystal elements that expand and contract at a high frequency shows energy propagation as a wave with the wavelength equal to the distance of one cycle. *Bottom*: Ultrasound propagates in the medium as a longitudinal wave. 📖 **F. 14-2**

■ **FIGURE 14-2** Ultrasound wavelength is determined by the frequency and the speed of sound in the propagation medium. Wavelengths in soft tissue are calculated for 2-, 5-, and 10-MHz ultrasound sources for soft tissue (*blue*). A comparison of wavelength in fat (*red*) to soft tissue at 5 MHz is also shown. 📖 **F. 14-3**

**TABLE 14-1 DENSITY, SPEED OF SOUND, AND ACOUSTIC IMPEDANCE FOR TISSUES AND MATERIALS RELEVANT TO MEDICAL ULTRASOUND**

| MATERIAL | DENSITY (kg/m³) | C (m/s) | Z (rayls)ᵃ |
|---|---|---|---|
| Air | 1.2 | 330 | $3.96 \times 10^2$ |
| Lung | 300 | 600 | $1.80 \times 10^3$ |
| Fat | 924 | 1,450 | $1.34 \times 10^6$ |
| Water | 1,000 | 1,480 | $1.48 \times 10^6$ |
| "Soft Tissue" | 1,050 | 1,540 | $1.62 \times 10^6$ |
| Kidney | 1,041 | 1,565 | $1.63 \times 10^6$ |
| Blood | 1,058 | 1,560 | $1.65 \times 10^6$ |
| Liver | 1,061 | 1,555 | $1.65 \times 10^6$ |
| Muscle | 1,068 | 1,600 | $1.71 \times 10^6$ |
| Skull bone | 1,912 | 4,080 | $7.8 \times 10^6$ |
| PZT | 7,500 | 4,000 | $3.0 \times 10^7$ |

ᵃAcoustic impedance is the product of density and speed of sound. The named unit, rayl, has base units of kg/(m²s) for values listed in the column. Acoustic impedance directly relates to the propagation characteristics of ultrasound in each medium and is the basis for echo formation.

    **d.** The *dB* scale logarithm function: compresses large and expands small ratios (Table 14-2)
        **(i)** Pressure is proportional to voltage, so Equation 14-2 compares induced voltages of echoes.
        **(ii)** Pressure or voltage comparisons have a factor of 2× higher values on *dB* scale relative to intensity.
        **(iii)** Intensity ratio of $10^6$ (*e.g.*, incident pulse intensity is $10^6$ greater than echo intensity) = 60 *dB* (Eq. 14-3).
        **(iv)** Change of 10 in the relative intensity *dB* scale = order of magnitude (10 times) change.
        **(v)** Change of 20 is equal to two orders of magnitude (100 times) change, and so forth.
        **(vi)** Intensity ratio greater than 1, *dB* scale is positive; less than 1, *dB* scale is negative.
        **(vii)** Loss of 3 *dB* (−3 *dB*) represents a 50% loss of signal intensity, the "half-value" thickness (*HVT*).
    **e.** Ultrasound energy imparted to the medium depends on the pressure amplitude variations generated by the degree of transducer expansion and contraction through transmit gain.

**TABLE 14-2  INTENSITY RATIO AND CORRESPONDING DECIBEL VALUES**

| INTENSITY RATIO | | DECIBELS (DB) |
|---|---|---|
| $I_2/I_1$ | $\text{LOG}(I_2/I_1)$ | $10 \times \text{LOG}(I_2/I_1)$ |
| 1 | 0 | 0 |
| 2 | 0.3 | 3 |
| 10 | 1 | 10 |
| 100 | 2 | 20 |
| 10,000 | 4 | 40 |
| 1,000,000 | 6 | 60 |
| 0.5 | −0.3 | −3 |
| 0.01 | −2 | −20 |
| 0.0001 | −4 | −40 |
| 0.000001 | −6 | −60 |

## 14.2  INTERACTIONS OF ULTRASOUND WITH TISSUES

Interactions of ultrasound are chiefly based on the *acoustic impedance* of tissues and result in *reflection, refraction, scattering,* and *absorption* of the ultrasound energy.

1. **Acoustic Impedance, Z:** a measure of tissue stiffness and flexibility
   a. Equal to the product of density and speed of sound: **Z = $\rho c$**
      (i)   $\rho$ is the density in kg/m$^3$; $c$ is the speed of sound in m/s.
      (ii)  $Z$ has the unit "rayl" with units of kg/(m$^2$s) and values in Table 14-1, **right column.**
   b. Sound energy transfer efficiency from one tissue to another is dependent on differences in Z.
      (i)   For similar Z, a large fraction of incident intensity will be transmitted through a boundary.
      (ii)  For wide differences in Z, most incident intensity will be reflected at the boundary.
      (iii) Most soft tissues have a similar Z, allowing ultrasound to penetrate deep into the body.
2. **Reflection back to the transducer**
   a. A beam traveling perpendicular (normal incidence = 90°) to boundary between two tissues (Fig. 14-3A).
   b. The fraction of incident intensity reflected at a boundary is the intensity reflection coefficient, $R_I$:

$$R_I = \frac{I_r}{I_i} = \left(\frac{Z_2 - Z_1}{Z_2 + Z_1}\right)^2 \qquad [14\text{-}4]$$

   Subscripts 1 and 2 represent tissues that are proximal and distal to the boundary, respectively.
   c. Intensity transmission coefficient $T_I$ is equal to $1 - R_I$.
   d. Example of reflection at fat/muscle interface, $Z_{fat} = 1.34$, $Z_{muscle} = 1.71$, 1.5% of intensity is reflected:

$$R_{I,(fat \to muscle)} = \frac{I_r}{I_i} = \left(\frac{1.71 - 1.34}{1.71 + 1.34}\right)^2 = 0.015; \quad T_{I,(fat \to muscle)} = 1 - R_{I,(fat \to muscle)} = 0.985$$

   e. With air, the reflection coefficient is 1, thus 100% of incident intensity is reflected.
   f. For nonnormal incidence, the reflected angle = incident angle relative to the normal direction.
3. **Refraction**
   a. A change in direction of the transmitted ultrasound pulse when the incident pulse is not perpendicular to the tissue boundary, and the speeds of sound in the two tissues are different (Fig. 14-3B).
   b. Angle of refraction determined by *Snell law:* $\frac{\sin\theta_t}{\sin\theta_i} = \frac{c_2}{c_1}$ ; approximated as $\frac{\theta_t}{\theta_i} \cong \frac{c_2}{c_1}$ .

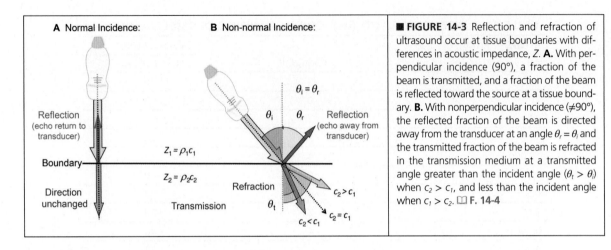

**■ FIGURE 14-3** Reflection and refraction of ultrasound occur at tissue boundaries with differences in acoustic impedance, $Z$. **A.** With perpendicular incidence (90°), a fraction of the beam is transmitted, and a fraction of the beam is reflected toward the source at a tissue boundary. **B.** With nonperpendicular incidence (≠90°), the reflected fraction of the beam is directed away from the transducer at an angle $\theta_r = \theta_i$ and the transmitted fraction of the beam is refracted in the transmission medium at a transmitted angle greater than the incident angle ($\theta_t > \theta_i$) when $c_2 > c_1$, and less than the incident angle when $c_1 > c_2$. 📖 **F. 14-4**

4. **Scattering**
   a. Arises from objects and interfaces within tissues with size on the order of ultrasound wavelength.
      (i)   Low frequencies (1 to 5 MHz) with longer λ, boundaries appear **specular** (mirror-like)
      (ii)  High frequencies (greater than 5 to 15 MHz) with shorter λ, boundaries are **nonspecular** (Fig. 14-4)
   b. Tissue *signatures* arise from different organs due to internal structure and echo correlation patterns.
   c. **Hypoechoic** and **hyperechoic** are terms describing characteristics of tissues in terms of the relative intensity of the backscattered signal.
5. **Absorption and Attenuation**
   a. Attenuation is the loss of US intensity with distance traveled from scattering and absorption.
   b. Expressed in decibels (dB), with an average attenuation of 0.5 dB/(cm-MHz) (See Table 14-4, textbook).
   c. Ultrasound attenuation occurs exponentially with depth and more rapidly with frequency (Fig. 14-5).
   d. Choice of ultrasound transducer frequency is strongly dependent on required depth of imaging.
   e. Example: calculate the relative ratio (incident pulse to returning echo) of a 5 MHz US wave traveling to a depth of 4 cm with a 100% reflective boundary. Answer: 5 MHz × 0.5 dB/(cm-MHz) = 2.5 dB/cm attenuation for a total travel distance of 8 cm (to and from reflector), loss of US intensity is thus 2.5 dB/cm × 8 cm = 20 dB. The relative ratio is thus 20 dB = 10 log ($I_{incident}/I_{echo}$); $I_{incident}$ = 100 $I_{echo}$.

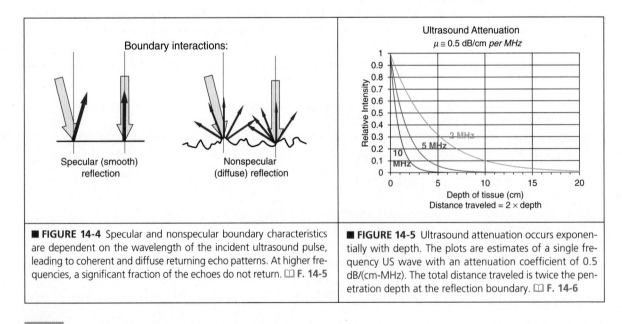

**■ FIGURE 14-4** Specular and nonspecular boundary characteristics are dependent on the wavelength of the incident ultrasound pulse, leading to coherent and diffuse returning echo patterns. At higher frequencies, a significant fraction of the echoes do not return. 📖 **F. 14-5**

**■ FIGURE 14-5** Ultrasound attenuation occurs exponentially with depth. The plots are estimates of a single frequency US wave with an attenuation coefficient of 0.5 dB/(cm-MHz). The total distance traveled is twice the penetration depth at the reflection boundary. 📖 **F. 14-6**

## 14.3   ULTRASOUND TRANSDUCERS

Ultrasound is transmitted and received by a *transducer array*, composed of hundreds of small ceramic elements with electromechanical (piezoelectric) properties, connected to controlling electronics and contained in a hand-held, plastic housing with other components essential to proper operation.

1. **Piezoelectric Materials**
   a. Lead zirconate titanate (PZT)—synthetic material composed of aligned dipole structure (Fig. 14-6).
   b. Electrodes attached to each surface of PZT thickness provide the ability to receive and produce US.
   c. Small mechanical displacements by returning waves in the receive mode create voltage differences of microvolts (µV).
   d. Externally applied voltage pulse (approximately 100 V) in the transmit mode reorients the PZT into crystal "thickness" contraction or expansion togenerate ultrasound energy.

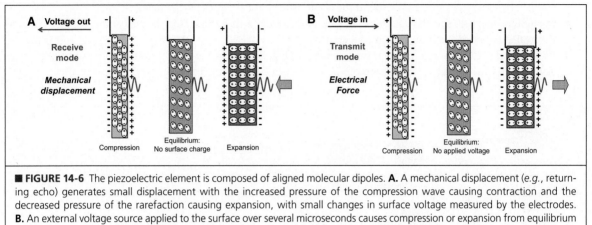

■ **FIGURE 14-6** The piezoelectric element is composed of aligned molecular dipoles. **A.** A mechanical displacement (*e.g.*, returning echo) generates small displacement with the increased pressure of the compression wave causing contraction and the decreased pressure of the rarefaction causing expansion, with small changes in surface voltage measured by the electrodes. **B.** An external voltage source applied to the surface over several microseconds causes compression or expansion from equilibrium in response to electrical attraction or repulsion force on the dipolar internal structure of the PZT. 📖 **F. 14-7**

   e. The US pulse is created using a short-duration voltage spike in the compression mode; the PZT vibrates at a natural frequency in the thickness mode of $\lambda/2$; crystal thickness determines frequency (Fig. 14-7).
2. **Resonance Frequency, Damping, Absorbing, and Matching Layers**
   a. Transducer arrays are composed of multiple elements, each attached with electrode wires.
   b. Excitation of undamped crystals will result in a long-duration, narrow bandwidth frequency (Fig. 14-8A).
      (i) "$Q$" factor represents the purity of produced sound: $Q = f_0/\text{bandwidth}$.
      (ii) A *damping layer* is required to shorten pulse width, which increases the bandwidth
      (iii) US imaging requires transducers with low $Q$ to obtain a short spatial pulse length.
   c. Compression in thickness mode causes expansion in the width and height of the elements (Fig. 14-8B).

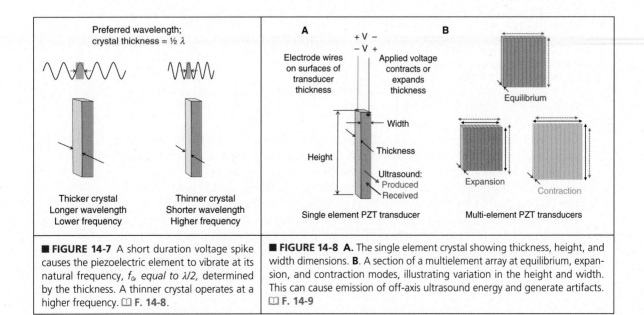

■ **FIGURE 14-7** A short duration voltage spike causes the piezoelectric element to vibrate at its natural frequency, $f_0$, equal to $\lambda/2$, determined by the thickness. A thinner crystal operates at a higher frequency. 📖 **F. 14-8.**

■ **FIGURE 14-8 A.** The single element crystal showing thickness, height, and width dimensions. **B**. A section of a multielement array at equilibrium, expansion, and contraction modes, illustrating variation in the height and width. This can cause emission of off-axis ultrasound energy and generate artifacts. 📖 **F. 14-9**

**d.** US is emitted in both directions upon PZT excitation, requiring the use of an adjacent *absorption layer*.

**e.** A *matching layer* provides the interface between the PZT and tissue to maximize transmission.

    **(i)** Matching layer thickness is equal to ¼ λ with a speed of sound between PZT and soft tissue.

    **(ii)** Acoustic coupling gel is also used to improve contact and eliminate air pockets.

**f.** The composite structure of the transducer element array and housing are shown in Figure 14-9.

## 3. Broad Bandwidth "Multifrequency" Transducer Operation

**a.** Transducer elements are manufactured with many small PZT rods backfilled with epoxy.

**b.** Properties of these elements provide a better acoustic impedance match with tissue and can be operated over a selectable range of frequencies due to the composite characteristics of the material.

**c.** Excitation pulses of specific square wave voltage pulses of 1 to 3 cycles selects the center frequency across the available bandwidths of the transducer array.

**d.** Broad bandwidth response of the transducer array (Fig. 14-10) permits reception of echoes at specific frequencies, useful for native tissue harmonic imaging (see Section 14.6.5).

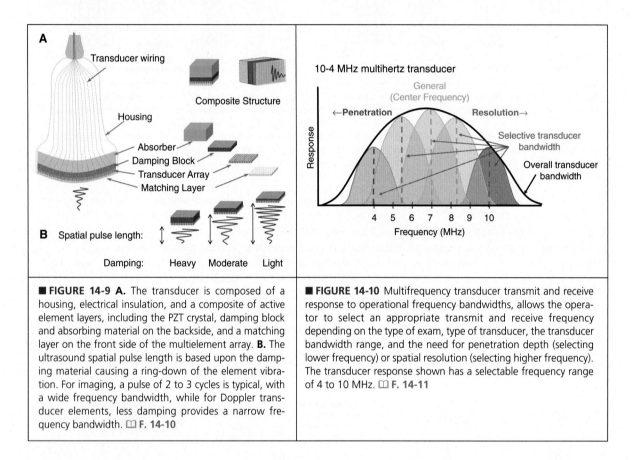

■ **FIGURE 14-9 A.** The transducer is composed of a housing, electrical insulation, and a composite of active element layers, including the PZT crystal, damping block and absorbing material on the backside, and a matching layer on the front side of the multielement array. **B.** The ultrasound spatial pulse length is based upon the damping material causing a ring-down of the element vibration. For imaging, a pulse of 2 to 3 cycles is typical, with a wide frequency bandwidth, while for Doppler transducer elements, less damping provides a narrow frequency bandwidth. 📖 **F. 14-10**

■ **FIGURE 14-10** Multifrequency transducer transmit and receive response to operational frequency bandwidths, allows the operator to select an appropriate transmit and receive frequency depending on the type of exam, type of transducer, the transducer bandwidth range, and the need for penetration depth (selecting lower frequency) or spatial resolution (selecting higher frequency). The transducer response shown has a selectable frequency range of 4 to 10 MHz. 📖 **F. 14-11**

## 4. Transducer Arrays

**a.** Linear, curvilinear, and phased array operation are most common for diagnostic ultrasound (Fig. 14-11).

**b.** Linear and curvilinear arrays activate a subset of elements producing a single transmit beam pulse.

    **(i)** Subsequent receive mode is activated to listen to echoes from depth

    **(ii)** Activation of a different subset of adjacent elements produces another beam pulse.

    **(iii)** This continues for all of the elements across the array, which is then repeated.

**c.** Phased transducer arrays activate all elements in the array, and with fine and ultrafine transmit delay timing, electronic steering of the beam can be achieved, producing a sector-scan format.

**d.** Intracavitary transducer arrays use both linear and phased array operation for imaging.

**e.** Mechanical/electronic array scanners are used for real-time 3D imaging (*e.g.*, fetal imaging, see text for details).

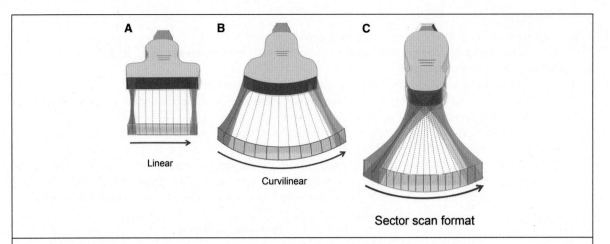

**■ FIGURE 14-11 A.** The linear array transducer activates a subgroup of transducer elements to produce an ultrasound beam directed perpendicular to the array, repeating with incremental shifting of the subgroup element by element. A rectangular field of view is produced. **B.** The curvilinear (also known as convex) array operates with subgroup transducer element excitation, like the linear array. A convex arrangement produces a trapezoidal field of view, with good coverage proximally and extended coverage distally. **C.** A phased array transducer produces a beam from the near-simultaneous excitation of all array elements. The beam can be electronically steered across the FOV using transmit delay excitation patterns. A sector scan format is produced with incremental time delay patterns to control the direction and number of lines across the FOV. □ F. 14-12A, F. 14-13A, F. 14-14B

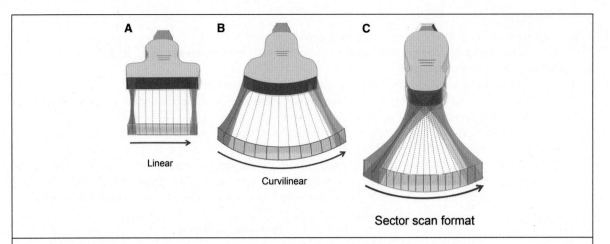

## 14.4  ULTRASOUND BEAM PROPERTIES

The transducer-generated US beam propagates as a longitudinal wave from the transducer surface into the propagation medium and exhibits two distinct beam patterns: a slightly converging beam out to a distance determined by the geometry and frequency of the transducer (*the near field*) and a diverging beam beyond that point (*the far field*). Other considerations include US beam focusing, the generation of side lobes and grating lobes, and the spatial resolution determinants in a US beam, including axial, lateral, and elevational.

**1. The Near Field**
   **a.** Also known as the Fresnel zone, is adjacent to the transducer face out to the minimum beam diameter.
      **(i)** A converging beam profile is due to interference patterns from the multiple US sources.
      **(ii)** "Huygens principle" describes the transducer as an infinite number of point sources.
   **b.** The near field depth increases with excitation radius, $r$, and inverse to US wavelength, $\lambda$: **length** = $r^2/\lambda$.
      **(i)** Lateral beam dimension for subarray of linear transducer is about ½ size of excitation footprint.
   **c.** Pressure amplitude changes are complex in the near field and vary rapidly (Fig. 14-12).

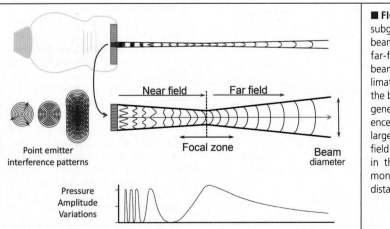

**■ FIGURE 14-12** A linear array transducer subgroup excitation (*top*) and the expanded beam profile (*middle*) shows the near-field and far-field characteristics of the ultrasound beam. The near field is characterized as a collimated beam, and the far-field begins when the beam diverges. Point emitters (*left middle*) generate constructive and destructive interference patterns that cause beam collimation and large pressure amplitude variations in the near field (*lower diagram*). Beam divergence occurs in the far-field, where pressure amplitude monotonically decreases with propagation distance. □ F. 14-16

2. **The Far Field**
   a. Also known as the Fraunhofer zone, begins at end of the near field
      (i) Characterized by diverging wave and monotonically decreasing pressure (Fig. 14-12)
3. **Transducer array beam focusing**
   a. Transmit focus is achieved by applying timing delays between transducer elements.
      (i) This occurs within the subgroup of elements for linear and curvilinear arrays and for all elements for phased array transducers (Fig. 14-13).
      (ii) Focal zones can occur at various depths depending on the delays between element excitations.
   b. Receive focus is dynamically applied to all active elements during the reception of the echoes.
      (i) Proximal echoes returning from a boundary interface are more concave—timing delays from central elements are longer relative to the peripheral elements to achieve phase coherence (Fig. 14-13).
      (ii) Distal echoes have a less concave echo pattern, and the variable timing circuitry adjusts accordingly.

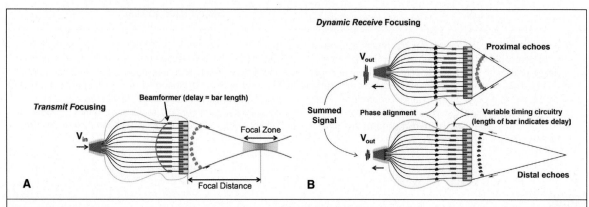

■ **FIGURE 14-13** Transmit and Receive focusing. **A.** Transmit focusing is achieved by implementing a programmable delay time (beamformer electronics) for the excitation of the individual transducer elements in a concave pattern with outer elements energized first. The individual ultrasound pulses converge to a minimum beam diameter (the focal distance) at a predictable depth in tissue. **B.** Dynamic receive focusing uses receive beamformer electronics to dynamically adjust delay times for processing the received echo signals. This compensates for differences in arrival time across the array as a function of time (depth of the echo) and results in phase alignment of the echo signals by all elements to achieve a good signal output as a function of time. ▭ **F. 14-17**

4. **Side Lobes and Grating Lobes**
   a. Side lobes represent US intensity created from the element width and height expansion and contraction.
      (i) Energy is directed adjacent to the main beam area in the forward direction (Fig. 14-14A).
      (ii) Side lobes can easily generate echoes that map into the main beam (see section on artifacts).
   b. Grating lobes result from the discrete excitations in multielement arrays.
      (i) US intensity is emitted at wide angles (Fig. 14-14B).
      (ii) The intensity of grating lobes is substantially less than side lobes.
   c. For both side lobes and grating lobes, intensity is diminished with low Q operation (see Section 14.3.2).

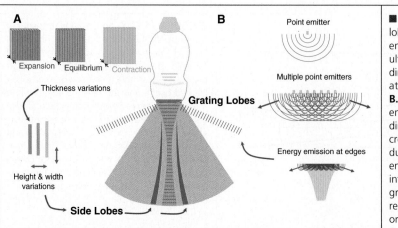

■ **FIGURE 14-14** Side lobes and grating lobes. **A.** Side lobes represent ultrasound energy produced outside of the main ultrasound beam along the same beam direction caused by height and width variations of the transducer elements. **B.** Grating lobes represent the emission of energy at large angles relative to the direction of the beam caused by the discrete nature of the multielement transducer array. At the edges of the array, energy is emitted that does not undergo interference as shown by the *inset* diagram. The grating lobe intensity is low relative to the intensity of the main beam or side lobes. ▭ **F. 14-18**

5. **Spatial Resolution**

US resolution has three separate components: *Axial, Lateral, and Elevational (Slice Thickness)* (Fig. 14-15). Visibility of detail in the image is determined by the volume and dimensions of the acoustic pulse.

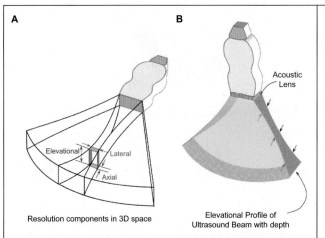

■ **FIGURE 14-15 A.** The axial, lateral, and elevational (slice-thickness) contributions in three dimensions are shown for a phased-array transducer ultrasound beam. Axial resolution, along the direction of the beam, is independent of depth; lateral resolution and elevational resolution are strongly depth-dependent. Lateral resolution is determined by transmit and receive focus electronics; elevational resolution is determined by the height of the transducer elements. At the focal distance, axial is better than lateral, and lateral is better than elevational resolution. **B.** Elevational resolution profile with an acoustic lens across the transducer array produces a weak focal zone in the slice thickness direction. ▭ **F. 14-19**

**a.** *Axial resolution* is also known as linear, range, longitudinal, or depth resolution.
  **(i)** The ability to distinguish closely spaced objects in the direction of the US beam.
  **(ii)** Is equal to ½ spatial pulse length (SPL), where SPL = product of wavelength and #cycles per pulse.
  **(iii)** Short SPL is achieved with higher damping of transducer elements, typically 2 to 3 cycles, and higher frequency of operation (shorter wavelength) (Fig. 14-16).
**b.** *Lateral resolution* is also known as azimuthal resolution.
  **(i)** The ability to distinguish closely spaced objects perpendicular to the direction of the US beam, and in the plane of the image.
  **(ii)** Beamwidth is the determining factor, which changes as a function of depth (Fig. 14-17).
  **(iii)** Lateral focal zones can be established to create a narrower beam diameter at a specified depth.
  **(iv)** Multiple focal zones can provide good resolution over a range of depths (Fig. 14-18).
  **(v)** Drawbacks of focal zone placement are a loss of temporal resolution and possible transition band artifacts (see section on Ultrasound Artifacts).

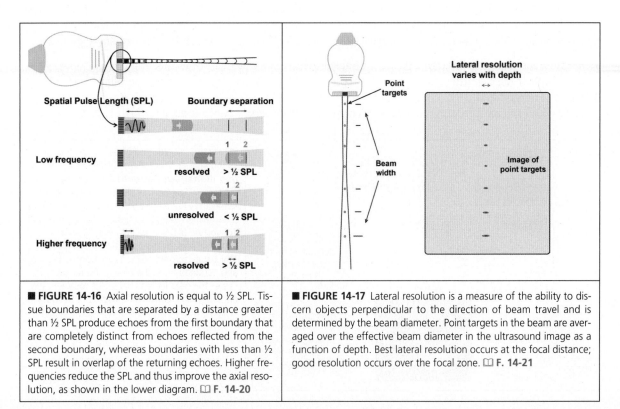

■ **FIGURE 14-16** Axial resolution is equal to ½ SPL. Tissue boundaries that are separated by a distance greater than ½ SPL produce echoes from the first boundary that are completely distinct from echoes reflected from the second boundary, whereas boundaries with less than ½ SPL result in overlap of the returning echoes. Higher frequencies reduce the SPL and thus improve the axial resolution, as shown in the lower diagram. ▭ **F. 14-20**

■ **FIGURE 14-17** Lateral resolution is a measure of the ability to discern objects perpendicular to the direction of beam travel and is determined by the beam diameter. Point targets in the beam are averaged over the effective beam diameter in the ultrasound image as a function of depth. Best lateral resolution occurs at the focal distance; good resolution occurs over the focal zone. ▭ **F. 14-21**

c. *Elevational resolution* is also known as slice thickness resolution.
   (i)   Like lateral resolution, elevational is depth dependent with a focal zone (Fig. 14-19).
   (ii)  "1.5D" arrays can provide multiple elevational focal zones.

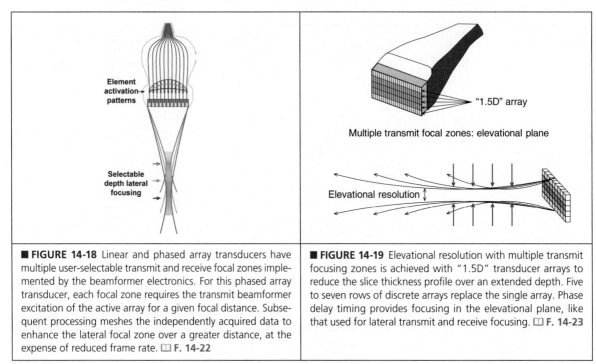

■ **FIGURE 14-18** Linear and phased array transducers have multiple user-selectable transmit and receive focal zones implemented by the beamformer electronics. For this phased array transducer, each focal zone requires the transmit beamformer excitation of the active array for a given focal distance. Subsequent processing meshes the independently acquired data to enhance the lateral focal zone over a greater distance, at the expense of reduced frame rate. 📖 **F. 14-22**

■ **FIGURE 14-19** Elevational resolution with multiple transmit focusing zones is achieved with "1.5D" transducer arrays to reduce the slice thickness profile over an extended depth. Five to seven rows of discrete arrays replace the single array. Phase delay timing provides focusing in the elevational plane, like that used for lateral transmit and receive focusing. 📖 **F. 14-23**

## 14.5  IMAGE DATA ACQUISITION AND PROCESSING

Images are acquired using a *pulse-echo* mode of ultrasound production and detection. Each pulse is directionally transmitted into the patient. Partial reflections from tissue boundaries at normal incidence create echoes that return to the transducer as a function of travel time and depth, along a corresponding line in the ultrasound image. The receiver detects the echoes, and the process is repeated incrementally across the field of view to sequentially construct the image line by line. Data acquisition and image formation using the pulse-echo approach requires several hardware components: the beamformer, pulser, receiver, amplifier, scan converter/image memory, and display system (Fig. 14-20).

1. Beamformer: generates electronic delays for transmit/receive focusing and beam steering
   a. Computer logic controls pulser, transmit/receive switch, preamps, analog to digital amplifiers
2. Pulser (Transmitter)
   a. Provides voltage for exiting transducer elements; controls output transmit power

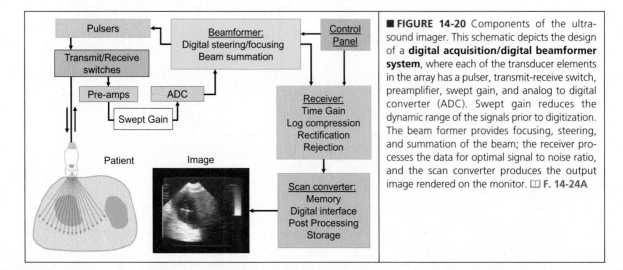

■ **FIGURE 14-20** Components of the ultrasound imager. This schematic depicts the design of a **digital acquisition/digital beamformer system**, where each of the transducer elements in the array has a pulser, transmit-receive switch, preamplifier, swept gain, and analog to digital converter (ADC). Swept gain reduces the dynamic range of the signals prior to digitization. The beam former provides focusing, steering, and summation of the beam; the receiver processes the data for optimal signal to noise ratio, and the scan converter produces the output image rendered on the monitor. 📖 **F. 14-24A**

3. Transmit/Receive Switch
   a. Isolates high-voltage associated with excitation (150 V) to voltage associated with echoes (approximately μV)
   b. "Ring-down" time—the time required for the transducer array to switch from excitation to reception
4. Pulse-Echo Operation
   a. Ultrasound intermittently transmits over a short period (approximately 1 μs) and then receives echoes (approximately 1,000 μs).
   b. Depth (D) of a received echo is determined by US speed and distance traveled = 2 × depth. Pertinent equations: (uses units of μs, cm, and speed of sound in cm/μs).

Time to receive echo after pulse: $T(\mu s) = \dfrac{2D(cm)}{c\left(\dfrac{cm}{\mu s}\right)} = \dfrac{2D\,cm}{0.154\dfrac{cm}{\mu s}} = \dfrac{13\ \mu s}{cm} \times D(cm)$

Round trip distance traveled: $D(cm) = \dfrac{0.154\dfrac{cm}{\mu s} \times T(\mu s)}{2} = 0.077 \times T(\mu s)$

   c. Number of pulses/s: pulse repetition frequency (PRF)
   d. Time between pulses: pulse repetition period (PRP) (Fig. 14-21)
   e. Pulse duration: ratio of the #cycles/pulse to the transducer frequency = "on" time—1 to 2 μs
   f. Duty cycle: fraction of "on" time = pulse duration/PRP = approximately 0.2% to 0.4%

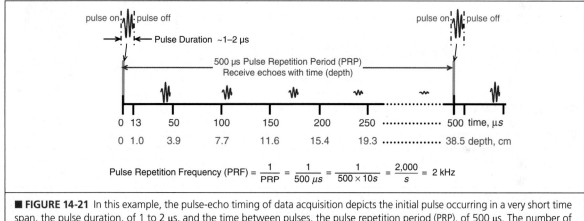

**FIGURE 14-21** In this example, the pulse-echo timing of data acquisition depicts the initial pulse occurring in a very short time span, the pulse duration, of 1 to 2 μs, and the time between pulses, the pulse repetition period (PRP), of 500 μs. The number of pulses per second, the pulse repetition frequency (PRF), is 2,000/s, or 2 kHz. The indicated depth is ½ of the total travel distance of the pulse/echo for the indicated time. 📖 **F. 14-25**

5. Preamplification and Analog-to-Digital Conversion
   a. Returning signals are preamplified prior to analog to digital conversion during swept gain step.
   b. Range of voltage amplitude changes can be as much as 120 dB (a factor of $10^6$ for pressure amplitude).

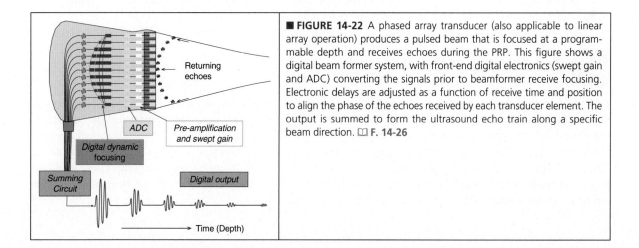

**FIGURE 14-22** A phased array transducer (also applicable to linear array operation) produces a pulsed beam that is focused at a programmable depth and receives echoes during the PRP. This figure shows a digital beam former system, with front-end digital electronics (swept gain and ADC) converting the signals prior to beamformer receive focusing. Electronic delays are adjusted as a function of receive time and position to align the phase of the echoes received by each transducer element. The output is summed to form the ultrasound echo train along a specific beam direction. 📖 **F. 14-26**

6. Beam Steering, Dynamic Focusing, and Signal Summation (Fig. 14-22)
    a. It is essential to orchestrate the acquisition to achieve a high SNR echo train during the PRP.
    b. A combination of preamplification and dynamic focusing produces a stream of reliable acoustic data.
7. Receiver accepts data from the beamformer during the PRP, with subsequent signal processing (Fig. 14-23): preamplification, time gain compensation, logarithmic compression, demodulation, and noise rejection
    a. Time gain compensation (Fig. 14-24) is a user-adjustable amplification of returning echoes versus time
        (i)   Ideal TGC curve makes all equally reflective boundaries at various depths have the same amplitude.
        (ii)  User adjustment is typical with multiple slider potentiometers or electronic calipers.
    b. Dynamic range/logarithmic compression reduces the echo amplitude range for the video display.
    c. Demodulation and envelope detection converts the detected signals into a positive, smooth pulse.
    d. Noise rejection sets the lower threshold signal level allowed to pass the scan converter.

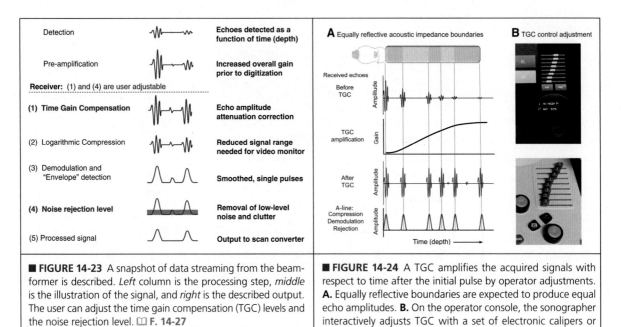

■ **FIGURE 14-23** A snapshot of data streaming from the beamformer is described. *Left* column is the processing step, *middle* is the illustration of the signal, and *right* is the described output. The user can adjust the time gain compensation (TGC) levels and the noise rejection level. ⬚ **F. 14-27**

■ **FIGURE 14-24** A TGC amplifies the acquired signals with respect to time after the initial pulse by operator adjustments. **A.** Equally reflective boundaries are expected to produce equal echo amplitudes. **B.** On the operator console, the sonographer interactively adjusts TGC with a set of electronic calipers or slide potentiometers to optimize the gain. ⬚ **F. 14-28**

    e. Processed signals are passed to the scan converter for gray scale image display.
8. Echo Signal Modes
    a. A-mode (amplitude) is the processed signal versus time as shown in Figure 14-23(**5**), where 1 A-line of data is produced per pulse for conventional line-by-line acquisition.
    b. B-mode (brightness) is the conversion of the A-mode amplitude into a B-mode gray scale values.
    c. M-mode (motion) is a technique using B-mode signals, a stationary beam, and deflecting the B-mode data as a function of time to evaluate anatomic motion; also known as T-M mode.
9. Scan Converter
    a. Generates 2D ultrasound images from B-mode data based on trajectory and time (depth), see Figure 14-20.
    b. Data interpolation is used to fill in empty or partially filled pixels in the matrix.

## 14.6   IMAGE ACQUISITION

The 2D ultrasound image is acquired by sweeping a pulsed ultrasound beam sequentially in a plane over the volume of interest to produce "video clips." The matrix size and frame rate are dependent on several factors including ultrasound frequency, pulse repetition frequency, the field of view, depth of penetration, number of lines per frame, and line density. Improvements in image acquisition rate are achievable with advanced techniques such as multiline acquisition (MLA), multiline transmission (MLT), plane, and diverging wave imaging. These advances provide frame rates that go well beyond conventional line-by-line acquisitions and create high temporal resolution imaging of several hundred to thousands of frames per second.

1. **Real-Time Imaging**: frame rate, FOV, depth, sampling tradeoffs (Fig. 14-25)
   a. Frame time depends on number of A-lines, maximum penetration depth, and time required for each line.

$$T_{\text{frame}} = N \times T_{\text{line}} = N \times 13 \ \mu s/cm \times D_{\text{max}} (cm)$$

   b. Frame rate is the reciprocal of the time required per frame.

$$\text{Frame rate} \left( s^{-1} \right) = \frac{1}{T_{\text{frame}}} = \frac{1}{N \times 13 \ \mu s \times D_{\text{max}} (cm)} = \frac{0.077 \ cm/\mu s}{N \times D_{\text{max}} (cm)} = \frac{77{,}000 \ cm/s}{N \times D_{\text{max}} (cm)}$$

   c. Line density (LD) is determined by $N$ and the field of view and impacts lateral resolution.
   d. For line by line imaging, the PRF of the acquisition is equal to $N$.
   e. Lateral focusing reduces frame rate by the inverse of the number of focusing zones set.

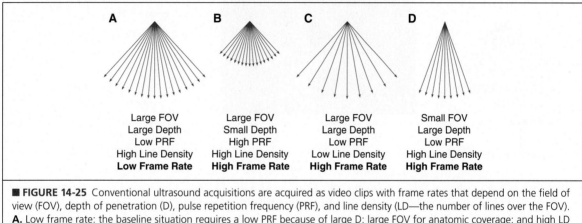

| A | B | C | D |
|---|---|---|---|
| Large FOV | Large FOV | Large FOV | Small FOV |
| Large Depth | Small Depth | Large Depth | Large Depth |
| Low PRF | High PRF | Low PRF | Low PRF |
| High Line Density | High Line Density | Low Line Density | High Line Density |
| **Low Frame Rate** | **High Frame Rate** | **High Frame Rate** | **High Frame Rate** |

■ **FIGURE 14-25** Conventional ultrasound acquisitions are acquired as video clips with frame rates that depend on the field of view (FOV), depth of penetration (D), pulse repetition frequency (PRF), and line density (LD—the number of lines over the FOV). **A.** Low frame rate: the baseline situation requires a low PRF because of large D; large FOV for anatomic coverage; and high LD for image quality. Ways to achieve high frame rate are **B.** Increased PRF with lower D (*e.g.*, with higher frequency transducer). **C.** Lower LD to maintain FOV. **D.** Small FOV to maintain LD. ▱ **F. 14-30**

2. **Multi-Line Acquisition** (linear transducer array) (Fig. 14-26)
   a. Transmit: Wide transmit beam with smaller excitation elements insonates a large volume of tissue.
   b. Receive: Groups of adjacent elements receive lines from specific subvolumes to form multiple lines in parallel (parallel beamforming).
   c. Number of parallel lines can be used to increase SNR, increase frame rate, or combination of both.

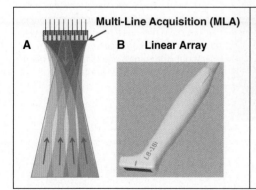

**Multi-Line Acquisition (MLA)**

A    B    **Linear Array**

■ **FIGURE 14-26 A.** Multiline acquisition (MLA) scheme shows a wide transmit beam profile (*orange*) generated by a small aperture excitation of a linear array transducer. The receive beams shown in shades of *blue* are generated in parallel from the single pulse; in this case, 4 lines are acquired. Thus, the image rate in this situation can be increased by 4 or can be used to increase the signal-to-noise ratio. **B.** A "hockey stick" linear array 8–18 MHz transducer has MLA capabilities. MLA can be applied to improve the frame rate but can also be applied to improve the signal-to-noise ratio of the images by averaging consecutive images acquired at higher temporal resolution. Also, a larger FOV can be imaged, where the gain in frame rate can be used to widen the area covered. Frame rates of 250 s$^{-1}$ and higher can be obtained. ▱ **F. 14-31**

3. **Spatial Compounding** (Fig. 14-27)
   a. Several angles (3 to 5) of insonation in consecutive excitations are averaged to produce an image.
   b. Pros: Increased SNR, reduced speckle noise, and enhance boundaries are achieved.
   c. Cons: Loss of temporal resolution, increased spatial blurring.

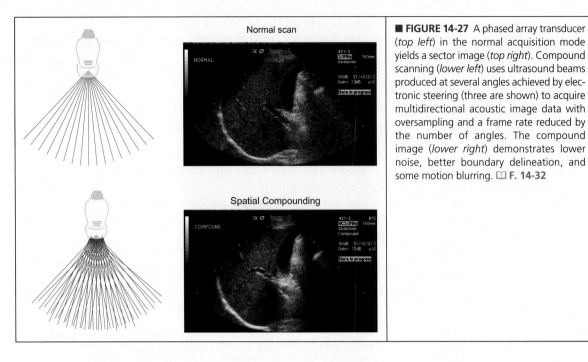

Normal scan

Spatial Compounding

■ **FIGURE 14-27** A phased array transducer (*top left*) in the normal acquisition mode yields a sector image (*top right*). Compound scanning (*lower left*) uses ultrasound beams produced at several angles achieved by electronic steering (three are shown) to acquire multidirectional acoustic image data with oversampling and a frame rate reduced by the number of angles. The compound image (*lower right*) demonstrates lower noise, better boundary delineation, and some motion blurring. **F. 14-32**

### 4. Contrast-Enhanced Ultrasound

   **a.** US contrast agents: gaseous compounds encapsulated in phospholipids of 3 to 5 $\mu$m diameter.

   **b.** Sulfur hexafluoride and perflurobutane are commonly used compounds.

   **c.** Injection of agents concentrate in vascular areas of the anatomy (Fig. 14-28).

   **d.** Acoustic impedance differences of the gas and soft tissue create large US reflections.

   **e.** Pulse-inversion "harmonic" imaging is possible from the nonlinear compressibility of bubbles, which can be used with multifrequency transducers to identify higher-order frequency harmonics of echoes.

   **f.** Destruction of microbubbles occurs with the incident ultrasound pulse.

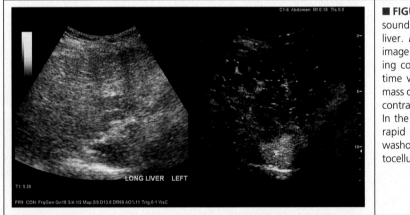

LONG LIVER    LEFT

■ **FIGURE 14-28** Contrast-enhanced ultrasound exam of the left upper lobe of the liver. *Left image* is the grayscale B-mode image and the *right image* is the corresponding contrast-processed image from a real-time video clip sequence. The hypoechoic mass on the gray scale image correlates with contrast uptake on the enhancement image. In the real-time video sequence, there was rapid contrast enhancement followed by washout of the mass, consistent with hepatocellular carcinoma. **F. 14-33**

### 5. Harmonic Imaging

   **a.** Nonlinear propagation of US in tissue produces higher integer frequency harmonics (Fig. 14-29).

      **(i)** Compression travels faster than rarefaction parts of the wave.

      **(ii)** Frequency harmonics build with distance traveled and concentrate in the center of the beam.

   **b.** Image acquisition is typically performed with a low frequency transmit beam (*e.g.*, 2 MHz).

   **c.** During echo reception, the receiver bandwidth is set to acquire the first-order harmonic (*e.g.*, 4 MHz).

   **d.** Outcome is reduced echo clutter for proximal echoes and improved spatial resolution (Fig. 14-30).

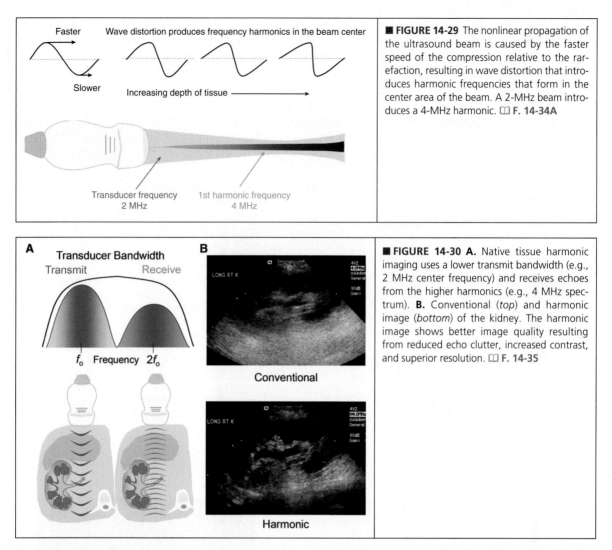

■ **FIGURE 14-29** The nonlinear propagation of the ultrasound beam is caused by the faster speed of the compression relative to the rarefaction, resulting in wave distortion that introduces harmonic frequencies that form in the center area of the beam. A 2-MHz beam introduces a 4-MHz harmonic. ▢ **F. 14-34A**

■ **FIGURE 14-30 A.** Native tissue harmonic imaging uses a lower transmit bandwidth (e.g., 2 MHz center frequency) and receives echoes from the higher harmonics (e.g., 4 MHz spectrum). **B.** Conventional (*top*) and harmonic image (*bottom*) of the kidney. The harmonic image shows better image quality resulting from reduced echo clutter, increased contrast, and superior resolution. ▢ **F. 14-35**

6. **US Elastography**
   a. Useful for analyzing tissue "stiffness" and to differentiate affected from normal tissues.
   b. Principles of elastography based on the tendency of tissues to resist deformation under an applied force.
   c. Measurements of "elastic moduli" include Young's modulus and shear modulus.
      (i) Measurable quantities generated from applied stress (force measured in pressure, kPa) and resultant strain, which manifests as expansion or compression per unit length of the tissue object.
      (ii) Young's modulus results from a normal (90°) stress: $E = \sigma_n/\varepsilon_n$ (stress/strain).
      (iii) Shear modulus results from tangential stress, generating shear waves in a perpendicular direction, where the measurable shear wave speed, $c_s$, is dependent on tissue density, $\rho$, and the stiffness, where stiffer tissues have a higher shear wave speed (see text book for details).
      (iv) The measurable shear modulus is related to Young's modulus as $E = 3\rho c_s^2$.
   d. *Strain elastography* measures displacement of tissues under an applied force (Fig. 14-31).

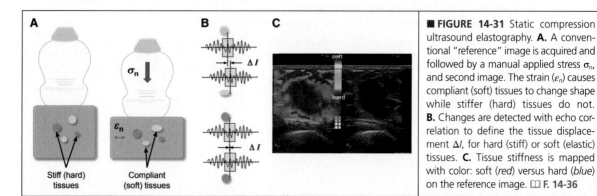

■ **FIGURE 14-31** Static compression ultrasound elastography. **A.** A conventional "reference" image is acquired and followed by a manual applied stress $\sigma_n$, and second image. The strain ($\varepsilon_n$) causes compliant (soft) tissues to change shape while stiffer (hard) tissues do not. **B.** Changes are detected with echo correlation to define the tissue displacement $\Delta l$, for hard (stiff) or soft (elastic) tissues. **C.** Tissue stiffness is mapped with color: soft (*red*) versus hard (*blue*) on the reference image. ▢ **F. 14-36**

e. *Transient shear wave elastography* uses a low-frequency external vibration source to measure the displacement of tissues by correlation of echos from 1D ultrasound measurements at approximately 5 MHz and 1 kHz pulses and estimating the shear wave speed to determine Young modulus.

f. *2D shear wave elastography (2D SWE)* (Figs. 14-32 and 14-33)

(i) Acoustic radiation force impulse (ARFI) excitations generate shear waves.

(ii) Multiple ARFI pulses are focused in a volume of interest to create a cylindrical shear wave cone.

(iii) Perpendicular directed shear waves create particle displacement, measured by high-speed plane wave imaging (greater than 1,000 frames/s) through speckle tracking to estimate the shear wave speed.

g. US elastography is important for evaluating liver, breast, thyroid, kidney, prostate, and lymph node disease.

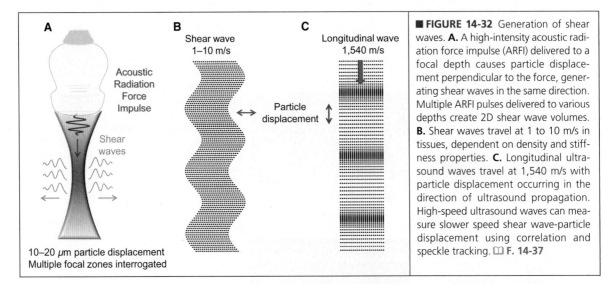

■ **FIGURE 14-32** Generation of shear waves. **A.** A high-intensity acoustic radiation force impulse (ARFI) delivered to a focal depth causes particle displacement perpendicular to the force, generating shear waves in the same direction. Multiple ARFI pulses delivered to various depths create 2D shear wave volumes. **B.** Shear waves travel at 1 to 10 m/s in tissues, dependent on density and stiffness properties. **C.** Longitudinal ultrasound waves travel at 1,540 m/s with particle displacement occurring in the direction of ultrasound propagation. High-speed ultrasound waves can measure slower speed shear wave-particle displacement using correlation and speckle tracking. ⌑ **F. 14-37**

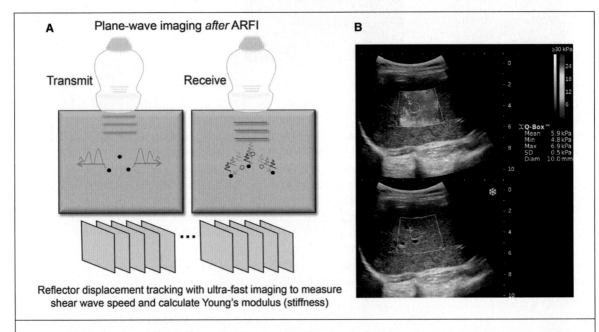

■ **FIGURE 14-33** Two-dimensional shear wave elastography. **A.** After several ARFI excitations are delivered, high frame rate imaging follows and uses plane wave transmit and receive to acquire thousands of frames/s. Displacement of particles is mapped by speckle tracking and corresponds to the local shear wave speed over the tissue volume. This allows the calculation of Young's modulus, a measure of tissue stiffness, in kPa, as a quantitative measure at the same tissue locations (see text). **B.** Example of a 2D-shear wave elastography evaluation of liver stiffness. ⌑ **F. 14-38**

7. **US Biopsy Guidance**
   a. Ultrasound-guided biopsy procedures of suspicious solid masses or signs of abnormal tissue change
   b. Fine needle or core needle biopsy occurs in real-time with excellent needle visibility due to the reflection and scattering of ultrasound.
   c. Common target organs include breast, prostate, thyroid, and abdominopelvic regions.
8. **Intravascular US**
   a. Transducers inside catheters provide an inside-out view of cross-sectional vessel anatomy.
   b. A single transducer with rotating reflector or multielement array transducers are used (Fig. 14-34).
   c. Short range radial images are produced.
   d. 10 to 60 MHz transducer frequency and 15 to 80 kHz PRF can provide 80 to 100 $\mu$m resolution.
   e. Vessel wall morphology, differentiation of plaques (fibrous-fatty-necrotic), and stenosis are performed.

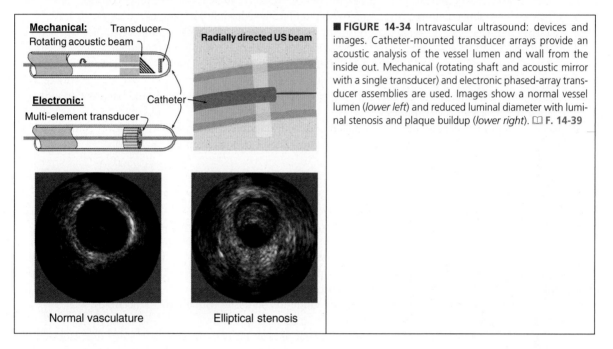

■ **FIGURE 14-34** Intravascular ultrasound: devices and images. Catheter-mounted transducer arrays provide an acoustic analysis of the vessel lumen and wall from the inside out. Mechanical (rotating shaft and acoustic mirror with a single transducer) and electronic phased-array transducer assemblies are used. Images show a normal vessel lumen (*lower left*) and reduced luminal diameter with luminal stenosis and plaque buildup (*lower right*). ▱ **F. 14-39**

9. **Three-Dimensional Imaging**
   a. Created with the acquisition of 2D tomographic B-scan image data over a volume of tissue.
   b. Location of the individual 2D images is determined by using known acquisition geometries.
   c. Volume sampling with a transducer array (Fig. 14-35) provides geometric alignment.

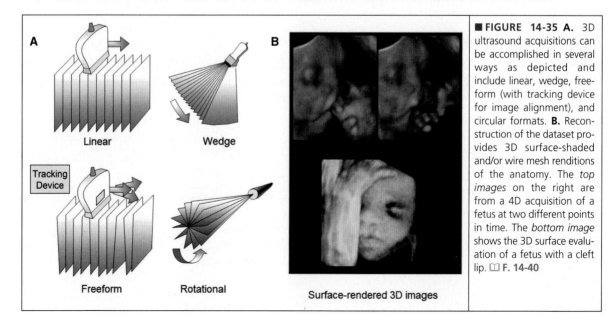

■ **FIGURE 14-35 A.** 3D ultrasound acquisitions can be accomplished in several ways as depicted and include linear, wedge, freeform (with tracking device for image alignment), and circular formats. **B.** Reconstruction of the dataset provides 3D surface-shaded and/or wire mesh renditions of the anatomy. The *top images* on the right are from a 4D acquisition of a fetus at two different points in time. The *bottom image* shows the 3D surface evaluation of a fetus with a cleft lip. ▱ **F. 14-40**

   **d.** Volume surface color rendering is achieved with opacity, lighting, and shading algorithms.

   **e.** 3D image acquisition as a function of time (4D) allows visualization of motion during the scan with real-time mechanical or electronic scanning transducer arrays.

   **f.** Applications of various 3D/4D techniques particularly in obstetric imaging to render features such as organ boundaries and surface features (*e.g.*, normal versus cleft lip).

## 14.7 IMAGE QUALITY, STORAGE, AND MEASUREMENTS

1. **Image Quality**
   - **a.** Dependent on US equipment, transducers, frequency, modes of imaging, positioning skills/protocols.
   - **b.** Often operator dependent, requiring experienced and knowledgeable sonographers.
   - **c.** Measures of image quality: spatial, contrast, and temporal resolution; image uniformity; noise; artifacts.
   - **d.** Spatial resolution includes axial, lateral, and elevational resolution, where axial > lateral > elevational.
   - **e.** Contrast resolution is the ability to discern differences in acoustic impedance assigned gray scale values.
   - **f.** Limits of contrast resolution: insufficient signal strength (transmit gain is too low); inappropriate TGC adjustments; anatomical clutter, excessive electronic noise; transducer malfunction; image artifacts; display calibration; poor viewing conditions.
   - **g.** *Image modifications* include gray scale adjustments with window width and window level controls; image processing, rescanning using "write zoom" to resample a volume with reduced FOV.

2. **Image Storage**
   - **a.** Video clips are now the standard method of acquiring ultrasound data.
   - **b.** Image matrix dimensions are manufacturer-dependent—600 × 800, 649 × 850, 748 × 982, 768 × 1024, 899 × 1442 are typical among many variations, stored with 8 bits per pixel (256 gray levels).
   - **c.** Grayscale uses 8 bits per pixel (256 gray levels); color encoding red-green-blue (RGB) uses 24 bits.
   - **d.** Image compression of video clips is typically lossy, using motion JPEG compression algorithms.
   - **e.** RGB color encoding of Doppler and Color Flow and elastography provides 8-bit data storage.
   - **f.** Ultrasound image storage, even with lossy compression, is significant (see Table 5-2, Pg. 129 of text book).

3. **Distance, Area, and Volume Measurements and Structured Reporting**
   - **a.** Measurements are possible due to the speed of sound in soft tissue with about 1% accuracy.
   - **b.** Distance is based on round-trip time between the pulse and the echo.
   - **c.** A notable example of distance measurement in fetal ultrasound is to measure fetal head diameter and circumference, femur length, and abdominal circumference as indicators of fetal age.
   - **d.** Distance measurements in axial direction are most accurate (better axial resolution along beam travel).
   - **e.** Errors in measurement occur more frequently in the lateral direction and when fatty tissue is present.
   - **f.** Translation of measurement data is aided electronically with the use of *Structured Reports* with templates to allow the automated download into specific fields, ensuring accurate information reporting.

## 14.8 DOPPLER ULTRASOUND

Doppler ultrasound assesses the velocity of moving reflectors, typically blood cells in the vasculature, based upon frequency shifts occurring with the incident pulse and returning echo (Fig. 14-36).

1. **Doppler Frequency Shift**
   - **a.** The *Doppler shift*, $f_D$, is the difference between the incident frequency $f_i$ and reflected frequency $f_r$ from moving objects (blood cells) for *parallel incidence*

$$f_D = f_i - f_r = 2 \times f_i \frac{\text{reflector speed}}{\text{reflector speed} + \text{speed of sound}} = 2 f_0 \frac{v}{c}$$

where $v$ is the velocity of the blood cells, $c$ is the velocity of ultrasound, and $f_0$ is the center frequency.
   - **b.** In the equation, the factor of 2 arises from reflection of US back to the source, simplification in the denominator is because the speed of sound $\gg$ speed of blood and $f_0$ is the same as $f_i$.

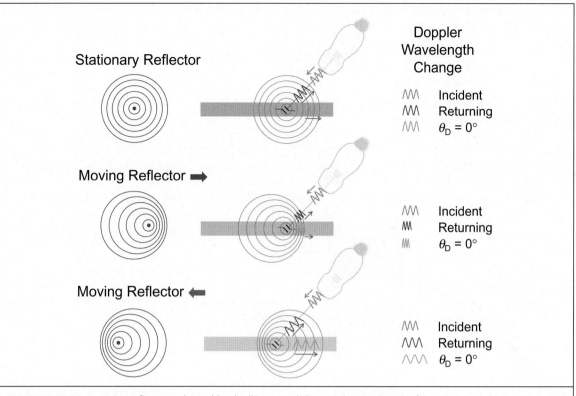

**FIGURE 14-36** A moving reflector such as a blood cell in a vessel changes the wavelength of the returning echo, and thus, the frequency, the degree to which is proportional to the velocity of motion and angle of the echo trajectory. For the reflector moving toward the transducer, the wavelength is shortened, and the frequency is increased (*middle illustration*), while the opposite occurs for the reflector moving away from the transducer (*bottom illustration*). When at an angle to the reflector direction, the measured wavelength (frequency) is not equal to that along the direction of the reflector, except in the case of a stationary reflector, where there is no change in wavelength or frequency (*top illustration*). $\theta_D$ is the Doppler angle. 📖 **F. 14-43**

**c.** Correction for Doppler angle, $\theta_D$, is made from trigonometric considerations (Fig. 14-37) with the modification:

$$f_D = 2f_0 \frac{v}{c} \cos(\theta_D)$$

**d.** The velocity of blood is solved as:

$$v = \frac{f_D}{\cos(\theta_D)} \times \frac{c}{2f_0}$$

where $1/cos(\theta_D)$ converts the Doppler frequency measured at angle $\theta_D$ to the Doppler frequency parallel to the vessel ($\theta_D = 0°$).

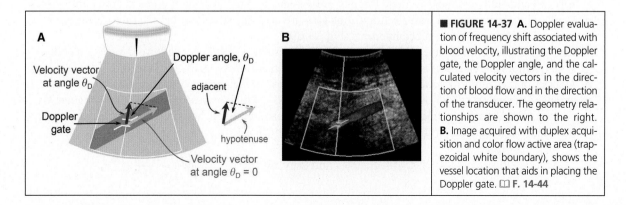

**FIGURE 14-37 A.** Doppler evaluation of frequency shift associated with blood velocity, illustrating the Doppler gate, the Doppler angle, and the calculated velocity vectors in the direction of blood flow and in the direction of the transducer. The geometry relationships are shown to the right. **B.** Image acquired with duplex acquisition and color flow active area (trapezoidal white boundary), shows the vessel location that aids in placing the Doppler gate. 📖 **F. 14-44**

**e.** Doppler shift occurs in the audible range (15 Hz to 20 kHz)—Example: Given: $f_0 = 5$ *MHz*, v = 35 *cm/s*, and $\theta_D = 45°$, calculate the Doppler shift frequency:

$$f_D = 2 \times 5 \times 10^6\,s^{-1} \times \frac{35\,cm\,s^{-1}}{154{,}000\,cm\,s^{-1}} \times \cos(45°) = 1.6 \times 10^3\,s^{-1} = 1.6\,kHz$$

**f.** The *preferred* Doppler angle is between 30° and 60° to minimize errors on the impact of angle estimates.

**2. Continuous Doppler Operation**
  **a.** Uses two transducers, one transmitting and one receiving, with overlapping beam areas (Fig. 14-38).
  **b.** Oscillator produces resonant frequency to drive the transmitting transducer and the demodulator.
  **c.** Receiver amplifies returning wave, mixes with the incident wave, and extracts Doppler shift frequency.
  **d.** Technique suffers from poor depth selectivity and overlying vessel interference.
  **e.** Major advantages are high accuracy due to narrow bandwidth and no aliasing of high-velocity blood.

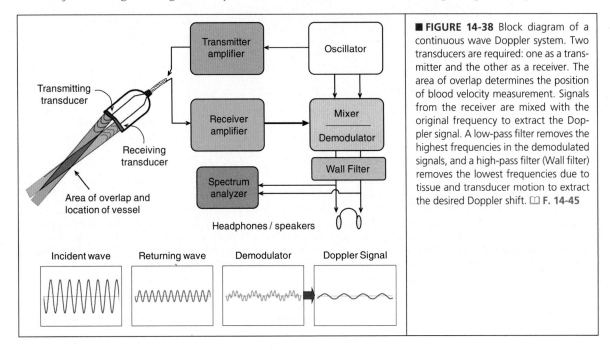

■ **FIGURE 14-38** Block diagram of a continuous wave Doppler system. Two transducers are required: one as a transmitter and the other as a receiver. The area of overlap determines the position of blood velocity measurement. Signals from the receiver are mixed with the original frequency to extract the Doppler signal. A low-pass filter removes the highest frequencies in the demodulated signals, and a high-pass filter (Wall filter) removes the lowest frequencies due to tissue and transducer motion to extract the desired Doppler shift. ⬚ **F. 14-45**

**3. Quadrature Detection**
  **a.** Demodulation measures the magnitude of the Doppler shift signal but does not reveal direction.
  **b.** Quadrature detection is phase sensitive and thus indicates the direction of flow toward or away from the transducers.

**4. Pulsed Doppler Operation**
  **a.** Combines velocity determination with range discrimination of pulse-echo imaging.
  **b.** User positions a "gate" area over the vessel of interest on a B-mode or color flow image (Fig. 14-39).
  **c.** A separate element group within the transducer array has a high Q factor (5 to 25 cycles/pulse) to achieve narrow bandwidth and more accurate Doppler measurements (axial resolution is not as important here).
  **d.** Depth selection is achieved with electronic time gate circuit—only signals within the gate are analyzed.
  **e.** Pulsed Doppler and system subcomponents (Fig. 14-39).
  **f.** Repeated echoes from the range gate are necessary to determine the Doppler shift from moving blood.
  **g.** A sample/hold circuit analyzes each echo train, and a Doppler signal is gradually built (Fig. 14-40).
  **h.** Analysis of the Doppler frequency is determined from phase change between subsequent echoes.
  **i.** Sampling occurs at the PRF of the Doppler transducer, $PRF_D$, which represents the sampling frequency
  **j.** Nyquist sampling theorem requires two samples of the maximum frequency shift, thus the maximum Doppler shift, $f_{Dmax}$, correlates with the maximum velocity of the blood, $v_{max}$:

$$f_{Dmax} = \frac{PRF_D}{2} = 2f_0 \frac{v_{max}}{c} \cos(\theta_D) \text{ and solving for } v_{max} = \frac{c}{4} \times \frac{PRF_D}{f_0 \cos(\theta_D)}$$

  **k.** To reduce or eliminate aliasing: increase $PRF_D$ (this is limited by range); increase Doppler angle $\theta_D$; or use a lower transducer frequency, $f_0$

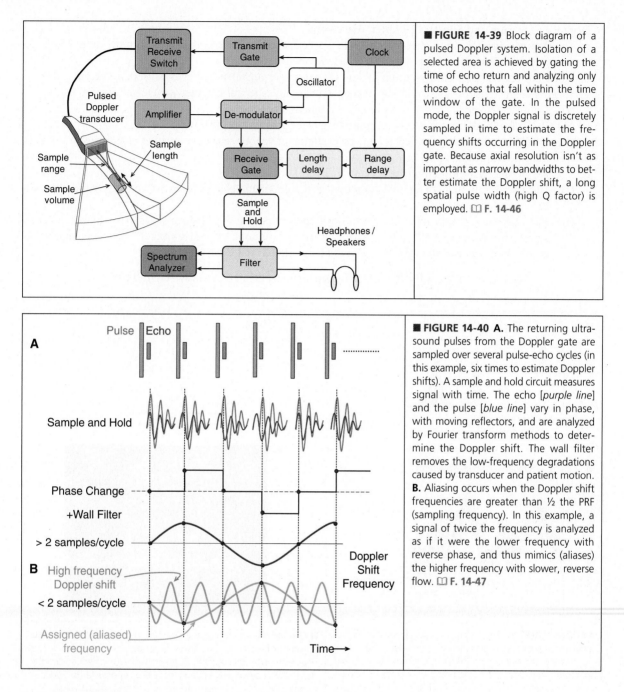

■ **FIGURE 14-39** Block diagram of a pulsed Doppler system. Isolation of a selected area is achieved by gating the time of echo return and analyzing only those echoes that fall within the time window of the gate. In the pulsed mode, the Doppler signal is discretely sampled in time to estimate the frequency shifts occurring in the Doppler gate. Because axial resolution isn't as important as narrow bandwidths to better estimate the Doppler shift, a long spatial pulse width (high Q factor) is employed. 📖 **F. 14-46**

■ **FIGURE 14-40 A.** The returning ultrasound pulses from the Doppler gate are sampled over several pulse-echo cycles (in this example, six times to estimate Doppler shifts). A sample and hold circuit measures signal with time. The echo [*purple line*] and the pulse [*blue line*] vary in phase, with moving reflectors, and are analyzed by Fourier transform methods to determine the Doppler shift. The wall filter removes the low-frequency degradations caused by transducer and patient motion. **B.** Aliasing occurs when the Doppler shift frequencies are greater than ½ the PRF (sampling frequency). In this example, a signal of twice the frequency is analyzed as if it were the lower frequency with reverse phase, and thus mimics (aliases) the higher frequency with slower, reverse flow. 📖 **F. 14-47**

## 5. Duplex Scanning

**a.** The combination of 2D B-mode imaging and pulsed Doppler data acquisition.

**b.** Positioning and sizing of the Doppler gate is aided by the gray scale image.

**c.** Doppler angle is determined from the trajectory of the US pulse and the long axis of the vessel.

**d.** Blood flow is determined from the cross-sectional vessel diameter to calculate area and combine with the velocity estimate.

**e.** Errors: vessel axis might not be within the scanned plane; vessel might be curved or flow altered from the perceived direction; beam-vessel axis (Doppler angle) could be in error, which is very problematic for angles greater than 60° (see Table 14-6 in text book on Pg. 297); Doppler gate could be mispositioned or of inappropriate size—which could affect average velocity measurements due to fast laminar (center of vessel) or slow turbulent (edge of vessel) flows.

**f.** Multigate pulsed Doppler acquisitions—several parallel channels closely spaced across vessel lumen.

## 6. Doppler Spectrum and Spectral Doppler Waveform

**a.** The Doppler signal is represented over a range (spectrum) of frequencies resulting from the range of velocities contained within the Doppler gate at a specific point in time.

**b.** Blood flow can be characterized as blunt laminar, vortex, or turbulent patterns, with periodic pulsatility.

**c.** Spectral characteristics vary with time, characterized by the spectral Doppler waveform (Fig. 14-41).

  **(i)** Doppler frequency (velocity) is plotted as a function of time.

  **(ii)** Pulsatile blood flow takes on the appearance of a choppy sinusoidal wave

  **(iii)** Waveform characteristics depend on vessel arterial or venous selection, location of the gate, and size of the gate within the vessel being analyzed.

**d.** Spectral Doppler waveform interpretation (Fig. 14-42)

  **(i)** Waveform is useful to determine the presence, direction, and characteristics of velocity, pulsatility, and turbulence associated with flow.

  **(ii)** Vascular pulsatile velocity changes can be tracked by spectral waveform analysis: *peak value* is the peak systolic frequency shift "*S*"; *minimum value* is the end diastolic frequency shift "*D*"; timed average value is "*A*"; these are used to assess hemodynamic function as follows:

$$\text{Resistive Index, RI} = (S-D)/S; \text{ Pulsatility Index, PI} = (S-D)/A; S/D \text{ ratio}$$

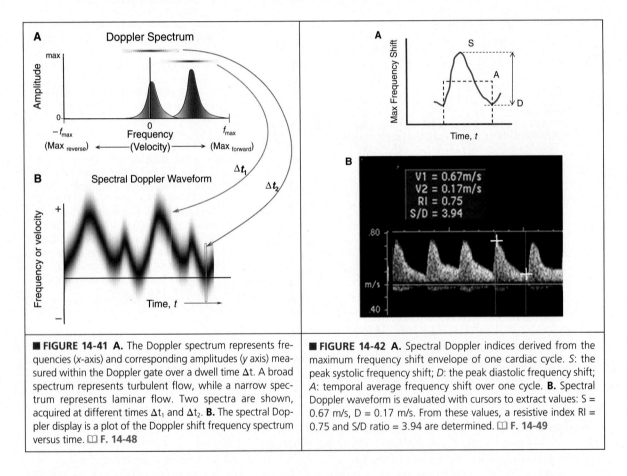

■ **FIGURE 14-41 A.** The Doppler spectrum represents frequencies (*x*-axis) and corresponding amplitudes (*y* axis) measured within the Doppler gate over a dwell time Δt. A broad spectrum represents turbulent flow, while a narrow spectrum represents laminar flow. Two spectra are shown, acquired at different times Δt$_1$ and Δt$_2$. **B.** The spectral Doppler display is a plot of the Doppler shift frequency spectrum versus time. ☐ **F. 14-48**

■ **FIGURE 14-42 A.** Spectral Doppler indices derived from the maximum frequency shift envelope of one cardiac cycle. *S:* the peak systolic frequency shift; *D:* the peak diastolic frequency shift; *A:* temporal average frequency shift over one cycle. **B.** Spectral Doppler waveform is evaluated with cursors to extract values: S = 0.67 m/s, D = 0.17 m/s. From these values, a resistive index RI = 0.75 and S/D ratio = 3.94 are determined. ☐ **F. 14-49**

## 7. Color Flow Imaging

**a.** 2D real-time display of moving blood superimposed on gray scale image (Fig. 14-43).

**b.** Uses a subregion of an image to evaluate velocity in coarse samples of the subregion with phase-shift autocorrelation or time-domain correlation techniques (text book, Pg. 606).

**c.** Velocities and directions are color-encoded (shades of red for blood moving toward the transducer and shades of blue for blood moving away from the transducer are typical color encoding).

**d.** Limitations: *noise and clutter; coarse spatial resolution; aliasing artifacts.*

## 8. Power Doppler

**a.** A signal processing method that relies on the total strength of the Doppler signal and not direction.

**b.** Sensitivity to slow blood flow is greatly enhanced; flash artifacts from patient motion are common.

**c.** Does *not* deliver more power, but processes signals with greater sensitivity by lowering the baseline.

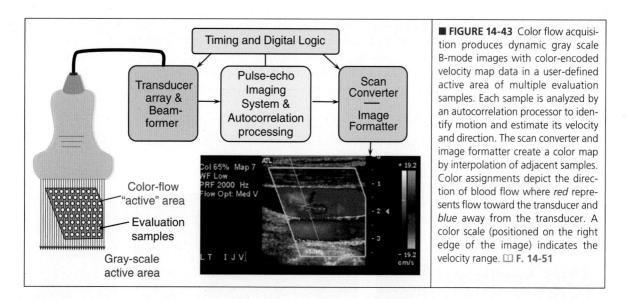

■ **FIGURE 14-43** Color flow acquisition produces dynamic gray scale B-mode images with color-encoded velocity map data in a user-defined active area of multiple evaluation samples. Each sample is analyzed by an autocorrelation processor to identify motion and estimate its velocity and direction. The scan converter and image formatter create a color map by interpolation of adjacent samples. Color assignments depict the direction of blood flow where *red* represents flow toward the transducer and *blue* away from the transducer. A color scale (positioned on the right edge of the image) indicates the velocity range. 📖 **F. 14-51**

## 14.9  ULTRASOUND ARTIFACTS

Most artifacts arise from violations of assumptions in the creation of the ultrasound image (Text book, Pg. 607–608).

1. **Refraction**
   a. Change in the direction of the transmitted ultrasound pulse at nonnormal incidence of a boundary
   b. Caused by a change in the speed of sound, resulting in a change in wavelength (frequency is constant)
   c. Misplaced anatomy or shadowing are the common results (Fig. 14-44)
2. **Shadowing and Enhancement** (Fig. 14-45)
   a. *Shadowing* occurs with objects of high attenuation or reflection and refraction.
   b. *Enhancement* or *through transmission* is the distal enhancement of gray scale beyond areas of low attenuation such as fluid-filled cysts and the bladder.

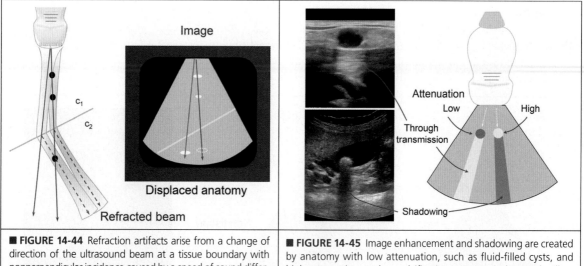

■ **FIGURE 14-44** Refraction artifacts arise from a change of direction of the ultrasound beam at a tissue boundary with nonperpendicular incidence caused by a speed of sound difference and a change in wavelength. *Left:* anatomy is displaced as the ultrasound beam sweeps over the field of view. *Right:* the actual colinear structures are incorrectly mapped. 📖 **F. 14-54**

■ **FIGURE 14-45** Image enhancement and shadowing are created by anatomy with low attenuation, such as fluid-filled cysts, and high attenuation, such as calcifications. Anatomical examples illustrate through transmission (enhancement) distal to a cyst and shadowing distal to a gallstone. 📖 **F. 14-55**

3. **Reverberation, Comet Tail, and Ringdown** (Figs. 14-46 and 14-47)
    a. *Reverberation*: Multiple echoes generated between highly reflective and parallel structures
    b. *Comet tail*: A form of reverberation between two closely spaced reflectors in the direction of the beam
    c. *Ringdown*: Arise from resonant vibrations within fluid trapped between a tetrahedron of air bubbles

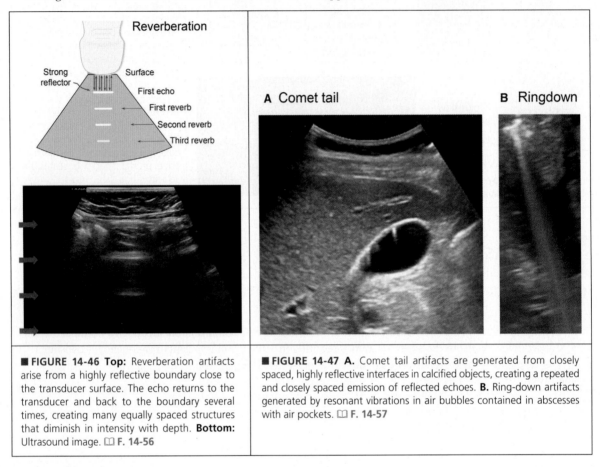

■ **FIGURE 14-46 Top:** Reverberation artifacts arise from a highly reflective boundary close to the transducer surface. The echo returns to the transducer and back to the boundary several times, creating many equally spaced structures that diminish in intensity with depth. **Bottom:** Ultrasound image. 📖 **F. 14-56**

■ **FIGURE 14-47 A.** Comet tail artifacts are generated from closely spaced, highly reflective interfaces in calcified objects, creating a repeated and closely spaced emission of reflected echoes. **B.** Ring-down artifacts generated by resonant vibrations in air bubbles contained in abscesses with air pockets. 📖 **F. 14-57**

4. **Speed Displacement**
    a. Caused by the lower speed of US in fatty tissue (1,450 m/s).
    b. Anatomical borders are displaced distally when US interacts in fatty tissues; for fatty replaced liver, soft tissue structures are displaced proximally (Fig. 14-48).
    c. Presence of fat also reduces distance accuracy measurements.

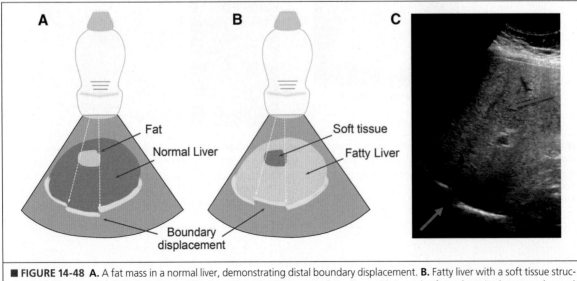

■ **FIGURE 14-48 A.** A fat mass in a normal liver, demonstrating distal boundary displacement. **B.** Fatty liver with a soft tissue structure, causing a proximal displacement of the boundary. **C.** Ultrasound of the liver with irregular fatty deposits (*upper red arrow*) and resultant distal displacement of the diaphragm due to the slower speed of sound in fat (*lower red arrow*). 📖 **F. 14-58**

### 5. Mirror Image and Multipath Reflection (Fig. 14-49)

**a.** US beam encounters a highly reflective nonperpendicular or curved boundary such as the diaphragm.

**b.** Redirected beam encounters reflector to produce echoes reflected along the same path to transducer.

**c.** Later echoes of the specular reflector of the redirected beam (double reflection) arrive at a later time.

**d.** Objects appear beyond the reflector as a mirror image.

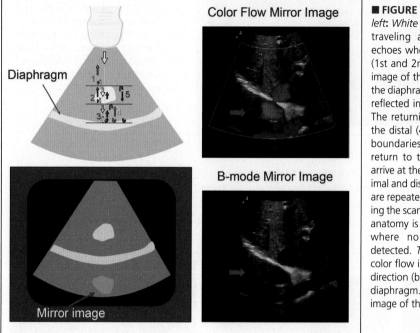

■ **FIGURE 14-49** Mirror image artifact. *Top left:* *White arrows* depict the ultrasound pulse traveling along the dashed path creating echoes when interacting at tissue boundaries (1st and 2nd echoes) generating the acoustic image of the anatomy in the normal mode. At the diaphragm, a large fraction of ultrasound is reflected indicated as a *red arrow* (3rd echo). The returning energy generates echoes from the distal (4th echo) and proximal (5th echo) boundaries of the anatomy. These echoes return to the diaphragm, are reflected, and arrive at the transducer later in time with proximal and distal boundaries reversed. The events are repeated along each ultrasound A-line during the scan. *Bottom left:* A mirror image of the anatomy is generated distal to the diaphragm where no ultrasound signals should be detected. *Top right:* Mirror image artifact of color flow image shows reversal of blood flow direction (blue to red) on opposite sides of the diaphragm. *Bottom right:* B-mode gray scale image of the mirror image artifact. ⌑ **F. 14-59**

### 6. Side Lobes and Grating Lobes

**a.** *Side lobes:* Energy outside of the main beam arises from width and height expansion of transducer elements, which travel adjacent to the main beam; *pseudo-sludge* is a common outcome (Fig. 14-50)

**b.** *Grating lobes:* energy released at wide angles relative to the main beam (see Fig. 14-14 in this chapter)

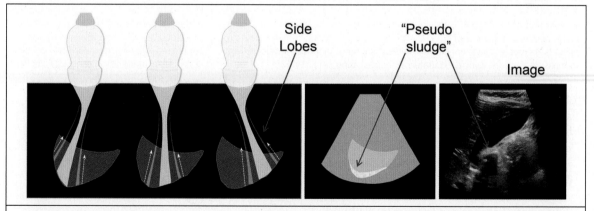

■ **FIGURE 14-50** Common side lobe artifacts are manifested when imaging curved hypoechoic structures such as the gallbladder, where the side lobe energy echoes adjacent to the beam are integrated within the beam. The example demonstrates artifactual "pseudo-sludge" in the gallbladder that can be ameliorated by scanning at a different angle. ⌑ **F. 14-60**

### 7. Ambiguity

**a.** Range ambiguity occurs with very high PRF that decreases the PRP as well as time to listen for echoes.

**b.** Returning echoes at greater depth are detected after the next pulse excitation and mismapped proximally.

**c.** Artifacts are most easily identified in regions of low attenuation such as cysts.

**d.** Decreasing PRF can reduce artifacts at the expense of reduced image quality.

**e.** Higher transducer frequency will reduce penetration depth, allowing higher PRF.

**8. Twinkling Artifact**

    **a.** In the presence of a calculus, occurs with color flow imaging, represented as a mixture of colors caused by narrowband ringing from the small reflectors (Fig. 14-51)

    **b.** May be used to identify small renal stones and differentiate echogenic foci from calcifications

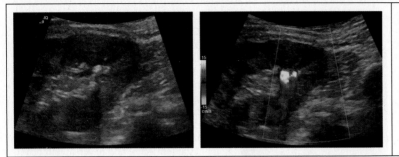

■ **FIGURE 14-51** *Left*: B-mode longitudinal image of the left kidney with a high-attenuation object and distal shadowing. *Right*: Color flow image with an obvious multicolor "twinkle" related to the object, due to ultrasound beam interactions with the calcified structure and associated narrow-band ringing. ▥ **F. 14-61**

**9. Doppler Spectrum and Color Flow Artifacts**

    **a.** Insufficient sampling of Doppler shift frequencies cause signal aliasing (not meeting Nyquist sampling).

    **b.** Higher frequencies "wrap around" and manifest as reverse flow from the Nyquist to lower frequencies.

    **c.** Doppler spectral waveforms with aliasing—and higher PRF to eliminate (Fig. 14-52).

    **d.** Alternate method to avoid aliasing is to adjust baseline for more sampling in the high-velocity direction.

    **e.** Aliasing in color flow acquisition with a high-velocity stenosis jet shows color reversal (Fig. 14-53).

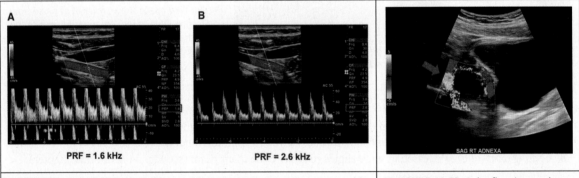

PRF = 1.6 kHz    PRF = 2.6 kHz    SAG RT ADNEXA

■ **FIGURE 14-52 A.** Aliasing in the Doppler spectral display is demonstrated by wraparound of the high-velocity signals (lower traces in the image). The Doppler pulse repetition frequency of 1.6 kHz was insufficient to provide an adequate sampling. **B.** A Doppler pulse repetition frequency of 2.6 kHz extends the velocity range to measure the peak velocity accurately without aliasing. ▥ **F. 14-62**

■ **FIGURE 14-53** Color flow image shows artifactual reverse blood flow in the center of a blood vessel of high velocity (*red arrow*: turquoise—see velocity color scale on the left) from insufficient sampling. ▥ **F. 14-63**

**10. BeamWidth and Slice Thickness**

    **a.** Artifacts result from the variable width of the beam diameter with depth (Fig. 14-64 textbook).

    **b.** Objects proximal and distal to the focal zone will have lateral "blurring."

    **c.** Solutions to this artifact are to implement multiple lateral focal zones, but downsides are lower temporal resolution due to requirements for multiple repeat acquisitions with different beamformer timing.

    **d.** Slice thickness is similarly affected—solutions are implementing 1.5 D and 2 D arrays (see Pg. 572, Fig. 14-23 in textbook).

**11. Equipment Settings and Equipment Failures**

    **a.** User-adjustable settings such as TGC can lead to artifactual image appearance (Fig. 14-65 textbook).

    **b.** Wall filter settings, when set too high, can lead to loss of spectral Doppler information.

    **c.** Loss of transducer element functionality (dropout) has an impact on image rendering that is mitigated by multielement transducers and acquisition techniques such as compound scanning.

    **d.** Focal zone banding occurs with multiple lateral focal zones when the timing is uncalibrated (Fig. 14-54).

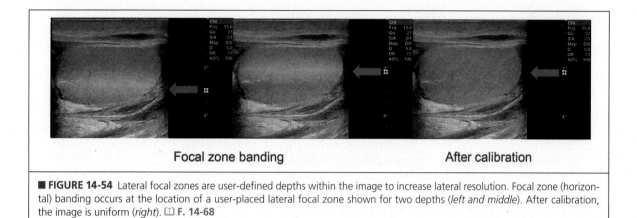

Focal zone banding                    After calibration

■ **FIGURE 14-54** Lateral focal zones are user-defined depths within the image to increase lateral resolution. Focal zone (horizontal) banding occurs at the location of a user-placed lateral focal zone shown for two depths (*left and middle*). After calibration, the image is uniform (*right*). ⬚ **F. 14-68**

### 12. Summary, Artifacts

Violations of the underlying assumptions used for acquiring and creating an ultrasound image, or improper equipment settings, or malfunctioning equipment lead to image artifacts. Some artifacts can reveal important information regarding tissue structure and composition that can assist in diagnosis. Periodic quality control is an important and useful activity to identify component failure effects on the ultrasound images and to direct repair and replacement by service engineers to maintain optimal image quality.

## 14.10  ULTRASOUND SYSTEM PERFORMANCE AND QUALITY ASSURANCE

1. Ultrasound quality control—acceptance testing
   a. Testing procedures, frequency of testing, and passing criteria are important components of a QC program.
   b. Initial acceptance testing: verifies system performance specifications and sets baseline values for QC.
      (i)  All transducers evaluated and baseline performance documented
   c. Periodic QC testing should be adjusted to the probability of finding instabilities or maladjustments.
   d. US phantom description (Fig. 14-55A).

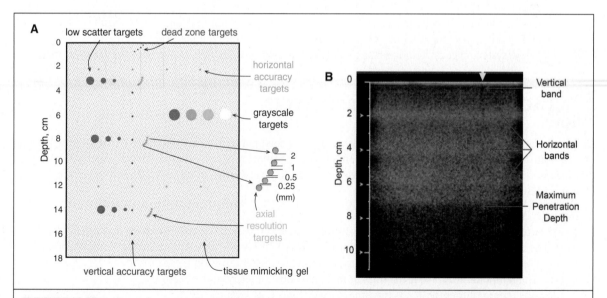

■ **FIGURE 14-55 A.** General purpose ultrasound quality assurance phantoms are composed of several scanning modules. System resolution targets (axial and lateral), dead zone depth, vertical and horizontal distance accuracy targets, contrast resolution (grayscale targets), and low scatter targets positioned at several depths (to determine penetration depths) are placed in a tissue-mimicking (acoustic scattering) gel. ⬚ **F. 14-69A. B.** The system uniformity module elucidates possible problems with image uniformity. Shown in this figure is a multifocal zone banding problem indicated by the horizontal bands. A transducer element dropout is indicated by the vertical band at the surface of the phantom, and the maximum penetration depth is identified with a dropoff of image intensity. ⬚ **F. 14-69C**

e. Spatial resolution, contrast resolution, and distance accuracy in tissue equivalent phantom.
   (i)   Axial resolution: resolve high-contrast targets separated by 2, 1, 0.5, and 0.25 mm at 3 depths
   (ii)  Lateral resolution: measuring lateral spread of high-contrast targets as a function of depth
   (iii) Contrast resolution: gray scale objects of low and high attenuation
   (iv)  Distance measurements: vertical targets of known distance—within 5% of known distance
f. Dead-zone (time that transducer can't receive echoes after excitation)—is determined with first high-contrast object observable at the phantom surface.
g. Elevational resolution and partial volume effects (measured by spherical phantom, see textbook Fig. 14-69B).
h. Uniformity and penetration depth—measured with uniformity phantom (Fig. 14-55B).
   (i)   Uniform response expected up to penetration depth of transducer array.
   (ii)  Power and gain settings are varied for test evaluation to identify operational limits.
i. Display monitor contrast and brightness settings—should conform to DICOM Grayscale Standard Display Function, part 14 (see Chapter 5 on display calibration).
j. Recommended QC tests and frequency (Table 14-3).

**TABLE 14-3 RECOMMENDED ROUTINE QC TESTS FOR AN ULTRASOUND PROGRAM**

| TEST (GRAY SCALE IMAGING MODE) FOR EACH SCANNER | FREQUENCY |
| --- | --- |
| System sensitivity and/or depth penetration capability | Semiannually |
| Image uniformity and artifact survey | Semiannually |
| Low-contrast detectability (optional) | Semiannually |
| Assurance of electrical and mechanical safety | Semiannually |
| Geometric accuracy (mechanically scanned transducers in the mechanically scanned direction) | Semiannually |
| Horizontal and vertical distance accuracy | At acceptance |
| Transducer ports/transducers (of different scan format) | Ongoing basis |
| Ultrasound scanner electronic image display performance | Semiannually |

📖 T. 14-7

2. Doppler Performance Measurements
   a. Dedicated flow phantoms assess the accuracy of blood velocity measurements.
   b. Blood mimicking fluids is pushed through tubes with calibrated pumps.
   c. Tests include maximum penetration depth at which flow can be measured; alignment of sample volume with duplex B-mode image, the accuracy of velocity measurements, and volume flow.
   d. Color flow system checks include sensitivity and alignment of color flow image with the B-mode image.

## 14.11 ACOUSTIC POWER AND BIOEFFECTS

Ultrasound acoustic power levels are strongly dependent on the operational characteristics of the system, including the transmit power, PRF, transducer frequency, and operation mode. Biological effects (bioeffects) are predominately related to the heating of tissues caused by high-intensity levels of ultrasound used to enhance image quality and functionality.

1. **Intensity Measures of Pulsed Ultrasound**
   a. Pressure measurements made with a hydrophone and show peak pulse compressions and rarefactions.
   b. Acoustic intensity is calculated as the square of pressure amplitude for a known acoustic impedance.
   c. In pulsed mode, instantaneous US intensity varies with time and position (Fig. 14-56).
      (i)   The temporal peak, $I_{TP}$, is the highest instantaneous intensity in the beam.
      (ii)  The temporal average, $I_{TA}$, is the time-averaged intensity over the PRP.
      (iii) The pulse average, $I_{PA}$, is the average intensity of the pulse.
      (iv)  The spatial peak, $I_{SP}$, is the highest intensity spatially in the beam.
      (v)   The spatial average, $I_{SA}$, is the average intensity over the beam area.

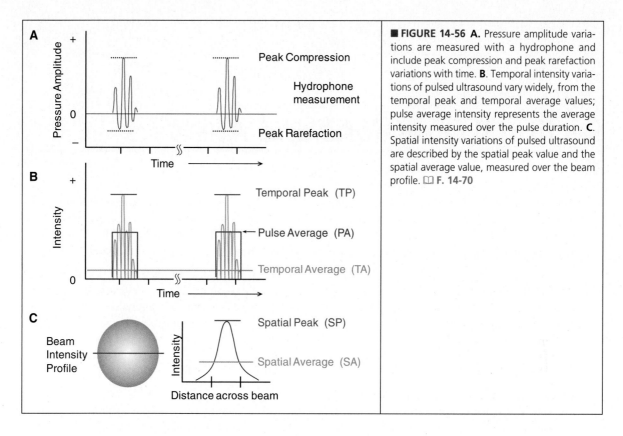

■ **FIGURE 14-56 A.** Pressure amplitude variations are measured with a hydrophone and include peak compression and peak rarefaction variations with time. **B.** Temporal intensity variations of pulsed ultrasound vary widely, from the temporal peak and temporal average values; pulse average intensity represents the average intensity measured over the pulse duration. **C.** Spatial intensity variations of pulsed ultrasound are described by the spatial peak value and the spatial average value, measured over the beam profile. ▢ **F. 14-70**

**d.** Combined temporal and spatial intensity measures are pertinent to energy deposition–acoustic power contained in the ultrasound beam (watts), averaged over at least one PRP and divided by the beam area is the spatial average–temporal average intensity $I_{SATA}$; other meaningful measures from $I_{SATA}$:

    **(i)** *The spatial average–pulse average intensity,* $I_{SAPA} = I_{SATA}/duty\ cycle,\ where\ I_{PA} = I_{TA}/duty\ cycle$

    **(ii)** The spatial peak–temporal average intensity, $I_{SPTA} = I_{SATA} \times [I_{SP}/I_{SA}]$, indicator of *thermal* US effects

    **(iii)** The spatial peak–pulse average intensity, $I_{SPPA} = I_{SATA} \times [I_{SP}/I_{SA}]/duty\ cycle$, indicator of *cavitation*

**e.** Thermal index, *TI*

    **(i)** The ratio of the acoustical power to the power required to raise tissue in the beam area by 1°C.

    **(ii)** Other thermal measures: *TIS* (*S* for soft tissue), *TIB* (*B* for bone), and *TIC* (*C* for cranial bone)—measures increased heat buildup at the bone to soft tissue interfaces (important for obstetrics).

    **(iii)** Doppler US has higher *TI* indices.

    **(iv)** *TI* is associated with $I_{SPTA}$ measure of intensity.

**f.** Mechanical index, *MI*

    **(i)** A value that estimates the likelihood of cavitation by the ultrasound beam.

    **(ii)** *MI* is directly proportional to the peak rarefactional (negative) pressure and inversely proportional to the square root of the ultrasound frequency (in *MHz*).

    **(iii)** *MI* values are associated with the $I_{SPPA}$ measure of intensity.

**2. Biological Mechanisms and Effects**

  **a.** At high intensities, ultrasound can cause biological effects by thermal and mechanical mechanisms.

  **b.** *Thermal effects* are dependent on the rate of heat deposition in a volume of the body and on how fast the heat is removed by blood flow and other means of heat conduction—*TI* is the useful value to monitor.

  **c.** *Nonthermal effects* include mechanical movement of the particles of the medium due to radiation pressure and acoustic streaming.

  **d.** *Cavitation*—sonically generated activity of highly compressible bodies.

    **(i)** *MI* is an estimate for producing cavitation.

    **(ii)** *Stable cavitation* refers to pulsation of persistent bubbles in the tissue at low to medium frequencies.

    **(iii)** *Transient cavitation*, related to the peak rarefactional pressure, can cause nonlinear bubble collapse and the formation of free radicals.

  **e.** Biological effects of US have been demonstrated at higher US power levels and longer duration.

  **f.** No bioeffects have been shown for $I_{SPTA}$ below 100 mW/cm² —for typical US imaging levels.

# Section II Questions and Answers

1. A change in which of the following ultrasound parameters is the cause of refraction at a tissue boundary?
   A. Absorption
   B. Speed
   C. Frequency
   D. Scatter

2. What is the definition of pulse repetition frequency?
   A. Number of multi-hertz bandwidths
   B. Number of cycles in the pulse
   C. Number of transducer excitations per unit time
   D. Number of A lines per image sector

3. What determines the resonance frequency of an ultrasonic transducer?
   A. Thickness of the piezoelectric crystal
   B. Frequency of the applied voltage pulse
   C. Epoxy material surrounding the electrodes
   D. Curie temperature of manufacturing process
   E. Backing block absorption and attenuation

4. Of the following tissues, which has the largest attenuation coefficient (decibels/cm)?
   A. Liver
   B. Fat
   C. Blood
   D. Skull bone

5. Which one of the following US system performance variables determines the maximum depth of visualization?
   A. Axial resolution
   B. Distance accuracy
   C. Image uniformity
   D. System sensitivity

6. In native tissue harmonic imaging, what characteristic of the returning echoes enhances image quality?
   A. Higher frequency
   B. Higher speed
   C. Higher spatial pulse length
   D. Higher acoustic impedance

7. Which combination of ultrasound power deposition descriptors indicates the thermal heating of tissues?
   A. SPTP (spatial peak temporal peak)
   B. SPTA (spatial peak temporal average)
   C. SATP (spatial average temporal peak)
   D. SPPA (spatial peak pulse average)
   E. SATA (spatial average temporal average)

8. Which ultrasound resolution component is unaffected by the depth of beam propagation?
   A. Temporal
   B. Lateral
   C. Elevational
   D. Axial

9. What is the primary parameter that determines the ultrasound reflection coefficient at a boundary interface between two materials?
   A. Acoustic impedance
   B. Speed of sound
   C. Tissue density
   D. Elastic variability
   E. Compressibility

10. Color flow imaging is based upon a change in which of the following parameters?
    A. Tissue density
    B. Frequency
    C. Speed
    D. Acoustic impedance

11. Which of the following factors limits the maximum PRF for an ultrasound imaging system?
    A. Depth of penetration
    B. Movement of the object
    C. Scan converter bandwidth
    D. Production of aliased signals

12. When an ultrasound pulse interacts with a moving object that is moving toward the transducer, what happens to the ultrasound frequency of the returning echo?
    A. Increases
    B. Decreases
    C. Remains the same

13. Decreasing the ultrasound pulse length by reducing the "Q" factor will most likely result in an improvement of which aspect of image resolution?
    A. Axial
    B. Lateral
    C. Elevational
    D. Azimuthal

14. When an ultrasound beam goes into a medium of high acoustic impedance from low acoustic impedance, what happens to the frequency of the beam?
    A. Increases
    B. Decreases
    C. Stays the same

15. Increasing which of the following parameters will increase acoustic exposure to the patient?
    A. Frame averaging
    B. TGC settings
    C. Receiver gain
    D. Transmit gain
    E. Noise threshold

16. Of the following choices, what parameter can the operator increase to minimize the possibility of aliasing in blood velocity determinations?
    A. Doppler angle
    B. Noise rejection
    C. Time gain compensation
    D. Transmit power
    E. Wall filter threshold

17. When an Ultrasound system is configured for M-mode acquisition, what is being displayed?
    A. Multiple compound angles
    B. Extended field of view of B-mode image
    C. Moving anatomy as a function of time
    D. Metastable harmonic frequencies
    E. Frequency distribution of spectral blood flow

18. If the number of ultrasound scan lines in a real-time frame is doubled, which of the following is improved?
    A. Axial resolution
    B. Lateral resolution
    C. Sensitivity
    D. Temporal resolution
    E. Elevational resolution

19. Of the following, what is the most likely benefit of spatial compounding compared with conventional B-mode imaging?
    A. Faster frame rate
    B. Improved dynamic range
    C. Increased maximum depth of penetration
    D. Reduced speckle and clutter artifacts

20. An ultrasound pulse that travels a distance equal to the half-value tissue thickness has lost an intensity corresponding to how many dB?
    A. −1          C. −10
    B. −3          D. −30

21. What material in the ultrasound transducer contributes to the efficient coupling of ultrasound from the piezoelectric elements to the skin?
    A. Backing material
    B. Electrical insulator
    C. Matching layer
    D. Radiofrequency shield
    E. Transmit crystal

22. What is the chief mechanism related to the MI indicator in an ultrasound system?
    A. Acoustic streaming at tissue boundaries
    B. Cavitation during rarefaction
    C. Heating effects in a tissue volume
    D. Piezoelectric disruption
    E. Side-lobe energy dissipation

23. Which of the following is most likely to occur when switching to a higher frequency operation of a multihertz transducer?
    A. Increased speed of sound
    B. Increased wavelength
    C. Increased maximum depth of penetration
    D. Increased attenuation

24. When the ultrasound beam encounters fatty tissue surrounded by soft tissue with normal incidence, in which direction does displacement of the tissue boundary occur?
    A. Distal          C. Medial
    B. Lateral          D. Proximal

25. For a 10-MHz ultrasound beam in the near field, what characteristic of a tissue boundary at normal incidence results in diffusion and loss of the returning echo?
    A. Nonspecular
    B. Impedance mismatch
    C. Reverberation
    D. Through transmission

26. Which electronic component steers and focuses the ultrasound in a phased array transducer?
    A. Pulser
    B. Transmitter
    C. Receiver
    D. Beamformer
    E. Scan converter

27. Which of the following is an advantage of Power Doppler relative to spectral Doppler?
    A. Provides accurate measurement of flow velocity
    B. Is unaffected by patient motion
    C. Allows detection of slow flow
    D. Can discriminate direction of blood flow

28. What mode of ultrasound operation is being used when the twinkling artifact appears?
    A. B mode
    B. Doppler
    C. M-mode
    D. Harmonic
    E. Color flow

# Answers

1. **B** Refraction in ultrasound is chiefly dependent on the change in speed of sound (velocity) of two tissues at a boundary, as the frequency of the pulse does not change. This causes a change in the wavelength of the ultrasound, which in turn causes a change in the direction at the boundary. Speed is an amplitude quantity; velocity is a vector, with amplitude and direction. *(Pg. 555)*

2. **C** Definition of PRF. The unit of time is per second, and the typical PRF is in kHz (1,000 pulses/s). Other distractors describe US operational details. *(Pg. 575)*

3. **A** The transducer crystal resonates in the thickness mode, where the emitted wavelength is equal to twice the crystal thickness, or crystal thickness = $\lambda/2$. The frequency is selected by choosing the crystal thickness: higher frequency is attained with a thinner crystal. *(Pg. 560, Fig. 14-8)*

4. **D** Bone has a large difference in acoustic impedance relative to soft tissue and therefore attenuates the ultrasound beam greater than the other tissues listed. An outcome is shadowing distal to the bone (*e.g.*, calcifications) causing a shadowing artifact. *(Pg. 557, Table 14-4)*

5. **D** The system sensitivity determines the maximum depth of useful US beam penetration and is mainly determined by the transmit gain (also known as transmit power). Other parameters (gain compensation) can also impact the depth as visualized on the system monitor. *(Pg. 619–621, Table 14-7)*

6. **A** Native tissue harmonic imaging arises as a result of the compressional part of the ultrasound wave traveling faster than the rarefactional part of the wave, introducing "harmonics," which are integer multiples of the carrier ultrasound frequencies. The higher harmonic frequencies build with distance and are chiefly located in the center area of the beam. In order to effectively use the harmonic components of the returning echoes, a broadband transducer with the ability to transmit lower frequencies (*e.g.*, 2 MHz) and receive higher frequencies (*e.g.*, 4 MHz) is necessary. The benefits of native tissue harmonic imaging include improved resolution (shorter wavelength of the received echoes) and removal of low-frequency echoes from proximal interfaces, which improves contrast resolution. *(Pg. 585–586)*

7. **B** Thermal heating mechanisms are dependent on the temporal average of energy deposition. The thermal index, TI, is the "real-time" estimate of ultrasound thermal effects, indicating the ratio of the acoustic power produced by the transducer to the power required to raise the tissue in the beam area by 1°C. Operationally, this is dependent on the spatial peak temporal average (SPTA) intensity. *(Pg. 624)*

8. **D** Axial resolution is dependent on the spatial pulse length (SPL), which is dependent on the transducer frequency and transducer Q factor (related to the damping of the transducer vibration). It is therefore independent of depth. Lateral and elevational (slice thickness) resolution change considerably with depth and can be controlled by beamformer electronics. Axial resolution is better (higher detail) than lateral or elevational resolution by a factor of 2 to 3 ×. *(Pg. 569–570, Fig. 14-20)*

9. **A** The difference in acoustic impedance at normal incidence gives rise to the returning echoes used in the ultrasound image formation process. *(Pg. 554–570, Eq 14-4)*

10. **B** Color flow imaging (also known as Color Doppler imaging) detects the frequency changes caused by moving tissues (chiefly blood cell reflectors in moving blood). This is achieved over a subarea of the B-mode image and using time-correlation or cross-correlation algorithms to detect the change. An average velocity is estimated along with the direction toward or away from the transducer. Colors encode the direction toward (typically red) or away (typically blue) from the transducer. *(Pg. 604–606, Fig. 14-51)*

11.  **A**  The maximum pulse repetition frequency (PRF) is limited by the time that must be spent listening for echoes (PRP), which is inversely equal to the PRF. Thus, as the PRF increases, the PRP shrinks. If insufficient time is allocated to the PRP, echoes at depth will still be traveling to the transducer during the time the next pulse is created, leading to an ambiguity of the depth from which the echo was generated. Aliasing in Doppler evaluations is associated with PRF but does not limit the maximum PRF that can be used. *(Pg. 575–576, Fig. 14-25)*

12.  **A**  The returning echo from a moving object such as a blood cell toward the transducer will compress the wavelength. The shorter wavelength results in a higher frequency. *(Pg. 595–596, Fig. 14-43)*

13.  **A**  The "Q" factor is a measure of the frequency "purity" of the ultrasound pulse. Numerically, it is defined as the center operating frequency, $f_0$, divided by the bandwidth, BW, of the ultrasound pulse. By dampening the transducer vibration, the spatial pulse length is reduced, improving axial resolution, but the BW is broadened, thus reducing the Q factor. *(Pg. 560–561)*

14.  **C**  Ultrasound frequency does not change when the medium of propagation has a different speed of sound. The wavelength changes according to c = lf or l = c/f. However, for moving reflectors, the frequency will change. *(Pg. 550–551)*

15.  **D**  The transmit gain is achieved by how much voltage is applied to the transducer, from which the amount of compression and rarefaction (mechanical displacement) is imparted to the tissues. All of the other choices are postprocessing adjustments to improve the image uniformity, noise properties, and gray scale rendition. *(Pg. 573–574; 622)*

16.  **A**  The Doppler shift is dependent on the pulse repetition frequency, the center operating frequency, and *the Doppler angle* for pulse-echo instrumentation. Aliasing occurs when the sampling frequency is less than 2 times the frequency contained in the Doppler signal, which is dependent on the maximum velocity of the blood. Frequency aliasing can be reduced by increasing the PRF (pulse repetition frequency), decreasing the PRP (pulse repetition period), or increasing the Doppler angle to reduce the apparent Doppler shift. This is mathematically described in the following equations by solving for Vmax and determining parameters that can be changed to increase this value. Therefore, increasing PRF, decreasing the transducer operating frequency, or increasing the Doppler angle toward 90° [cos(q) gets smaller approaching 90°] will reduce the measured (apparent) Doppler shift, which is then corrected to the actual Doppler shift. *(Pg. 599–601)*

17.  **C**  M-mode is Motion or Time-Motion mode, which uses an ultrasound beam that is positioned and fixed over a specific anatomy (*e.g.*, valve leaflets). The A-line data are brightness modulated and deflected as a function of time to demonstrate motion. Periodic and a-periodic motion can readily be determined. *(Pg. 579–580, Fig. 14-29)*

18.  **B**  The lateral resolution in real-time imaging is partially a function of the # lines/frame; increasing the number of lines over the FOV decreases the lateral sampling distance and thus improves lateral resolution. *(Pg. 581–582, Fig. 14-30)*

19.  **D**  Spatial compounding is a technique to employ multiple ultrasound beam directions in the insonated volume so that there is a greater possibility of normal incidence to tissue boundaries. This requires multiple passes of the ultrasound beam that reduces the frame rate but improves SNR and boundary detection. The increased averaging reduces speckle and clutter. Dynamic range is unaffected. *(Pg. 583–584, Fig. 14-32)*

20.  **B**  Intensity in dB is given by 10 log ($I_1/I_2$). When $I_1/I_2$ = 0.5, then 10 log (0.5) = −3 dB. Therefore, −3 dB is the loss of intensity resulting from traveling through a half-value thickness of tissue. *(Pg. 557–558, Example 1)*

21.  **C**  The matching layer ensures the best energy transfer from the transducer material to soft tissue (and vice-versa). It is composed of a material with acoustic impedance between that of the skin and the transducer material. It happens that the thickness of the material equal to ¼ wavelength is the most efficient in transferring mechanical energy. *(Pg. 560–561, Fig. 14-9)*

22.  **B**  MI is the mechanical index, an indication that the tissues can be disrupted by high-intensity ultrasound delivery and is chiefly related to the likelihood of cavitation of microbubbles during the rarefaction (lower pressure part of the ultrasound beam). This results in an implosion of the gas in the local area and a release of concentrated energy over a small region with the potential formation of free radicals. It is related to the $I_{SPPA}$ intensity measure for pulsed ultrasound acquisitions. *(Pg. 622–624)*

23. **D**   The relationship of speed of sound, wavelength, and frequency is C = lf. In a specific tissue, C is constant, thus l is inversely related to ƒ, and a higher frequency will result in a shorter wavelength. As the frequency increases, the attenuation exponentially increases, and the maximum depth of penetration decreases. *(Pg. 556–558, Fig. 14-6)*

24. **A**   Since the speed of sound in fat is 1,450 m/s, the ultrasound travels slower, causing the pulse to lag behind an adjacent pulse in soft tissue. This results in boundaries displaced distally compared to ultrasound pulses traveling in soft tissue only. *(Pg. 610–611, Fig. 14-58)*

25. **A**   Higher frequency ultrasound pulses have much shorter wavelengths, resulting in the boundaries of tissues becoming "nonspecular" and rough compared to a similar ultrasound pulse at a lower frequency. This increases the diffusion of the returning intensity of the ultrasound. The other distractors are not associated with diffusion of the returning signal. *(Pg. 556, Fig. 14-5)*

26. **D**   The beamformer is the component of the ultrasound instrumentation that generates electronic delays during transmit/receive for focusing and steering of the beam for a phased array transducer. *(Pg. 573–574, Fig. 14-17)*

27. **C**   Power Doppler uses an adjustment of postprocessing that enhances the sensitivity to motion by eliminating the ability to discriminate the direction of blood flow by color flow (color Doppler) acquisitions. This type of processing is very sensitive to transducer motion and "flash" artifacts. *(Pg. 606–607, Fig. 14-53)*

28. **E**   Twinkling artifacts occur when using color flow imaging, causing a rapidly changing mixture of colors, distal to a strong reflector such as a calculus, caused by changes in frequency due to the wide bandwidth of the initial pulse and the narrow band "ringing" that cause continuing echoes deep to the reflector. Other distractors: A is associated with speed artifact; C is associated with reverberation; D is associated with extreme attenuation; D is not related to artifacts per se. *(Pg. 614–615, Fig. 14-63)*

# Section III Key Equations and Symbols

| QUANTITY | EQUATION | EQ NO./PAGE/COMMENTS |
|---|---|---|
| Speed, frequency, wavelength relationship for ultrasound | $c = \lambda f$ | Eq. 14-1/Pg. 550. |
| Speed of sound relationship to material bulk modulus, $B$ and density | $c = \sqrt{\dfrac{B}{\rho}}$ | Pg. 550 (Eq), Table 14-1, Pg. 551—speed for tissues and materials. Equation indicates that speed of sound is dependent on material stiffness/compressibility |
| Relative pressure and intensity | Relative pressure (dB) $= 20 \log \dfrac{P_1}{P_2}$ <br><br> Relative intensity (dB) $= 10 \log \dfrac{I_1}{I_2}$ | Eqs. 14-2 and 14-3/Pg. 552/Table 14-2, Pg. 553. Relative measure of pressure and intensity measures; Note $I \propto P^2$ |
| Acoustic impedance | $Z = \rho c$ | Pg. 553 and Table 14-1. $Z$ is the product of density and speed, with units of rayls ($kg/(m^2s)$) |
| Reflection coefficient, normal incidence | $R_i = \dfrac{I_r}{I_i} = \left( \dfrac{Z_2 - Z_1}{Z_2 + Z_1} \right)^2$ | Eq. 14-4/Pg. 554—$R_i$ is the fraction of US reflected at a boundary; $1 - R_i = T_i$, the fraction of US transmitted |
| Refraction, nonnormal incidence—described by Snell Law | $\dfrac{\sin \theta_t}{\sin \theta_i} = \dfrac{c_2}{c_1}$ | Pg. 554–555. With speed of sound change, US transmission angle changes across boundary; $\theta_t$ is transmission, $\theta_i$ is incident angle |
| Attenuation of US | 0.5 ($dB/cm$)/MHz | Pg. 556–557—"rule of thumb" for average attenuation of US in tissue; 10 Mz has attenuation of ~5 dB/cm |
| Thickness, $T_{PZT}$, resonant frequency of PZT transducer element | $T_{PZT} = \dfrac{1}{2} \lambda_{PZT} = \dfrac{c_{PZT}}{2f_r}$ | Figure 14-8. $f_r$ is resonant frequency; thus for $c_{PZT}$ = 4 mm/μs, then $T_{PZT}(mm) = 2/f_r$ (MHz); A 4 MHz $f_r$ is created with a 0.5 mm $T_{PZT}$ |
| Transducer element "Q" factor | $Q = \dfrac{f_0}{\text{bandwidth}}$ | Pg. 561. $f_0$ is the center transducer frequency; bandwidth is width of distribution with damping |
| Axial resolution and spatial pulse length (SPL) | Axial resolution = ½ SPL | Figure 14-20, Pg. 570. Axial resolution is function of frequency (inverse wavelength) and damping factor |
| Lateral resolution | ~½ beamwidth | Figure 14-21, Pg. 571. The beamwidth varies with depth, narrow at focus |
| Time, $T$(ms), US travel to depth, $D$ (cm) and return to transducer | $T(\mu s) = 13 \times D(cm)$ <br><br> $D(cm) = 0.077 \times T(\mu s)$ | Pg. 575. These equations are for 2× distance traveled to a depth D |
| Pulse repetition frequency and pulse repetition period | PRF = 1/PRP | Pg. 575. PRF and PRP are inversely equal; PRP(s) is time for echo reception, PRF is #pulses/s |
| Pulse duration and duty cycle | Duty cycle = pulse duration/PRP | Pg. 576. Pulse duration is the length of pulse (1–2 ms); duty cycle is a fraction of PRP (Table 14-5) |
| US frames per second (FPS) | $FPS = \dfrac{77,000 \text{ cm/s}}{N \times D_{max}}$ | Pg. 581. Maximum frame rate as function of $N$, # lines/frame, and max depth (cm), for 1 line/pulse |

*(Continued)*

| QUANTITY | EQUATION | EQ NO./PAGE/COMMENTS |
|---|---|---|
| Tissue stiffness by Young's modulus, *E*, tissue density, r, and shear wave speed $c_s$ | $E = 3\rho c_s^2$ | Pg. 588–589. Measurement of shear wave speed provides estimate of tissue stiffness |
| Doppler frequency shift $f_D$ at an insonation angle $\theta_D$ | $f_D = 2f_0 \dfrac{v}{c} \cos(\theta_D)$ | Eq. 14-5, Pg. 596. $f_0$ is transducer frequency, *v* is blood velocity, *c* is speed of sound, $\theta_D$ is Doppler angle |
| Maximum Doppler shift frequency, $f_{Dmax}$, determined by PRF/2 | $f_{Dmax} = \dfrac{PRF_D}{2} = 2f_0 \dfrac{v_{max}}{c} \cos(\theta_D)$ | Pg. 600. Equation relates PRF to max Doppler shift and max velocity without aliasing according to the Nyquist sampling theorem |

| SYMBOL | QUANTITY | UNITS |
|---|---|---|
| *c* | Speed of sound | *m/s; cm/s; mm/μs* |
| λ | Wavelength | *mm* |
| *f* | Frequency | cycles/second, Hz, kHz, MHz |
| *B* | Bulk modulus | *Newton/m²; kg/m-s²* |
| ρ | Density (of tissue) | *kg/m³* |
| dB | Decibel | unitless |
| P | Pressure | *Newton/m², Pascals (Pa), kPa* |
| I | Intensity | *W/cm², mW/cm²* |
| Z | Acoustic impedance | *rayl—kg/m²s* |
| $\theta_i$, $\theta_r$, $\theta_t$ | Angle of incidence, reflection, transmission | *degrees* |
| $R_I$ | Intensity reflection coefficient | unitless |
| $T_I$ | Intensity transmission coefficient | unitless |
| *m* | Attenuation | *~0.5 dB/(cm-MHz)* |
| HVT | Half value thickness | *cm tissue* |
| Q | Q factor | unitless |
| SPL | Spatial pulse length | *mm* |
| PRF | Pulse repetition frequency | *pulses/s; kHz* |
| PRP | Pulse repetition period | *seconds, s; microseconds, ms* |
| *E* | Young's modulus | *N/m²; kg/m-s²* |
| *G* | Shear modulus | *N/m²; kg/m-s²* |
| *s* | Stress | *N/m²; kPa* |
| *e* | Strain | unitless |
| $f_D$ | Doppler shift frequency | *Hz, kHz* |
| $\theta_D$ | Doppler angle | *degrees* |
| $I_{SPTA}$ | Spatial peak temporal average intensity | *mW/cm²* |
| $I_{SPPA}$ | Spatial peak pulse average intensity | *mW/cm²* |
| TI | Thermal index | unitless |
| MI | Mechanical index | unitless |

SECTION

III

# Nuclear Medicine

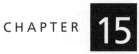

# Radioactivity and Nuclear Transformation

## 15.0 INTRODUCTION

The nuclei of unstable atoms undergo a transformation during which ionizing radiation (which can be in the form of particles or waves or both) is emitted from the nucleus. This process is referred to as *radioactive decay* following which the atomic nucleus is in a less unstable (still radioactive) or stable (not radioactive) state. The *radioactivity* of a material refers to the rate at which it emits radiation. The terms and equations that describe the process of radioactive decay are discussed in this chapter along with the different types of decay processes that are common to radionuclides utilized in nuclear medicine.

## 15.1 DEFINITIONS

1. **Activity**
   a. The quantity of radioactive material is expressed as the number of radioactive atoms undergoing nuclear transformation per unit time ($t$).
      (i) Activity is equal to the change ($dN$) in the total number of radioactive atoms ($N$) in a given time interval ($dt$), or

$$A = -dN/dt$$

[15-1]

      (ii) Activity has traditionally been expressed in units of curies (Ci), in honor of Marie Curie, one of the most accomplished women in the history of science. One Ci is defined as $3.70 \times 10^{10}$ disintegrations per second (dps), approximately the rate of disintegrations from 1 g of radium-226 (Ra-226).
      (iii) In honor of Henri Becquerel, the discoverer of radioactivity, the official SI-derived unit of activity was given the special name of becquerel (Bq), which is equal to 1 dps.
      (iv) Multiply mCi "millicurie" by 37 to obtain MBq "megabecquerel" or divide MBq by 37 to obtain mCi (*e.g.*, 1 mCi = 37 MBq).

2. **Decay constant**
   a. The decay constant ($\lambda$) is equal to the fraction of the number of radioactive atoms remaining in a sample that decay per unit time.

$$-dN/dt = \lambda N$$

[15-2]

   Note that the minus sign indicates that the number of radioactive atoms decaying per unit time (the decay rate or activity of the sample) decreases with time.
   b. The relationship between activity $A$ and the decay constant $\lambda$ can be seen by considering Equation 15-1 and substituting $A$ for $-dN/dt$ in Equation 15-2.

$$A = \lambda N$$

[15-3]  📖 Eq. 15-4

3. **Physical half-life**
   a. The time required for the number of radioactive atoms remaining in a sample to decrease by one half.
      (i) From an initial number of radioactive atoms ($N_0$), the number remaining in the sample ($N$) after ($n$) half-lives have elapsed is given by Equation 15-4.

$$N = N_0/2^n$$

[15-4]  📖 Eq. 15-5

**TABLE 15-1 PHYSICAL HALF-LIFE ($T_p\frac{1}{2}$) AND DECAY CONSTANT ($\lambda$) FOR RADIONUCLIDES COMMONLY USED IN NUCLEAR MEDICINE**

| RADIONUCLIDE | $T_p\frac{1}{2}$ | $\lambda$ |
|---|---|---|
| Rubidium-82 ($^{82}$Rb) | 75 s | 0.0092 s$^{-1}$ |
| Fluorine-18 ($^{18}$F) | 110 min | 0.0063 min$^{-1}$ |
| Technetium-99m ($^{99m}$Tc) | 6.02 h | 0.1151 h$^{-1}$ |
| Iodine-123 ($^{123}$I) | 13.27 h | 0.0522 h$^{-1}$ |
| Samarium-153 ($^{153}$Sm) | 1.93 d | 0.3591 d$^{-1}$ |
| Yttrium-90 ($^{90}$Y) | 2.69 d | 0.2575 d$^{-1}$ |
| Molybdenum-99 ($^{99}$Mo) | 2.75 d | 0.2522 d$^{-1}$ |
| Indium-111 ($^{111}$In) | 2.81 d | 0.2466 d$^{-1}$ |
| Thallium-201 ($^{201}$Tl) | 3.04 d | 0.2281 d$^{-1}$ |
| Gallium-67 ($^{67}$Ga) | 3.26 d | 0.2126 d$^{-1}$ |
| Xenon-133 ($^{133}$Xe) | 5.24 d | 0.1323 d$^{-1}$ |
| Lutetium-177 ($^{177}$Lu) | 6.7 d | 0.1034 d$^{-1}$ |
| Iodine-131 ($^{131}$I) | 8.02 d | 0.0864 d$^{-1}$ |
| Radium-223 ($^{223}$Ra) | 11.4 | 0.0608 d$^{-1}$ |
| Strontium-82 ($^{82}$Sr) | 25.60 d | 0.0271 d$^{-1}$ |
| Cobalt-57 ($^{57}$Co) | 271.79 d | 0.0117 d$^{-1}$ |

(ii) After 10 half-lives, the number of radioactive atoms in a sample is reduced by approximately a factor of 1,000. After 20 half-lives, it is reduced to about one millionth.

b. The decay constant and the physical half-life are related as follows:

$$\lambda = \ln 2 / T_p \frac{1}{2} = 0.693 / T_p \frac{1}{2}$$

[15-5]   📖 Eq. 15-6

where ln 2 denotes the natural logarithm of 2. Note that the derivation of this relationship is identical to that between the half-value layer (HVL) and the linear attenuation coefficient ($\mu$) in Chapter 3 (Eq. 3-7). 📖 Eq. 3-9

4. **Fundamental decay equation**

a. The relationship between $N_t$ (the number of radioactive atoms) or $A_t$ (activity) remaining in a sample at time ($t$) is given by the following equation:

$$N_t = N_0 e^{-\lambda t} \text{ or } A_t = A_0 e^{-\lambda t}$$

[15-6]   📖 Eq. 15-7

b. Examples of $T_p\frac{1}{2}$ and $\lambda$ for radionuclides commonly used in nuclear medicine are listed in Table 15-1.

c. A plot of activity as a function of time on a linear scale results in a curvilinear exponential relationship in which the total activity asymptotically approaches zero (Fig. 15-1). If the logarithm of the activity is plotted versus time (semilog plot), this exponential relationship appears as a straight line (Fig. 15-2).

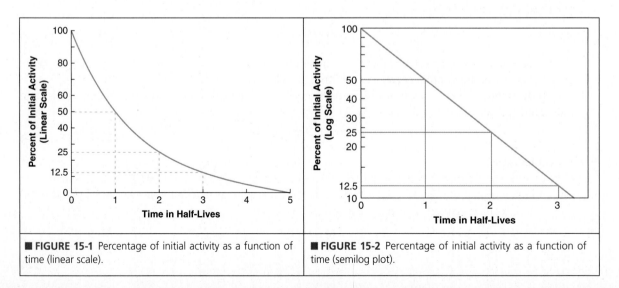

■ **FIGURE 15-1** Percentage of initial activity as a function of time (linear scale).

■ **FIGURE 15-2** Percentage of initial activity as a function of time (semilog plot).

## 15.2 NUCLEAR TRANSFORMATION

When an unstable (*i.e.*, radioactive) atomic nucleus undergoes the spontaneous transformation, called radioactive decay, radiation is emitted. If the decay product nucleus is stable, this spontaneous transformation ends. If the decay product is also unstable, the process continues until a stable nuclide is reached. Most radionuclides decay in one or more of the following ways: (1) alpha decay ($\alpha^{++}$), (2) beta-minus emission ($\beta^{-}$), (3) beta-plus (positron) emission ($\beta^{+}$), (4) electron capture ($\varepsilon$), or (5) isomeric transition via gamma-ray ($\gamma$) emission.

**1. Alpha decay**

    **a.** Alpha particles (*i.e.*, helium nucleus) are emitted from the atomic nucleus of heavy unstable nuclides ($A >$ 150) with discrete energies in the range of 2 to 10 MeV, often followed by $\gamma$ and characteristic x-ray emissions and sometimes $\beta$ emissions, Figure 15-3. The photon emissions are often accompanied by the competing processes of internal conversion and Auger electron emission discussed in Chapter 2.

    **b.** Alpha particles are not used in imaging as their ranges are limited to approximately 1 cm/MeV in air and typically less than 100 μm in tissue. Even the most energetic alpha particles cannot penetrate the dead layer of the skin. However, their ability to produce intense ionization tracks make them a potentially serious health hazard should sufficient quantities of alpha-emitting radionuclides enter the body via ingestion, inhalation, or a wound.

    **c.** One alpha-emitting radionuclide radium-223 (Ra-223) is in clinical therapeutic use for the treatment of metastatic prostate cancer while others are being evaluated for therapeutic potential such as astatine-212, bismuth-212, and bismuth-213 (At-211, Bi-212, and Bi-213) chelated to monoclonal antibodies to produce stable radioimmunoconjugates directed against tumors as radioimmunotherapeutic agents.

**2. Beta-minus decay**

    **a.** Beta-minus decay characteristically occurs with radionuclides that have an excess number of neutrons compared with the number of protons (*i.e.*, a high $N/Z$ ratio).

    **b.** The decay results in the conversion of a neutron into a proton with the simultaneous ejection of a $\beta^{-}$ particle and an antineutrino ($\overline{\nu}$) (Fig. 15-4).

    **c.** Except for their origin (the nucleus), $\beta^{-}$ particles are identical to and behave as ordinary electrons. However, compared to the $\beta^{-}$, the $\overline{\nu}$ has an infinitesimal mass and is electrically neutral making them very difficult to detect because they rarely interact with matter.

    **d.** Beta decay increases the number of protons by 1 and transforms the atom into a different element with an atomic number $Z +1$; however, the neutron number is decreased by one thus the mass number remains unchanged. Decay modes in which the mass number remains constant are called *isobaric transitions*.

    **e.** Radionuclides produced by nuclear fission are "neutron-rich," and therefore, most decay by $\beta^{-}$emission. The $\beta^{-}$ decay decreases the $N/Z$ ratio, bringing the decay product closer to the line of stability (see Chapter 2).

    **f.** Depending on the radionuclide one or more, $\beta^{-}$ particles may be emitted during each decay event. While each $\beta^{-}$ will have a characteristic maximal possible kinetic energy ($E_{max}$), that is specific to the radionuclide; almost all are emitted with energies lower than the maximum. The average energy of the $\beta^{-}$ particles is approximately 1/3 $E_{max}$. The balance of the energy is given to the $\overline{\nu}$.

    **g.** Any excess energy in the nucleus after beta decay is emitted as $\gamma$-rays, internal conversion electrons, and other associated radiations.

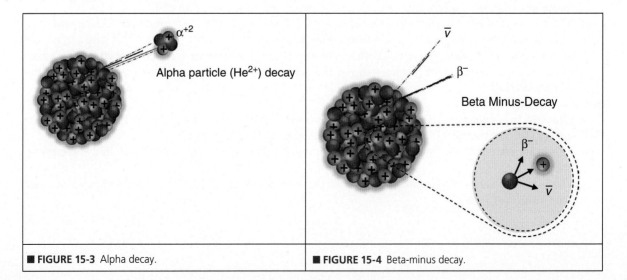

■ **FIGURE 15-3** Alpha decay.    ■ **FIGURE 15-4** Beta-minus decay.

3. **Beta-plus decay (positron emission)**
   a. Another unstable configuration of the atomic nucleus is when the ratio of the number of neutrons to protons is in a state opposite to that which favors $\beta^-$ decay (*i.e.*, "neutron poor," low $N/Z$ ratio). In many cases, increase nuclear stability is achieved by the beta-plus (positron) emission decay process.
   b. The decay result is the conversion of a proton into a neutron with the simultaneous ejection of a positron ($\beta^+$) and a neutrino ($\nu$) (Fig. 15-5).
   c. However, in this case, the fate of the $\beta^+$ is much different than that of its counterpart emitted during beta-minus decay ($\beta^-$). While positrons undergo a similar process of energy deposition via excitation and ionization, when they come to rest, they react violently with their antiparticles (electrons). This process results in the entire rest mass of both particles being instantaneously converted to energy and emitted as two oppositely directed (*i.e.*, approximately 180° apart) 511-keV *annihilation radiation* photons (Fig. 15-6). Medical imaging of annihilation radiation from positron-emitting radiopharmaceuticals, called positron emission tomography (PET), is discussed in Chapter 19.
   d. Beta-plus decay decreases the number of protons by one and thus transforms the atom into a different element with an atomic number $Z - 1$; however, the neutron number is increased by one thus the mass number remains unchanged making this decay mode isobaric.
   e. The energy distribution between the positron and the neutrino is similar to that between the $\beta^-$ and the antineutrino in beta-minus decay; thus, positrons are polyenergetic with average kinetic energy equal to approximately $1/3\ E_{max}$. As with $\beta^-$ decay, excess energy following positron decay is released as $\gamma$-rays and other associated radiation.
   f. For positron decay to occur, there is an inherent energy threshold between the unstable nucleus and its decay product that must exist that is equal to or greater than the sum of the rest mass energy equivalent of two electrons (*i.e.*, $2 \times 511$ keV, or 1.02 MeV).

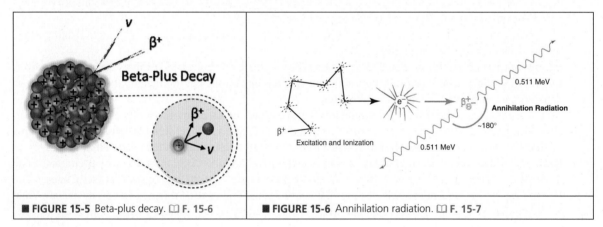

■ **FIGURE 15-5** Beta-plus decay. ▯ F. 15-6     ■ **FIGURE 15-6** Annihilation radiation. ▯ F. 15-7

4. **Electron capture decay**
   a. Electron capture (E) is an alternative to positron decay for neutron-deficient radionuclides.
   b. In this decay mode, the nucleus captures an orbital (usually a K- or L-shell) electron, with the conversion of a proton into a neutron and the simultaneous ejection of a neutrino ($\nu$) (Fig. 15-7).
   c. The net effect of electron capture is the same as positron emission: the atomic number is decreased by 1, creating a different element; the mass number remains unchanged (isobaric); increase $N/Z$ ratio and nuclear stability (Fig. 15-8). The capture of an orbital electron creates a vacancy in the electron shell, which is filled by an electron cascade from higher-energy shells resulting in the emission of characteristic x-rays and/or Auger electrons.
5. **Isomeric transition**
   a. Often during radioactive decay, a decay product is formed in an "excited state" (*i.e.*, an intermediate nuclear energy state between that of the parent and that of the final decay product).
   b. $\gamma$-Rays are emitted as the nucleus undergoes an internal transition from its excited state to a lower-energy state.
   c. Once created, most excited states transition almost instantaneously ($<10^{-12}$ s) to lower-energy states with the emission of $\gamma$-rays.

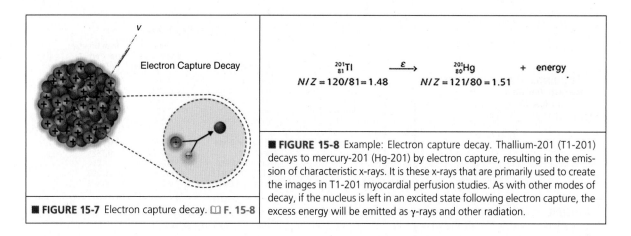

**■ FIGURE 15-7** Electron capture decay. ▢ F. 15-8

**■ FIGURE 15-8** Example: Electron capture decay. Thallium-201 (T1-201) decays to mercury-201 (Hg-201) by electron capture, resulting in the emission of characteristic x-rays. It is these x-rays that are primarily used to create the images in T1-201 myocardial perfusion studies. As with other modes of decay, if the nucleus is left in an excited state following electron capture, the excess energy will be emitted as γ-rays and other radiation.

    **d.** However, some excited states persist for longer periods, with half-lives ($T_p\frac{1}{2}$) ranging from nanoseconds ($10^{-9}$ s) to more than 30 years. Those with $T_p\frac{1}{2} > 10^{-3}$ s are called *metastable* and are denoted by the letter "m" after the mass number (*e.g.*, Tc-99m).

    **e.** Isomeric transition is a decay process that yields γ-rays without the emission or capture of a particle by the nucleus. There is no change in Z, A, or neutron number. Thus, this decay is isobaric and isotonic, and it occurs between two nuclear energy states with no change in the N/Z ratio.

**6. Decay schemes**

    **a.** Each radionuclide's decay process is a unique characteristic of that radionuclide. The majority of the pertinent information about the decay process and its associated radiation can be summarized in a line diagram called a decay scheme (Fig. 15-9).

    **b.** Decay schemes identify the parent, decay product (*i.e.*, progeny or daughter), mode of decay, energy levels including those of excited and metastable states, radiation emissions, and sometimes physical half-life and other characteristics of the decay sequence,

    **c.** The top horizontal line represents the parent, and the bottom horizontal line represents the decay product as well as their half-lives or notation if the decay product is stable. Horizontal lines between those two represent intermediate excited or metastable states.

    **d.** By convention, a diagonal arrow to the right indicates an increase in Z, which occurs with beta-minus decay. A diagonal arrow to the left indicates a decrease in Z such as decay by electron capture.

    **e.** A vertical line followed by a diagonal arrow to the left is used to indicate alpha decay and in some cases to indicate positron emission when a radionuclide decays by both electron capture and positron emission (*e.g.*, F-18). Vertical down-pointing arrows indicate γ-ray emission, including those emitted during isomeric transition.

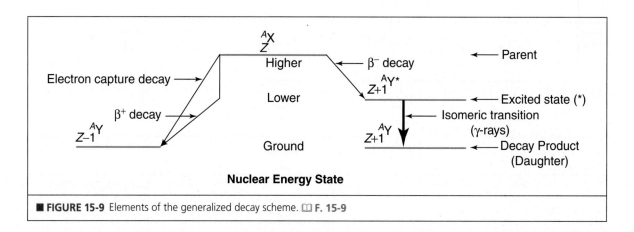

**■ FIGURE 15-9** Elements of the generalized decay scheme. ▢ F. 15-9

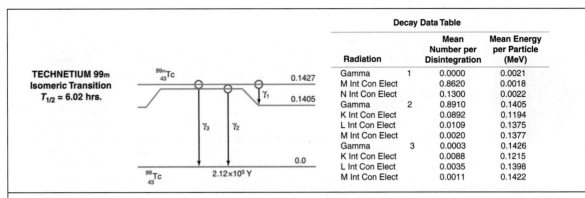

| | Decay Data Table | | |
|---|---|---|---|
| **Radiation** | | **Mean Number per Disintegration** | **Mean Energy per Particle (MeV)** |
| Gamma | 1 | 0.0000 | 0.0021 |
| M Int Con Elect | | 0.8620 | 0.0018 |
| N Int Con Elect | | 0.1300 | 0.0022 |
| Gamma | 2 | 0.8910 | 0.1405 |
| K Int Con Elect | | 0.0892 | 0.1194 |
| L Int Con Elect | | 0.0109 | 0.1375 |
| M Int Con Elect | | 0.0020 | 0.1377 |
| Gamma | 3 | 0.0003 | 0.1426 |
| K Int Con Elect | | 0.0088 | 0.1215 |
| L Int Con Elect | | 0.0035 | 0.1398 |
| M Int Con Elect | | 0.0011 | 0.1422 |

**TECHNETIUM 99m**
**Isomeric Transition**
$T_{1/2}$ = 6.02 hrs.

$^{99m}_{43}$Tc — 0.1427
— 0.1405 $\gamma_1$
$\gamma_3$ $\gamma_2$
— 0.0
$^{99}_{43}$Tc   $2.12 \times 10^5$ Y

■ **FIGURE 15-10** Principal decay scheme of technetium-99m. Auger electron nomenclature: KXY Auger Elect is an Auger electron emitted from the "Y" shell as a result of a transition of an electron of the "X" shell to a vacancy in the K-shell. "X" and "Y" are shells higher than the K-shell. For example, KLL Auger Elect is an Auger electron emitted from the L-shell as a result of a transition of another L-shell electron to a vacancy in the K-shell. ▭ **F. 15-13**

f. The process of γ-ray emission by isomeric transition is of primary importance to nuclear medicine because most procedures performed depend on the emission and detection of γ-rays.

g. Figure 15-10 shows the decay scheme for Tc-99m. There are three γ-ray transitions as Tc-99m decays to Tc-99. The low-energy (2.2 keV) gamma 1 ($\gamma_1$) transition occurs very infrequently because 99.2% of the time this energy is internally converted resulting in the emission of either an M-shell internal conversion electron (86.2%) with a mean energy of 1.8 keV or an N-shell internal conversion electron (13.0%) with a mean energy of 2.2 keV.

h. After internal conversion, the nucleus is left in an excited state, which is followed almost instantaneously by gamma 2 ($\gamma_2$) transition at 140.5 keV to ground state. This transition occurs 89.1% of the time and is the principal photon imaged in nuclear medicine.

i. Vacancies created in orbital electron shells following internal conversion result in the production of characteristic x-rays and Auger electrons.
A summary of the characteristics of radionuclide decay modes previously discussed is provided in Table 15-2. ▭ **T. 15-4**

### TABLE 15-2 SUMMARY OF RADIONUCLIDE DECAY

| TYPE OF DECAY | PRIMARY RADIATION EMITTED | OTHER RADIATION EMITTED | NUCLEAR TRANSFORMATION | CHANGE IN | | NUCLEAR CONDITION PRIOR TO TRANSFORMATION |
|---|---|---|---|---|---|---|
| | | | | **Z** | **A** | |
| Alpha | $^4_2$He$^{+2}$ | γ-rays / C x-rays / AE, ICE | $^A_Z X \rightarrow ^A_Z X \rightarrow ^{-2} + ^4_2 He^{2+} + energy$ | −2 | −4 | Z > 83 |
| Beta minus | β$^{-1}$ | γ-rays / C x-rays / AE, ICE, $\bar{\nu}$ | $^A_Z X \rightarrow ^A_{Z+1} Y + \beta^- + \bar{\nu} + energy$ | +1 | 0 | N/Z too large |
| Beta plus | β$^{+1}$ | γ-rays / C x-rays / AE, ICE, $\nu$ | $^A_Z X \rightarrow ^A_{Z-1} Y + \beta^+ + \nu + energy$ | −1 | 0 | N/Z too small |
| Electron capture | C x-rays | γ-rays / AE, ICE, $\nu$ | $^A_Z X + e^- \rightarrow ^A_{Z-1} Y + \nu + energy$ | −1 | 0 | N/Z too small |
| Isomeric transition | γ-rays | C x-rays / AE, ICE | $^{Am}_Z X \rightarrow ^A_Z X + energy$ | 0 | 0 | Excited or metastable nucleus |

ICE, internal conversion electron; AE, Auger electron; C x-rays, characteristic x-rays; γ-rays, gamma rays; $\bar{\nu}$, antineutrino; $\nu$, neutrino.

# Section II Questions and Answers

1. Following beta-minus decay, the resultant nucleus has:
   A. one more proton and one more neutron than the "parent" nucleus
   B. one less proton and one less neutron than the "parent" nucleus
   C. one less proton and one more neutron than the "parent" nucleus.
   D. one more proton and one less neutron than the "parent" nucleus
   E. two fewer protons and two fewer neutrons than the "parent" nucleus

2. The *N/Z* ratio increases following which two decay modes?
   A. Alpha and beta minus
   B. Beta minus and isomeric transition
   C. Isomeric transition and election capture
   D. Election capture and position emission
   E. Positron emission and beta minus

3. Which of the following radionuclides has the smallest decay constant?
   A. F-18                 D. I-131
   B. Mo-99                E. Tl-201
   C. Tc-99m

4. The decay constant ($\lambda$) of a radionuclide is related to its physical half-life by:
   A. $\lambda = 1.44T_{1/2}$          D. $\lambda = 0.693T_{1/2}$
   B. $\lambda = 1.44/T_{1/2}$         E. $\lambda = 0.693/T_{1/2}$
   C. $\lambda = T_{1/2}/1.44$

5. The fraction of the initial number of radioactive atoms present after a period of time *t* is:
   A. $\lambda$             D. $e^{-\lambda t}$
   B. $\lambda t$           E. $1 - e^{-\lambda t}$
   C. $-\lambda t$

6. With regard to the decay of Tc-99m, which statement is most correct.
   A. The decay product is Mo-98.
   B. The decay product is Tc-99.
   C. The decay product is Tc-99* (excited state).
   D. The decay Tc-99 that is stable.
   E. The decay product is Tc-99, which decays to Ru-99.

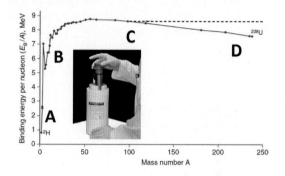

7. Where on the graph on the image above would you find the source material used to produce Mo-99 by nuclear fission?
   A. A
   B. B
   C. C
   D. D

8. Concerning the image above, where on the graph would you find the daughter of Mo-99, and what radionuclide is it?
   A. B, Tc-99m
   B. B, Mo-98
   C. C, Tc-99m
   D. D, Mo-98

9. Regarding antineutrino emitted from a radiopharmaceutical and absorbed dose, which statement is most correct?
   A. They are of no consequence because they instantaneously interact with a neutrino where their mass is converted to energy photons that escape the body.
   B. They are of no consequence because of their infinitesimal mass and because they are electrically neutral thus rarely interacting with matter.
   C. On average, they are responsible for 1/3 of the dose following beta-minus decay.
   D. On average, they are responsible for 1/3 of the dose following beta-plus decay.

10. Which of the following statements is most correct?

    A. A becquerel (Bq) is equal to exactly 1 nuclear disintegration per second (dps).

    B. A becquerel (Bq) is the unit used to describe the "activity" of radioactivity (*i.e.*, how likely the next nuclear disintegration will occur per second [dps]).

    C. The amount of radioactivity remaining in a sample after time (*t*) can be calculated by multiplying the initial activity in becquerel (Bq) by the radionuclides physical half-life and dividing by 0.0693.

    D. The becquerel (Bq) replaced the previous unit curie (Ci), although their numerical values are the same (*i.e.*, 1 Bq = 1 Ci).

    E. The becquerel (Bq) replaced the previous unit curie (Ci), although their numerical values are not the same (*i.e.*, 1 Bq = 100 Ci).

# Answers

1. **D** During beta-decay a neutron is transformed into its proton energy state thus increasing the number of protons by 1, and transforming the atom into a different element with one less neutron thus the mass number remains unchanged making the transition isobaric. *(Pg. 635)*

2. **D** Neutron-deficient radionuclides can decay by electron capture and/or positron emission. In both cases, the proton number is decreased by 1, increasing the $N/Z$ ratio, while the mass number remains unchanged (isobaric). *(Pg. 636–638)*

3. **D** $\lambda = 0.693/T_{1/2}$. Thus, the radionuclide with the smallest decay constant has the longest half-life. F-18 has a half-life of about 110 minutes, Tc-99m has a half-life of about 6 hours, and Mo-99 and Tl-201 have half-lives of about 3 days. I-131 has the longest $T_{1/2}$ of about 8 days. *(Pg. 631 and Eq. 15-6 and Table 15-3)*

4. **E** $\lambda = 0.693/T_{1/2}$. The fundamental decay equation Eq. 15-6 is $N = N_0 e^{-\lambda t}$ Setting $t$ equal to one half-life, we get $N_0/2 = N_0 e^{-\lambda T_{1/2}}$. After canceling terms, we have $1/2 = e^{-\lambda T_{1/2}}$, and after taking the natural log (ln) of both sides of the equation, we have $-0.693 = -\lambda T_{1/2}$. Finally after rearranging terms, we have $\lambda = 0.693/T_{1/2}$. *(Pg. 631 and Eq. 15-6)*

5. **D** $A_t = A_0 e^{-\lambda t}$, where $e^{-\lambda t}$ is the fraction of the initial number of radioactive atoms present after a period of time $t$, and $1 - e^{-\lambda t}$ is the fraction of the initial number of radioactive atoms that have decayed after time $t$. *(Pg. 632 and Fig. 15-13)*

6. **E** While Answer B is correct, a more complete answer is E. While Tc-99 is radioactive, its half-life of 212,000 years means very few (if any) Tc-99 atoms will decay to Ru-99 during the average lifetime of the patient. *(Pg. 643, Fig. 15-12)*

7. **D** When uranium is mined, it consists of approximately 99.3% uranium-238 (U-238) and a very small amount of U-235 (0.7%). Uranium is enriched to increase the percentage of U-235 to make it suitable to use as nuclear fuel capable of sustaining a nuclear fission chain reaction. A number of the fission products produced are radionuclides useful to nuclear medicine including Mo-99 and I-131. *(Pg. 642, Fig. 15-12)*

8. **C** Tc-99m is the daughter of Mo-99 with a mass number of 99. *(Pg. 641-642, Fig. 15-12)*

9. **B** The 1/3 refers to the average energy (relative to the maximum kinetic energy) of the beta particle emitted. *(Pgs. 635, 637)*

10. **A** The becquerel is the SI-derived unit of radioactivity. One becquerel is defined as the activity of a quantity of radioactive material in which one nucleus decays per second (dps). The conversion between Bq and Ci common in nuclear medicine is 37 MBq per mCi. The factor of 100 applies to the conversion from rad to Gray and rem to sievert (*e.g.*, 100 rad = 1 Gy and 100 rem = 1 Sv). *(Pg. 630)*

# Section III Key Equations and Symbols

| QUANTITY | EQUATION | EQ NO./PAGE/COMMENTS |
|---|---|---|
| Activity | $A = -\,dN/dt$ | Eq. 15-1/Pg. 630/Activity ($A$) is the change ($dN$) in the total number of radioactive atoms ($N$) in a given time interval ($dt$) |
| Decay constant | $\lambda = \ln 2 / T_p\tfrac{1}{2} = 0.693 / T_p\tfrac{1}{2}$ | Eq. 15-6/Pg. 631/It is the fraction of the number of radioactive atoms remaining in a sample that decay per unit time |
| Physical half-life | $T_p\tfrac{1}{2}$ | Eq. 15-5/Pg. 631/$T_p\tfrac{1}{2}$ is the physical half-life |
| Fundamental decay equation | $A_t = A_0 e^{-\lambda t}$ | Eq. 15-7/Pg. 632/The relationship between the initial activity $A_0$ and the (activity) remaining $A_t$ in a sample at time ($t$) |

| SYMBOL | QUANTITY | UNITS |
|---|---|---|
| $T_p\tfrac{1}{2}$ | Physical half-life | Any time unit |
| $\lambda$ | Decay constant | 1/Any time unit |
| $A$ | Activity | Bq |
| $\alpha^{++}$ | Alpha particle | NA |
| $\beta^-$ | Beta-minus particle | NA |
| $\beta^+$ | Beta-plus particle (positron) | NA |
| $\varepsilon$ | Electron capture | NA |
| $\gamma$ | Gamma-ray | NA |
| $\bar{v}$ | Antineutrino | NA |
| $v$ | Neutrino | NA |
| $E_{max}$ | Maximum kinetic energy | keV |
| $N/Z$ | Neutron/proton ratio in the atomic nucleus | NA |
| $A$ | Atomic mass number (number of protons and neutrons in the atomic nucleus) | NA |

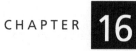

# CHAPTER 16

# Radionuclide Production, Radiopharmaceuticals, and Internal Dosimetry

## 16.0  INTRODUCTION

This chapter presents the various forms by which radionuclides are produced for use in radiopharmaceuticals to include cyclotrons, fission reactors, and parent-progeny generators. Radiopharmaceuticals are discussed next to include their ideal characteristics for imaging, requirements for use in therapy, mechanisms for tissue localization, and production quality control. Computation of patient organ dose is then discussed via the MIRD and ICRP schema, along with the role of dosimetry in both diagnostic imaging and therapy. The chapter closes with an overview of regulatory issues.

## 16.1  RADIONUCLIDE PRODUCTION

Methods of production of radionuclides for use in medical imaging and therapy include the following:

1. Particle accelerators (element transmutation by absorption of a charged particle)
2. Nuclear reactor (fission product extraction or induced activity by neutron activation)
3. Radionuclide generators (device that includes the parent radionuclide from which the daughter radionuclide is extracted) (Table 16-1)

**TABLE 16-1  COMPARISON OF RADIONUCLIDE PRODUCTION METHODS**

| | PRODUCTION METHOD | | | |
|---|---|---|---|---|
| **CHARACTERISTIC** | *Linear Accelerator/ Cyclotron* | *Nuclear Reactor (Fission)* | *Nuclear Reactor (Neutron Activation)* | *Radionuclide Generator* |
| Bombarding particle | Proton, alpha | Neutron | Neutron | Production by decay of parent |
| Product | Neutron poor | Neutron excess | Neutron excess | Neutron poor or excess |
| Typical decay pathway | Positron emission, electron capture | Beta minus | Beta minus | Several modes |
| Typically carrier free | Yes | Yes | No | Yes |
| High specific activity | Yes | Yes | No | Yes |
| Relative cost | High | Low | Low | Low ($^{99m}$Tc) |
| | | | | High ($^{82}$Rb) |
| Radionuclides for nuclear medicine applications | $^{11}$C, $^{13}$N, $^{15}$O, $^{18}$F, $^{57}$Co, $^{67}$Ga, $^{68}$Ge, $^{111}$In, $^{123}$I, $^{201}$Tl | $^{99}$Mo, $^{131}$I, $^{133}$Xe | $^{32}$P, $^{51}$Cr, $^{89}$Sr, $^{125}$I, $^{153}$Sm | $^{68}$Ga, $^{81m}$Kr, $^{82}$Rb, $^{90}$Y, $^{99m}$Tc |

## Cyclotron-Produced Radionuclides

1. Charged particles must be accelerated to high kinetic energies to overcome and penetrate the repulsive coulombic barrier of the target atoms' nuclei.
2. A cyclotron has a vacuum chamber between the poles of an electromagnet. Inside the vacuum chamber is a pair of hollow, semicircular electrodes, each shaped like the letter D and thus referred to as "dees." An alternating high voltage is applied between the two dees.
3. When positive ions are injected into the center of the cyclotron, they are attracted to and accelerated toward the negatively charged dee. The static magnetic field constrains the ions to travel in a circular path, whereby the radius of the circle increases as the ions gain kinetic energy (Fig. 16-1).

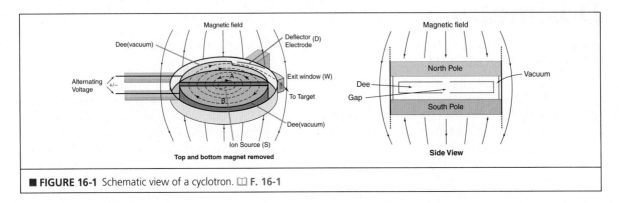

■ **FIGURE 16-1** Schematic view of a cyclotron. ▭ F. 16-1

4. Halfway around the circle, the ions approach the gap between the dees; at this time, the polarity of the electrical field between the two dees is reversed, causing the ions to be accelerated toward the negative dee. This cycle is repeated again and again, with the particles accelerated each time they cross the gap, acquiring additional kinetic energy and sweeping out larger and larger circles. The cyclic nature of these events led to the name "cyclotron."
5. The accelerated ions collide with the target nuclei, causing nuclear reactions. An incident particle may leave the target nucleus after interacting, transferring some of its energy to it, or it may be completely absorbed.
6. The specific reaction depends on the type and energy of the bombarding particle as well as the composition of the target. In either case, target nuclei are left in an excited state, and this excitation energy is disposed of through the emission of particulate (protons and neutrons) and electromagnetic (γ-rays) radiations. Depending on the design of the cyclotron, particle energies can range from a few million electron volts (MeV) to several hundred MeV.
7. In the first example below, an accelerated proton (p) is absorbed by a stable atom of zinc-68 ($^{68}$Zn) after which two neutrons are emitted, leaving an atom of gallium-67 as the reaction product.

*Example reactions of industrial cyclotron-produced radionuclides used in nuclear medicine imaging:*

| RADIONUCLIDE | CHARGED-PARTICLE PRODUCTION REACTION |
|---|---|
| Gallium-67 | $^{68}$Zn (p, 2n)$^{67}$Ga |
| Iodine-123 | $^{127}$I(p,5n)$^{123}$Xe $\xrightarrow[T_{1/2}\,2h]{EC}$ $^{123}$I   or |
|  | $^{124}$Xe(p,2n) $^{123}$Cs $\xrightarrow[T_{1/2}\,1s]{EC\,or\,\beta^+}$ $^{123}$Xe $\xrightarrow[T_{1/2}\,2h]{EC}$ $^{123}$I |
| Indium-111 | $^{109}$Ag (α, 2n)$^{111}$In   or $^{111}$Cd (p, n)$^{111}$In   or $^{112}$Cd (p, 2n)$^{111}$In |
| Cobalt-57 | $^{56}$Fe (d, n)$^{57}$Co |
| Thallium-201 | $^{203}$Tl(p,3n)$^{201}$Pb $\xrightarrow[T_{1/2}\,9.4h]{EC\,or\,\beta^+}$ $^{201}$Tl |

8. Industrial cyclotron facilities that produce large activities of clinically useful radionuclides are very expensive and require substantial cyclotron and radiochemistry support staff and facilities. Cyclotron-produced radionuclides are usually more expensive than those produced by other technologies.

9. Much smaller, specialized cyclotrons, installed in commercial radiopharmacies serving metropolitan areas or in hospitals, produce positron-emitting radionuclides for positron emission tomography (PET).

10. These cyclotrons operate at lower energies (10 to 30 MeV) than industrial cyclotrons and commonly accelerate H⁻ ions, which is a proton with two orbital electrons. The beam is extracted by passing it through a carbon stripping foil, which removes the electrons thus creating an H⁺ ion (proton) beam.

11. The medical cyclotrons are usually located near the PET imaging system because of the short half-lives of the radionuclides produced. In the interests of design simplicity and cost, some medical cyclotrons accelerate only protons. These advantages may be offset for particular productions such as $^{15}$O when an expensive rare isotope $^{15}$N that requires proton bombardment must be used in place of the cheap and abundant $^{14}$N isotope that requires deuteron bombardment.

12. Fluorine-18 (F-18) is an exception to this generalization owing to its longer half-life (110 min). Regional production and distribution of $^{18}$F is thus an option for this commonly used PET radionuclide.

*Example reactions of medical center cyclotron-produced radionuclides used in nuclear medicine imaging:*

| RADIONUCLIDE | CHARGED PARTICLE PRODUCTION REACTIONS/RADIONUCLIDE PHYSICAL HALF-LIFE | |
|---|---|---|
| Fluorine-18 | $^{18}$O (p, n)$^{18}$F | ($T_{1/2}$ = 110 min) |
| Nitrogen-13 | $^{16}$O(p, α)$^{13}$N | ($T_{1/2}$ = 10 min) |
| Oxygen-15 | $^{14}$N(d, n)$^{15}$O or $^{15}$N (p, n)$^{15}$O | ($T_{1/2}$ = 2.0 min) |
| Carbon-11 | $^{14}$N (p, α)$^{11}$C | ($T_{1/2}$ = 20.4 min) |

## Nuclear Reactor-Produced Radionuclides

Nuclear reactors are another major source of clinically used radionuclides. Neutrons, being uncharged, have an advantage in that they can penetrate the nucleus without being accelerated to high energies. There are two principal methods by which radionuclides are produced in a reactor: *nuclear fission* and *neutron activation*.

## Nuclear Reactors and the Nuclear Chain Reaction

1. Fission is the splitting of an atomic nucleus into two smaller nuclei. Whereas some unstable nuclei fission spontaneously, others require the input of energy to overcome the nuclear binding forces. This energy is often provided by the absorption of neutrons.

2. Neutrons can induce fission only in certain very heavy nuclei. Whereas high-energy neutrons can induce fission in several such nuclei, there are only three nuclei of reasonably long half-life that are fissionable by neutrons of all energies; these are called fissile nuclides.

3. The most widely used fissile nuclide is uranium-235 (U-235). Elemental uranium exists in nature primarily as U-238 (99.3%) with a small fraction of U-235 (0.7%). U-235 has a high fission cross section (*i.e.*, high fission probability); therefore, its concentration is usually enriched (typically to 3% to 5%) to make the fuel used in nuclear reactors.

4. When a U-235 nucleus absorbs a neutron, the resulting nucleus (U-236) is in an extremely unstable excited energy state that usually promptly fissions into two smaller nuclei called fission fragments. The fission fragments separate with very high kinetic energies, with the simultaneous emission of γ radiation and the ejection of two to five neutrons per fission:

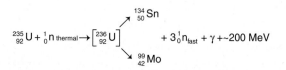

$$^{235}_{92}\text{U} + {}^{1}_{0}\text{n}_{\text{thermal}} \rightarrow \left[ {}^{236}_{92}\text{U} \right] \underset{{}^{99}_{42}\text{Mo}}{\overset{{}^{134}_{50}\text{Sn}}{\nearrow}} + 3{}^{1}_{0}\text{n}_{\text{fast}} + \gamma + \sim 200 \text{ MeV}$$

5. The fission of uranium creates fission fragment nuclei having a wide range of mass numbers. More than 200 radionuclides with mass numbers between 70 and 160 are produced (Fig. 16-2). These fission products are neutron-rich, and therefore, almost all of them decay by beta-minus (β−) particle emission.

6. The energy released by the nuclear fission of a uranium atom is more than 200 MeV. Under the right conditions, this reaction can be perpetuated if the fission neutrons interact with other U-235 atoms, causing additional fissions and leading to a self-sustaining nuclear chain reaction (Fig. 16-3).

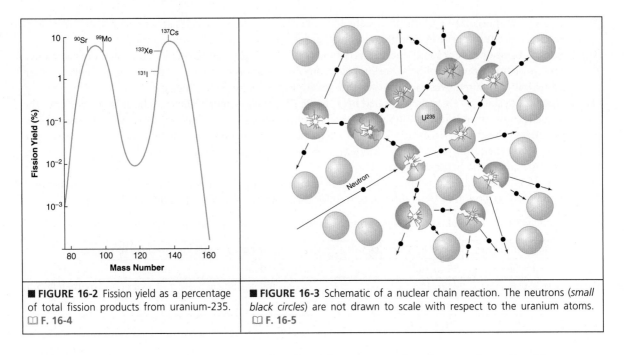

■ **FIGURE 16-2** Fission yield as a percentage of total fission products from uranium-235. □ F. 16-4

■ **FIGURE 16-3** Schematic of a nuclear chain reaction. The neutrons (*small black circles*) are not drawn to scale with respect to the uranium atoms. □ F. 16-5

7. The probability of fission with U-235 is greatly enhanced as neutrons slow down or thermalize. The neutrons emitted from fission are very energetic (called fast neutrons) and are slowed (moderated) to thermal energies (approximately 0.025 eV) as they scatter in water in the reactor core. Good moderators are low-Z materials that slow the neutrons without absorbing a significant fraction of them. Water is the most commonly used moderator.

## Nuclear Fission–Produced Medical Radionuclides

1. The fission products most often used in nuclear medicine are molybdenum-99 (Mo-99), iodine-131 (I-131), and xenon-133 (Xe-133). These products can be chemically separated from other fission products with essentially no stable isotopes (carrier) of the radionuclide present.
2. The concentration or specific activity (measured in MBq or Ci per gram) of these "carrier-free" fission-produced radionuclides is very high. High-specific-activity, carrier-free nuclides are preferred in radiopharmaceutical preparations to increase the labeling efficiency and minimize the mass and volume of the injected material.

## Neutron Activation–Produced Medical Radionuclides

1. Neutrons produced by the fission of uranium in a nuclear reactor can be used to create radionuclides by bombarding stable target material placed in the reactor. Ports exist in the reactor core between the fuel elements where samples to be irradiated are inserted. This process, called neutron activation, involves the capture of neutrons by stable nuclei, which results in the production of radioactive nuclei.
2. The most common neutron capture reaction for thermal (slow) neutrons is the (n,γ) reaction, in which the capture of the neutron by a nucleus is immediately followed by the emission of a γ-ray.
3. Other thermal neutron capture reactions include the (n,p) and (n,α) reactions, in which the neutron capture is followed by the emission of a proton or an alpha particle, respectively. Almost all radionuclides produced by neutron activation decay by beta-minus particle emission.

*Example neutron activation methods of producing radionuclides used in nuclear medicine imaging:*

| RADIONUCLIDE | NEUTRON ACTIVATION PROCESS/RADIONUCLIDE PHYSICAL HALF-LIFE | |
|---|---|---|
| Phosphorus-32 | $^{31}P(n, \gamma)^{32}P$ | $(T_{1/2} = 14.3 \text{ days})$ |
| Chrominum-51 | $^{50}Cr(n, \gamma)^{51}Cr$ | $(T_{1/2} = 27.8 \text{ days})$ |
| Iodine-125 | $^{124}Xe(n, \gamma)^{125}Xe \xrightarrow[T_{1/2} 17 \text{ h}]{EC \text{ or } \beta^+} {}^{125}I$ | $(T_{1/2} = 60.2 \text{ days})$ |

## Radionuclide Generators

Since the mid-1960s, technetium-99m (Tc-99m) has been the most important radionuclide used in nuclear medicine for a wide variety of radiopharmaceutical applications. However, its relatively short half-life (6 h) makes it impractical to store even a weekly supply. This supply problem is overcome by obtaining the parent Mo-99, which has a longer half-life (67 h) and continually produces Tc-99m. The Tc-99m is collected periodically in sufficient quantities for clinical operations. A system for holding the parent in such a way that the daughter can be easily separated for clinical use is called a radionuclide generator.

1. In a molybdenum-99/technetium-99m radionuclide generator, Mo-99 (produced by nuclear fission of U-235 to yield a high-specific-activity, carrier-free parent) is loaded, in the form of ammonium molybdate ($NH4+$) ($MoO_4^-$), onto a porous column containing 5 to 10 g of an alumina ($Al_2O_3$) resin.
2. As with all radionuclide generators, the chemical properties of the parent and daughter are different. In the Mo-99/Tc-99m or "moly" generator, the Tc-99m is much less tightly bound than the Mo-99. The daughter is removed (eluted) by the flow of isotonic saline (the "eluant") through the column.
3. When the saline solution is passed through the column, the chloride ions easily exchange with the $TcO_4^-$ (but not the $MoO_4^-$) ions, producing sodium pertechnetate, $Na+(^{99m}TcO_4^-)$. Technetium-99m pertechnetate ($^{99m}TcO_4^-$) is produced in a sterile, pyrogen-free form with high specific activity and a pH (approximately 5.5) that is ideally suited for radiopharmaceutical preparations.
4. Commercially, moly generators have a large reservoir of oxygenated saline (the eluant) connected by tubing to one end of the column and a vacuum extraction vial to the other. On insertion of the vacuum collection vial (contained in a shielded elution tool), saline is drawn through the column and the eluate is collected during elution, which takes about 1 to 2 min (Fig. 16-4).
5. Moly generators are typically delivered with approximately 37 to 740 GBq (1 to 20 Ci) of Mo-99, depending on the workload of the department. The larger activity generators are typically used by commercial radiopharmacies supplying radiopharmaceuticals to multiple nuclear medicine departments. The generators are shielded by the manufacture with lead, tungsten, or, in the case of higher activity, depleted uranium.
6. The activity of the daughter at the time of elution depends on the following:
   a. The activity of the parent
   b. The rate of formation of the daughter, which is equal to the rate of decay of the parent
   c. The decay rate of the daughter
   d. The time since the last elution
   e. The elution efficiency (typically 80% to 90%)

## Transient Equilibrium

1. Between elutions, the daughter (Tc-99m) builds up or "grows in" as the parent (Mo-99) continues to decay. After approximately 23 h, the Tc-99m activity reaches a maximum, at which time the production rate and the decay rate are equal and the parent and daughter are said to be in transient equilibrium. Once transient equilibrium has been achieved, the daughter activity decreases, with an apparent half-life equal to the half-life of the parent.
2. Transient equilibrium occurs when the half-life of the parent is greater than that of the daughter by a factor of approximately 10. In the general case of transient equilibrium, the daughter activity will exceed the parent at equilibrium.
3. If all of the (Mo-99) decayed to Tc-99m, the Tc-99m activity would slightly exceed (approximately 10% higher) that of the parent at equilibrium. However, approximately 12% of Mo-99 decays directly to Tc-99 without first producing Tc-99m (Fig. 16-5). Therefore, at equilibrium, the Tc-99m activity will be only approximately 97% (1.1 × 0.88) that of the parent (Mo-99) activity.
4. Moly generators (sometimes called "cows") are usually delivered weekly and eluted (a process referred to as "milking the cow") each morning, allowing maximal yield of the daughter. The elution process is approximately 90% efficient. This fact, together with the limitations on Tc-99m yield in the Mo-99 decay scheme, results in a maximum elution yield of approximately 85% of the Mo-99 activity at the time of elution.

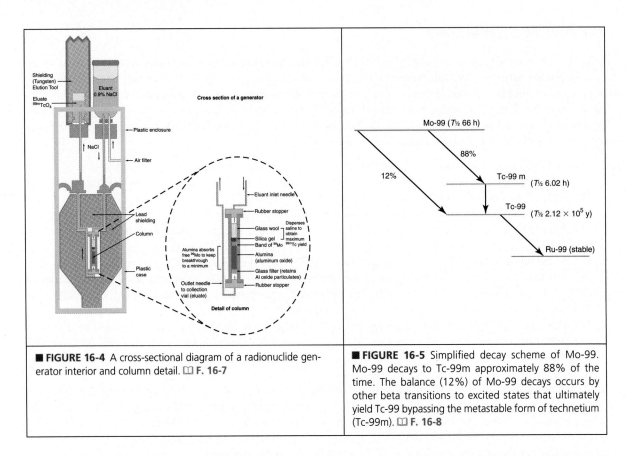

■ **FIGURE 16-4** A cross-sectional diagram of a radionuclide generator interior and column detail. 🕮 **F. 16-7**

■ **FIGURE 16-5** Simplified decay scheme of Mo-99. Mo-99 decays to Tc-99m approximately 88% of the time. The balance (12%) of Mo-99 decays occurs by other beta transitions to excited states that ultimately yield Tc-99 bypassing the metastable form of technetium (Tc-99m). 🕮 **F. 16-8**

5. Therefore, a typical elution on Monday morning from a moly generator with 55.5 GBq (1.5 Ci) of Mo-99 yields approximately 47.2 GBq (1.28 Ci) of Tc-99m in 10 mL of normal saline (a common elution volume). By Friday morning of that same week, the same generator would be capable of delivering only about 17.2 GBq (0.47 Ci). The moly generator can be eluted more frequently than every 23 h; however, the Tc-99m yield will be less. Approximately half of the maximal yield will be available 6 h after the last elution. Figure 16-6 shows a typical time-activity curve for a moly generator.

## Secular Equilibrium

1. Although the moly generator is by far the most widely used in nuclear medicine, other generator systems produce clinically useful radionuclides. When the half-life of the parent is much longer than that of the daughter (*i.e.*, more than about 100 times longer), secular equilibrium occurs after approximately five to six half-lives of the daughter. In secular equilibrium, the activity of the parent and the daughter are the same if all of the parent atoms decay directly to the daughter.
2. Once secular equilibrium is achieved, the daughter will have an apparent half-life equal to that of the parent. The strontium-82/rubidium-82 (Sr-82/Rb-82) generator, with parent and daughter half-lives of 25.5 days and 75 s, respectively, reach secular equilibrium within approximately 7.5 min after elution. Figure 16-7 shows a time-activity curve demonstrating secular equilibrium (Table 16-2).

## Quality Control

1. The users of moly generators are required to perform molybdenum and alumina breakthrough tests. Mo-99 contamination in the Tc-99m eluate is called molybdenum breakthrough. Mo-99 is an undesirable contaminant because its long half-life and highly energetic betas increase the radiation dose to the patient without providing any clinical information.
2. The high-energy γ-rays (approximately 740 and 780 keV) are very penetrating and cannot be efficiently detected by scintillation cameras. The U.S. Pharmacopeia (USP) and the U.S. Nuclear Regulatory Commission (NRC) limit the Mo-99 contamination to 0.15 $\mu$Ci of Mo-99 per mCi of Tc-99m or (0.15 kBq/MBq) at the time of administration.
3. Contaminant limits are specified in 10CFR35.204 and include those for the Rb-82 generators: 0.02 $\mu$Ci of Sr-85 per mCi of Rb-82 or (0.02 kBq/MBq).

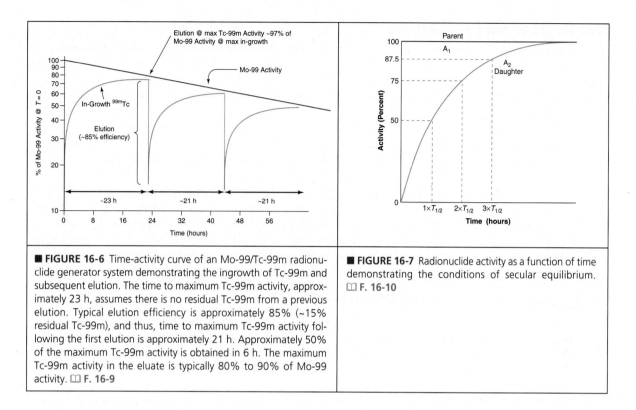

■ **FIGURE 16-6** Time-activity curve of an Mo-99/Tc-99m radionu-clide generator system demonstrating the ingrowth of Tc-99m and subsequent elution. The time to maximum Tc-99m activity, approx-imately 23 h, assumes there is no residual Tc-99m from a previous elution. Typical elution efficiency is approximately 85% (~15% residual Tc-99m), and thus, time to maximum Tc-99m activity fol-lowing the first elution is approximately 21 h. Approximately 50% of the maximum Tc-99m activity is obtained in 6 h. The maximum Tc-99m activity in the eluate is typically 80% to 90% of Mo-99 activity. 📖 **F. 16-9**

■ **FIGURE 16-7** Radionuclide activity as a function of time demonstrating the conditions of secular equilibrium. 📖 **F. 16-10**

**TABLE 16-2 CLINICALLY USED RADIONUCLIDE GENERATOR SYSTEMS IN NUCLEAR MEDICINE**

| PARENT | DECAY MODE AND (HALF-LIFE) | DAUGHTER | TIME OF MAXIMAL INGROWTH (EQUILIBRIUM) | DECAY MODE AND (HALF-LIFE) | DECAY PRODUCT |
|---|---|---|---|---|---|
| $^{68}$Ge | EC (271 d) | $^{68}$Ga | ~6.5 h (S) | $\beta^+$ EC (68 min) | $^{68}$Zn (stable) |
| $^{90}$Sr | $\beta^-$ (28.8 y) | $^{90}$Y | ~1 mo (S) | $\beta^-$ (2.67 d) | $^{90}$Zr (stable) |
| $^{81}$Rb | $\beta^+$ EC (4.6 h) | $^{81m}$Kr | ~80 s (S) | IT (13.5 s) | $^{81}$Kr$^a$ |
| $^{82}$Sr | EC (25.5 d) | $^{82}$Rb | ~7.5 min (S) | $\beta^+$ (75 s) | $^{82}$Kr (stable) |
| $^{99}$Mo | $\beta^-$ (67 h) | $^{99m}$Tc | ~24 h (T) | IT (6 h) | $^{99}$Tc$^a$ |

*Note:* Decay modes: EC, electron capture; $\beta^+$, positron emission; $\beta^-$, beta minus; IT, isometric transition (*i.e.*, $\gamma$-ray emission). Radionuclide equilibrium: T, transients; S, secular.
$^a$These nuclides have half-lives greater than $10^5$ years and for medical applications can be considered to be essentially stable.

## 16.2 RADIOPHARMACEUTICALS

## Characteristics of Ideal Radiopharmaceuticals for Diagnostic Imaging

### Low Radiation Dose

1. It is important to minimize radiation exposure to patients while preserving the diagnostic quality of the image. Radionuclides can be selected that have few particulate emissions and a high abundance of clinically useful photons.
2. Most modern scintillation cameras are optimized for photon energies close to 140 keV, which is a compromise among patient attenuation, spatial resolution, and detection efficiency. Photons whose energies are too low are largely attenuated by the body, increasing the patient dose without contributing to image formation. High-energy photons are more likely to escape the body but have poor detection efficiency and easily penetrate col-limator septa of scintillation cameras.
3. A radiopharmaceutical should have an effective half-life long enough to complete the study with an adequate concentration in the tissues of interest but short enough to minimize the patient dose.

## High Target-to-Nontarget Activity

1. The ability to detect and evaluate lesions depends largely on the concentration of the radiopharmaceutical in the organ, tissue, or lesion of interest or on a clinically useful uptake and clearance pattern. Maximizing the concentration of the radiopharmaceutical in the target tissues of interest while minimizing the uptake in surrounding (nontarget) tissues and organs improves contrast and the ability to detect subtle abnormalities in the radiopharmaceutical's biodistribution.

2. Maximizing this target/nontarget ratio is characteristic of all clinically useful radiopharmaceuticals and is improved by observing the recommended interval between injection and imaging for the specific agent. This interval is a compromise between the uptake of the activity in the target tissue, washout of the activity in the background (nontarget) tissues, and practical considerations of clinic operations.

3. With some radiopharmaceuticals such as the bone scanning agent, Tc-99m–labeled methylene diphosphonate (99mTc-MDP), instructions to the patient, needed both to improve image quality and to reduce radiation dose to patient and technologist, might include the request to be well hydrated and to void the urinary bladder just prior to imaging.

4. Disassociation of the radionuclide from the radiopharmaceutical alters the desired biodistribution, thus degrading image quality. Good-quality control over radiopharmaceutical preparation helps to ensure that the radionuclide continues to be chemically bound to the pharmaceutical throughout the imaging session.

## Safety, Convenience, and Cost-Effectiveness

1. Low chemical toxicity is enhanced by the use of high-specific-activity, carrier-free radionuclides that also facilitate radiopharmaceutical preparation and minimize the required amount of the isotope.

2. For example, 3.7 GBq (100 mCi) of I-131 contains only 0.833 $\mu$g of iodine. Radionuclides should also have a chemical form, pH, concentration, and other characteristics that facilitate rapid complexing with the pharmaceutical under normal laboratory conditions.

3. The compounded radiopharmaceutical should be stable, with a shelf life compatible with clinical use, and should be readily available from several manufacturers to minimize cost.

## Characteristics of Ideal Radiopharmaceuticals for Therapy

1. Radiopharmaceuticals are also used for the treatment of a number of diseases. The goal of radiopharmaceutical therapy is to deliver a sufficiently large dose to the target organ, tissue, or cell type while limiting the dose to nontargeted tissues to minimize deterministic effects such as bone marrow suppression and to minimize the risk of cancer.

2. Prior to 2013, all approved therapeutic radiopharmaceuticals were based radionuclides that decayed either through beta-particle emission ($^{32}$P, $^{89}$Sr, $^{90}$Y, $^{124}$I, $^{131}$I, $^{153}$Sm, $^{177}$Lu, $^{186}$Re, and $^{188}$Re) or Auger electron emission ($^{103}$Pd, $^{111}$In, $^{117m}$Sn, $^{123}$I, $^{125}$I, $^{193m}$Pt, or $^{195m}$Pt).

3. In May of 2013, the U.S. FDA approved the first therapy radiopharmaceutical using an alpha-particle emitter: Xofigo (radium Ra-223 dichloride) for the treatment of patients with castration-resistant prostate cancer (CRPC), symptomatic bone metastases, and no known visceral metastatic disease.

4. Since that milestone, there has been significant research activities and ongoing clinical trials in the development of other alpha-emitter therapy radiopharmaceuticals across a variety of cancer types such as breast, prostate, neuroendocrine tumors, and leukemia. Alpha emitters of current interest in radiopharmaceutical therapy include $^{211}$At, $^{212}$Pb, $^{212}$Bi, $^{213}$Bi, $^{223}$Ra, $^{225}$Ac, and $^{227}$Th.

## Radiopharmaceutical Mechanisms of Localization

| MECHANISM | DESCRIPTION/EXAMPLE RADIOPHARMACEUTICALS |
| --- | --- |
| a. Compartmental localization/leakage | Compartmental localization refers to the introduction of the radiopharmaceutical into a well-defined anatomic compartment. Examples include Xe-133 gas inhalation into the lung, intraperitoneal instillation of P-32 chromic phosphate, and Tc-99m–labeled RBCs injected into the circulatory system. |
| b. Cell sequestration | To evaluate splenic morphology and function, red blood cells are withdrawn from the patient, labeled with Tc-99m, and slightly damaged by in vitro heating in a boiling water bath for ~30 min. After they have been reinjected, the spleen's ability to recognize and remove the damaged RBCs is evaluated. |
| c. Phagocytosis | The cells of the reticuloendothelial system are distributed in the liver (~85%), spleen (~10%), and bone marrow (~5%). These cells recognize small foreign substances in the blood and remove them by phagocytosis. In a liver scan, for example, Tc-99m–labeled sulfur colloid particles (~100 nm) are recognized and are rapidly removed from circulation. |

| MECHANISM | DESCRIPTION/EXAMPLE RADIOPHARMACEUTICALS |
|---|---|
| d. Passive diffusion | Passive diffusion is simply the free movement of a substance from a region of high concentration to one of lower concentration. Anatomic and physiologic mechanisms exist in the brain tissue and surrounding vasculature that allow essential nutrients, metabolites, and lipid-soluble compounds to pass freely between the plasma and brain tissue while many water-soluble substances (including most radiopharmaceuticals) are prevented from entering healthy brain tissue. This system, called the blood-brain barrier, protects and regulates access to the brain. Disruptions of the blood-brain barrier permits radiopharmaceuticals such as Tc-99m diethylenetriaminepentaacetic acid (DTPA), which is normally excluded by the blood-brain barrier, to follow the concentration gradient and enter the affected brain tissue. |
| e. Active transport | Active transport involves cellular metabolic processes that expend energy to concentrate the radiopharmaceutical into a tissue against a concentration gradient and above plasma levels. The classic example in nuclear medicine is the trapping and organification of radioactive iodide. Trapping of iodide in the thyroid gland occurs by transport against a concentration gradient into follicular cells, where it is oxidized to a highly reactive iodine by a peroxidase enzyme system. Organification follows, resulting in the production of radiolabeled triiodothyronine (T3) and thyroxine (T4). F-18 FDG is a glucose analog that concentrates in cells that rely upon glucose as an energy source or in cells whose dependence on glucose increases under pathophysiological conditions. F-18 FDG is actively transported into the cell where it is phosphorylated and trapped for several hours as FDG-6-phosphate. The retention and clearance of FDG reflect glucose metabolism in a given tissue. F-18 FDG is used to assist in the evaluation of malignancy in patients with known or suspected cancer. |
| f. Capillary blockade | When particles slightly larger than RBCs are injected intravenously, they become trapped in the capillary beds. A common example in nuclear medicine is in the assessment of pulmonary perfusion by the injection of Tc-99m-MAA, which is trapped in the pulmonary capillary bed. Imaging the distribution of Tc-99m-MAA provides a representative assessment of pulmonary perfusion. The "microemboli" created by this radiopharmaceutical do not pose a significant clinical risk because only a very small percentage of the pulmonary capillaries are blocked and the MAA is eventually removed by biodegradation. |
| g. Perfusion | Relative perfusion of a tissue or organ system is an important diagnostic element in many nuclear medicine procedures. For example, the perfusion phase of a three-phase bone scan helps to distinguish between an acute process (*e.g.*, osteomyelitis) and remote fracture. Perfusion is also an important diagnostic element in examinations such as renograms, cerebral and hepatic blood flow studies, and myocardial perfusion studies. |
| h. Chemotaxis | Chemotaxis describes the movement of a cell such as a leukocyte in response to a chemical stimulus. [111]In- and [99m]Tc–labeled leukocytes respond to products formed in immunologic reactions by migrating and accumulating at the site of the reaction as part of an overall inflammatory response. |
| i. Antibody-antigen complexation | An antigen is a biomolecule (typically a protein) that is capable of inducing the production of, and binding to, an antibody in the body. The antibody has a strong and specific affinity for the antigen. Antigen-antibody complexation is also used in diagnostic imaging with such agents as In-111–labeled monoclonal antibodies for the detection of colorectal carcinoma. This class of immunospecific radiopharmaceuticals promises to provide an exciting new approach to diagnostic imaging. In addition, a variety of radiolabeled (typically with I-131 or Y-90) monoclonal antibodies directed toward tumors are being used in an attempt to deliver tumoricidal radiation doses. This procedure, called radioimmunotherapy, has proven effective in the treatment of some non-Hodgkin lymphomas and is under clinical investigation for other malignancies. |
| j. Receptor binding | This class of radiopharmaceuticals is characterized by their high affinity to bind to specific receptor sites. For example, the uptake of In-111-octreotide, used for the localization of neuroendocrine and other tumors, is based on the binding of a somatostatin analog to receptor sites in tumors. |
| k. Physiochemical adsorption | The localization of methylene diphosphonate (MDP) occurs primarily by adsorption in the mineral phase of the bone. MDP concentrations are significantly higher in amorphous calcium than in mature hydroxyapatite crystalline structures, which helps to explain its concentration in areas of increased osteogenic activity. |

## Radiopharmaceutical Quality Control

1. Aside from the radionuclidic purity quality control performed on the [99m]Tc-pertechnetate generator eluate, the most common radiopharmaceutical quality control procedure is the test for radiochemical purity. The radiochemical purity assay identifies the fraction of the total radioactivity that is in the desired chemical form.

2. Radiochemical impurity can occur as the result of temperature changes, presence of unwanted oxidizing or reducing agents, pH changes, or radiation damage to the radiopharmaceutical (called autoradiolysis). The presence of radiochemical impurities compromises the diagnostic utility of the radiopharmaceutical by reducing uptake in the organ of interest and increasing background activity, thereby degrading image quality. In addition to lowering the diagnostic quality of the examination, radiochemical impurities unnecessarily increase patient dose.

3. The two principal radiochemical impurities in technetium-labeled radiopharmaceuticals are free (*i.e.*, unbound) Tc-99m-pertechnetate and hydrolyzed Tc-99m. The Tc-99m radiopharmaceutical complex and its associated impurities will, depending upon the solvent, either remain at the origin or move with the solvent front to a location near the end of the strip.

## 16.3  INTERNAL DOSIMETRY

1. Radiation doses to patients from diagnostic imaging procedures are an important issue and, in the absence of a medical physicist at an institution (*e.g.*, private practice radiology), radiologists and nuclear medicine physicians are often consulted as the local experts. Radiation dosimetry is primarily of interest because radiation dose quantities serve as indices of the risk from diagnostic imaging procedures using ionizing radiation.

2. Dosimetry also plays an important role in radiopharmaceutical therapy where estimates of activity necessary to produce tumoricidal doses must be weighed against potential radiotoxicity to healthy tissue. In nuclear medicine procedures, the chemical form of the radiopharmaceutical, its route of administration (*e.g.*, intravenous injection, ingestion, inhalation), the administered activity, the radionuclide, and patient-specific disease states and pharmacokinetics determine the patient dose.

### MIRD and ICRP schema

1. The original mathematical methods, models, equations, nuclear decay data, and biokinetic parameters needed for computing radiation absorbed dose to internal organs were developed by the Medical Internal Radiation Dose (or MIRD) Committee of the Society of Nuclear Medicine and Molecular Imaging (SNMMI) in the late 1950s to early 1960s.

2. The most recent revision of the MIRD schema for internal organ dosimetry was published in 2009 as MIRD Pamphlet No. 21 in the *Journal of Nuclear Medicine*. In the 1970s, the International Commission on Radiological Protection (ICRP) developed its own set of expression, quantities, and terminology for the same purpose—estimating dose to internal organs following intake of both radionuclides and radiopharmaceuticals.

3. With the issue of ICRP Publication 130 (in 2015) and ICRP Publication 133 (in 2016), however, a harmonization of the dosimetry schema for internal organ dosimetry was made, thus providing a consistent terminology and approach to the field of internal dosimetry.

### Mean Absorbed Dose Rate

1. The mean absorbed dose $D(r_T)$ is defined as the mean energy imparted to target tissue (or region) $r_T$ per unit tissue mass. The rate at which the absorbed dose is delivered to target tissue $r_T$ within a patient from a radiopharmaceutical distributed uniformly within source tissue $r_S$ at time $t$ following radiopharmaceutical administration is given as:

$$\dot{D}(r_T, t) = \sum_{r_S} A(r_S, t) S(r_T \leftarrow r_S, t) \qquad \text{[16-1] ⬚ Eq. 16-7}$$

where $A(r_S, t)$ is the time-dependent activity of the radiopharmaceutical in source tissue $r_S$ and $S(r_T \leftarrow r_S, t)$ is a quantity called the radionuclide $S$ value (or $S$ coefficient).

2. The expression involves a summation over all possible source regions $r_S$ that might contribute absorbed dose to the target region $r_T$ (Fig. 16-8).

3. For short-range radiations emitted by the radionuclide, the relevant source tissue may only be the target tissue itself (*i.e.*, $r_T = r_S$).

4. For source tissues that emit photons (gamma-rays or x-rays), the relevant source tissues may be adjacent to or even at a distance from the target tissue (*i.e.*, $r_T \neq r_S$) and may also include the target tissue itself (*i.e.*, $r_T = r_S$).

**5.** The time-dependent activity $A(r_S, t)$ represents the rate of nuclear decays in the source tissue $r_S$ at time $t$, while the $S$ value represents the absorbed dose rate to the target tissue $r_T$ per radionuclide activity in source region tissue $r_S$.

**6.** The $S$ value is characteristic of the radionuclide and the anatomic model chosen to represent the internal body anatomy of the patient. In many cases, "reference" anatomic models are used to compute the $S$ value. These may be anatomic models of either the averaged sized male or female patients at fixed ages—newborn, 1-, 5-, 10-, 15-year-old, and the adult (see Fig. 16-9).

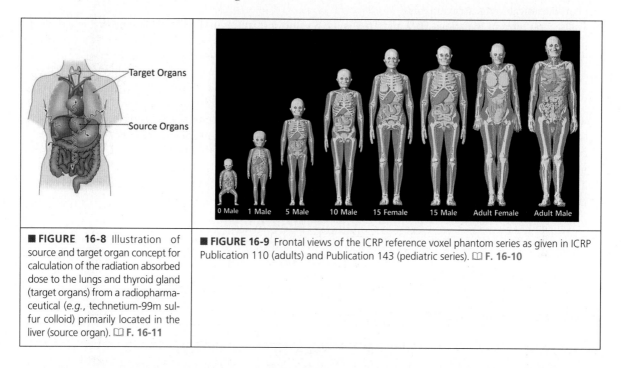

■ **FIGURE 16-8** Illustration of source and target organ concept for calculation of the radiation absorbed dose to the lungs and thyroid gland (target organs) from a radiopharmaceutical (*e.g.*, technetium-99m sulfur colloid) primarily located in the liver (source organ). 📖 **F. 16-11**

■ **FIGURE 16-9** Frontal views of the ICRP reference voxel phantom series as given in ICRP Publication 110 (adults) and Publication 143 (pediatric series). 📖 **F. 16-10**

## Mean Absorbed Dose—Time-Independent Formulation

**1.** The mean absorbed dose to a target tissue $r_T$ is thus obtained by time integrating the mean absorbed dose rate:

$$D(r_T, \tau) = \int_0^\tau \dot{D}(r_T, t)dt = \sum_{r_S} \tilde{A}(r_S, \tau)\, S(r_T \leftarrow r_S) \qquad \text{[16-2]} \;\text{📖 Eq. 16-8}$$

$$\tilde{A}(r_S, \tau) = \int_0^\tau A(r_S, t)dt \qquad \text{[16-3]} \;\text{📖 Eq. 16-9}$$

where $\tilde{A}(r_S, \tau)$ is the time-integrated activity (TIA) in source tissue $r_S$ over dose integration period $\tau$.

**2.** The time-integrated activity represents the total number of decays with the source tissue. The magnitude of the organ dose $D(r_T, \tau)$ is directly proportional to the activity of the radiopharmaceutical administered to the patient, $A_0$. Thus, doubling or tripling $A_0$ will then double or triple the organ doses resulting from that nuclear medicine study.

**3.** It is then convenient to normalize organ dose by the value of $A_0$, thus reporting the organ dose per activity administered (mGy per MBq). If the ratio of $A(r_S, t)$ to the administrated activity $A_0$ is denoted as $a(r_S, t)$, then we can define the absorbed dose coefficient $d(r_T, \tau)$ in the target tissue $r_T$ as:

$$d(r_T, \tau) = \sum_{r_S} \tilde{a}(r_S, \tau)\, S(r_T \leftarrow r_S) \qquad \text{[16-4]} \;\text{📖 Eq. 16-10}$$

$$\tilde{a}(r_S, \tau) = \int_0^\tau \frac{A(r_S, t)}{A_0}dt = \int_0^\tau a(r_S, t)dt \qquad \text{[16-5]} \;\text{📖 Eq. 16-11}$$

where $a(r_S, t)$ is the fraction of administered activity in the source tissue $r_S$ at time $t$ after administration, and the quantity $\tilde{a}(r_S, \tau)$ is the time-integrated activity coefficient (TIAC).

**4.** The time-dependent activity in source tissues of the patient may be obtained directly via quantitative imaging, including 2D planar imaging, 3D SPECT, 3D PET, or by tissue sampling (*e.g.*, blood or urine collection). In the case of preclinical animal studies, this may also be determined by the counting of individual organs or tissues of the experimental animals.

5. Alternatively, in the absence of direct measurement, the time-dependent activity in the source tissue may be obtained by numeric solution of a set of first-order coupled differential equations defined by compartment models for all organs and suborgan tissues of interest.

6. In earlier forms of the MIRD schema, the quantity $\tilde{a}(r_S, \tau)$ was referred to as the residence time of the radiopharmaceutical in the source tissue.

7. The second term in Equations 16-2 and 16-4 is the $S$ value, a quantity in the MIRD schema that is specific to the radionuclide and to the computational anatomic model defining the spatial relationship and tissue compositions of $r_S$ and $r_T$, as well as their intervening tissues. In equation form, the $S$ value is defined as:

$$S(r_T \leftarrow r_S) = \frac{1}{m(r_T)} \sum_i E_i Y_i \phi(r_T \leftarrow r_S, E_i) = \frac{1}{m(r_T)} \sum_i \Delta_i \phi(r_T \leftarrow r_S, E_i) \qquad \text{[16-6]} \ \square \ \text{Eq. 16-12}$$

where $E_i$ is the mean (or individual) energy per particle of the ith radiation emitted; $Y_i$ is number of the ith radiation emitted per nuclear decay; $\Delta_i$ is their product (mean energy of the ith radiation emitted per nuclear decay); $\phi(r_T \leftarrow r_S, E_i)$ is the absorbed fraction (fraction of $E_i$ emitted in $r_S$ absorbed in target tissue $r_T$); and $m(r_T)$ is the mass of the target tissue $r_T$ in the model.

8. The specific absorbed fraction $\Phi(r_T \leftarrow r_S, E_i)$ is further defined as the ratio of the absorbed fraction and the target mass (Table 16-3):

$$\Phi(r_T \leftarrow r_S, E_i) = \frac{\phi(r_T \leftarrow r_S, E_i)}{m(r_T)} \qquad \text{[16-7]} \ \square \ \text{Eq. 16-13}$$

$$S(r_T \leftarrow r_S) = \sum_i \Delta_i \Phi(r_T \leftarrow r_S, E_i) \qquad \text{[16-8]} \ \square \ \text{Eq. 16-14}$$

## TABLE 16-3 Tc-99m S-VALUES (mGy/MBq-s) $\square$ T. 16-5

| TARGET ORGANS | Adrenals | Brain | LLI Contents | SI Content | Stomach Contents | ULI Contents | Heart Contents | Heart Wall | Kidneys | Liver | Lungs |
|---|---|---|---|---|---|---|---|---|---|---|---|
| Adrenals | 1.80E−04 | 4.18E−10 | 2.25E−08 | 7.46E−08 | 2.73E−07 | 9.58E−08 | 2.53E−07 | 2.85E−07 | 7.24E−07 | 4.35E−07 | 2.33E−07 |
| Brain | 4.18E−10 | 4.23E−06 | 1.57E−11 | 3.91E−11 | 4.27E−10 | 4.68E−11 | 3.14E−09 | 2.54E−09 | 1.58E−10 | 8.16E−10 | 7.63E−09 |
| Breasts | 5.05E−08 | 3.17E−09 | 2.28E−09 | 7.35E−09 | 5.73E−08 | 8.00E−09 | 2.41E−07 | 2.61E−07 | 1.99E−08 | 6.82E−08 | 2.33E−07 |
| Gallbladder wall | 3.57E−07 | 1.54E−10 | 6.49E−08 | 4.38E−07 | 3.05E−07 | 7.53E−07 | 1.03E−07 | 1.22E−07 | 4.09E−07 | 8.70E−07 | 7.46E−08 |
| LLI wall | 1.98E−08 | 1.32E−11 | 1.23E−05 | 5.92E−07 | 9.10E−08 | 2.14E−07 | 4.06E−09 | 4.90E−09 | 5.50E−08 | 1.44E−08 | 3.29E−09 |
| Small intestine | 7.46E−08 | 3.91E−11 | 7.16E−07 | 4.22E−06 | 2.08E−07 | 1.25E−06 | 1.57E−08 | 2.06E−08 | 2.13E−07 | 1.16E−07 | 1.35E−08 |
| Stomach wall | 2.85E−07 | 2.52E−10 | 1.24E−07 | 2.13E−07 | 8.53E−06 | 2.86E−07 | 1.66E−07 | 2.65E−07 | 2.53E−07 | 1.48E−07 | 1.19E−07 |
| ULI wall | 9.41E−08 | 4.76E−11 | 3.10E−07 | 1.36E−06 | 2.65E−07 | 8.37E−06 | 2.12E−08 | 2.65E−08 | 2.12E−07 | 1.88E−07 | 1.81E−08 |
| Heart wall | 2.85E−07 | 2.54E−09 | 5.42E−09 | 2.06E−08 | 2.33E−07 | 2.97E−08 | 5.48E−06 | 1.19E−05 | 8.22E−08 | 2.33E−07 | 4.40E−07 |
| Kidneys | 7.24E−07 | 1.58E−10 | 7.10E−08 | 2.13E−07 | 2.73E−07 | 2.12E−07 | 6.45E−08 | 8.22E−08 | 1.32E−05 | 2.93E−07 | 6.66E−08 |
| Liver | 4.35E−07 | 8.16E−10 | 1.80E−08 | 1.16E−07 | 1.47E−07 | 1.87E−07 | 2.13E−07 | 2.33E−07 | 2.93E−07 | *3.16E−06* | 1.97E−07 |
| Lungs | 2.33E−07 | 7.63E−09 | 4.50E−09 | 1.35E−08 | 1.10E−07 | 1.77E−08 | 4.59E−07 | 4.40E−07 | 6.66E−08 | 2.09E−07 | 3.57E−06 |
| Muscle | 1.12E−07 | 2.21E−08 | 1.23E−07 | 1.12E−07 | 9.96E−08 | 1.07E−07 | 8.83E−08 | 9.20E−08 | 9.79E−08 | 7.52E−08 | 9.34E−08 |
| Ovaries | 3.14E−08 | 1.52E−11 | 1.26E−06 | 9.23E−07 | 5.85E−08 | 7.71E−07 | 4.55E−09 | 6.15E−09 | 7.02E−08 | 3.81E−08 | 5.39E−09 |
| Pancreas | 1.09E−06 | 4.15E−10 | 5.21E−08 | 1.42E−07 | 1.23E−06 | 1.62E−07 | 2.65E−07 | 3.57E−07 | 4.97E−07 | 3.86E−07 | 1.74E−07 |
| Red marrow | 2.53E−07 | 1.01E−07 | 2.01E−07 | 1.79E−07 | 7.50E−08 | 1.43E−07 | 1.11E−07 | 1.11E−07 | 1.71E−07 | *8.32E−08* | 1.11E−07 |
| Osteogenic cells | 2.67E−07 | 2.99E−07 | 1.82E−07 | 1.49E−07 | 1.03E−07 | 1.27E−07 | 1.60E−07 | 1.60E−07 | 1.62E−07 | 1.24E−07 | 1.66E−07 |
| Skin | 3.41E−08 | 3.97E−08 | 3.62E−08 | 3.01E−08 | 3.41E−08 | 3.09E−08 | 3.41E−08 | 3.70E−08 | 3.79E−08 | 3.62E−08 | 4.02E−08 |
| Spleen | 4.58E−07 | 5.19E−10 | 6.53E−08 | 1.01E−07 | 7.83E−07 | 1.05E−07 | 1.24E−07 | 1.67E−07 | 6.63E−07 | 7.22E−08 | 1.64E−07 |
| Tests | 1.54E−09 | 1.46E−12 | 1.40E−07 | 2.61E−08 | 2.90E−09 | 1.92E−08 | 5.16E−10 | 6.16E−10 | 3.10E−09 | *1.57E−09* | 3.67E−10 |
| Thymus | 5.66E−08 | 6.88E−09 | 2.04E−09 | 4.66E−09 | 3.65E−08 | 5.43E−09 | 8.87E−07 | 7.35E−07 | 1.73E−08 | 5.93E−08 | 2.85E−07 |
| Thyroid | 8.11E−09 | 1.35E−07 | 2.48E−10 | 4.87E−10 | 2.62E−09 | 7.69E−10 | 5.17E−08 | 4.33E−08 | 2.95E−09 | 8.64E−09 | 8.82E−08 |
| Urinary bladder wall | 7.55E−09 | 6.02E−12 | 4.98E−07 | 2.12E−07 | 1.73E−08 | 1.61E−07 | 2.22E−09 | 2.17E−09 | 1.87E−08 | 1.16E−08 | 1.33E−09 |
| Uterus | 1.89E−08 | 1.31E−11 | 5.17E−07 | 8.37E−07 | 5.05E−08 | 3.97E−07 | 4.87E−09 | 5.47E−09 | 6.42E−08 | 3.29E−08 | 4.10E−09 |
| Total body | 1.72E−07 | 1.25E−07 | 1.49E−07 | 1.59E−07 | 1.17E−07 | 1.41−07 | 1.17E−07 | 1.65E−07 | 1.58E−07 | 1.59E−07 | 1.44E−07 |

## Time-Dependent Models of Activity in Source Regions

1. Radiopharmaceuticals may be introduced into the body via a variety of routes, including intravenous, intra-arterial, or intrathecal injection, or oral or inhaled administration. The tissue regions that incorporate the radioactivity become source regions.

2. Once introduced into the body, the radiopharmaceutical undergoes biological uptake and clearance in various source organs and tissues of the body. The kinetics of biological uptake (bu) and biological clearance (bc) are often of an exponential form with half-times denoted as $T_{bu}$ and $T_{bc}$, respectively.

3. Similarly, the rate constants for biological uptake and biological clearance are denoted as $\lambda_{bu}$ and $\lambda_{bc}$, respectively, with $\lambda = \ln2/T$. Biological uptake and biological clearance, coupled with physical radionuclide decay, result in values of effective uptake and effective clearance rate constants ($\lambda_{eu}$ and $\lambda_{ec}$) and effective uptake and effective clearance half-times ($T_{eu}$ and $T_{ec}$) as given by the following expressions:

$$\lambda_{eu} = \lambda_{bu} + \lambda_p \ \text{ and } \ T_{eu} = \frac{T_{bu}T_p}{T_{bu}+T_p} \qquad \text{[16-9]} \ \square \ \text{Eq. 16-18}$$

$$\lambda_{ec} = \lambda_{bc} + \lambda_p \ \text{ and } \ T_{ec} = \frac{T_{bc}T_p}{T_{bc}+T_p} \qquad \text{[16-10]} \ \square \ \text{Eq. 16-19}$$

4. The time-dependent activity in source region $A(r_S, t)$ can thus be given as the product of the administered activity $A_0$, the fraction $f_s$ of the total administered activity taken up by a single identified source region $r_S$, and the difference of time-dependent exponential terms for radiopharmaceutical clearance and uptake, respectively:

$$A(r_S, t) = A_0 f_s \left[ e^{-\lambda_{ec}t} - e^{-\lambda_{eu}t} \right] \qquad \text{[16-11]} \ \square \ \text{Eq. 16-20}$$

5. While radiopharmaceutical uptake to tissue source regions is, in general, adequately expressed by a single exponential term, there are frequently situations in which two or more exponential terms are required to sufficiently model radiopharmaceutical clearance from the source region.

6. As an example, Equation 16-12 would be modified to the following if radiopharmaceutical clearance were better expressed using two exponential terms:

$$A(r_S, t) = A_0 \left[ f_{s_1} e^{-\lambda_{ec_1}t} + f_{s_2} e^{-\lambda_{ec_2}t} - \left( f_{s_1} + f_{s_2} \right) e^{-\lambda_{eu}t} \right] \qquad \text{[16-12]} \ \square \ \text{Eq. 16-21}$$

where $\lambda_{ec_1}$ and $\lambda_{ec_2}$ are the effective clearance rate constants for the first and second compartment for radiopharmaceutical clearance, respectively, and $f_{s_1}$ and $f_{s_2}$ are the fractions of the administered activity, which localize within these same two compartments of source tissue region $r_S$.

7. The time-integrated activity within the source region, assuming the two-exponential model of Equation 16-12, is then given as:

$$\tilde{A}(r_S, \tau) = \int_0^\tau A(r_S, t)dt$$

$$= \frac{A_0 f_{s_1}}{\lambda_{ec_1}} \left[ 1 - e^{-\lambda_{ec_1}\tau} \right] + \frac{A_0 f_{s_2}}{\lambda_{ec_2}} \left[ 1 - e^{-\lambda_{ec_2}\tau} \right] - \frac{A_0 \left( f_{s_1} + f_{s_2} \right)}{\lambda_{eu}} \left[ 1 - e^{-\lambda_{eu}\tau} \right] \qquad \text{[16-13]} \ \square \ \text{Eq. 16-22}$$

## Role of Internal Dosimetry in Diagnostic Nuclear Medicine

Clinical applications of diagnostic nuclear medicine allow functional imaging of normal and diseased tissue. Although they may cover almost all clinical specialties, the localization of malignant tissue and its potential metastatic spread, as well as assessment of myocardial perfusion, are among the most common procedures.

1. Amount of administered activity in diagnostic nuclear medicine is very low.
2. Organ doses are thus below thresholds for deterministic radiation effects (*e.g.*, tissue reactions).
3. Organ doses are in the range where stochastic risks of cancer are possible, but these risks are extremely low and highly uncertain on an individual patient basis.
4. The role of internal dosimetry in diagnostic nuclear medicine is thus to provide the basis for stochastic risk quantification.
5. Once this risk is quantified, it may be used to optimize the amount of administered activity in order to maximize image quality while minimizing patient risk.

6. This optimization process is of particular importance for pediatric patients owing to their enhanced organ radiosensitivities and years over which any stochastic effects may become manifest. This optimization should consider, as much as possible, patient age, gender, and body morphometry, and pharmacokinetics, along with all available image acquisition and processing techniques.

7. Two options exist for quantification of $\tilde{A}$ in diagnostic nuclear medicine. The most patient-specific method entails serial imaging of the patient (2D planar, 3D SPECT, or 3D PET), data processing of these images to yield time-activity curves, and then integration of these time-activity curves.

8. In the development of new diagnostic imaging agents, this approach is required for regulatory approval and should be conducted under standardized protocols to yield the greatest amount of information on agent pharmacokinetics and patient dosimetry.

9. For existing diagnostic imaging agents, one may rely on reference biokinetic models, which when coupled to phantom-based radionuclide $S$ values via the MIRD schema, yield organ dose coefficients—organ dose per unit administered activity.

## Role of Internal Dosimetry in Therapeutic Nuclear Medicine

In many forms of radiation cancer therapy, to include external beam radiotherapy and brachytherapy, radiation dosimetry is an integral component to treatment planning, where the objective is to maximize the tumor absorbed dose while avoiding or minimizing normal tissue toxicities.

1. In therapeutic nuclear medicine, tumor dosimetry may be problematic owing to (1) lack of imaging data to define the tumor, especially for disseminated and diffuse disease; (2) the dynamic nature of radiopharmaceutical uptake, retention, and washout; (3) nonuniformities in the spatial distribution of the agent at the cellular level; and (4) time-dependent dose rates.

2. Consequently, there is a paucity of data on tumor dose-response relationships, upon which values of prescribed tumor dose may be assessed. Exceptions do occur, such as in treatment of solid tumors and malignant and benign thyroid disease, but even here, there are no standardized clinically accepted protocols for radionuclide treatment planning based upon delivery of a dose prescription to the tumor.

3. Resultantly, current dosimetry practice in therapeutic nuclear medicine is to assess the absorbed dose to radiosensitive tissues, and based upon a general understanding of toxicity thresholds (taken primarily from previous experience in external beam radiotherapy), adjust administered activities to the cancer patient to maximize uptake and dose to the tumor while avoiding normal organ toxicities. The dose to the tumor is neither quantified nor prescribed.

4. In current clinical practice in nuclear medicine therapy, treatment is delivered based upon an administered activity prescription. This prescribed activity is typically established in a Phase I clinical trial from the toxicity response of only three to six patients and is then applied to all subsequent patients.

5. The failure to account for patient variability will lead, in the majority of cases, to patient undertreatment. The relevant quantity for assuring therapeutic efficacy and avoiding organ toxicities is the radiation absorbed dose, and thus, patient-specific dosimetry is essential for optimal efficacy and patient safety.

6. Recent studies using patient-specific dosimetry have demonstrated the ability to establish dose-response relationships for toxicity avoidance. It is thus now clear that the application of patient-specific dosimetry is an essential element to optimizing radiopharmaceutical therapy.

## 16.4 REGULATORY ISSUES

### Investigational Radiopharmaceuticals

1. All pharmaceuticals for human use, whether radioactive or not, are regulated by the U.S. Food and Drug Administration (FDA). A request to evaluate a new radiopharmaceutical for human use is submitted to the FDA in an application called a "Notice of Claimed Investigational Exemption for a New Drug" (IND).

2. The IND can be sponsored by either an individual physician or a radiopharmaceutical manufacturer, who will work with a group of clinical investigators to collect the necessary safety and efficacy data. The IND application includes the names and credentials of the investigators, the clinical protocol, details of the research project, details of the manufacturing of the drug, and animal toxicology data.

3. The clinical investigation of the new radiopharmaceutical occurs in three stages. Phase I focuses on a limited number of patients and is designed to provide information on the pharmacologic distribution, metabolism, dosimetry, toxicity, optimal dose schedule, and adverse reactions.

4. For therapeutic pharmaceuticals, a maximum permissible dose (MPD) or recommended Phase II dose (RP2D) is determined for use in subsequent clinical Phase II studies. These studies include a limited number of patients with specific diseases and are conducted to begin the assessment of the drug's efficacy, to refine the dose schedule, and to collect more information on safety and efficacy.

5. Phase III clinical trials involve a much larger number of patients (and are typically conducted by several institutions) to provide more extensive (*i.e.*, statistically significant) information on efficacy, safety, and dose administration, often in a randomized, blinded fashion.

6. To obtain approval to market, a new radiopharmaceutical, a "New Drug Application" (NDA), must be submitted to and approved by the FDA. Approval of a new radiopharmaceutical typically requires 5 to 10 years from laboratory work to NDA.

7. The package insert of an approved radiopharmaceutical describes the intended purpose of the radiopharmaceutical, the suggested dose, dosimetry, adverse reactions, clinical pharmacology, and contraindications.

## By-Product Material, Authorized Users, Written Directives, and Medical Events

### Medical Use of By-Product Material

1. Although the production of radiopharmaceuticals is regulated by the FDA, the medical use of radioactive material is regulated under the terms of a license issued to a specific legal entity (such as a clinic or hospital, which is the *licensee*) by the U.S. Nuclear Regulatory Commission (NRC) or a comparable state agency (*i.e.*, an agreement state, which is discussed further in Chapter 21).

2. NRC regulations do not, however, specify permissible administered activities or patient radiation doses, as any such regulations would be considered as excessively intrusive on the practice of medicine. The NRC's regulations apply to the use of *by-product material*.

3. Until recently, the regulatory definition of by-product material included radionuclides that were the by-products of nuclear fission or nuclear activation but excluded others such as accelerator-produced radionuclides.

4. The current NRC's definition of by-product material, however, has been broadened to include virtually all radioactive material used in medicine. The regulations regarding the medical use of radioactive material are contained in Title 10, Part 35, of the *Code of Federal Regulations* (10 CFR 35).

### Authorized User

1. An *authorized user* (AU), in the context of the practice of nuclear medicine, is a physician who is responsible for the medical use of radioactive material and is designated by name on a license for the medical use of radioactive material or is approved by the radiation safety committee of a medical institution whose license authorizes such actions.

2. Such a physician may be certified by a medical specialty board, such as the American Board of Radiology, whose certification process includes all of the requirements identified in Part 35 for the medical use of unsealed sources of radioactive materials for diagnosis and therapy.

3. Alternatively, a physician can apply to the NRC or comparable state agency for AU status by providing documentation of the specific education, training, and experience requirements contained in 10 CFR 35.

### Written Directive

1. The NRC requires that, before the administration of a dosage of I-131 sodium iodide greater than 1.11 MBq (30 mCi) or any therapeutic dosage of unsealed by-product material, a *written directive* must be signed and dated by an authorized user.

2. The written directive must contain the patient or human research subject's name and must describe the radioactive drug, the activity, and (for radionuclides other than I-131) the route of administration.

3. In addition, the NRC requires the implementation of written procedures to provide, for each administration requiring a written directive, high confidence that the patient or human research subject's identity is verified before the administration and that each administration is performed in accordance with the written directive.

### Medical Events

1. The NRC defines certain errors in the administration of radiopharmaceuticals as *medical events* and requires specific actions to be taken within specified time periods following the recognition of the error. The initial report to the NRC (or, in an agreement state, the comparable state agency) must be made by telephone no later than the next calendar day after the discovery of the event and must be followed by a written report within 15 days.

2. This report must include specific information such as a description of the incident, the cause of the medical event, the effect (if any) on the individual or individuals involved, and proposed corrective actions.

3. The referring physician must be notified of the medical event, and the patient must also be notified, unless the referring physician states that he or she will inform the patient or that, based on medical judgment, notification of the patient would be harmful. Additional details regarding these reporting requirements can be found in 10 CFR 35.

## NRC Definition of a Medical Event

1. A medical event is defined by the NRC as the administration of NRC-licensed radioactive material that results in one of the following conditions (2, 3, 4, or 5), unless its occurrence was as the direct result of a patient intervention (*e.g.*, an I-131 therapy patient takes only one half of the prescribed treatment and then refuses to take the balance of the prescribed dosage):

2. A dose that differs from the prescribed dose or dose that would have resulted from the prescribed *dosage* (*i.e.*, administered activity) by more than 0.05 Sv (5 rem) effective dose equivalent, 0.5 Sv (50 rem) to an organ or tissue, or 0.5 Sv (50 rem) shallow dose equivalent to the skin, and one of the following conditions (a or b) has also occurred.

   a. The total dose delivered differs from the prescribed dose by 20% or more.

   b. The total dosage delivered differs from the prescribed dosage by 20% or more or falls outside the prescribed dosage range. Falling outside the prescribed dosage range means the administration of activity that is greater or less than a predetermined range of activity for a given procedure that has been established by the licensee.

3. A dose that exceeds 0.05 Sv (5 rem) effective dose equivalent, 0.5 Sv (50 rem) to an organ or tissue, or 0.5 Sv (50 rem) shallow dose equivalent to the skin from any of the following:

   a. An administration of a wrong radioactive drug containing by-product material

   b. An administration of a radioactive drug containing by-product material through the wrong route of administration

   c. An administration of a dose or dosage to the wrong individual or human research subject

4. A dose to the skin or an organ or tissue other than the treatment site that exceeds by 0.5 Sv (50 rem) and 50% or more of the dose expected from the administration defined in the written directive.

5. Any event resulting from intervention of a patient or human research subject in which the administration of by-product material or radiation from by-product material results or will result in unintended permanent functional damage to an organ or a physiological system, as determined by a physician.

# Section II Questions and Answers

1. Which of the following positron-emitting radio-nuclides can be produced in a regionally based cyclotron facility as opposed to one located at the medical facility where PET imaging is performed?
   A. F-18
   B. N-13
   C. C-11
   D. O-15

2. Fission fragments, the primary products of the fission reaction following absorption of a thermal neutron by the radionuclide U-235, almost always undergo radioactive decay by what process?
   A. Alpha particle decay
   B. Beta-minus decay
   C. Beta-plus decay
   D. Orbital electron capture

3. How is the U-235 fission reaction (Eq. 16-4) sustained in the form of a steady-state chain reaction?
   A. Additional neutrons are created from emitted γ-rays.
   B. Fast neutrons emitted in fission are thermalized.
   C. Fission fragments reform additional U-235 atoms.
   D. Emitted neutrons are immediately captured by U-235.

4. Medical radionuclides derived from fission fragments produced in a nuclear reactor have high specific activity. What are the units of specific activity?
   A. MBq or Ci per $m^2$
   B. MBq or Ci per hour
   C. MBq or Ci per $m^3$
   D. MBq or Ci per gram

5. I-123 is used in pretherapy scans of patients with thyroid cancer to provide information on the amount of thyroid remnant present. By what production mechanism do we obtain I-123?
   A. Radionuclide generator
   B. Nuclear reactor—neutron activation
   C. Nuclear reactor—fission product
   D. Linear accelerator/cyclotron

6. A radiopharmacy delivers a Mo-99/Tc-99m generator early Monday morning. The initial activity of the parent is 700 GBq. How much Mo-99 is still available in the generator 48 h later?
   A. 123 GBq
   B. 223 GBq
   C. 323 GBq
   D. 423 GBq

7. In transient equilibrium, the daughter activity will build up and exceed that of the parent at equilibrium (steady-state conditions). However, this is not the case for Mo-99/Tc-99m as shown in Figure 16-9. Why?
   A. Only 88% of Mo-99 decays yield Ru-99.
   B. Only 12% of Mo-99 decays yield Tc-99m.
   C. Only 88% of Mo-99 decays yield Tc-99m.
   D. Only 12% of Mo-99 decays yield Ru-99.

8. Under secular equilibrium, if there is no daughter activity present at $t = 0$, what percentage of the parent activity has the daughter established by 4 daughter half-lives?
   A. 96.5%
   B. 93.8%
   C. 90.8%
   D. 87.5%

9. There are two quality control tests performed routinely on Mo-99/Tc-99m radionuclide generators. These are:
   A. Ru-99 via test strips/Mo-99 via dose calibrator
   B. Mo-99 via dose calibrator/alumina via test strips
   C. Ru-99 via dose calibrator/alumina via test strips
   D. Mo-99 via test strips/Ru-99 via dose calibrator

10. Which of the following reasons is **not** associated with the wide-spread use of Tc-99m in more than 85% of diagnostic imaging radiopharmaceuticals?
    A. High yield of intermediate energy 140-keV γ-ray
    B. Stable daughter Ru-99
    C. Moderate physical half-life of 6.02 h
    D. Robust options for radiolabeling of pharmaceuticals

11. Which of the following radiopharmaceutical characteristics increases radiation dose to nontargeted tissues?
    A. Long blood circulation times
    B. Short blood circulation times
    C. High target tissue uptake fractions
    D. Short imaging times

12. If chemical dissociation from a radiopharmaceutical occurs in the patient, what happens to the released radionuclide?
    A. Tissue uptake given by physical half-life
    B. Tissue uptake given by pharmaceutical biokinetics
    C. Tissue uptake given by radioisotopic biokinetics
    D. Tissue uptake given by elemental biokinetics

13. Which of the following is **not** a desired feature of diagnostic imaging radiopharmaceuticals?
    A. High specific activity
    B. Radionuclides that are carrier free
    C. Multiple photons in the emission spectrum
    D. Shelf life that is compatible with clinical use

14. The U.S. FDA approved the very first alpha-particle–emitting radiopharmaceutical in 2013 for an advanced form of prostate cancer. The alpha-emitting radionuclide was which one of the following?
    A. At-211          C. Ra-223
    B. Bi-212          D. Th-227

15. The radiopharmaceutical Tc-99m-MAA is used for imaging of pulmonary perfusion. Of which mechanism of tissue localization is this an example?
    A. Compartmental localization and leakage
    B. Capillary blockage
    C. Receptor binding
    D. Physiochemical adsorption

16. Tc-99m–labeled red blood cells injected into the circulatory system is an example of which mechanism of tissue localization?
    A. Perfusion
    B. Compartmental localization and leakage
    C. Chemotaxis
    D. Active transport

17. Tc-99m diethylenetriaminepentaacetic acid (DTPA) for brain imaging is an example of which mechanism of tissue localization?
    A. Phagocytosis
    B. Perfusion
    C. Passive diffusion
    D. Active transport

18. F-18 fluorodeoxyglucose (or FDG) used in metastatic cancer screening is an example of which mechanism of tissue localization?
    A. Physiochemical adsorption
    B. Receptor binding
    C. Passive diffusion
    D. Active transport

19. What does the acronym MIRD stand for?
    A. Method for Individual Radiation Dose
    B. Medical Internal Radiation Dose
    C. Method of Internal Radiation Dosimetry
    D. Medical Internal Radiopharmaceutical Dosimetry

20. The MIRD schema is given by the expression: $\dot{D}(r_T, t) = \sum_{r_S} A(r_S, t) S(r_T \leftarrow r_S, t)$. Which of the terms denote the absorbed dose rate to the target tissue per activity of the radiopharmaceutical in the source tissue?
    A. $\dot{D}(r_T, t)$
    B. $A(r_S, t)$
    C. $S(r_T \leftarrow r_S, t)$
    D. $\sum_{r_S} A(r_S, t) S(r_T \leftarrow r_S, t)$

21. A new Tc-99m–labeled radiopharmaceutical uniformly distributes throughout the brain. Given that the brain self-dose $S$ value for Tc-99m $[S(\text{brain} \leftarrow \text{brain})]$ is $4.23 \times 10^{-6}$ mGy/MBq-s, how many total decays of Tc-99m would be required to give a mean absorbed dose to the brain of 50 $\mu$Gy?
    A. 11.8 decays
    B. 11.8 thousand decays
    C. 11.8 billion decays
    D. 11.8 trillion decays

22. A new Tc-99m–labeled radiopharmaceutical for kidney evaluation delivers 90% of injected activity to the target organ ($f_s$). Subsequent biokinetic analysis gives a biological uptake half-time $T_{bu}$ of 2 h and a biological clearance half-time $T_{bc}$ of 8 h. At 10 h post-injection, what percentage of the administered activity $A_0$ is still present in the kidneys?
    A. 1.1%          C. 50%
    B. 11%           D. 100%

23. What **percent error** would be introduced in the answer to Question 22 if the uptake phase was ignored? (Assume at $t = 0$, the radiopharmaceutical immediately was taken up by the kidneys and then activity decreased only through biological clearance and physical decay.)
    A. −8%           C. −4%
    B. +8%           D. +4%

24. In Question 22, for an administered activity $A_0 =$ 500 MBq, what is the total absorbed dose to the kidneys (assuming $\tau = \infty$) under the conditions of no biological uptake and a single exponential decline in activity due to biological clearance and physical decay? (Use a simplified version of Eq. 16-22 for $\tilde{A}$ (kidneys) and the Tc-99m $S$ value for kidney self-dose from Table 16-5.)
    A. 2.9 $\mu$Gy          C. 10.6 mGy
    B. 29 $\mu$Gy           D. 106 mGy

25. In Questions 22 to 24, the radiopharmaceutical uptake in the kidneys is 90% of $A_0$. If the remaining 10% of $A_0$ is localized in the neighboring liver with instantaneous uptake and a biological clearance half-time $T_{bc}$ of 8 h ($\lambda_{bc}$ is the same for both organs), what percent increase in kidney

dose is expected for γ-ray cross-fire from the liver Tc-99m activity to the kidney target organ?

A. 0.25%          C. 25%

B. 2.5%          D. No increase

26. In the ICRP Publication 137 compartmental model for systemic iodine, which sets of organs have separate subcompartments for the presence of both inorganic and organic forms of iodine?
    A. Urinary bladder, thyroid, blood, and kidneys
    B. Liver, thyroid, salivary glands, blood
    C. Thyroid, liver, kidneys, blood
    D. Thyroid, liver, stomach contents, kidneys

27. All pharmaceuticals for human use, whether radioactive or not, are regulated by which agency?
    A. CDC—Centers for Disease Control and Prevention
    B. NIH—National Institutes of Health
    C. NRC—Nuclear Regulatory Agency
    D. FDA—Food and Drug Administration

28. In addition to the IND (investigational new drug) and NDA (new drug application) process, an additional mechanism for limited use of radio-pharmaceuticals is the RDRC protocol. RDRC stands for:
    A. Radioactive Drug Research Committee
    B. Radiation Dose Research Concurrence
    C. Radioactive Drug Retrospective Compliance
    D. Radiation Determination for Research Compliance

29. Which of the following does **not** define an *authorized user* (AU)?
    A. Physician responsible for the medical use of the agent
    B. Designated on a license for medical use of the agent
    C. Listed on the radiopharmaceutical patent
    D. Is approved by the radiation safety committee

30. Which federal agency defines certain errors in the administration of radiopharmaceuticals as a *medical event*?
    A. CDC—Centers for Disease Control and Prevention
    B. NIH—National Institutes of Health
    C. NRC—Nuclear Regulatory Agency
    D. FDA—Food and Drug Administration

# Answers

1. **A**  PET is short for positron emission tomography whereby the radiopharmaceutical is labeled with a radio-nuclide that decays via positron emission (see Section 15.2.3). There are four primary radionuclides that are used for radiolabeling pharmaceuticals in PET imaging. These are F-18, N-13, O-15, and C-11. Their physical half-lives are, respectively, 110, 10, 2, and 20 min. The latter three thus decay too quickly to be produced regionally (that is away from the PET imaging center), and thus, they must be produced by a cyclotron (proton accelerator) colocated at the imaging facility. The slightly longer physical half-life of F-18, however, permits production outside the imaging center with daily shipping to the PET imaging center without excessive loss by physical decay before radiopharmaceutical preparation. *(Pg. 649)*

2. **B**  Nuclear fission of U-235 by thermal neutrons yields a release of energy (approximately 200 MeV), prompt gamma-rays, additional neutrons (needed to sustain the chain reaction after they are slowed by moderation), and two nuclear "fragments." These fragments typically are "neutron rich" ($N/P$ ratio is too high to balance nuclear attractive and repulsive forces), and thus, the vast majority of these fission-produced radionuclides must undergo beta-minus decay (see Section 15.2.2). The three other forms of radioactive decay are associated with radioactive nuclei that are "neutron poor." *(Pg. 650)*

3. **B**  In the nuclear fission of U-235, four products are formed: large fragments of the "split" U-235 atom, approximately 3 neutrons emitted at high energy (fast neutrons), gamma-ray photons, and approximately 200 MeV of energy, which typically heats the surrounding water in a nuclear reactor (which eventually produces steam which runs turbines which generates electricity). The emitted neutrons cannot immediately cause additional fission reactions—they must be slowed down through elastic collisions with hydrogen (or oxygen) nuclei in the surrounding water (same water that is absorbed as heat energy from fission). This process is called "neutron moderation" thus moving an emitted fast neutron down to thermal energies where it can begin the fission process again through absorption by another U-235 atom. *(Pg. 650)*

4. **D**  Specific activity of a radionuclide is the amount of radioactivity (SI units of MBq [$10^6$ decays per second] or Ci [$3.7 \times 10^{10}$ decays per second]) per unit mass (*e.g.*, gram) of that radionuclide. A high specific activity thus implies that mass concentration of radioactive atoms is large within your sample. *(Pg. 653)*

5. **D**  I-123 is produced in a linear or cyclotron accelerator in which protons irradiate stable I-127, which yields radioactive Xe-123 (2-h physical half-life). Following electron capture decay of Xe-123, we get the desired radionuclide I-123. *(Pg. 619, Eq. 16-2; Pg. 654, Table 16-1)*

6. **D**  We need to use the fundamental decay equation given in Section 15.1.4 (Eq. 15-7). The physical half-life ($T_p$ or $T_{1/2}$) of Mo-99 is 66 h (Fig. 16-8) and thus the physical decay constant $\lambda_p = \ln(2)/T_p = (0.693)/(66\ h)$ = 0.01050 $h^{-1}$. Using Equation 15-7, we thus have $A = A_0 e^{-\lambda t} = (700\ GBq)\ \exp[-(0.01050\ h^{-1})(48\ h)] = (700\ GBq) \times (0.60411) = 423\ GBq$. Thus, after 48 h (2 full days), some 40% of the parent radionuclide Mo-99 has decayed and only 60% of the original 700 GBq remains or 423 GBq. Note that 1 GBq = $10^9$ Bq or one billion decays per second. *(Pg. 623, 656)*

7. **C**  If 100% of Mo-99 decays yielded the single daughter radionuclide Tc-99m, then transient equilibrium would be established such that at steady state, the activity of the Tc-99m daughter will exceed that of the Mo-99 by approximately 10%. This is not the case (Tc-99m activity will at most be only 97% of that of the parent Mo-99) because only 88% of all Mo-99 decays (not 100%) give the daughter Tc-99m. The remaining 12% of Mo-99 decays yield a different daughter radionuclide Tc-99 (without the "m"). The difference between Tc-99m and Tc-99 is that the former is left in an excited nuclear state ("m" means metastable) and must release that energy in the form of a 140-keV $\gamma$-ray (the same $\gamma$-ray with which we image the patient in nuclear medicine using Tc-99m—labeled radiopharmaceuticals). *(Pg. 656–657)*

**8.** **B**  As shown in graphically in Figure 16-10, the daughter activity exponentially approaches the activity of the parent under the condition of secular equilibrium. Here, we see that after one, two, and three physical half-lives of the daughter radionuclide, the daughter activity achieves 50%, 75%, and then 87.5% of the parent activity (assuming no daughter at $t = 0$). In each case, we see that the percentage increase in daughter activity is one half the prior gain for each additional one half-life increase in time. The percent increase in daughter activity is shown to be 87.5% − 75% or 12.5% over the time interval $t = 2T_P$ and $t = 3T_P$. Thus, the next percent increase between $t = 3T_P$ and $t = 4T_P$ would be 12.5%/2 or 6.25%. The final answer is thus 87.5% + 6.25% or 93.75% (rounded to 93.8%). Recall that physical half-life is given by either the symbol $T_{1/2}$ or $T_P$. *(Pg. 657–658, Fig. 16-10)*

**9.** **B**  Under ideal conditions, the eluant from an Mo-99/Tc-99m radionuclide generator should only contain the intended radioactive daughter Tc-99m, which is captured at approximately 85% efficiency. In a radiopharmacy quality control program, two different impurities should be monitored in the eluant. The first is the presence of the parent radionuclide Mo-99, which ideally will remain on a porous column of ammonium molybdate. To detect for the presence of the parent, the eluant is placed within a thick lead container, which is in turn placed within a dose calibrator—a well-geometry ion chamber filled with pressurized argon gas (see Fig. 17-27). The 140-keV γ-rays from Tc-99m are thus absorbed in the lead container, but if any Mo-99 is present, their higher-energy γ-rays (740 and 780 keV) will penetrate that container and register detection counts in the dose calibrator. The second potential contaminant is the alumina of the column material itself. $Al^{3+}$ ion can be readily measured colorimetrically. *(Pg. 656–657)*

**10.** **B**  There are three primary reasons for the fact that approximately 85% of all radiopharmaceuticals for diagnostic nuclear medicine imaging use Tc-99m as the radionuclide for pharmaceutical labeling. First, the single high-yield (88%) 140-keV γ-ray is ideal for nuclear medicine imaging as it is energetic enough to make it out of the patient's body without substantial body absorption yet not too high to potentially be missed by the detector array surrounding the patient in the imaging system. Second, the 6.02-h physical half-life is also just right for nuclear medicine imaging. With shorter half-lives, radiopharmaceutical decays predominant in blood circulation before sufficient time permits target tissue accumulation for imaging. With longer half-lives, the discharged patient become a source of medical staff and family member exposures, thus potentially delaying patient release. Finally, technetium is an element that is readily chelated to many different forms of pharmaceuticals thus allowing reasonable efforts in radiochemistry for radiopharmaceutical production. The production of stable Ru-99 following Tc-99m decay is not a factor in its widespread use in nuclear medicine. *(Pg. 659)*

**11.** **A**  To lower radiation dose to nontargeted tissues (those for which radiopharmaceutical uptake was not desired nor intended), the radiopharmaceutical should be present in circulating blood for only a period of time needed for maximum uptake to the imaged organ or tissue. The residual fraction of the administered activity that is not taken up by the target tissue should (1) have a relatively short time in general blood circulation, (2) should be only minimally taken up by other unintended organs and tissues, and (3) should be readily excreted from the body via the urinary pathway. *(Pg. 665)*

**12.** **D**  In the event that the chemical bond between the radionuclide and the pharmaceutical (drug component of the radiopharmaceutical) does not hold while in blood circulation, the pharmaceutical moiety will most likely continue to undergo uptake within the intended organ for nuclear medicine imaging (although loss of the radionuclide might additionally alter that fate). The radionuclide, however, will most likely not be taken up within the intended organ for imaging as that feature of localization was driven by the pharmaceutical, not the radionuclide portion of the radiopharmaceutical. Free radionuclides in circulating blood will thus have their own unique biokinetics—processes entailing the organs of radionuclide uptake and the time course of that uptake. Furthermore, it is only the element of the radionuclide that drives this process. For example, the biokinetics of free iodine are the same regardless of the isotope of iodine—I-131 versus I-125, for example. Both will be taken up primarily by the thyroid gland. *(Pg. 665)*

**13.** **C**  Key and desirable features of a radiopharmaceutical would include (1) high specific activity—so that a given administered activity is associated with a small injection of radiolabeled drug mass; (2) carrier-free radionuclides, that is, without other radionuclides present in the injected radiopharmaceutical administration, which will most likely lead to additional patient dose with no imaging benefit, and (3) a shelf life that conforms to the frequency and patient load of the imaging center (thus avoiding undue disposal of unused radiopharmaceutical). Imaging of the radiopharmaceutical is significantly enhanced technically with more simple (ideally single-energy) photon emissions in the radionuclide decay scheme. *(Pg. 665)*

14. **C**  In May of 2013, the U.S. FDA approved the first therapy radiopharmaceutical using an alpha-particle emitter: Xofigo (radium Ra 223 dichloride) for the treatment of patients with castration-resistant prostate cancer (CRPC), symptomatic bone metastases, and no known visceral metastatic disease. Since that milestone, there has been significant research activities and ongoing clinical trials in the development of other alpha-emitter therapy radiopharmaceuticals across a variety of cancer types such as breast, prostate, neuroendocrine tumors, and leukemia. Alpha-emitters of current interest in radiopharmaceutical therapy include At-211, Pb-212, Bi-212, Bi-213, Ra-223, Ac-225, and Th-227. *(Pg. 666)*

15. **B**  When particles slightly larger than RBCs are injected intravenously, they become trapped in the capillary beds. A common example in nuclear medicine is in the assessment of pulmonary perfusion by the injection of Tc-99m-MAA (microaggregated albumin), which is trapped in the pulmonary capillary bed. Imaging the distribution of Tc-99m-MAA provides a representative assessment of pulmonary perfusion. *(Pg. 666–668)*

16. **B**  Compartmental localization refers to the introduction of the radiopharmaceutical into a well-defined anatomic compartment. Examples include Xe-133 gas inhalation into the lung, intraperitoneal instillation of P-32 chromic phosphate, and Tc-99m–labeled RBCs injected into the circulatory system. Compartmental leakage is used to identify an abnormal opening in an otherwise closed compartment, as when labeled RBCs are used to detect gastrointestinal bleeding. *(Pg. 666–668)*

17. **C**  Passive diffusion is simply the free movement of a substance from a region of high concentration to one of lower concentration. Anatomic and physiologic mechanisms exist in the brain tissue and surrounding vasculature that allow essential nutrients, metabolites, and lipid-soluble compounds to pass freely between the plasma and brain tissue while many water-soluble substances (including most radiopharmaceuticals) are prevented from entering healthy brain tissue. Disruptions of the blood-brain barrier can be produced by trauma, neoplasms, and inflammation. The disruption permits radiopharmaceuticals such as Tc-99m diethylenetriaminepentaacetic acid (DTPA), which is normally excluded by the blood-brain barrier, to follow the concentration gradient and enter the affected brain tissue. *(Pg. 666–668)*

18. **D**  Active transport involves cellular metabolic processes that expend energy to concentrate the radiopharmaceutical into a tissue against a concentration gradient and above plasma levels. The classic example in nuclear medicine is the trapping and organification of radioactive iodide. F-18 FDG is a glucose analog that concentrates in cells that rely upon glucose as an energy source or in cells whose dependence on glucose increases under pathophysiological conditions. F-18 FDG is actively transported into the cell where it is phosphorylated and trapped for several hours as FDG-6-phosphate. The retention and clearance of FDG reflect glucose metabolism in a given tissue. F-18 FDG is used to assist in the evaluation of malignancy in patients with known or suspected diagnoses of cancer. *(Pg. 666–668)*

19. **B**  The original mathematical methods, models, equations, nuclear decay data, and biokinetic parameters needed for computing radiation absorbed dose to internal organs were developed by the Medical Internal Radiation Dose (or MIRD) Committee of the Society of Nuclear Medicine and Molecular Imaging (SNMMI) in the late 1950s to early 1960s. The most recent revision of the MIRD schema for internal organ dosimetry was published in 2009 as MIRD Pamphlet No. 21 in the *Journal of Nuclear Medicine*. *(Pg. 670)*

20. **C**  The time-dependent activity $A(r_s, t)$ represents the rate of nuclear decays in the source tissue $r_s$ at time $t$, while the $S$ value represents the absorbed dose rate to the target tissue $r_T$ per radionuclide activity in the source region $r_s$ also at time $t$. *(Pg. 671)*

21. **C**  This example is a simple application of the MIRD schema equation (Eqs. 16-8 and 16-9) where the absorbed dose to the target tissue $D(r_T = \text{brain})$ is given as the product of the time-integrated activity is the brain $\tilde{A}(r_s = \text{brain})$ and the radionuclide $S$ values for Tc-99m in the brain for the brain as both the source and target region $S$ (brain ← brain). Note that we are not given information as to the time $\tau$ over which the dose is delivered—it can be assumed to be to $\tau = \infty$. We know $D$ and $S$, but not $\tilde{A}$. We compute $\tilde{A}$ as the ratio of $D$ to $S$ or as the product of $D$ and $(1/S)$.

$$\tilde{A}(\text{brain}) = (50 \ \mu\text{Gy}) \times \left( \frac{\text{mGy}}{1000 \ \mu\text{Gy}} \right) \times \left( \frac{\text{MBq-s}}{4.23 \times 10^{-6} \ \text{mGy}} \right) \times \left( \frac{10^6 \ \text{Bq}}{\text{MBq}} \right)$$
$$= 1.18 \times 10^{10} \ \text{Bq-s}$$

Comments: Here, we can to make sure that all units were consistent. First, the absorbed dose in microgray ($\mu$Gy) had to be converted to units of milligray (mGy) to be consistent with the given units of the $S$ value.

Also, one nuclear decay can be written using the combined unit Bq-s as 1 Bq is a 1 decay per second (and thus implicitly the seconds and per second cancel each other leaving us with decays). However, the $S$ value was given as the absorbed dose in mGy per million decays—MBq-s. Thus, we had to convert MBq to Bq to give us our final answer in just units of Bq-s (or decays). The answer $1.18 \times 10^{10}$ decays is also equivalent to 11.8 billion decays. Final note—in this problem, we assumed that the brain was the only source of the Tc-99m radiopharmaceutical. If there were uptake in other source organs, we would have to account for their contribution to brain dose (via the 140-keV emitted γ-rays) by looking up additional $S$ values from Table 16-5 for what is called cross-dose irradiation (simulations where the brain is the target but other organs are additional sources). *(Pg. 672–673, 679–680; Table 16-5)*

22. **B**  To solve this problem, we use Eqs. 16-18, 16-19, and then 16-20. The physical half-life of Tc-99m is 6.02 h and thus the value of $\lambda_P$ = ln(2)/6.02 h = 0.11514 $h^{-1}$. The biological uptake rate constant for this radio-pharmaceutical is $\lambda_{bu}$ = ln(2)/$T_{bu}$ = ln(2)/2 h = 0.34657 $h^{-1}$. The biological clearance rate constant is given as $\lambda_{bc}$ = ln(2)/$T_{bc}$ = ln(2)/8 h = 0.08664 $h^{-1}$. The corresponding effective uptake and clearance rate constants are then $\lambda_{eu}$ = $\lambda_{bu}$ + $\lambda_P$ = 0.34657 $h^{-1}$ + 0.11514 $h^{-1}$ = 0.46171 $h^{-1}$ and $\lambda_{ec}$ = $\lambda_{bc}$ + $\lambda_P$ = 0.08664 $h^{-1}$ + 0.11514 $h^{-1}$ = 0.20178 $h^{-1}$. The fraction of administered activity $A_0$ that goes to the kidneys is 90% and thus $f_s$ = $f_{kidneys}$ = 0.9. Using Eq. 16-20 and evaluating that equation at $t$ = 10 h, then gives:

$$\frac{A(t=10\text{ h})}{A_0} = (0.9)\left[ e^{-(0.20178h^{-1})(10h)} - e^{-(0.46171h^{-1})(10h)} \right] = (0.9)[0.13295 - 0.00988] = 0.11076$$

The fraction of administered radiopharmaceutical activity still present in the kidneys 10 h after that administration is approximately 11%. Note—in this solution, we use the expression $\lambda_P$ = ln(2)/$T_P$ = ln(2)/6.02 h = 0.11514 $h^{-1}$. If the natural logarithm of 2 [ln(2)] were approximated by the fractional numeral 0.693, then $\lambda_P$ = 0.693/$T_P$ = 0.693/6.02 h = 0.11516 $h^{-1}$—a slight change in the 5th significant digit. *(Pg. 674)*

23. **B**  If you ignored the uptake phase of the radiopharmaceutical in Question 22, that is mathematically equivalent to changing the biological uptake half-time from $T_{bu}$ = 2 h to $T_{bu}$ = 0 h. In this case, we revise our value of $\lambda_{bu}$ = ln(2)/$T_{bu}$ = ln(2)/0 h = ∞ $h^{-1}$. Next, the second exponential term in Eq. 16-20 then goes to zero (as $e^{-\lambda t} \to 0$ as $\lambda \to \infty$). The revised answer to Question 22 is then computed by changing the second term in the brackets (0.00988) to zero. The new solution is then $A/A_0$ = (0.9) × (0.13295) = 0.11966, which is 12% expressed as a percentage and rounded to two significant figures. Your percent error by ignoring the biological uptake phase is then (0.11966 − 0.11076)/(0.11076) = 0.08035 or 8% error. Note that by ignoring biological uptake and instead assuming instantaneous organ uptake from blood, your estimate of organ activity 10 h postadministration is 8% higher than it would be with a more time-dependent (noninstantaneous) organ uptake. *(Pg. 674)*

24. **D**  We use the MIRD schema to compute the kidney absorbed dose. By setting the dose integration period $\tau$ = ∞, we get the highest estimate of organ dose. In Equation 16-22, there are three terms. In this problem, we can ignore (set to zero) the third term as we are asked to ignore biological uptake of the radiopharmaceutical to the kidneys. Additionally, we are told that the kidney clearance of the radiopharmaceutical follows a single exponential decrease. Equation 16-22 allows for a two-exponential fit to the radiopharmaceutical clearance (hence the subscripts 1 and 2). Thus, in this problem, we can set the second term to zero (the 2nd compartment) and work only with the first term. Our modified form of Equation 16-22 is thus:

$$\tilde{A}(r_s, \infty) = \frac{A_0 f_S}{\lambda_{ec}}\left[1 - e^{-\lambda_{ec}(\infty)}\right] = \frac{A_0 f_S}{\lambda_{ec}}[1 - 0] = \frac{A_0 f_S}{\lambda_{ec}} \quad \text{since} \, e^{-\infty} \to 0.$$

Thus, we can compute the time-integrated activity in the kidneys as $\tilde{A}$(kidneys) = [$A_0$ × $f_s$]/$\lambda_{ec}$ = [500 MBq × 0.9]/(0.20178 $h^{-1}$) = 2.23015 × $10^3$ MBq-h × (3,600 s/h) = 8.02855 × $10^6$ MBq-s. Note that we had to convert MBq-h to MBq-s as the radionuclide $S$ values is typically given in units of mGy per MBq-s. In Table 16-5, we see that the $S$ value for kidney self-dose for Tc-99m–labeled radiopharmaceuticals is $S$(kidney ← kidney) = 1.32 × $10^{-5}$ mGy/MBq-s. The total absorbed dose to the kidneys for this imaging agent would then be given by the MIRD schema as $D$(kidneys) = $\tilde{A}$(kidneys) × $S$(kidneys ← kidneys) = (8.02855 × $10^6$ MBq-s) × (1.32 × $10^{-5}$ mGy/MBq-s) = 106 mGy. *(Pg. 675, Eq. 16-22)*

25. **A**  As before, we need to use the MIRD schema to compute, in this case, the cross-dose from radiopharma-ceutical activity in the liver (additional source organ) to the kidney (original target organ). As in Question 24, we first compute the time-integrated activity as $\tilde{A}$(liver) = [$A_0$ × $f_s$]/$\lambda_{ec}$ where the $A_0$ is the same (500 MBq), $f_s$ is

now 0.1, and $\lambda_{ec}$ is the same as that computed for the kidneys. Thus, $\bar{A}$(liver) = [500 MBq × 0.1]/(0.20178 h$^{-1}$) = 2.47795 × 10$^2$ MBq-h × (3,600 s/h) = 8.92061 × 10$^5$ MBq-s. Note that due to the lower value of fraction uptake ($f_s$ = 0.1 and not 0.9), the time-integrated activity in the liver is approximately a factor of 10 lower than that in the kidneys. Next, we go to Table 16-5 and find the value for S(kidneys ← liver) = 2.93 × 10$^{-7}$ mGy/MBq-s. Again, note that S(kidneys ← liver) for kidney cross-dose is lower than S(kidney ← kidney) for kidney self-dose for Tc-99m. It is lower by factor of approximately 45. This is always the case, as organ self-dose is generally dominated by charged-particle emissions (alpha particles, beta particles, conversion, and Auger electrons), which only (generally) contribute to organ self-dose. Only the radionuclide's photon component of the emission spectrum (γ-rays, characteristic x-rays, and possibly bremsstrahlung x-rays) can contribute to organ dose when $r_S \neq r_T$. The value of the absorbed dose to the kidneys from Tc-99m radiopharmaceutical activity in the liver is thus computed as D(kidneys) = $\bar{A}$(liver) × S(kidneys ← liver) = (8.92061 × 10$^5$ MBq-s) × (2.93 × 10$^{-7}$ mGy/MBq-s) = 0.261 mGy. The percent increase in kidney dose from liver photon cross-fire is thus (0.261 mGy/106 mGy) × 100% or 0.25%. It is very small and in this case may be ignored. (*Pg. 675, Eq. 16-22*)

26. **C** As shown in Figure 16-13, the organs in which both organic and inorganic iodine are given as separate subcompartments are the thyroid, liver, kidneys, and blood. Other organs are given by only a single compartment in this systemic biokinetic model. (*Pg. 676, Fig. 16-13*)

27. **D** All pharmaceuticals for human use, whether radioactive or not, are regulated by the U.S. Food and Drug Administration (FDA). A request to evaluate a new radiopharmaceutical for human use is submitted to the FDA in an application called a "Notice of Claimed Investigational Exemption for a New Drug" (IND). (*Pg. 682–685*)

28. **A** An additional mechanism for limited investigational use of radiopharmaceuticals is a Radioactive Drug Research Committee (RDRC) protocol. An institution can form its own RDRC or request another institution's RDRC to review a protocol. RDRC approval places a number of limitations on the types of human investigational studies that are allowed. The intent is to allow the collection of data for basic research studies regarding the agent (*e.g.*, to obtain an understanding of the metabolism, pharmacokinetics, and dosimetry of the agent). (*Pg. 682–685*)

29. **C** An authorized user (AU), in the context of the practice of nuclear medicine, is a physician who is responsible for the medical use of radioactive material and is designated by name on a license for the medical use of radioactive material or is approved by the radiation safety committee of a medical institution whose license authorizes such actions. (*Pg. 682–685*)

30. **C** The NRC defines certain errors in the administration of radiopharmaceuticals as medical events and requires specific actions to be taken within specified time periods following the recognition of the error. The initial report to the NRC (or, in an agreement state, the comparable state agency) must be made by telephone no later than the next calendar day after the discovery of the event and must be followed by a written report within 15 days. (*Pg. 682–685*)

# Section III Key Equations and Symbols

| QUANTITY | EQUATION(S) | EQ NO./PAGE/COMMENTS |
|---|---|---|
| Production of medical radionuclide Ga-67 | $^{68}Zn\,(p,\,2n)^{67}Ga$ | Eq. 16-1/Pg. 647/Cyclotron-facilitated proton irradiation of Zn-68 |
| Production of the medical radionuclide I-123 | $^{127}I\,(p,\,5n)^{123}Xe$ <br> $^{123}Xe \xrightarrow[T_{1/2}2h]{EC} {}^{123}I$ | Eq. 16-2/Pg. 647/Cyclotron-facilitated proton irradiation of I-127 followed by electron capture decay to I-123 |
| Alternative production of the medical radionuclide I-123 | $^{124}Xe(p,\,2n)^{123}Cs$ <br> $^{123}Cs \xrightarrow[T_{1/2}1s]{EC\,or\,\beta^+} {}^{123}Xe$ <br> $^{123}Xe \xrightarrow[T_{1/2}2h]{EC} {}^{123}I$ | Eq. 16-2/Pg. 647/Cyclotron-facilitated proton irradiation of Xe-124 with subsequent electron capture or positron decay to Xe-123 with further electron capture decay to I-123 |
| Production of the medical radionuclide In-111 | $^{109}Ag\,(\alpha,\,2n)^{111}In$ | Eq. 16-2/Pg. 647/Cyclotron-facilitated alpha-particle irradiation of Ag-109 |
| Alternative production of the medical radionuclide In-111 | $^{111}Cd\,(p,\,n)^{111}In$ | Eq. 16-2/Pg. 647/Cyclotron-facilitated proton irradiation of Cd-111 |
| Alternative production of the medical radionuclide In-111 | $^{112}Cd\,(p,\,2n)^{111}In$ | Eq. 16-2/Pg. 647/Cyclotron-facilitated proton irradiation of Cd-112 |
| Production of the medical radionuclide Co-57 | $^{56}Fe\,(d,\,n)^{57}Co$ | Eq. 16-2/Pg. 647/Cyclotron-facilitated deuteron irradiation of Fe-56 |
| Production of the medical radionuclide Tl-201 | $^{203}Tl\,(p,\,3n)^{201}Pb$ <br> $^{201}Pb \xrightarrow[T_{1/2}9.4h]{EC\,or\,\beta^+} {}^{201}Tl$ | Eq. 16-2/Pg. 647/Cyclotron-facilitated proton irradiation of Tl-203 followed by electron capture or positron decay of Pb-201 |
| Production of the positron-emitting radionuclide F-18 | $^{18}O\,(p,\,n)^{18}F$ | Eq. 16-3/Pg. 649/Cyclotron-facilitated proton irradiation of O-18 |
| Production of the positron-emitting radionuclide N-13 | $^{16}O(p,\,\alpha)^{13}N$ | Eq. 16-3; Pg. 649. Cyclotron-facilitated proton irradiation of O-16 |
| Production of the positron-emitting radionuclide O-15 | $^{14}N(d,\,n)^{15}O$ | Eq. 16-3/Pg. 649/Cyclotron-facilitated deuteron irradiation of N-14 |
| Alternative production of the positron-emitting radionuclide O-15 | $^{15}N\,(p,\,n)^{15}O$ | Eq. 16-3/Pg. 649/Cyclotron-facilitated proton irradiation of N-15 |
| Production of the positron-emitting radionuclide C-11 | $^{14}N\,(p,\,\alpha)^{11}C$ | Eq. 16-3/Pg. 649/Cyclotron-facilitated proton irradiation of N-14 |

*(Continued)*

*(Continued)*

| QUANTITY | EQUATION(S) | EQ NO./PAGE/COMMENTS |
|---|---|---|
| Example of U-235 fission | $${}^{235}_{92}U + {}^{1}_{0}n_{thermal} \rightarrow \left[ {}^{236}_{92}U \right] \begin{array}{c} {}^{134}_{50}Sn \\ \\ {}^{99}_{42}Mo \end{array} + 3{}^{1}_{0}n_{fast} + \gamma + \sim 200\,MeV$$ | Eq. 16-4/Pg. 649/In this example, the fragments produced Sn-134 and Mo-99 are produced (the latter being the parent of Tc-99m) |
| Production of the medical radionuclide P-32 | $^{31}P(n, \gamma)^{32}P$ | Eq. 16-5/Pg. 653/Neutron activation of P-31 |
| Production of the medical radionuclide Cr-51 | $^{50}Cr(n, \gamma)^{51}Cr$ | Eq. 16-5/Pg. 653/Neutron activation of Cr-50 |
| Production of the medical radionuclide I-125 | $^{124}Xe(n, \gamma)^{125}Xe$ <br><br> $^{125}Xe \xrightarrow[T_{1/2}17\,hr]{EC\ or\ \beta^+} {}^{125}I$ | Eq. 16-6/Pg. 653/Neutron activation of Xe-124 followed by electron capture or positron decay of Xe-125 |
| *MIRD schema:* Mean absorbed dose rate to target tissue $r_T$ at time $t$ postadministration | $\dot{D}(r_T,t) = \sum_{r_S} A(r_S,t)\, S(r_T \leftarrow r_S,t)$ | Eq. 16-7/Pg. 671/Tissue dose rate is the product of the activity in each source tissue and the corresponding $S$ value for that source/target pair. The summation is over all possible source tissues |
| *MIRD schema:* Mean absorbed dose to target tissue $r_T$ over time interval (0 to $\tau$) | $D(r_T,\tau) = \int_0^{\tau} \dot{D}(r_T,t)dt = \sum_{r_S} \tilde{A}(r_S,\tau)\, S(r_T \leftarrow r_S)$ | Eq. 16-8/Pg. 672/Total mean absorbed dose to target tissue given as the time integration of the corresponding dose rate |
| *MIRD schema:* Time-integrated activity (or TIA) | $\tilde{A}(r_S,\tau) = \int_0^{\tau} A(r_S,t)dt$ | Eq. 16-9/Pg. 672/Time-integrated activity (or total number of nuclear decays) is given as the integral of the time-dependent activity in the source region $r_S$. *Historically, this was called the cumulative activity* |
| *MIRD schema:* Absorbed dose coefficient for target tissue $r_T$ | $d(r_T,\tau) = \sum_{r_S} \tilde{a}(r_S,\tau)\, S(r_T \leftarrow r_S)$ | Eq. 16-10/Pg. 672/The dose coefficient is the ratio of the tissue absorbed dose and the administered activity |
| *MIRD schema:* Time-integrated activity coefficient (or TIAC) | $\tilde{a}(r_S,\tau) = \int_0^{\tau} \frac{A(r_S,t)}{A_0}dt = \int_0^{\tau} a(r_S,t)dt$ | Eq. 16-11/Pg. 672/The TIAC is the ratio of the TIA and the administered activity. *Historically, this was called the residence time* |
| *MIRD schema:* Radionuclide $S$ value for a given source/target tissue combination in the patient anatomic model | $S(r_T \leftarrow r_S) = \dfrac{1}{m(r_T)} \sum_i E_i\, Y_i\, \phi(r_T \leftarrow r_S, E_i)$ <br><br> $= \dfrac{1}{m(r_T)} \sum_i \Delta_i\, \phi(r_T \leftarrow r_S, E_i)$ | Eq. 16-12/Pg. 673/The $S$ value is the absorbed dose to target tissue $r_T$ per radionuclide decay in source tissue $r_S$ |
| *MIRD schema:* Specific absorbed fraction (absorbed fraction divided by the target tissue mass) | $\Phi(r_T \leftarrow r_S, E_i) = \dfrac{\phi(r_T \leftarrow r_S, E_i)}{m(r_T)}$ | Eq. 16-13/Pg. 673/The specific absorbed fraction $\Phi$ is computed as the ratio of the absorbed fraction $\phi$ (fraction of particle energy emitted in source tissue $r_S$ that is deposited in target tissue $r_T$) and the mass of the target tissue $m(r_T)$ |
| *MIRD schema:* Alternative expression for the $S$ value for a given source tissue $r_S$ and target tissue $r_T$ combination in the anatomical model of the patient | $S(r_T \leftarrow r_S) = \sum_i \Delta_i\, \Phi(r_T \leftarrow r_S, E_i)$ | Eq. 16-14/Pg. 673/$S$ value given as the product of the total energy emitted per decay for particle or photon $i$ ($\Delta_i$) and the corresponding specific absorbed fraction ($\Phi$), and summed over all radionuclide emissions (particles and photons) |

**(Continued)**

| QUANTITY | EQUATION(S) | EQ NO./PAGE/COMMENTS |
|---|---|---|
| *MIRD schema:* Expression for the absorbed dose to target tissue $r_T$ when both the source tissue activity and the radionuclide $S$ value are time dependent | $$D(r_T, \tau) = \int_0^\tau \dot{D}(r_T, t)\, dt$$ $$= \sum_{r_S} \int_0^\tau A(r_S, t)\, S(r_T \leftarrow r_S, t)\, dt$$ | Eq. 16-15/ Pg. 673 |
| *MIRD schema:* Expression for the absorbed dose coefficient to target tissue $r_T$ when both the source tissue activity and the radionuclide $S$-value are time dependent | $$d(r_T, \tau) = \frac{D(r_T, \tau)}{A_0} = \sum_{r_S} \int_0^\tau a(r_S, t)\, S(r_T \leftarrow r_S, t)\, dt$$ | Eq. 16-16/Pg. 673 |
| *MIRD schema:* The full expressions for the radionuclide $S$ value in its time-dependent form | $$S(r_T \leftarrow r_S, t) = \frac{1}{m(r_T, t)} \sum_i E_i\, Y_i\, \phi(r_T \leftarrow r_S, E_i, t)$$ $$= \frac{1}{m(r_T, t)} \sum_i \Delta_i\, \phi(r_T \leftarrow r_S, E_i, t)$$ | Eq. 16-17/Pg. 673 |
| *MIRD schema:* Effective uptake rate constant | $$\lambda_{eu} = \lambda_{bu} + \lambda_p \quad \text{and} \quad T_{eu} = \frac{T_{bu} T_p}{T_{bu} + T_p}$$ | Eq. 16-18/Pg. 674/For exponential model of the radiopharmaceutical uptake, the effective uptake rate constant is the sum of the biological uptake rate constant of the *radiopharmaceutical* and the physical decay constant of the *radionuclide*. This also leads to an expression of the effective uptake half-time in terms of the corresponding biological uptake half-time of the *radiopharmaceutical* and the physical half-life of the *radionuclide* |
| *MIRD schema:* Effective clearance rate constant | $$\lambda_{ec} = \lambda_{bc} + \lambda_p \quad \text{and} \quad T_{ec} = \frac{T_{bc} T_p}{T_{bc} + T_p}$$ | Eq. 16-19/Pg. 674/For exponential model of the radiopharmaceutical clearance from the source tissue $r_S$, the effective clearance rate constant is the sum of the biological clearance rate constant of the *radiopharmaceutical* and the physical decay constant of the *radionuclide*. This also leads to an expression of the effective clearance half-time in terms of the corresponding biological clearance half-time of the *radiopharmaceutical* and the physical half-life of the *radionuclide* |
| *MIRD schema:* Expression for the time dependent activity of the radiopharmaceutical in a given source tissue $r_S$ | $$A(r_S, t) = A_0\, f_s \left[ e^{-\lambda_{ec} t} - e^{-\lambda_{eu} t} \right]$$ | Eq. 16-20/Pg. 674/Exponential model of both source tissue uptake and source tissue clearance of the radiopharmaceutical |

*(Continued)*

| QUANTITY | EQUATION(S) | EQ NO./PAGE/COMMENTS |
|---|---|---|
| *MIRD schema:* Expression for the time-dependent activity of the radiopharmaceutical in a given source tissue $r_S$ with one uptake compartment and two clearance compartments | $A(r_S,t) = A_0 \left[ f_{S_1} e^{-\lambda_{ec_1}t} + f_{S_2} e^{-\lambda_{ec_2}t} - \left( f_{S_1} + f_{S_2} \right) e^{-\lambda_{eu}t} \right]$ | Eq. 16-21/Pg. 674/Expansion of the Eq. 16-20 model to now include two exponential compartments for radiopharmaceutical clearance from the source tissue $r_S$ |
| *MIRD schema:* Time-integrated activity of the radiopharmaceutical in source tissue $r_S$ for the two-compartment clearance model of Eq. 16-21 | $\tilde{A}(r_S,\tau) = \int_0^\tau A(r_S,t)dt = \dfrac{A_0 f_{S_1}}{\lambda_{ec_1}} \left[ 1 - e^{-\lambda_{ec_1}\tau} \right]$ $+ \dfrac{A_0 f_{S_2}}{\lambda_{ec_2}} \left[ 1 - e^{-\lambda_{ec_2}\tau} \right] - \dfrac{A_0 \left( f_{S_1} + f_{S_2} \right)}{\lambda_{eu}} \left[ 1 - e^{-\lambda_{eu}\tau} \right]$ | Eq. 16-22/Pg. 676./TIA of the source tissue $r_S$ for the time-dependent exponential model of radiopharmaceutical activity given by Eq. 16-21 |

| SYMBOL | QUANTITY | UNITS[A] |
|---|---|---|
| $r_S$ | Source region (or tissue) | No units |
| $r_T$ | Target region (or tissue) | No units |
| $A_0$ | Activity of the radiopharmaceutical administered to the patient—administered activity (AA) | Bq; MBq (mCi; μCi) |
| $A(r_S, t)$ | Radiopharmaceutical activity in source region $r_S$ at time $t$ postadministration | Bq; MBq (mCi; μCi) |
| $\tilde{A}(r_S, \tau)$ | Time-integrated activity (TIA) in source region $r_S$ over time interval 0 to $\tau$ | Bq-s; MBq-s (mCi-h) |
| $\tilde{a}(r_S, \tau)$ | Time-integrated activity coefficient (TIAC) for source region $r_S$ over time interval 0 to $\tau$ | s; h |
| $\dot{D}(r_T, t)$ | Absorbed dose rate to target region $r_T$ at time $t$ postadministration | Gy/s; mGy/min; mGy/h |
| $D(r_T, \tau)$ | Absorbed dose to target region $r_T$ assessed over time interval 0 to $\tau$ postadministration | Gy; mGy |
| $d(r_T, \tau)$ | Absorbed dose coefficient for target region $r_T$ over time interval 0 to $\tau$ postadministration | Gy/Bq; mGy/MBq |
| $S(r_T \leftarrow r_S, t)$ | Radionuclide $S$ value—absorbed dose to target region $r_T$ per decay in source region $r_S$ at time $t$ postadministration | Gy/Bq-s; mGy/MBq-s |
| $S(r_T \leftarrow r_S)$ | Radionuclide $S$ value—absorbed dose to target region $r_T$ per decay in source region $r_S$ (assuming no time dependence) | Gy/Bq-s; mGy/MBq-s |
| $E_i$ | Energy of radiation particle or photon $i$ | MeV; keV |
| $Y_i$ | Yield of radiation particle or photon $i$ | $(Bq\text{-}s)^{-1}$ |
| $\Delta_i$ | Energy released by particle or photon $i$ per radionuclide decay | MeV/Bq-s; keV/Bq-s |
| $m(r_T, t)$ | Mass of target region $r_T$ at time $t$ postadministration | g; kg |
| $m(r_T)$ | Mass of the target region $r_T$ (assuming no time dependence) | g; kg |
| $\phi(r_T \leftarrow r_S, E_i, t)$ | Absorbed fraction (AF)—fraction of particle energy $E_i$ emitted within source region $r_S$ that is deposited to target region $r_T$ at time $t$ postadministration. | Unitless—ratio of energy absorbed to energy emitted |
| $\phi(r_T \leftarrow r_S, E_i)$ | Absorbed fraction (AF)—fraction of particle energy $E_i$ emitted within source region $r_S$ that is deposited to target region $r_T$ (assuming no time dependence) | Unitless—ratio of energy absorbed to energy emitted |

**(Continued)**

| SYMBOL | QUANTITY | UNITS[A] |
|---|---|---|
| $\Phi(r_T \leftarrow r_s, E_i)$ | Specific absorbed fraction (SAF)—fraction of particle energy $E_i$ emitted within source region $r_s$ that is deposited per unit mass to target region $r_T$ (assuming no time dependence) | $g^{-1}$; $kg^{-1}$ |
| $\Phi(r_T \leftarrow r_s, E_i, t)$ | Specific absorbed fraction (SAF)—fraction of particle energy $E_i$ emitted within source region $r_s$ that is deposited per unit mass to target region $r_T$ at time $t$ postadministration | $g^{-1}$; $kg^{-1}$ |
| $T_p$ or $T_{1/2}$ | Physical half-life of the radionuclide | s; h |
| $\lambda_p$ | Physical decay constant of the radionuclide $\lambda_p = \ln(2)/T_p$ | $s^{-1}$; $h^{-1}$ |
| $T_{bu}$ | Biological uptake half-time | s; h |
| $\lambda_{bu}$ | Biological uptake rate constant $\lambda_{bu} = \ln(2)/T_{bu}$ | $s^{-1}$; $h^{-1}$ |
| $T_{eu}$ | Effective uptake half-time | s; h |
| $\lambda_{eu}$ | Effective uptake rate constant $\lambda_{eu} = \lambda_{bu} + \lambda_p$ | $s^{-1}$; $h^{-1}$ |
| $T_{bc}$ | Biological clearance half-time | s; h |
| $\lambda_{bc}$ | Biological clearance rate constant $\lambda_{bc} = \ln(2)/T_{bc}$ | $s^{-1}$; $h^{-1}$ |
| $T_{ec}$ | Effective clearance half-time | s; h |
| $\lambda_{ec}$ | Effective clearance rate constant $\lambda_{ec} = \lambda_{bc} + \lambda_p$ | $s^{-1}$; $h^{-1}$ |
| $\lambda_{ec_1}$ | Effective clearance rate constant for compartment 1 $\lambda_{ec_1} = \lambda_{bc_1} + \lambda_p$ | $s^{-1}$; $h^{-1}$ |
| $\lambda_{ec_2}$ | Effective clearance rate constant for compartment 2 $\lambda_{ec_2} = \lambda_{bc_2} + \lambda_p$ | $s^{-1}$; $h^{-1}$ |
| $f_s$ | Fraction of administered activity $A_0$ that localizes within source region $r_s$ | Unitless |
| $f_{s_1}$ | Fraction of administered activity $A_0$ that localizes within compartment 1 of source region $r_s$ | Unitless |
| $f_{s_2}$ | Fraction of administered activity $A_0$ that localizes within compartment 2 of source region $r_s$ | Unitless |

[a]SI units are given. For quantities related to radiopharmaceutical activity, traditional units are given in parentheses.

# Radiation Detection and Measurements

## 17.0 INTRODUCTION

The detection and measurement of ionizing radiation are the basis for the majority of diagnostic imaging. In this chapter, the basic concepts of radiation detection and measurement are introduced, followed by a discussion of the characteristics of specific types of detectors.

1. *Ionization* is the removal of electrons from atoms or molecules. (An atom or molecule stripped of an electron has a net positive charge and is called a *cation*. In many gases, the free electrons become attached to uncharged atoms or molecules, forming negatively charged *anions*. An ion pair consists of a cation and its associated free electron or anion.)
2. *Excitation* is the elevation of electrons to excited states in atoms, molecules, or a crystal. Excitation and ionization may produce chemical changes or the emission of visible light or ultraviolet (UV) radiation. Most energy deposited by ionizing radiation is ultimately converted into thermal energy.

## 17.1 TYPES OF DETECTORS AND BASIC PRINCIPLES

Radiation detectors may be classified by their detection method.

1. A *gas-filled detector* consists of a volume of gas between two electrodes. Ions produced in the gas by the radiation are collected by the electrodes, resulting in an electrical signal.
2. The interaction of ionizing radiation with certain materials produces UV radiation and/or visible light. These materials are called *scintillators*. They are commonly attached to or incorporated in devices that convert UV radiation and light into an electrical signal.
3. *Semiconductor detectors* are especially pure crystals of silicon, germanium, or other semiconductor materials to which trace amounts of impurity atoms have been added so that they act as diodes. A diode is an electronic device with two terminals that permits a large electrical current to flow when a voltage is applied in one direction, but very little current when the voltage is applied in the opposite direction.

Detectors may also be classified by the type of information produced.

1. Detectors, such as Geiger-Müeller (GM) detectors, that indicate the number of interactions occurring in the detector are called *counters*.
2. Detectors that yield information about the energy distribution of the incident radiation, such as NaI scintillation detectors, are called *spectrometers*.
3. Detectors that indicate the net amount of energy deposited in the detector by multiple interactions are called *dosimeters*.

### Pulse and Current Modes of Operation

1. Many radiation detectors produce an electrical signal after each interaction of a particle or photon. The signal generated by the detector passes through a series of electronic circuits, each of which performs a function such as signal amplification, signal processing, or data storage.
2. A detector and its associated electronic circuitry form a *detection system*. There are two fundamental ways that the circuitry may process the signal—pulse mode and current mode. In *pulse mode*, the signal from each interaction is processed individually. In *current mode,* the electrical signals from individual interactions are averaged together, forming a net current signal.

3. There are advantages and disadvantages to each method of handling the signal. GM detectors are operated in pulse mode, whereas most ionization chambers, including ion chamber survey meters and the dose calibrators used in nuclear medicine, are operated in current mode.

4. Scintillation detectors are operated in pulse mode in nuclear medicine applications, but in current mode in direct digital radiography, fluoroscopy, and x-ray computed tomography (CT).

5. In this chapter, the term *interaction* typically refers to the interaction of a single photon or charged particle, such as the interaction of a gamma-ray by the photoelectric effect or Compton scattering.

6. The term *event* may refer to a single interaction, or it may refer to something more complex, such as two nearly simultaneous interactions in a detector. In instruments that process the signals from individual interactions or events in pulse mode, an interaction or event that is registered is referred to as a *count*.

## Effect of Interaction Rate on Detectors Operated in Pulse Mode

1. The main problem with using a radiation detector or detection system in pulse mode is that two interactions must be separated by a finite amount of time if they are to produce distinct signals. This interval is called the *dead time* of the system.

2. If a second interaction occurs during this time interval, its signal will be lost; furthermore, if it is close enough in time to the first interaction, it may even distort the signal from the first interaction. The fraction of counts lost from dead-time effects is smallest at low interaction rates and increases with increasing interaction rate.

3. The dead time of a detection system is largely determined by the component in the series with the longest dead time. For example, the detector usually has the longest dead time in GM counter systems, whereas in multi-channel analyzer (MCA) systems (see later discussion), the analog-to-digital converter (ADC) generally has the longest dead time.

4. The dead times of different types of systems vary widely. GM counters have dead times ranging from tens to hundreds of microseconds, whereas most other systems have dead times of less than a few microseconds. It is important to know the count-rate behavior of a detection system; if a detection system is operated at too high an interaction rate, an artificially low count rate will be obtained.

5. There are two mathematical models describing the behavior of detector systems operated in pulse mode—paralyzable and nonparalyzable. Although these models are simplifications of the behavior of real detection systems, real systems may behave like one or the other model. In a *paralyzable* system, an interaction that occurs during the dead time after a previous interaction extends the dead time; in a *nonparalyzable* system, it does not.

6. Figure 17-1 shows the count rates of paralyzable and nonparalyzable detector systems as a function of the interaction rate in the detector.

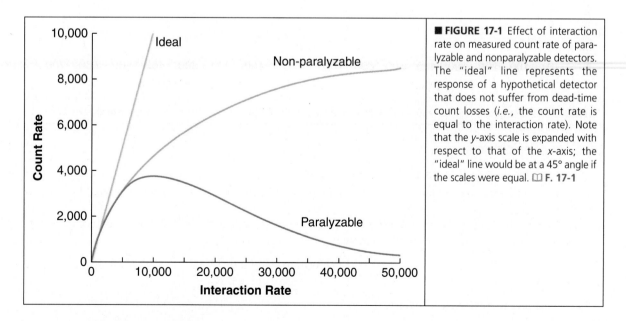

■ **FIGURE 17-1** Effect of interaction rate on measured count rate of paralyzable and nonparalyzable detectors. The "ideal" line represents the response of a hypothetical detector that does not suffer from dead-time count losses (*i.e.*, the count rate is equal to the interaction rate). Note that the y-axis scale is expanded with respect to that of the x-axis; the "ideal" line would be at a 45° angle if the scales were equal. 📖 **F. 17-1**

## Current Mode of Operation

1. When a detector is operated in current mode, all information regarding individual interactions is lost. For example, neither the interaction rate nor the energies deposited by individual interactions can be determined.

2. However, if the amount of electrical charge collected from each interaction is proportional to the energy deposited by that interaction, then the net electrical current is proportional to the dose rate in the detector material.
3. Detectors subject to very high interaction rates are often operated in current mode to avoid dead-time information losses. Image-intensifier tubes and flat-panel image receptors in fluoroscopy, detectors in x-ray CT machines, direct digital radiographic image receptors, ion chambers used in phototimed radiography, and most nuclear medicine dose calibrators are operated in current mode.

## Spectroscopy

1. The term *spectroscopy,* literally the viewing of a spectrum, is commonly used to refer to measurements of the energy distributions of radiation fields, and a *spectrometer* is a detection system that yields information about the energy distribution of the incident radiation.
2. Most spectrometers are operated in pulse mode, and the amplitude of each pulse is proportional to the energy deposited in the detector by the interaction causing that pulse.
3. *The energy deposited by an interaction, however, is not always the total energy of the incident particle or photon.* For example, a gamma-ray may interact with the detector by Compton scattering, with the scattered photon escaping the detector. In this case, the deposited energy is the difference between the energies of the incident and scattered photons.
4. A *pulse height spectrum* is usually depicted as a graph of the number of interactions depositing a particular amount of energy in the spectrometer as a function of energy (Fig. 17-2). Because the energy deposited by an interaction may be less than the total energy of the incident particle or photon and also because of random variations in the detection process, *the pulse height spectrum produced by a spectrometer is not identical to the actual energy spectrum of the incident radiation.*
5. The energy resolution of a spectrometer is a measure of its ability to differentiate between particles or photons of different energies. Pulse height spectroscopy is discussed later in this chapter.

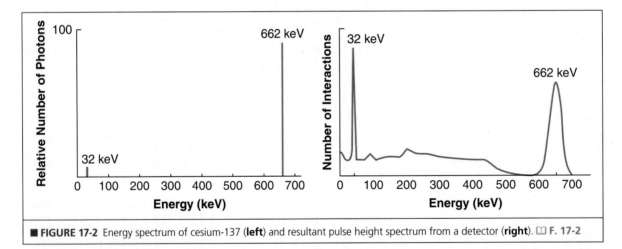

■ **FIGURE 17-2** Energy spectrum of cesium-137 (**left**) and resultant pulse height spectrum from a detector (**right**). ▥ F. 17-2

## Detector Efficiency

1. The *efficiency* (or *sensitivity*) of a detector is a measure of its ability to detect radiation. The efficiency of a detection system operated in pulse mode is defined as the probability that a particle or photon emitted by a source will be detected.
2. It is measured by placing a source of radiation in the vicinity of the detector and dividing the number of particles or photons detected by the number emitted:

$$\text{Efficiency} = \frac{\text{Number detected}}{\text{Number emitted}} \qquad [17\text{-}1a] \quad \text{▥ E. 17-1}$$

This equation can be written as follows:

$$\text{Efficiency} = \frac{\text{Number reaching detector}}{\text{Number emitted}} \times \frac{\text{Number detected}}{\text{Number reaching detector}} \qquad [17\text{-}1b] \quad \text{▥ E. 17-1}$$

3. Therefore, the detection efficiency is the product of two terms: the geometric efficiency and the intrinsic efficiency:

$$\text{Efficiency} = \text{Geometric efficiency} \times \text{Intrinsic efficiency} \qquad [17\text{-}2] \quad \square\,\text{E. 17-2}$$

where the *geometric efficiency* of a detector is the fraction of emitted particles or photons that reach the detector and the *intrinsic efficiency* is the fraction of those particles or photons reaching the detector that are detected. Because total, geometric, and intrinsic efficiencies are all probabilities, each ranges from 0 to 1.

4. The geometric efficiency is determined by the geometric relationship between the source and the detector (Fig. 17-3). It increases as the source is moved toward the detector and approaches 0.5 when a point source is placed against a flat surface of the detector because in that position-half of the photons or particles are emitted into the detector.

5. For a source inside a well-type detector, the geometric efficiency approaches 1, because most of the particles or photons are intercepted by the detector. A well-type detector is a detector containing a cavity for the insertion of samples.

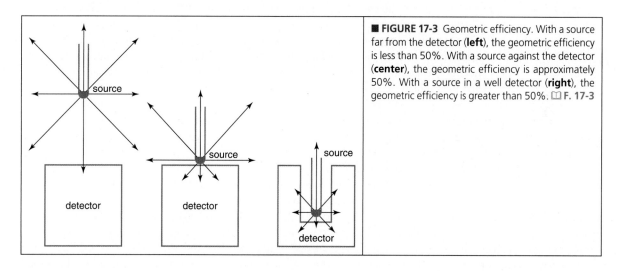

■ **FIGURE 17-3** Geometric efficiency. With a source far from the detector (**left**), the geometric efficiency is less than 50%. With a source against the detector (**center**), the geometric efficiency is approximately 50%. With a source in a well detector (**right**), the geometric efficiency is greater than 50%. $\square$ **F. 17-3**

6. The intrinsic efficiency of a detector in detecting photons also called the *quantum detection efficiency* (QDE) is determined by the energy of the photons and the atomic number, density, and thickness of the detector.

7. If a parallel beam of monoenergetic photons is incident upon a detector of uniform thickness, the intrinsic efficiency of the detector is given by the following equation:

$$\text{Intrinsic efficiency} = 1 - e^{-\mu x} = 1 - e^{-(\mu/\rho)\rho x} \qquad [17\text{-}3] \quad \square\,\text{E. 17-3}$$

where $\mu$ is the linear attenuation coefficient of the detector material, $\rho$ is the density of the material, $\mu/\rho$ is the mass attenuation coefficient of the material, and $x$ is the thickness of the detector.

8. This equation shows that the intrinsic efficiency for detecting x-rays and gamma rays increases with the thickness of the detector and the density and the mass attenuation coefficient of the detector material. The mass attenuation coefficient increases with the atomic number of the material and, within the range of photon energies used in diagnostic imaging, decreases with increasing photon energy, with the exception of absorption edges.

## 17.2  GAS-FILLED DETECTORS

### Basic Principles

1. As shown in Figure 17-4, a gas-filled detector consists of a volume of gas between two electrodes, with an electric potential difference (voltage) applied between the electrodes.

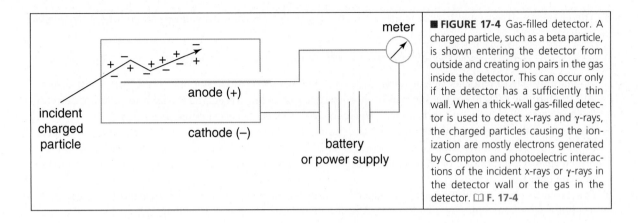

■ **FIGURE 17-4** Gas-filled detector. A charged particle, such as a beta particle, is shown entering the detector from outside and creating ion pairs in the gas inside the detector. This can occur only if the detector has a sufficiently thin wall. When a thick-wall gas-filled detector is used to detect x-rays and γ-rays, the charged particles causing the ionization are mostly electrons generated by Compton and photoelectric interactions of the incident x-rays or γ-rays in the detector wall or the gas in the detector. 📖 **F. 17-4**

2. Ionizing radiation forms ion pairs in the gas. The positive ions (cations) are attracted to the negative electrode (cathode), and the electrons or anions are attracted to the positive electrode (anode). In most detectors, the cathode is the wall of the container that holds the gas or a conductive coating on the inside of the wall, and the anode is a wire inside the container. After reaching the anode, the electrons travel through the circuit to the cathode, where they recombine with the cations. This electrical current can be measured with a sensitive ammeter or other electrical circuitry.

3. There are two types of gas-filled detectors in common use—ionization chambers and GM counters. The type of detector is determined primarily by the voltage applied between the two electrodes.
   **a.** In an ionization chamber, the two electrodes can have almost any configuration: they may be two parallel plates, two concentric cylinders, or a wire within a cylinder.
   **b.** In GM counters, the anode must be a thin wire.

4. Figure 17-5 shows the amount of electrical charge collected after a single interaction as a function of the electrical potential difference (voltage) applied between the two electrodes.

5. Ionizing radiation produces ion pairs in the gas of the detector. If no voltage is applied between the electrodes, no current flows through the circuit because there is no electric field to attract the charged particles to the electrodes; the ion pairs merely recombine in the gas. When a small voltage is applied, some of the cations are attracted to the cathode and some of the electrons or anions are attracted to the anode before they can recombine. As the voltage is increased, more ions are collected, and fewer recombine. This region, in which the current increases as the voltage is raised, is called the *recombination region* of the curve.

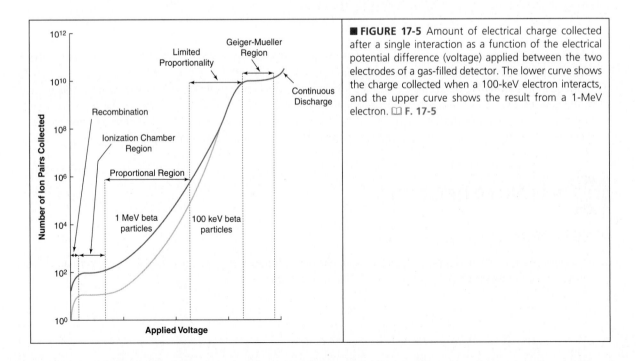

■ **FIGURE 17-5** Amount of electrical charge collected after a single interaction as a function of the electrical potential difference (voltage) applied between the two electrodes of a gas-filled detector. The lower curve shows the charge collected when a 100-keV electron interacts, and the upper curve shows the result from a 1-MeV electron. 📖 **F. 17-5**

6. As the voltage is increased further, a plateau is reached in the curve. In this region, called the *ionization chamber region*, the applied electric field is sufficiently strong to collect almost all ion pairs; additional increases in the applied voltage do not significantly increase the current.

7. Beyond the ionization region, the collected current again increases as the applied voltage is raised. In this region, called the *proportional region*, electrons approaching the anode are accelerated to such high kinetic energies that they cause additional ionization. This phenomenon, called *gas multiplication*, amplifies the collected current; the amount of amplification increases as the applied voltage is raised. At any voltage through the ionization chamber region and the proportional region, the amount of electrical charge collected from each interaction is *proportional* to the amount of energy deposited in the gas of the detector by the interaction. For example, the amount of charge collected after an interaction depositing 100 keV is one tenth of that collected from an interaction depositing 1 MeV.

8. Beyond the proportional region is a region in which the amount of charge collected from each event is the same, regardless of the amount of energy deposited by the interaction. In this region, called the *Geiger-Müeller region* (GM region), the gas multiplication spreads the entire length of the anode. The size of a pulse in the GM region tells nothing about the energy deposited in the detector by the interaction causing the pulse.

## Gas-Filled Detectors

1. Because gas multiplication does not occur at the relatively low voltages applied to ionization chambers, the amount of electrical charge collected from a single interaction is very small and would require huge amplification to be detected. For this reason, ionization chambers are seldom used in pulse mode. The advantage to operating them in current mode is the almost complete freedom from dead-time effects, even in very intense radiation fields.

2. Almost any gas can be used to fill the chamber. If the gas is air and the walls of the chamber are of a material whose effective atomic number is similar to air, the amount of current produced is proportional to the *exposure rate* (exposure is the amount of electrical charge produced per mass of air).

3. Air-filled ion chambers are used in portable survey meters and can accurately indicate exposure rates from less than 1 mR/h to tens or hundreds of roentgens per hour. Air-filled ion chambers are also used for performing quality assurance testing of diagnostic and therapeutic x-ray machines, and they are the detectors in most x-ray machine phototimers.

4. Measurements using an air-filled ion chamber that is open to the atmosphere are affected by the density of the air in the chamber, which is determined by ambient air pressure and temperature. Measurements using such chambers that require great accuracy must be corrected for these factors.

5. Gas-filled detectors tend to have low intrinsic efficiencies for detecting x-rays and gamma rays because of the low densities of gases and the low atomic numbers of most common gases. The sensitivity of ion chambers to x-rays and gamma rays can be enhanced by filling them with a gas that has a high atomic number, such as argon ($Z = 18$) or xenon ($Z = 54$), and pressurizing the gas to increase its density. Well-type ion chambers called dose calibrators are used in nuclear medicine to assay the activities of dosages of radiopharmaceuticals to be administered to patients; many are filled with pressurized argon. Xenon-filled pressurized ion chambers were formerly used as detectors in some CT machines.

6. Air-filled ion chambers are commonly used to measure the related quantities air kerma and exposure rate. *Air kerma* is the *initial kinetic energy transferred to charged particles* (in this case electrons), liberated in air by the radiation, per mass air, while *exposure* is the *amount of electrical charge* created by these electrons in air caused by ionization, per mass air.

7. There is a problem measuring the ionization in the small volume of air in an ionization chamber of reasonable size. The energetic electrons released by interactions in the air have long ranges in air, and many of them would escape the air in the chamber and cause much of their ionization elsewhere.

8. This problem can be partially solved by building the ion chamber with thick walls of a material whose effective atomic number is similar to that of air. In this case, the number of electrons escaping the volume of air is approximately matched by a similar number of electrons released in the chamber wall entering the air in the ion chamber. This situation, if achieved, is called *electronic equilibrium*.

9. For this reason, most ion chambers for measuring exposure or air kerma have thick *air equivalent* walls or are equipped with removable *air equivalent buildup caps* to establish electronic equilibrium. The thickness of material needed to establish electronic equilibrium increases with the energy of the x- or gamma rays.

10. However, thick walls or buildup caps may significantly attenuate low energy x- and gamma rays. Many ion chamber survey meters have windows that may be opened in the thick material around the ion chamber to permit more accurate measurement of low energy x- and gamma rays.

## Geiger-Müeller Counters

1. GM counters must also contain gases with specific properties. Because gas multiplication produces billions of ion pairs after an interaction, the signal from a GM detector requires little additional amplification. For this reason, GM detectors are often used for inexpensive survey meters.

2. GM detectors have high efficiencies for detecting charged particles that penetrate the walls of the detectors; almost every such particle reaching the interior of a detector is counted. Many GM detectors are equipped with thin windows to allow beta particles and conversion electrons to reach the gas and be detected.

3. Very weak charged particles, such as the beta particles emitted by tritium ($^3$H, $E_{max}$ = 18 keV), which is extensively used in biomedical research, cannot penetrate the windows; therefore, contamination by $^3$H cannot be detected with a GM survey meter. Flat, thin-window GM detectors, called "pancake"-type detectors, are very useful for finding radioactive contamination.

4. The size of the voltage pulse from a GM tube is independent of the energy deposited in the detector by the interaction causing the pulse: an interaction that deposits 1 keV causes a voltage pulse of the same size as one caused by an interaction that deposits 1 MeV. Therefore, GM detectors cannot be used as spectrometers or precise dose-rate meters.

5. Many portable GM survey meters display measurements in units of milliroentgens per hour. However, the GM counter cannot truly measure exposure rates, and so its reading must be considered only an approximation.

6. If a GM survey meter is calibrated to indicate exposure rate for 662-keV gamma rays from $^{137}$Cs (commonly used for calibrations), it may overrespond by as much as a factor of 5 for photons of lower energies, such as 80 keV. If an accurate measurement of exposure rate is required, an air-filled ionization chamber survey meter should be used.

7. GM detectors suffer from extremely long dead times, ranging from tens to hundreds of microseconds. For this reason, GM counters are seldom used when accurate measurements are required of count rates greater than a few hundred counts per second. A portable GM survey meter may become paralyzed in a very high radiation field and yield a reading of zero. Ionization chamber instruments should always be used to measure high-intensity x-ray and gamma-ray fields.

## 17.3  SCINTILLATION DETECTORS

### Basic Principles

1. *Scintillators* are materials that emit visible light or UV radiation after the interaction of ionizing radiation with the material. Scintillators are used in conventional film-screen radiography, many direct digital radiographic image receptors, fluoroscopy, scintillation cameras, CT scanners, and positron emission tomography (PET) scanners.

2. Although the light emitted from a single interaction can be seen if the viewer's eyes are dark-adapted, most scintillation detectors incorporate a means of signal amplification. In conventional film-screen radiography, photographic film is used to amplify and record the signal. In other applications, electronic devices such as photomultiplier tubes (PMTs), photodiodes, or image-intensifier tubes convert the light into electrical signals. PMTs and image-intensifier tubes amplify the signal as well.

3. A *scintillation detector* consists of a scintillator and a device, such as a PMT, that converts the light into an electrical signal.

4. When ionizing radiation interacts with a scintillator, electrons are raised to an excited energy level. Ultimately, these electrons fall back to a lower energy state, with the emission of visible light or UV radiation.

5. Most scintillators have more than one mode for the emission of visible light or UV radiation, and each mode has its characteristic decay constant. *Luminescence* is the emission of light after excitation. *Fluorescence* is the prompt emission of light, whereas *phosphorescence* (also called *afterglow*) is the delayed emission of light.

6. When scintillation detectors are operated in current mode, the prompt signal from an interaction cannot be separated from the phosphorescence caused by previous interactions. When a scintillation detector is operated in pulse mode, afterglow is less important because electronic circuits can separate the rapidly rising and falling components of the prompt signal from the slowly decaying delayed signal resulting from previous interactions. *Properties that are desirable in a scintillator:*

   a. The *conversion efficiency*, the fraction of deposited energy that is converted into light or UV radiation, should be high. (Conversion efficiency should not be confused with detection efficiency).

   b. For many applications, the decay times of excited states should be short. (Light or UV radiation is emitted promptly after an interaction.)

   c. The material should be transparent to its own emissions. (Most emitted light or UV radiation escapes reabsorption.)

   d. The frequency spectrum (color) of emitted light or UV radiation should match the spectral sensitivity of the light receptor (PMT, photodiode, or film).

   e. If used for x-ray and gamma-ray detection, the attenuation coefficient ($\mu$) should be large, so that detectors made of the scintillator have high detection efficiencies. Materials with large atomic numbers and high densities have large attenuation coefficients.

   f. The material should be rugged, unaffected by moisture, and inexpensive to manufacture.

7. In all scintillators, the amount of light emitted after an interaction increases with the energy deposited by the interaction. Therefore, scintillators may be operated in pulse mode as spectrometers. When a scintillator is used for spectroscopy, its energy resolution (ability to distinguish between interactions depositing different energies) is primarily determined by its conversion efficiency.

8. There are several categories of materials that scintillate. Many organic compounds exhibit scintillation. In these materials, scintillation is a property of the molecular structure. Solid organic scintillators are used for timing experiments in particle physics because of their extremely prompt light emission. Organic scintillators include the liquid scintillation fluids that are used extensively in biomedical research. Organic scintillators are not used for medical imaging because the low atomic numbers of their constituent elements and their low densities make them poor x-ray and gamma-ray detectors. When photons in the diagnostic energy range do interact with organic scintillators, it is primarily by Compton scattering.

9. Many inorganic crystalline materials exhibit scintillation. In these materials, the scintillation is a property of the crystalline structure: if the crystal is dissolved, the scintillation ceases. Many of these materials have much larger average atomic numbers and higher densities than organic scintillators and therefore are excellent photon detectors. They are widely used for radiation measurements and imaging in radiology.

10. Most inorganic scintillation crystals are deliberately grown with trace amounts of impurity elements called *activators*. The atoms of these activators form preferred sites in the crystals for the excited electrons to return to the ground state. The activators modify the frequency (color) of the emitted light, the promptness of the light emission, and the proportion of the emitted light that escapes reabsorption in the crystal.

## Inorganic Crystalline Scintillators in Radiology

1. No one scintillation material is best for all applications in radiology. Sodium iodide activated with thallium [NaI(Tl)] is used for most nuclear medicine applications. It is coupled to PMTs and operated in pulse mode in scintillation cameras, thyroid probes, and gamma well counters.

2. NaI(Tl) high content of iodine ($Z = 53$) and high density provides a high photoelectric absorption probability for x-rays and gamma rays emitted by common nuclear medicine radiopharmaceuticals (70 to 365 keV).

3. NaI(Tl) has a very high conversion efficiency; approximately 13% of deposited energy is converted into light. Because a light photon has an energy of about 3 eV, approximately one light photon is emitted for every 23 eV absorbed by the crystal. This high conversion efficiency gives it a very good energy resolution.

4. NaI(Tl) emits light very promptly (decay constant, 250 ns), permitting it to be used in pulse mode at interaction rates greater than 100,000/s. Very large crystals can be manufactured; for example, the rectangular crystals of one modern scintillation camera are 59 cm (23 inches) long, 44.5 cm (17.5 inches) wide, and 0.95 cm thick. Unfortunately, NaI(Tl) crystals are fragile; they crack easily if struck or subjected to rapid temperature change. Also, they are hygroscopic (*i.e.*, they absorb water from the atmosphere) and therefore must be hermetically sealed.

5. Positron emission tomography (PET), discussed in Chapter 19, requires high detection efficiency for 511-keV annihilation photons and a prompt signal from each interaction because the signals must be processed in pulse mode at high interaction rates. PET detectors are thick crystals of high-density, high atomic number scintillators optically coupled to PMTs.

6. For many years, bismuth germanate ($Bi_4Ge_3O_{12}$, often abbreviated as "BGO") was the preferred scintillator. The high atomic number of bismuth ($Z = 83$) and the high density of the crystal yield a high intrinsic efficiency for the 511-keV positron annihilation photons. The primary component of the light emission is sufficiently prompt (decay constant, 300 ns) for PET. NaI(Tl) was used in early and some less-expensive PET scanners.

7. Today, lutetium oxyorthosilicate ($Lu_2SiO_4O$, abbreviated LSO), lutetium-yttrium oxyorthosilicate ($Lu_xYSiO_4O$, abbreviated LYSO), and gadolinium oxyorthosilicate ($Gd_2SiO_4O$, abbreviated GSO), all activated with cerium, are used in newer PET scanners. Their densities and effective atomic numbers are similar to those of BGO, but their conversion efficiencies are much larger, and they emit light much more promptly.

8. Calcium tungstate ($CaWO_4$) is used in CT scanners. It was also used for many years in intensifying screens in film-screen radiography. It was largely replaced by rare earth phosphors, such as gadolinium oxysulfide activated with terbium. The intensifying screen is an application of scintillators that does not require very prompt light emission because the film usually remains in contact with the screen for at least several seconds after exposure.

9. Cesium iodide activated with thallium is used as the phosphor layer of many indirect-detection thin-film transistor radiographic and fluoroscopic image receptors, described in Chapters 7 and 9. Cesium iodide activated with sodium is used as the input phosphor, and zinc cadmium sulfide activated with silver is used as the output phosphor of image-intensifier tubes in fluoroscopes.

Table 17-1 lists the properties of several inorganic scintillators of importance in radiology and nuclide medicine.

**TABLE 17-1 INORGANIC SCINTILLATORS USED IN MEDICAL IMAGING**

| MATERIAL | ATOMIC NUMBERS | DENSITY (g/cm³) | WAVELENGTH OF MAXIMAL EMISSION (nm) | CONVERSION EFFICIENCY[a] (%) | DECAY CONSTANT (µS) | AFTER GLOW (%) | USES |
|---|---|---|---|---|---|---|---|
| NaI(Tl) | 11, 53 | 3.67 | 415 | 100 | 0.25 | 0.3–5 at 6 ms | Scintillation cameras |
| $Bi_4Ge_3O_{12}$ | 83, 32, 8 | 7.13 | 480 | 12–14 | 0.3 | 0.005 at 3 ms | PET scanners |
| $Lu_2SiO_4O(Ce)$ | 71, 14, 8 | 7.4 | 420 | 75 | 40 | | PET scanners |
| CsI(Na) | 55, 53 | 4.51 | 420 | 85 | 0.63 | | Input phosphor of image-intensifier tubes |
| CsI(Tl) | 55, 53 | 4.51 | 550 | 45[b] | 1.0 | 0.5–5 at 6 ms | Thin-film transistor radiographic and fluoroscopic image receptors |
| ZnCdS(Ag) | 30, 48, 16 | – | – | – | – | – | Output phosphor of image-intensifier tubes |
| $CdWO_4$ | 48, 74, 8 | 7.90 | 475 | 40 | 14 | 0.1 at 3 ms | Computed tomographic (CT) scanners |
| $CaWO_4$ | 20, 74, 8 | 6.12 | – | 14–18 | 0.9–20 | – | Radiographic screens |
| $Gd_2O_2S(Tb)$ | 64, 8, 16 | 7.34 | – | – | 560 | – | Radiographic screens |

[a]Relative to NaI(Tl), using a PMT to measure light.

[b]The light emitted by CsI(Tl) does not match the spectral sensitivity of PMTs very well; its conversion efficiency is much larger if measured with a photodiode.

*Source:* Data on NaI(Tl), BGO, CsI(Na), CsI(Tl), and $CdWO_4$ courtesy of Saint-Gobain Crystals, Hiram, OH. Data on LSO from Ficke DC, Hood JT, Ter-Pogossian MM. A spheroid positron emission tomograph for brain imaging: a feasibility study. *J Nucl Med.* 1996;37:1222.

## Conversion of Light into an Electrical Signal

### The Photomultiplier Tube (PMT)

1. PMTs perform two functions—conversion of UV and visible light photons into an electrical signal and signal amplification, on the order of millions to billions.

2. As shown in Figure 17-6, a PMT consists of an evacuated glass tube containing a *photocathode*, typically 10 to 12 electrodes called *dynodes*, and an *anode*. The photocathode is a very thin electrode, located just inside the

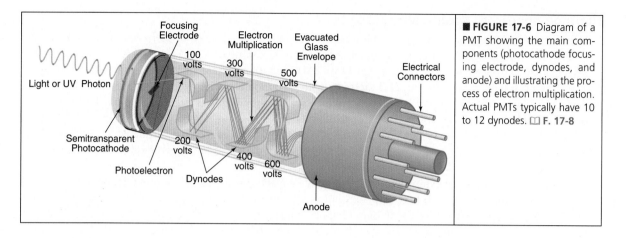

■ **FIGURE 17-6** Diagram of a PMT showing the main components (photocathode focusing electrode, dynodes, and anode) and illustrating the process of electron multiplication. Actual PMTs typically have 10 to 12 dynodes. □ **F. 17-8**

glass entrance window of the PMT, which emits electrons when struck by visible light. Photocathodes are inefficient; approximately one electron is emitted from the photocathode for every five UV or light photons incident upon it.

3. A high-voltage power supply provides a voltage of approximately 1,000 V, and a series of resistors divide the voltage into equal increments. The first dynode is given a voltage of about +100 V with respect to the photocathode; successive dynodes have voltages that increase by approximately 100 V per dynode. The electrons emitted by the photocathode are attracted to the first dynode and are accelerated to kinetic energies equal to the potential difference between the photocathode and the first dynode. (If the potential difference is 100 V, the kinetic energy of each electron is 100 eV.)

4. When these electrons strike the first dynode, about five electrons are ejected from the dynode for each electron hitting it. These electrons are then attracted to the second dynode, reaching kinetic energies equal to the potential difference between the first and second dynodes, and causing about five electrons to be ejected from the second dynode for each electron hitting it.

5. This process continues down the chain of dynodes, with the number of electrons being multiplied by a factor of 5 at each stage. The total amplification of the PMT is the product of the individual multiplications at each dynode.

## Photodiodes

1. Photodiodes are semiconductor diodes that convert light into electrical signals. In use, photodiodes are reverse biased. *Reverse bias* means that the voltage is applied with the polarity such that essentially no electrical current flows.

2. When the photodiode is exposed to light, an electrical current is generated that is proportional to the intensity of the light. Photodiodes are sometimes used with scintillators instead of PMTs.

3. Photodiodes produce more electrical noise than PMTs do, but they are smaller and less expensive. Most photodiodes, unlike PMTs, do not amplify the signal. However, a type of photodiode called an avalanche photodiode does provide signal amplification, although not as much as a PMT.

4. Photodiodes coupled to $CdWO_4$ or other scintillators are used in current mode in CT scanners. Photodiodes are also essential components of indirect-detection thin-film transistor radiographic and fluoroscopic image receptors, which use scintillators to convert x-ray energy into light.

### Multi-Pixel Photon Counters—Silicon Photomultipliers (SiPMs)

1. Another solid-state electronic device that can detect and measure visible light and/or UV radiation from a scintillator is a rectangular array of tiny (typically 10 to 100 μm) avalanche photodiodes operated in Geiger mode, with the outputs summed.

2. Such diode arrays have been given several names, including multi-pixel photon counters, but perhaps are most commonly referred to as silicon photomultipliers (SiPMs).

### Scintillators with Trapping of Excited Electrons

In most applications of scintillators, the prompt emission of light after an interaction is desirable. However, there are inorganic scintillators in which electrons become trapped in excited states after interactions with ionizing radiation. These trapped electrons can be released by heating or exposure to light; the electrons then fall to their ground state with the emission of light, which can be detected by a PMT or other sensor. These trapped electrons, in effect, store information about the radiation exposure.

## Thermoluminescent Dosimeters (TLDs)

1. Scintillators with electron trapping can be used for dosimetry. In the case of *thermoluminescent dosimeters* (TLDs), to read the signal after exposure to ionizing radiation, a sample of TLD material is heated, the light is detected and converted into an electrical signal by a PMT, and the resultant signal is integrated and displayed.
2. The amount of light emitted by the TLD increases with the amount of energy absorbed by the TLD but may deviate from proportionality, particularly at higher doses. After the TLD has been read, it may be baked in an oven to release the remaining trapped electrons and reused.
3. Lithium fluoride (LiF) is one of the most useful TLD materials. It is commercially available in forms with different trace impurities (Mg and Ti or Mg, Cu, and P), giving differences in properties such as sensitivity and linearity of response with dose.
4. LiF has trapping centers that exhibit almost negligible release of trapped electrons at room temperature, so there is little loss of information with time from exposure to the reading of the TLD. The effective atomic number of LiF is close to that of tissue, so the amount of light emission is almost proportional to the tissue dose over a wide range of x-ray and gamma-ray energies. It is commonly used instead of photographic film for personnel dosimetry.

## Optically Stimulated Luminescent Dosimeters (OSLDs)

1. In optically stimulated luminescence (OSL), the trapped excited electrons are released by exposure to light, commonly produced by a laser, of a frequency optimal for releasing the trapped electrons. The most commonly used OSL material is aluminum oxide ($Al_2O_3$) activated with a small amount of carbon.
2. The effective atomic number of aluminum oxide is significantly higher than that of soft tissue, and so the dose to this material is not proportional to the dose to soft tissue over the full range of energies used in medical imaging.

## Photostimulable Phosphors

1. *Photostimulable phosphors* (PSPs), like TLDs, are scintillators in which a fraction of the excited electrons become trapped. PSP plates are used in radiography as image receptors, instead of film-screen cassettes.
2. Although the trapped electrons could be released by heating, a laser is used to scan the plate and release them. The electrons then fall to the ground state, with the emission of light.
3. Barium fluorohalide activated with europium is commonly used for PSP imaging plates. In this material, the wavelength that is most efficient in stimulating luminescence is in the red portion of the spectrum, whereas the stimulated luminescence itself is in the blue-violet portion of the spectrum.
4. The stimulated emissions are converted into an electrical signal by PMTs. After the plate is read by the laser, it may be exposed to light to release the remaining trapped electrons that can be reused.

## 17.4 SEMICONDUCTOR DETECTORS

1. Semiconductors are crystalline materials whose electrical conductivities are less than those of metals but more than those of crystalline insulators. Silicon and germanium are common semiconductor materials.
2. In crystalline materials, electrons exist in energy bands, separated by forbidden gaps. In metals (*e.g.*, copper), the least tightly bound electrons exist in a partially occupied band, called the conduction band. The conduction-band electrons are mobile, providing high electrical conductivity.
3. In an insulator or a semiconductor, the valence electrons exist in a filled valence band. In semiconductors, these valence-band electrons participate in covalent bonds and so are immobile. The next higher energy band, the conduction band, is empty of electrons.
4. However, if an electron is placed in the conduction band, it is mobile, as are the upper band electrons in metals. The difference between insulators and semiconductors is the magnitude of the energy gap between the valence and conduction bands. In insulators, the band gap is greater than 5 eV, whereas in semiconductors, it is about 1 eV or less (Fig. 17-7).
5. In semiconductors, valence-band electrons can be raised to the conduction band by ionizing radiation, visible light or UV radiation, or thermal energy.

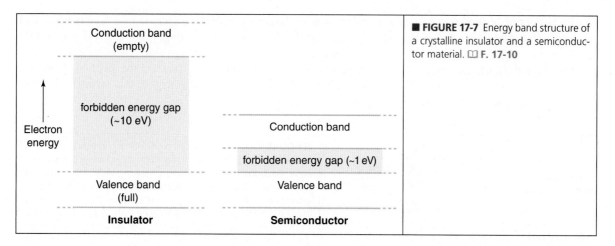

■ **FIGURE 17-7** Energy band structure of a crystalline insulator and a semiconductor material. 📖 **F. 17-10**

6. When a valence-band electron is raised to the conduction band, it leaves behind a vacancy in the valence band. This vacancy is called a *hole*. Because a hole is the absence of an electron, it is considered to have a net positive charge, equal but opposite to that of an electron.

7. When another valence-band electron fills the hole, a hole is created at that electron's former location. Thus, holes behave as mobile positive charges in the valence band even though positively charged particles do not physically move in the material.

8. The hole-electron pairs formed in a semiconductor material by ionizing radiation are analogous to the ion pairs formed in a gas by ionizing radiation.

9. A crystal of a semiconductor material can be used as a radiation detector. A voltage is placed between two terminals on opposite sides of the crystal. When ionizing radiation interacts with the detector, electrons in the crystal are raised to an excited state, permitting an electrical current to flow, similar to a gas-filled ionization chamber. Unfortunately, the radiation-induced current, unless it is very large, is masked by a larger current induced by the applied voltage.

10. To reduce the magnitude of the voltage-induced current so that the signal from radiation interactions can be detected, the semiconductor crystal is "doped" with a trace amount of impurities so that it acts as a diode. The impurity atoms fill sites in the crystal lattice that would otherwise be occupied by atoms of the semiconductor material.

11. If atoms of the impurity material have more valence electrons than those of the semiconductor material, the impurity atoms provide mobile electrons in the conduction band. A semiconductor material containing an electron-donor impurity is called an *n-type material* (Fig. 17-8). N-type material has mobile electrons in the conduction band.

12. On the other hand, an impurity with fewer valence electrons than the semiconductor material provides sites in the valence band that can accept electrons. When a valence-band electron fills one of these sites, it creates a hole at its former location. Semiconductor material doped with a hole-forming impurity is called *p-type material*. P-type material has mobile holes in the valence band (Fig. 17-8).

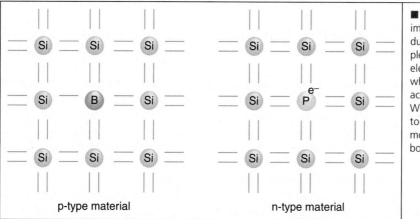

■ **FIGURE 17-8** P-type and n-type impurities in a crystal of a semiconductor material, silicon in this example. N-type impurities provide mobile electrons in the conduction band, whereas p-type impurities provide acceptor sites in the valence band. When filled by electrons, these acceptor sites create holes that act as mobile positive charges. Si, silicon; B, boron; P, phosphorus. 📖 **F. 17-11**

13. A semiconductor diode consists of a crystal of semiconductor material with a region of n-type material that forms a junction with a region of p-type material (Fig. 17-9). If an external voltage is applied with the positive polarity on the p-type side of the diode and the negative polarity on the n-type side, the holes in the p-type material and the mobile conduction-band electrons of the n-type material are drawn to the junction. There, the mobile electrons fall into the valence band to fill holes. Applying an external voltage in this manner is referred to as *forward bias*. Forward bias permits a current to flow with little resistance.

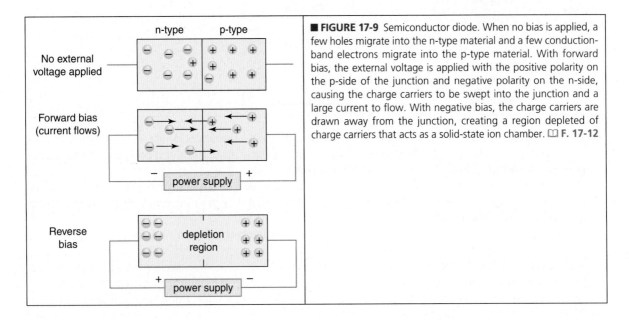

■ **FIGURE 17-9** Semiconductor diode. When no bias is applied, a few holes migrate into the n-type material and a few conduction-band electrons migrate into the p-type material. With forward bias, the external voltage is applied with the positive polarity on the p-side of the junction and negative polarity on the n-side, causing the charge carriers to be swept into the junction and a large current to flow. With negative bias, the charge carriers are drawn away from the junction, creating a region depleted of charge carriers that acts as a solid-state ion chamber. ⊞ **F. 17-12**

14. On the other hand, if an external voltage is applied with the opposite polarity—that is, with the negative polarity on the p-type side of the diode and the positive polarity on the n-type side—the holes in the p-type material and the mobile conduction-band electrons of the n-type material are drawn away from the junction. Applying the external voltage in this polarity is referred to as *reverse bias*. Reverse bias draws the charge carriers away from the n-p junction, forming a region depleted of current carriers. Very little electrical current flows when a diode is reverse biased.

15. A reverse-biased semiconductor diode can be used to detect visible light and UV radiation or ionizing radiation. The photons of light or ionization and excitation produced by ionizing radiation can excite lower energy electrons in the depletion region of the diode to higher energy bands, producing hole-electron pairs. The electrical field in the depletion region sweeps the holes toward the p-type side and the conduction-band electrons toward the n-type side, causing a momentary pulse of current to flow after the interaction.

16. *Semiconductor detectors* are semiconductor diodes designed for the detection of ionizing radiation. The amount of charge generated by an interaction is proportional to the energy deposited in the detector by the interaction; therefore, semiconductor detectors are spectrometers. Because thermal energy can also raise electrons to the conduction band, many types of semiconductor detectors used for x-ray and gamma-ray spectroscopy must be cooled with liquid nitrogen.

17. The energy resolution of germanium semiconductor detectors is greatly superior to that of NaI(Tl) scintillation detectors. Liquid nitrogen–cooled germanium detectors are widely used for the identification of individual gamma-ray–emitting radionuclides in mixed radionuclide samples because of their superb energy resolution.

18. Semiconductor detectors are seldom used for medical imaging devices because of high expense, because of low quantum detection efficiencies in comparison to scintillators such as NaI(Tl) (Z of iodine = 53, Z of germanium = 32, Z of silicon = 14), because they can be manufactured only in limited sizes, and because many such devices require cooling.

19. Efforts are being made to develop semiconductor detectors of higher atomic numbers than germanium that can be operated at room temperature. A leading candidate to date is cadmium zinc telluride (CZT). A small field-of-view nuclear medicine camera using CZT detectors has been developed.

20. A layer of semiconductor material, amorphous selenium (Z = 34), is used in some radiographic image receptors, including those in some mammography systems. The selenium is commonly referred to as a "photoconductor." In these image receptors, the selenium layer is electrically coupled to a rectangular array of thin-film transistor detector elements, which collect and store the mobile electrical charges produced in the selenium by x-ray interactions during image acquisition.

## 17.5 PULSE HEIGHT SPECTROSCOPY

1. Many radiation detectors, such as scintillation detectors, semiconductor detectors produce electrical pulses whose amplitudes are proportional to the energies deposited in the detectors by individual interactions.
2. *Pulse height analyzers* (PHAs) are electronic systems that may be used with these detectors to perform pulse height spectroscopy and energy-selective counting. In energy-selective counting, only interactions that deposit energies within a certain energy range are counted.
3. Energy-selective counting can be used to reduce the effects of background radiation, to reduce the effects of scatter, or to separate events caused by different radionuclides in a sample containing multiple radionuclides.
4. Two types of PHAs are *single-channel analyzers* (SCAs) and *multichannel analyzers* (MCAs). Pulse height discrimination circuits are incorporated in scintillation cameras, and other nuclear medicine imaging devices to reduce the effects of scatter on the images.

### Single-Channel Analyzer Systems

1. Figure 17-10 depicts an SCA system. Although the system is shown with a NaI(Tl) crystal and PMT, it could be used with any pulse-mode spectrometer. The high-voltage power supply typically provides 800 to 1,200 V to the PMT. The series of resistors divide the total voltage into increments that are applied to the dynodes and anode of the PMT. Raising the voltage increases the magnitude of the voltage pulses from the PMT.
2. The detector is often located some distance from the majority of the electronic components. The pulses from the PMT are usually routed to a preamplifier (preamp), which is connected to the PMT by as short a cable as possible. The function of the preamp is to amplify the voltage pulses further, so as to minimize distortion and attenuation of the signal during transmission to the remainder of the system. The pulses from the preamp are routed to the amplifier, which further amplifies the pulses and modifies their shapes. The gains of most amplifiers are adjustable.
3. The pulses from the amplifier then proceed to the SCA. The user is allowed to set two voltage levels, a lower level, and an upper level. If a voltage pulse whose amplitude is less than the lower level or greater than the upper level is received from the amplifier, the SCA does nothing. If a voltage pulse whose amplitude is greater than the lower level but less than the upper level is received from the amplifier, the SCA produces a single logic pulse. A logic pulse is a voltage pulse of fixed amplitude and duration.
4. Figure 17-11 illustrates the operation of an SCA. The counter counts the logic pulses from the SCA for a time interval set by the timer.

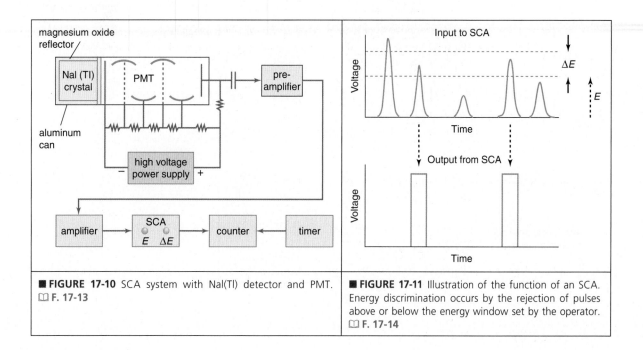

■ **FIGURE 17-10** SCA system with NaI(Tl) detector and PMT.
📖 F. 17-13

■ **FIGURE 17-11** Illustration of the function of an SCA. Energy discrimination occurs by the rejection of pulses above or below the energy window set by the operator.
📖 F. 17-14

## Multichannel Analyzer Systems

1. An MCA system permits an energy spectrum to be automatically acquired much more quickly and easily than does an SCA system. Figure 17-12 is a diagram of a counting system using an MCA. The detector, high-voltage power supply, preamp, and amplifier are the same as were those described for SCA systems.
2. The MCA consists of an analog-to-digital converter (ADC), a memory containing many storage locations called *channels,* control circuitry, and a timer. The memory of an MCA typically ranges from 256 to 8,192 channels, each of which can store a single integer. When the acquisition of a spectrum begins, all of the channels are set to zero. When each voltage pulse from the amplifier is received, it is converted into a binary digital signal, the value of which is proportional to the amplitude of the analog voltage pulse.
3. This digital signal designates a particular channel in the MCA's memory. The number stored in that channel is then incremented by 1. As many pulses are processed, a spectrum is generated in the memory of the MCA. Figure 17-13 illustrates the operation of an MCA. Today, most MCAs are interfaced to digital computers that store, process, and display the resultant spectra.

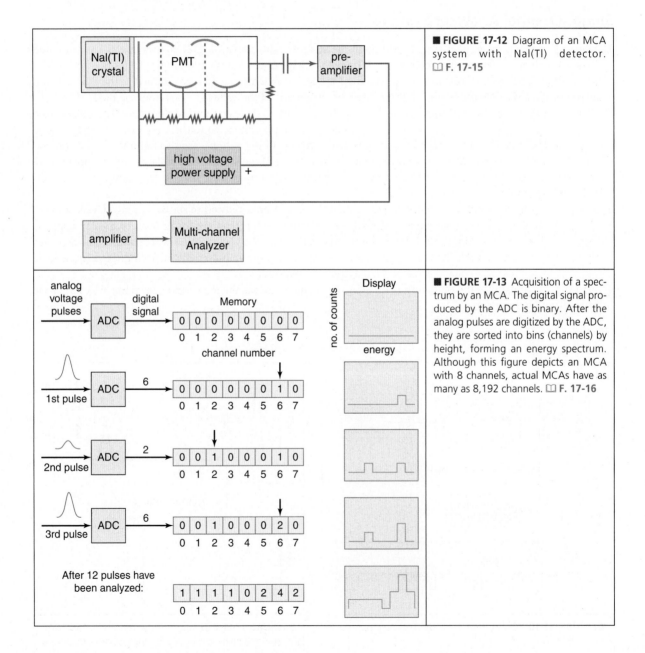

■ **FIGURE 17-12** Diagram of an MCA system with NaI(Tl) detector. 📖 **F. 17-15**

■ **FIGURE 17-13** Acquisition of a spectrum by an MCA. The digital signal produced by the ADC is binary. After the analog pulses are digitized by the ADC, they are sorted into bins (channels) by height, forming an energy spectrum. Although this figure depicts an MCA with 8 channels, actual MCAs have as many as 8,192 channels. 📖 **F. 17-16**

## Interactions of Photons with a Spectrometer

1. There are several mechanisms by which an x-ray or gamma-ray can deposit energy in the detector, several of which deposit only a fraction of the incident photon energy.

2. As illustrated in Figure 17-14, an incident photon can deposit its full energy by a photoelectric interaction (A) or by one or more Compton scatters followed by a photoelectric interaction (B). However, a photon will deposit only a fraction of its energy if it interacts by Compton scattering, and the scattered photon escapes the detector (C). In that case, the energy deposited depends on the scattering angle, with larger angle scatters depositing larger energies. Even if the incident photon interacts by the photoelectric effect, less than its total energy will be deposited if the inner-shell electron vacancy created by the interaction results in the emission of a characteristic x-ray that escapes the detector (D).

3. Most detectors are shielded to reduce the effects of natural background radiation and nearby radiation sources. Figure 17-14 shows two ways by which an x-ray or gamma-ray interaction in the shield of the detector can deposit energy in the detector. The photon may Compton scatter in the shield, with the scattered photon striking the detector (E), or a characteristic x-ray from the shield may interact with the detector (F).

4. Most interactions of x-rays and gamma rays with a NaI(Tl) detector are with iodine atoms because iodine has a much larger atomic number than sodium does. Although thallium has an even larger atomic number, it is only a trace impurity.

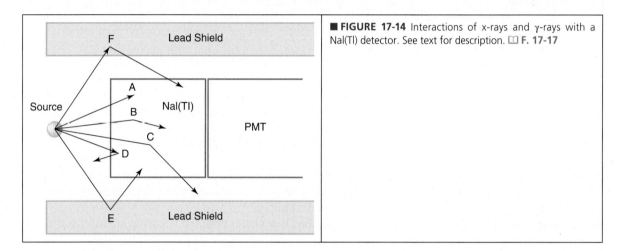

■ **FIGURE 17-14** Interactions of x-rays and γ-rays with a NaI(Tl) detector. See text for description. 📖 **F. 17-17**

## Spectrum of Cesium-137

1. The spectrum of $^{137}$Cs is often used to introduce pulse height spectroscopy because of the simple decay scheme of this radionuclide. As shown at the top of Figure 17-15, $^{137}$Cs decays by beta particle emission to $^{137m}$Ba, whose nucleus is in an excited state. The $^{137m}$Ba nucleus attains its ground state by the emission of a 662-keV gamma-ray 90% of the time.

2. In 10% of the decays, a conversion electron is emitted instead of a gamma-ray. The conversion electron is usually followed by the emission of an approximately 32-keV K-shell characteristic x-ray as an outer-shell electron fills the inner-shell vacancy.

3. In the left in Figure 17-15 is the actual energy spectrum of $^{137}$Cs, and on the right is its pulse height spectrum obtained with the use of a NaI(Tl) detector. There are two reasons for the differences between the spectra.

   a. First, there are several mechanisms by which an x-ray or gamma-ray can deposit energy in the detector, several of which deposit only a fraction of the incident photon energy.

   b. Second, there are random variations in the processes by which the energy deposited in the detector is converted into an electrical signal. In the case of a NaI(Tl) crystal coupled to a PMT, there are random variations in the fraction of deposited energy converted into light, the fraction of the light that reaches the photocathode of the PMT, and the number of electrons ejected from the back of the photocathode per unit energy deposited by the light.

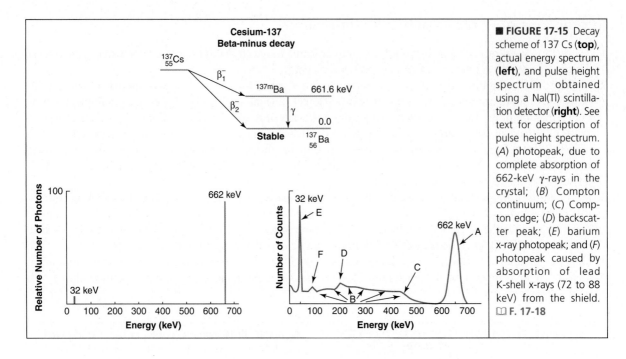

**FIGURE 17-15** Decay scheme of 137 Cs (**top**), actual energy spectrum (**left**), and pulse height spectrum obtained using a NaI(Tl) scintillation detector (**right**). See text for description of pulse height spectrum. (*A*) photopeak, due to complete absorption of 662-keV γ-rays in the crystal; (*B*) Compton continuum; (*C*) Compton edge; (*D*) backscatter peak; (*E*) barium x-ray photopeak; and (*F*) photopeak caused by absorption of lead K-shell x-rays (72 to 88 keV) from the shield. F. 17-18

c. These factors cause random variations in the size of the voltage pulses produced by the detector, even when the incident x-rays or gamma rays deposit exactly the same energy. The energy resolution of a spectrometer is a measure of the effect of these random variations on the resultant spectrum.

4. In the pulse height spectrum of $^{137}$Cs, on the right in Figure 17-14, the photopeak (A) is caused by interactions in which the energy of an incident 662-keV photon is entirely absorbed in the crystal. This may occur by a single photoelectric interaction or by one or more Compton scattering interactions followed by a photoelectric interaction.

5. The Compton continuum (B) is caused by 662-keV photons that scatter in the crystal, with the scattered photons escaping the crystal. Each portion of the continuum corresponds to a particular scattering angle. The Compton edge (C) is the upper limit of the Compton continuum.

6. The backscatter peak (D) is caused by 662-keV photons that scatter from the shielding around the detector into the detector.

7. The barium x-ray photopeak (E) is a second photopeak caused by the absorption of barium K-shell x-rays (31 to 37 keV), which are emitted after the emission of conversion electrons.

8. Another photopeak (F) is caused by lead K-shell x-rays (72 to 88 keV) from the shield.

## Spectrum of Technetium-99m

1. The decay scheme of $^{99m}$Tc is shown at the top in Figure 17-16. $^{99m}$Tc is an isomer of $^{99}$Tc that decays by isomeric transition to its ground state, with the emission of a 140.5-keV gamma-ray. In 11% of the transitions, a conversion electron is emitted instead of a gamma-ray.

2. The pulse height spectrum of $^{99m}$Tc is shown at the bottom of Figure 17-16. The photopeak (A) is caused by the total absorption of the 140-keV gamma rays.

3. The escape peak (B) is caused by 140-keV gamma rays that interact with the crystal by the photoelectric effect but with the resultant iodine K-shell x-rays (28 to 33 keV) escaping the crystal.

4. There is also a photopeak (C) caused by the absorption of lead K-shell x-rays from the shield. The Compton continuum is quite small, unlike the continuum in the spectrum of $^{137}$Cs, because the photoelectric effect predominates in iodine at 140 keV.

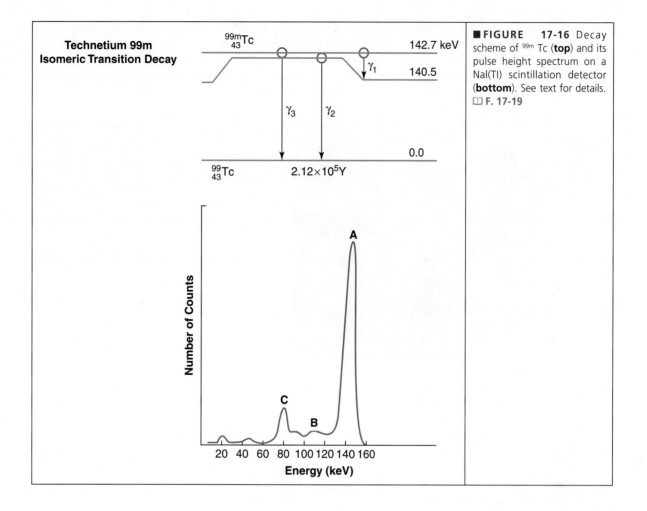

**Technetium 99m
Isomeric Transition Decay**

$^{99m}_{43}Tc$    142.7 keV

$\gamma_1$    140.5

$\gamma_3$    $\gamma_2$

0.0

$^{99}_{43}Tc$    $2.12 \times 10^5 Y$

Number of Counts

A

C

B

20 40 60 80 100 120 140 160
**Energy (keV)**

■**FIGURE  17-16** Decay scheme of $^{99m}$ Tc (**top**) and its pulse height spectrum on a NaI(Tl) scintillation detector (**bottom**). See text for details. 📖 **F. 17-19**

## Energy Resolution

1. The energy resolution of a spectrometer is a measure of its ability to differentiate between particles or photons of different energies. It can be determined by irradiating the detector with monoenergetic particles or photons and measuring the width of the resultant peak in the pulse height spectrum.
2. Statistical effects in the detection process cause the amplitudes of the pulses from the detector to randomly vary about the mean pulse height, giving the peak a gaussian shape. A wider peak implies a poorer energy resolution.
3. The width is usually measured at half the maximal height of the peak, as illustrated in Figure 17-17. This is called the full width at half maximum (FWHM).
4. The FWHM is then divided by the pulse amplitude corresponding to the maximum of the peak:

$$\text{Energy resolution} = \frac{\text{FWHM}}{\text{Pulse amplitude at center of peak}} \times 100\%  \quad [17\text{-}4] \quad 📖 \text{E. 17-4}$$

5. For example, the energy resolution of a 5-cm-diameter and 5-cm-thick cylindrical NaI(Tl) crystal, coupled to a PMT and exposed to the 662-keV gamma rays of $^{137}$Cs, is typically about 7% to 8%.

## 17.6  NONIMAGING DETECTOR APPLICATIONS

## Sodium Iodide Thyroid Probe and Well Counter

### Thyroid Probe

1. A nuclear medicine department typically has a thyroid probe for measuring the uptake of $^{123}$I or $^{131}$I by the thyroid glands of patients and for monitoring the activities of $^{131}$I in the thyroid glands of staff members who handle large activities of $^{131}$I.

2. A thyroid probe, as shown in Figures 17-17 and 17-18, usually consists of a 5.1-cm (2-inch)-diameter and 5.1-cm-thick cylindrical NaI(Tl) crystal coupled to a PMT, which in turn is connected to a preamplifier. The probe is shielded on the sides and back with lead and is equipped with a collimator so that it detects photons only from a limited portion of the patient. The thyroid probe is connected to a high-voltage power supply and either an SCA or an MCA system.

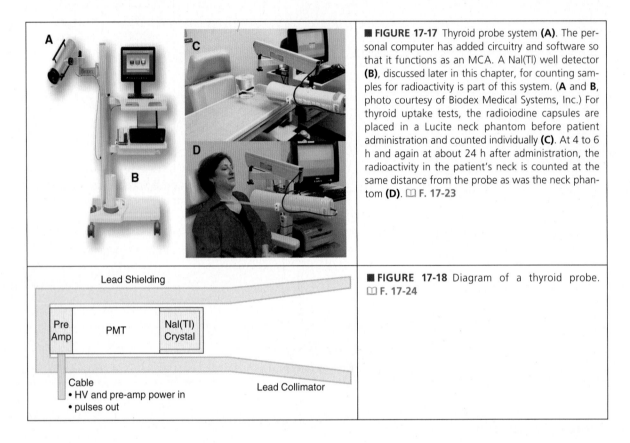

■ **FIGURE 17-17** Thyroid probe system **(A)**. The personal computer has added circuitry and software so that it functions as an MCA. A NaI(Tl) well detector **(B)**, discussed later in this chapter, for counting samples for radioactivity is part of this system. (**A** and **B**, photo courtesy of Biodex Medical Systems, Inc.) For thyroid uptake tests, the radioiodine capsules are placed in a Lucite neck phantom before patient administration and counted individually **(C)**. At 4 to 6 h and again at about 24 h after administration, the radioactivity in the patient's neck is counted at the same distance from the probe as was the neck phantom **(D)**. ▭ F. 17-23

■ **FIGURE 17-18** Diagram of a thyroid probe. ▭ F. 17-24

3. Thyroid uptake measurements may be performed using one or two capsules of $^{123}$I or $^{131}$I sodium iodide. A neck phantom, consisting of a Lucite cylinder of a diameter similar to the neck and containing a hole parallel to its axis for a radioiodine capsule, is required.
4. In the two-capsule method, the capsules should have almost identical activities. Each capsule is placed in the neck phantom and counted separately. Then, one capsule is swallowed by the patient. The other capsule is called the "standard."
5. Next, the emissions from the patient's neck are counted, typically at 4 to 6 h after administration and again at 24 h after administration. Each time that the patient's thyroid is counted, the patient's distal thigh is also counted for the same length of time, to approximate nonthyroidal activity in the neck, and a background count is obtained.
6. All counts are performed with the NaI crystal at the same distance, typically 20 to 30 cm, from the thyroid phantom or the patient's neck or thigh. (This distance reduces the effects of small differences in distance between the detector and the objects being counted.)
7. Furthermore, each time that the patient's thyroid is counted, the remaining capsule is placed in the neck phantom and counted. Finally, the uptake is calculated for each neck measurement:

$$\text{Uptake} = \frac{(\text{Thyroid count} - \text{Thigh count})}{(\text{Count of standard in phantom} - \text{Background count})} \times \frac{\text{Initial count of standard in phantom}}{\text{Initial count of patient capsule in phantom}}$$

[17-5]

8. Some nuclear medicine laboratories instead use a method that requires only one capsule. In this method, a single capsule is obtained, counted in the neck phantom, and swallowed by the patient. As in the previous method, the patient's neck and distal thigh are counted, typically at 4 to 6 h and again at 24 h after administration. The times of the capsule administration and the neck counts are recorded. Finally, the uptake is calculated for each neck measurement:

$$\frac{\left(\text{Thyroid count} - \text{Thigh count}\right)}{\left(\text{Count of capsule in phantom} - \text{Background count}\right)} \times e^{0.693t/T_{1/2}} \qquad [17\text{-}6]$$

where $T_{1/2}$ is the physical half-life of the radionuclide and $t$ is the time elapsed between the count of the capsule in the phantom and the thyroid count.

9. The single-capsule method avoids the cost of the second capsule and requires fewer measurements, but it is more susceptible to instability of the equipment, technologist error, and dead-time effects.

## Sodium Iodine Well Counter

1. A nuclear medicine department also usually has a NaI(Tl) well counter, shown in Figure 17-19. The NaI(Tl) well counter may be used for clinical tests such as Schilling tests (a test of vitamin $B_{12}$ absorption), plasma or red blood cell volume determinations, and radioimmunoassays, although radioimmunoassays have been largely replaced by immunoassays that do not use radioactivity.

2. The well counter is also commonly used to assay wipe test samples to detect radioactive contamination. The well counter usually consists of a cylindrical NaI(Tl) crystal, either 5.1 cm (2 inches) in diameter and 5.1 cm thick or 7.6 cm (3 inches) in diameter and 7.6 cm thick, with a hole in the crystal for the insertion of samples. This configuration gives the counter an extremely high efficiency, permitting it to assay samples containing activities of less than 1 nCi ($10^{-3}$ $\mu$Ci).

3. The crystal is coupled to a PMT, which in turn is connected to a preamplifier. A well counter in a nuclear medicine department should have a thick lead shield because it is used to count samples containing nanocurie activities in the vicinity of mCi activities of high-energy gamma-ray emitters such as $^{67}$Ga, $^{111}$In, and $^{131}$I.

4. The well counter is connected to a high-voltage power supply and either an SCA or an MCA system. Departments that perform large numbers of radioimmunoassays often use automatic well counters, such as the one shown in Figure 17-20, to count large numbers of samples.

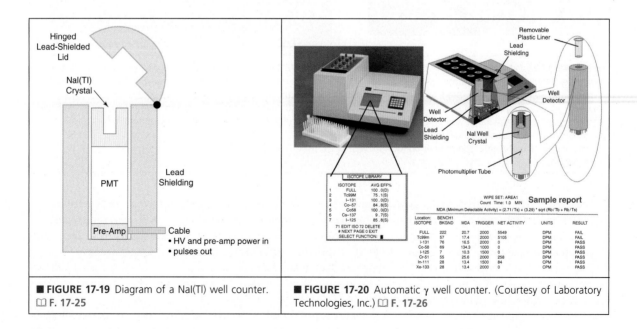

■ **FIGURE 17-19** Diagram of a NaI(Tl) well counter. 📖 **F. 17-25**

■ **FIGURE 17-20** Automatic γ well counter. (Courtesy of Laboratory Technologies, Inc.) 📖 **F. 17-26**

## The Dose Calibrator

1. A dose calibrator, shown in Figure 17-21, is used to measure the activities of dosages of radiopharmaceuticals to be administered to patients. The U.S. Nuclear Regulatory Commission (NRC) and state regulatory agencies require that dosages of x-ray–emitting and gamma-ray–emitting radiopharmaceuticals be determined before administration to patients.

2. NRC allows administration of a "unit dosage" (an individual patient dosage prepared by a commercial radio-pharmacy, without any further manipulation of its activity by the nuclear medicine department that administers it) without measurement. It also permits the determination of activities of nonunit dosages by volumetric measurements and mathematical calculations.

3. Most dose calibrators are well-type ionization chambers that are filled with argon ($Z = 18$) and pressurized to maximize sensitivity. Most dose calibrators have shielding around their chambers to protect users from the radioactive material being assayed and to prevent nearby sources of radiation from affecting the measurements.

4. A dose calibrator cannot directly measure activity. Instead, it measures the intensity of the radiation emitted by a dosage of a radiopharmaceutical. The manufacturer of a dose calibrator determines calibration factors relating the magnitude of the signal from the detector to activity for specific radionuclides commonly used in nuclear medicine.

5. The user pushes a button or turns a dial on the dose calibrator to designate the radionuclide being measured, thereby specifying a calibration factor, and the dose calibrator displays the measured activity.

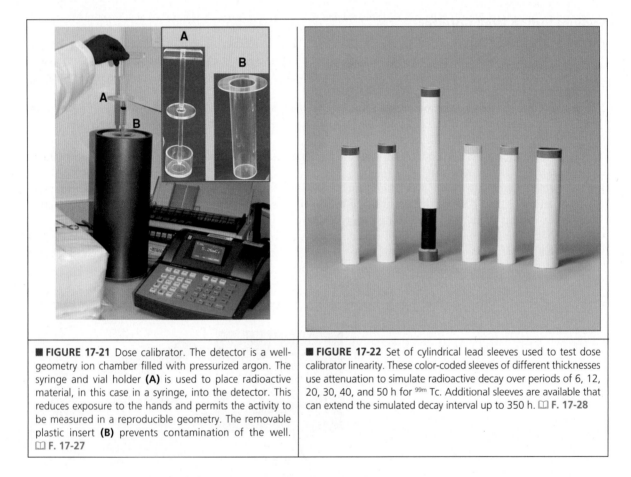

■ **FIGURE 17-21** Dose calibrator. The detector is a well-geometry ion chamber filled with pressurized argon. The syringe and vial holder **(A)** is used to place radioactive material, in this case in a syringe, into the detector. This reduces exposure to the hands and permits the activity to be measured in a reproducible geometry. The removable plastic insert **(B)** prevents contamination of the well. 📖 **F. 17-27**

■ **FIGURE 17-22** Set of cylindrical lead sleeves used to test dose calibrator linearity. These color-coded sleeves of different thicknesses use attenuation to simulate radioactive decay over periods of 6, 12, 20, 30, 40, and 50 h for $^{99m}$Tc. Additional sleeves are available that can extend the simulated decay interval up to 350 h. 📖 **F. 17-28**

6. Because the assay of activity using the dose calibrator is often the only assurance that the patient is receiving the prescribed activity, quality assurance testing of the dose calibrator is required by the NRC and state regulatory agencies. The NRC requires the testing to be in accordance with nationally recognized standards or the manufacturer's instructions. The following set of tests is commonly performed to satisfy this requirement.

7. The device should be tested for *accuracy* upon installation and annually thereafter. Two or more sealed radioactive sources (often $^{57}$Co and $^{137}$Cs) whose activities are known within 5% are assayed. The measured activities must be within 10% of the actual activities.

8. The device should also be tested for *linearity* (a measure of the effect that the amount of activity has on the accuracy) upon installation and quarterly thereafter. The most common method requires a vial of $^{99m}$Tc containing the maximal activity that would be administered to a patient.

9. The vial is measured two or three times daily until it decays to less than 30 µCi; the measured activities and times of the measurements are recorded. One measurement is assumed to be correct, and from this measurement, activities are calculated for the times of the other measurements. No measurement may differ from the corresponding calculated activity by more than 10%.

**10.** An alternative to the decay method for testing linearity is the use of commercially available lead cylindrical sleeves of different thicknesses that simulate radioactive decay via attenuation (Fig. 17-22). These devices must be calibrated prior to first use by comparing their simulated decay with the decay method described above.

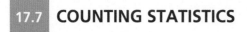

## 17.7 COUNTING STATISTICS

## Introduction

### Sources of Error

**1.** There are three types of errors in measurements.
  **a.** The first is *systematic error*. Systematic error occurs when measurements differ from the correct values in a systematic fashion. For example, a systematic error occurs in radiation measurements if a detector is used in pulse mode at too high an interaction rate; dead-time count losses cause the measured count rate to be lower than the actual interaction rate.
  **b.** The second type of error is *random error*. Random error is caused by random fluctuations in whatever is being measured or in the measurement process itself.
  **c.** The third type of error is the *blunder* (*e.g.*, setting the single-channel analyzer window incorrectly for a single measurement).

### Random Error in Radiation Detection

**1.** The processes by which radiation is emitted and interacts with matter are random in nature. Whether a particular radioactive nucleus decays within a specified time interval, the direction of an x-ray emitted by an electron striking the target of an x-ray tube, whether a particular x-ray passes through a patient to reach the film cassette of an x-ray machine, and whether a gamma-ray incident upon a scintillation camera crystal is detected are all random phenomena.
**2.** Therefore, all radiation measurements, including medical imaging, are subject to random error. Counting statistics enable judgments of the validity of measurements that are subject to random error.

## Characterization of Data

### Accuracy and Precision

**1.** If a measurement is close to the correct value, it is said to be *accurate*.
**2.** If measurements are reproducible, they are said to be *precise*.
**3.** Precision does not imply accuracy; a set of measurements may be very close together (precise) but not close to the correct value (*i.e.*, inaccurate). If a set of measurements differs from the correct value in a systematic fashion (systematic error), the data are said to be *biased*.

### Measures of Central Tendency—Mean and Median

**1.** Two measures of central tendency of a set of measurements are the *mean* (average) and the median. The mean ($x$) of a set of measurements is defined as follows:

$$\bar{x} = \frac{x_1 + x_2 + \ldots + x_N}{N}$$

[17-7]  📖 E. 17-6

where $N$ is the number of measurements.
**2.** To obtain the *median* of a set of measurements, they must first be put in order by size. The median is the middle measurement if the number of measurements is odd, and it is the average of the two midmost measurements if the number of measurements is even.
**3.** For example, to obtain the median of the five measurements 8, 14, 5, 9, and 12, they are first sorted by size: 5, 8, 9, 12, and 14. The median is 9. The advantage of the median over the mean is that the median is less affected by outliers. An outlier is a measurement that is much greater or much less than the others.

## Measures of Variability—Variance and Standard Deviation

1. The variance and standard deviation are measures of the variability (spread) of a set of measurements. The variance ($\sigma^2$) is determined from a set of measurements by subtracting the mean from each measurement, squaring the differences, summing the squares, and dividing by one less than the number of measurements:

$$\sigma^2 = \frac{\left(x_1 - \overline{x}\right)^2 + \left(x_2 - \overline{x}\right)^2 + \cdots + \left(x_N - \overline{x}\right)^2}{N-1}$$   [17-8]   📖 E. 17-7

   where $N$ is the total number of measurements and $\overline{x}$ is the sample mean.

2. The *standard deviation* ($\sigma$) is the square root of the variance:

$$\sigma = \sqrt{\sigma^2}$$   [17-9]   📖 E. 17-8

3. The *fractional standard deviation* (also referred to as the *fractional error* or *coefficient of variation*) is the standard deviation divided by the mean:

$$\text{Fractional standard deviation} = \sigma / \overline{x}$$   [17-10]   📖 E. 17-9

## Binary Processes

1. A *trial* is an event that may have more than one outcome. A *binary process* is a process in which a trial can only have two outcomes, one of which is arbitrarily called a *success*.
2. A toss of a coin is a binary process. The toss of a die can be considered a binary process if, for example, a "two" is selected as a success and any other outcome is considered to be a failure.
3. Whether a particular radioactive nucleus decays during a specified time interval is a binary process. Whether a particular x-ray or gamma-ray is detected by a radiation detector is a binary process. Table 17-2 lists examples of binary processes.
4. A measurement consists of counting the number of successes from a specified number of trials. Tossing 10 coins and counting the number of "heads" is a measurement. Placing a radioactive sample on a detector and recording the number of events detected is a measurement.

**TABLE 17-2  BINARY PROCESSES**

| TRIAL | DEFINITION OF A SUCCESS | PROBABILITY OF A SUCCESS |
|---|---|---|
| Toss of a coin | "Heads" | 1/2 |
| Toss of a die | "A four" | 1/6 |
| Observation of a radioactive nucleus for a time "$t$" | It decays | $1 - e^{-\lambda t}$ |
| Observation of a detector of efficiency $E$ placed near a radioactive nucleus for a time "$t$" | A count | $E(1 - e^{-\lambda t})$ |

Adapted from Knoll GF. *Radiation Detection and Measurement*. 4th ed. Copyright © 2010, John Wiley and Sons.

## Estimating the Uncertainty of a Single Measurement

### Estimated Standard Deviation

1. The standard deviation can be estimated by making several measurements and applying Equations 17-8 and 17-9. Nevertheless, if the process being measured is binary, the standard deviation can be estimated from a single measurement.
2. The single measurement is probably close to the mean. Because the standard deviation is approximately the square root of the mean (in binary processes as described by the binomial, Poisson, and Gaussian functions), it is also approximately the square root of the single measurement:

$$\sigma \approx \sqrt{x}$$   [17-11]   📖 E. 17-14

   where $x$ is the single measurement.

3. The fractional standard deviation of a single measurement may also be estimated as

$$\text{Fractional error} = \frac{\sigma}{x} \approx \frac{\sqrt{x}}{x} = \frac{1}{\sqrt{x}}$$   [17-12]   📖 E. 17-15

4. For example, a single measurement of a radioactive source yields 1,256 counts. The estimated standard deviation is

$$\sigma \approx \sqrt{1,256\,\text{cts}} = 35.4\,\text{cts}$$

5. The fractional standard deviation is estimated as

$$\text{Fractional error} = 35.4\,\text{cts}/1,256\,\text{cts} = 0.028 = 2.8\%$$

6. Table 17-3 lists the estimated fractional errors for various numbers of counts. The fractional error decreases with increasing number of counts.

**TABLE 17-3 FRACTIONAL ERRORS (PERCENT STANDARD DEVIATIONS) FOR SEVERAL NUMBERS OF COUNTS**

| COUNT | FRACTIONAL ERROR (%) |
|---|---|
| 100 | 10.0 |
| 1,000 | 3.2 |
| 10,000 | 1.0 |
| 100,000 | 0.32 |

## Confidence Intervals

1. Table 17-4 lists intervals about a measurement, called *confidence intervals*, for which the probability of containing the true mean is specified.
2. There is a 68.3% probability that the true mean is within one standard deviation ($1\sigma$) of a measurement, a 95% probability that it is within $2\sigma$ of a measurement, and a 99.7% probability that it is within $3\sigma$ of a measurement, assuming that the measurements follow a gaussian distribution.
3. For example, let us assume that a count of 853 is obtained. What is the interval about this count in which there is a 95% probability of finding the true mean? First, the standard deviation is estimated as

$$\sigma \approx \sqrt{853\,\text{cts}} = 29.2\,\text{cts}$$

4. From Table 17-4, the 95% confidence interval is determined as follows: 853 cts ± 1.96 $\sigma$ = 853 cts ± 1.96 (29.2 cts) = 853 cts ± 57.2 cts. So, the 95% confidence interval ranges from 796 to 910 counts.

**TABLE 17-4 CONFIDENCE INTERVALS**

| INTERVAL ABOUT MEASUREMENT | PROBABILITY THAT MEAN IS WITHIN INTERVAL (%) |
|---|---|
| $\pm 0.674\sigma$ | 50.0 |
| $\pm 1\sigma$ | 68.3 |
| $\pm 1.64\sigma$ | 90.0 |
| $\pm 1.96\sigma$ | 95.0 |
| $\pm 2.58\sigma$ | 99.0 |
| $\pm 3\sigma$ | 99.7 |

Adapted from Knoll GF. *Radiation Detection and Measurement*. 4th ed. Copyright © 2010, John Wiley and Sons.

## Propagation of Error

1. In nuclear medicine, calculations are frequently performed using numbers that incorporate random error. It is often necessary to estimate the uncertainty in the results of these calculations.
2. Although the standard deviation of a count may be estimated by simply taking its square root, it is incorrect to calculate the standard deviation of the result of a calculation by taking its square root.
3. Instead, the standard deviations of the actual counts must first be calculated and entered into propagation of error equations to obtain the standard deviation of the result.

## Multiplication or Division of a Number with Error by a Number without Error

1. It is often necessary to multiply or divide a number containing random error by a number that does not contain random error. For example, to calculate a count rate, a count (which incorporates random error) is divided by a counting time (which does not involve significant random error).
2. If a number x has a standard deviation $\sigma$ and is multiplied by a number $c$ without random error, the standard deviation of the product $cx$ is $c\sigma$. If a number $x$ has a standard deviation $\sigma$ and is divided by a number $c$ without random error, the standard deviation of the quotient $x/c$ is $\sigma/c$.
3. For example, a 5-min count of a radioactive sample yields 952 counts (cts). The count rate is 952 cts/5 min = 190 cts/min. The standard deviation and percent standard deviation of the count are

$$\sigma \approx \sqrt{952 \text{ cts}} = 30.8 \text{ cts}$$
$$\text{Fractional error} = 30.8 \text{ cts}/952 \text{ cts} = 0.032 = 3.2\%$$

4. The standard deviation of the count rate is $\sigma$ = 30.8 cts/5 min = 6.16 cts/min and the fractional error = 6.16 cts/190 cts = 3.2%. Notice that the percent standard deviation is not affected when a number is multiplied or divided by a number without random error.

## Additional or Subtraction of Numbers with Error

1. It is often necessary to add or subtract numbers with random error. For example, a background count may be subtracted from a count of a radioactive sample. Whether two numbers are added or subtracted, the same equation is used to calculate the standard deviation of the result, as shown in Table 17-5.

### TABLE 17-5 PROPAGATION OF ERROR EQUATIONS

| DESCRIPTION | OPERATION | STANDARD DEVIATION |
|---|---|---|
| Multiplication of a number with random error by a number without random error | $cx$ | $c\sigma$ |
| Division of a number with random error by a number without random error | $x/c$ | $\sigma/c$ |
| Addition of two numbers containing random errors | $x_1 + x_2$ | $\sqrt{\sigma_1^2 + \sigma_2^2}$ |
| Subtraction of two numbers containing random errors | $x_1 - x_2$ | $\sqrt{\sigma_1^2 + \sigma_2^2}$ |

*Note:* c is a number without random error, $\sigma$ is the standard deviation of x, $\sigma_1$ is the standard deviation of $x_1$, and $\sigma_2$ is the standard deviation of $x_2$.

2. For example, let us assume that a count of a radioactive sample yields 1,952 counts, and a background count with the sample removed from the detector yields 1,451 counts. The count of the sample, corrected for background, is 1,952 cts −1,451 cts = 501 cts.
3. The standard deviation and percent standard deviation of the original sample count are

$$\sigma_{s+b} \approx \sqrt{1,952 \text{ cts}} = 44.2 \text{ cts}$$
$$\text{Fractional error} = 44.2 \text{ cts}/1,952 \text{ cts} = 2.3\%$$

4. The standard deviation and percent standard deviation of the background count are

$$\sigma_b \approx \sqrt{1,451 \text{ cts}} = 38.1 \text{ cts}$$
$$\text{Fractional error} = 38.1 \text{ cts}/1,451 \text{ cts} = 2.6\%$$

5. The standard deviation and percent standard deviation of the sample count corrected for background are

$$\sigma_s \approx \sqrt{(44.4 \text{ cts})^2 + (38.3 \text{ cts})^2} = 58.3 \text{ cts}$$
$$\text{Fractional error} = 58.1 \text{ cts}/501 \text{ cts} = 11.6\%$$

6. Note that the fractional error of the difference is much larger than the fractional error of either count. The fractional error of the difference of two numbers of similar magnitude can be much larger than the fractional errors of the two numbers.

## Combination Problems

1. It is sometimes necessary to perform mathematical operations in series, for example, to subtract two numbers and then to divide the difference by another number. The standard deviation is calculated for each intermediate result in the series by entering the standard deviations from the previous step into the appropriate propagation of error equation in Table 17-5.

2. For example, a 5-min count of a radioactive sample yields 1,290 counts and a 5-min background count yields 451 counts. What is the count rate due to the sample alone and its standard deviation?

3. First, the count is corrected for background: count = 1,290 cts − 451 cts = 839 cts.

4. The estimated standard deviation of each count and the difference are calculated as

$$\sigma_{s+b} \approx \sqrt{1,290 \text{ cts}} = 35.9 \text{ cts and } \sigma_b \approx \sqrt{451 \text{ cts}} = 21.2 \text{ cts}$$

$$\sigma_2 \approx \sqrt{(35.9 \text{ cts})^2 + (21.2 \text{ cts})^2} = 41.7 \text{ cts}$$

5. Finally, the count rate due to the source alone and its standard deviation are calculated as

$$\text{Count rate} = 839 \text{ cts}/5 \text{ min} = 168 \text{ cts}/\text{min}$$

$$\sigma_2/c = 41.7 \text{ cts}/5 \text{ min} = 8.3 \text{ cts}/\text{min}$$

# Section II Questions and Answers

1. Radiation detectors that yield information on the energy distribution of incident radiation particles are called:
   A. Counters
   B. Dosimeters
   C. Spectrometers
   D. Survey meters

2. Which one of the following statements is true regarding scintillation detectors and their mode of operation?
   A. Operated in pulse mode in digital radiography
   B. Operated in pulse mode in computed tomography
   C. Operated in current mode in nuclear medicine
   D. Operated in pulse mode in nuclear medicine

3. Two mathematical models of detector dead time include paralyzable and nonparalyzable. In a very high-intensity radiation field, which type of detector might result in the incorrect reporting of a zero count rate?
   A. Both paralyzable and nonparalyzable detectors
   B. Neither paralyzable nor nonparalyzable detectors
   C. Only paralyzable detectors
   D. Only nonparalyzable detectors

4. The absolute efficiency for a photon detector operated in pulse mode is defined by which ratio?
   A. (Number reaching detector)/(number emitted)
   B. (Number detected)/(number reaching detector)
   C. (Number detected)/(number emitted)
   D. (Number emitted)/(number detected)

5. The intrinsic efficiency of a photon detector is a function of what properties?
   A. Photon energy and detector thickness
   B. Atomic number $Z$ and mass density $\rho$ of the detector
   C. Photon energy
   D. Photon energy and $Z$, $\rho$, and thickness of the detector

6. For a gas-filled photon detector, what component of the detector collects the free electrons?
   A. Anode wire
   B. Cathode wall
   C. Anode wall
   D. Cathode wire

7. For a generic gas-filled photon detector, the number of ion pairs collected increases with increasing applied voltage. As that voltage increases, transitions occur across six different operating regions. What are the *first* three regions starting at zero applied voltage?
   A. Recombination, ion saturation, proportional
   B. Proportional, limited proportional, GM
   C. Limited proportional, GM, continuous discharge
   D. Recombination, ion saturation, GM

8. For a generic gas-filled photon detector, the number of ion pairs collected increases with increasing applied voltage. As that voltage increases, one transitions across six different operating regions. What are the *last* three regions?
   A. Recombination, ion saturation, proportional
   B. Proportional, limited proportional, GM
   C. Limited proportional, GM, continuous discharge
   D. Recombination, ion saturation, GM

9. Why do the ion pairs collected in a gas-filled photon detector increase with increasing applied voltage in the recombination region (no. 1) but are constant with increasing applied voltage in the ion saturation region (no. 2)?
   A. Gas multiplication becomes stable in no. 2.
   B. As voltage increases, more ion pairs are produced in no. 1.
   C. Gas multiplication ends as you transition from no. 1 to no. 2.
   D. Only at a high enough voltage are all ion pairs produced by the radiation event fully collected in no. 2.

10. Regarding the design of the walls of gas-cavity ion chambers, what is meant by the term *electronic equilibrium*?
    A. The applied voltage is set at an equilibrium value
    B. The electrical anode wire current is set at an equilibrium value.
    C. Secondary electrons are equilibrated to positive gas ions
    D. Secondary electrons born in the gas cavity and lost to the detector walls are compensated by secondary electrons born in the walls that enter the gas cavity.

11. In an ion chamber proportional region, the number of ion pairs increases with increasing applied voltage due to a phenomenon called *gas multiplication*, defined as:
    A. Positively charged gas molecules release additional orbital electrons on their way to the cathode wall.
    B. Electrons gain sufficient kinetic energy during anode wire collection, cause additional gas ionization events, and thus additional ion pairs.
    C. The original gas molecules are split into smaller gas molecules during electron collisions.
    D. Electrons recombine with positive gas molecules at higher rates as applied voltage increases.

12. In the Geiger-Müller (or GM) region, a chain reaction of gas multiplication avalanches are generated. This chain reaction extends to a size proportional to the applied voltage, but it is not in any way related to the original number of ion pairs created by the radiation event. What triggers and sustains this chain reaction in the GM counter?
    A. Collection of the first electron avalanche
    B. Collection of the last electron avalanche
    C. Characteristic x-rays from excited gas molecules
    D. Collection of the first positive gas molecule

13. Which of the following is **not** a desired feature of a scintillation detector?
    A. The conversion efficiency (fraction of deposited energy converted to light photons) should be low.
    B. Decay times of excited states should be short.
    C. Material should be transparent to its own scintillation photon emissions.
    D. Color of emitted light should match the spectral sensitivity of the light receptor (PMT).

14. A variety of inorganic scintillators are used in medical imaging detectors. Which scintillator is primarily used in computed tomography scanners?
    A. NaI(Tl)—sodium iodide thallium-activated
    B. CsI(Na)—cesium iodide sodium-activated
    C. BaFBr—barium fluoro bromide
    D. $CdWO_4$—cadmium tungstate

15. A variety of inorganic scintillators are used in medical imaging detectors. Which scintillator is typically used as the input phosphor for image intensifier tubes used in fluoroscopy?
    A. NaI(Tl)—sodium iodide thallium-activated
    B. CsI(Na)—cesium iodide sodium-activated
    C. BaFBr—barium fluoro bromide
    D. $CdWO_4$—cadmium tungstate

16. A variety of inorganic scintillators are used in medical imaging detectors. What is the primary scintillator used in the nuclear medicine scintillation gamma-camera?
    A. NaI(Tl)—sodium iodide thallium-activated
    B. CsI(Na)—cesium iodide sodium-activated
    C. BaFBr—barium fluoro bromide
    D. $CdWO_4$—cadmium tungstate

17. The conversion of scintillation photons to an electrical signal can be accomplished in which device?
    A. Photomultiplier tube
    B. Photodiode
    C. Multi-pixel photon counters
    D. All the above

18. What is the distinguishing feature between the thermoluminescent dosimeter (TLD) and the optically stimulated luminescent dosimeter (OSLD)?
    A. Method by which radiation exposure results in the trapping of electrons
    B. Method by which energy is delivered to release trapped electrons following radiation exposure
    C. Method by which the material is deployed for personnel dosimetry
    D. Method by which scintillation photons are emitted

19. Which inorganic scintillator is commonly used in the optically stimulated luminescent dosimeter (OSLD)?
    A. $Al_2O_3$(C)—aluminum oxide carbon-activated
    B. LiF(Mg)—lithium fluoride manganese-activated
    C. NaI(Tl)—sodium iodide thallium-activated
    D. CsI(Tl)—cesium iodine thallium-activated

20. What is the primary distinction between an insulator and a semiconductor?
    A. Lack of a conduction band in the insulator
    B. Lack of a conduction band in the semiconductor
    C. Presence of intermediate energy states in the forbidden energy gap in the semiconductor
    D. Forbidden energy gap size (in eV) between the valence and conduction band for electrons

21. In a silicon-based semiconductor, which of the following elements might be substituted for a silicon atom to form a p-type semiconductor?
    A. Beryllium—Be
    B. Boron—B
    C. Sulfur—S
    D. Phosphorus—P

22. In a silicon-based semiconductor, which of the following elements might be substituted for a silicon atom to form an n-type semiconductor?
    A. Beryllium—Be
    B. Boron—B
    C. Sulfur—S
    D. Phosphorus—P

23. The sensitive volume of a semiconductor radiation detector coincides with the depletion region located at the interface between a p-type and an n-type semiconductor. How is this depletion region is formed?
    A. Power supply is connected under reverse bias.
    B. Power supply is connected under forward bias.
    C. No external voltage is applied.
    D. Power supply is rapidly alternated between reverse bias and forward bias connections.

24. A single-channel analyzer (SCA) is used to produce counts of Tc-99m gamma-rays in a scintillation counter. The lower-level discriminator is set at 130 keV and the upper-level discriminator is set at 150 keV. Ten energy deposition events occur in the scintillation detector: 159, 151, 132, 137, 130, 154, 152, 121, 153, and 160 keV. How many counts are registered by the SCA?
    A. 1
    B. 3
    C. 7
    D. 10

25. The pulse height spectrum from a NaI(Tl) scintillation detector exposed to Cs-137 decay photons registers an array of pulses between 32 and 662 keV. Which events would **not** contribute to these intermediate pulse heights?
    A. Compton scattered electrons
    B. Gamma-rays that backscatter from the Pb shield

C. Single-escape peaks following pair production
    D. X-rays from ionized Pb atoms in the detector shield

26. In a NaI(Tl) scintillation detector, the distribution of pulse heights for a fixed energy deposition from Tc-99m is Gaussian. Which of the following statistical variations does **not** contribute to this spread?
    A. Variations in the number of promoted electrons from the valence to the conduction band
    B. Variations in the emitted gamma-ray energy from Tc-99m decay
    C. Variations in the numbers of scintillation photons generated
    D. Variations in the number of photoelectrons generated at the detector-PMT interface

27. A dose calibrator is used for what purpose?
    A. Comparing the efficiency of a TLD and an OSLD
    B. Assessing the relationship between channels in a multichannel analyzer and the size of energy deposition pulse heights
    C. Confirming the activity of a radiopharmaceutical prior to administration to the patient
    D. Assessing the relationship between count rates of a GM detector and radiation dose rates of a source

28. Which probability distribution is **not** relevant to binary processes (like the flip of a coin to yield heads or tails)?
    A. Gaussian or normal distribution
    B. Exponential distribution
    C. Binominal distribution
    D. Poisson distribution

29. A radioactive sample gives the following results:
    G = 1,000 counts (gross counts) in $t_G$ = 2 min
    B = 500 counts (background counts) in $t_B$ = 10 min
    What is the net count rate ($r = g - b$)?

    A. 100 cpm
    B. 250 cpm
    C. 450 cpm
    D. 500 cpm

30. A radioactive sample gives the following results:
    G = 1,000 counts (gross counts) in $t_G$ = 2 min
    B = 500 counts (background counts) in $t_B$ = 10 min
    What is the standard error of the net count rate?

    A. 16 cpm
    B. 20 cpm
    C. 30 cpm
    D. 45 cpm

# Answers

1. **C** Spectrometers are radiation detectors that are operated in pulse mode (electrical signal is generated for each detectable radiation interaction event) in which the size of the resulting voltage pulse (following proper calibration) is directly proportional to the energy deposition in the detector's sensitive volume. Under conditions in which there are no secondary radiations that escape the detector, that voltage pulse is thus a direct measure of the incident radiation particle or photon. For example, the voltage pulse will match the energy of an incident photon provided that the very last interaction of that photon is a photoelectric absorption event (possibly preceded by Compton scattering events). If, however, a Compton scatter photon leaves the detector, the voltage pulse does not measure the incident photon energy, but only the total of the energies of Compton electrons released in the detector volume. Counters (like GM detectors) provide a measure of radiation field intensity but with no energy distribution information. Dosimeters provide a measure of radiation absorbed dose, generally without information on the energies of incident radiations depositing that dose. Survey meters are a general category of detectors that are either counters or dosimeters, not spectrometers. *(Pg. 688)*

2. **D** Scintillation detectors are operated in current mode in direct digital radiography, fluoroscopy, and x-ray computed tomography. However, they are operated in pulse mode in nuclear medicine detection. *(Pg. 688)*

3. **C** In a paralyzable detector, a radiation interaction that occurs during the detector dead time after a previous interaction extends the overall detector dead time. In a nonparalyzable system, this dead time extension does not occur (subsequent interactions are simply lost). As shown in Figure 17-1, the measured count rate for a paralyzable system continues to fall with increasing interaction rate. *(Pg. 689)*

4. **C** The absolute detector efficiency is a product of two other efficiencies—the geometric efficiency (ratio of the number of photons reaching the detector to the number emitted by the source) and the intrinsic efficiency (ratio of the number of photons detected to the number reaching the detector). Thus, the absolute detector efficiency is the ratio of the number of photons detected to the number emitted by the source. *(Pg. 690)*

5. **D** The intrinsic efficiency of a photon detector is defined as the ratio of the number of detected photons relative to the number of photons reaching the detector from the source. It is primarily a function of the size of the detector relative to the incident photon direction (*e.g.*, detector thickness) and the linear attenuation coefficient $\mu$. The linear attenuation coefficient in turn is a function of the photon energy, the effective atomic number $Z$ of the detector material, and the mass density of the detector material. *(Pg. 691 and Eq. 17-3)*

6. **A** Free electrons released in the ionization of the detector counting gas are collected on a central wire running through the gas cavity. This wire is positively charged and thus called the anode. Conversely, the positively charged gas molecules are collected at the inner surface of the detector wall which is negatively charged, and thus called the cathode. *(Pg. 692 Fig. 17-4)*

7. **A** The six regions of operation of a gas-filled detector are shown in Figure 17-5. They are (1) recombination region, (2) ion saturation region, (3) proportional region, (4) region of limited proportionality, (5) GM or Geiger-Müller region, and (6) region of continuous discharge. *(Pg. 693, Fig. 17-5)*

8. **C** The six regions of operation of a gas-filled detector are shown in Figure 17-5. They are (1) recombination region, (2) ion saturation region, (3) proportional region, (4) region of limited proportionality, (5) GM or Geiger-Müller region, and (6) region of continuous discharge. *(Pg. 693, Fig. 17-5)*

9. **D** Once the photon interacts with the gas-filled detector, a fixed amount of energy is deposited which leads to a fixed number of ion pairs (free electrons and ionized gas molecules). The goal of an ion chamber is thus to collect all free electrons at the wire anode and all positive gas molecules at the cathode wall. In the ion saturation region (no. 2), the applied voltage is sufficient to accomplish full ion pair collection. With increas-

ing voltage in region no. 2, one simply collects all radiation-produced ion pairs more rapidly, but there is no gas multiplication of those ion pairs. At lower applied voltage (region no. 1), the ion pairs are collected at very low velocities such that electron-positive ion recombination is possible. The amount of recombination decreases with increasing collection efficiency driven by increasing applied voltage. *(Pg. 693–695)*

10. **D**   The energetic secondary electrons are released by photon interactions in the gas cavity (typically air for ionization chambers), and thus, many of them will escape the air cavity and cause ionization elsewhere. This problem can be partially solved by building the ion chamber with thick walls of a material whose effective atomic number is similar to that of air. In this case, the number of electrons escaping the air volume is approximately matched by a similar number of electrons released in the chamber wall that enter the air cavity. This compensating situation is called *electronic equilibrium*. *(Pg. 695)*

11. **B**   In the ion saturation region, only those ion pairs produced by the original photon energy deposition event are collected at the anode/cathode, and with increasing applied voltage, they are collected at greater velocities. At some point, however, accelerated free electrons (which are collected earlier at the wire anode than are the positive gas ion at the cathode wall) will have sufficient kinetic energy that exceeds the ionization threshold of the counting gas molecules. At that point, each originally produced electron will create a small avalanche of additional ion pairs. As the applied voltage increases within the proportional region, the number (*i.e.*, magnitude) of secondary ionization avalanches will increase. As such, each original electron will create perhaps 100, or 1,000, or even 10,000 new secondary electrons, which are collected at the wire anode. The size of the avalanche—which grows with increasing applied voltage—is called the multiplication factor. *(Pg. 695)*

12. **C**   The voltage pulse generated in a GM counter is produced by a process referred to as the GM discharge. At the applied voltages used in GM counters, each original electron from each original ion pair will cause secondary gas ionizations during their travel to the wire anode. As the excited gas molecules de-excite through the emission of characteristic x-rays, these x-rays will travel through the detector gas volume and can create new ion pairs through photoelectric absorption with either other gas molecules or with atoms along the inner surface of the GM counter wall. This process—avalanche formation, x-ray production, new avalanche formation, etc.—continues in a chain reaction fashion giving us a very large voltage pulse. The voltage pulse produced by this GM discharge is excellent for "counting" photon interactions, but the magnitude of the voltage pulse is decoupled to the original number of ion pairs produced by the incident radiation interaction event. Thus, all energy deposition information is lost. The chain reaction eventually terminates with the buildup of slowly collected positive gas molecules (space charge), which electronically screens the applied voltage and thus lowers and eventually stops further internal gas multiplication. *(Pg. 695–697)*

13. **A**   Answers B, C, and D are true statements regarding desirable characteristics of a photon scintillation detector. However, answer A is incorrect. The ideal situation would be for the conversion efficiency to be high, not low. For a given amount of energy deposition, we want to maximize the number of scintillation photons, which will then lead to a maximum number of photoelectrons entering the photomultiplier tube and finally the maximal voltage pulse for that detection event. *(Pg. 698)*

14. **D**   A primary inorganic scintillator used in computed tomography (CT) scanners is cadmium tungstate $CdWO_4$ as shown in Table 17-1, although many proprietary ceramic scintillators are now used in modern systems. *(Pg. 699–700 and Table 17-1)*

15. **B**   The primary inorganic scintillator composing the input phosphor for image-intensifier tubes used in fluoroscopy is cesium iodide sodium-activated: CsI(Na). *(Pg. 699–700 and Table 17-1)*

16. **A**   The primary inorganic scintillator used in scintillation gamma cameras for nuclear medicine imaging is sodium iodide thallium-activated: NaI(Tl). *(Pg. 699–700 and Table 17-1)*

17. **D**   As noted in Section 17.3.3, the conversion of scintillation photons to an electrical signal may be accomplished by the photomultiplier tube, the photodiode, or the multi-pixel photon counter. The latter is also called a silicon photomultiplier. *(Pg. 701–702)*

18. **B**   The distinguishing feature between the thermoluminescent dosimeter (TLD) and the optically stimulated luminescent dosimeter (OSLD) is the method by which energy is delivered to the device to release trapped electrons. Thermal energy is used in the TLD while laser light is used for the OSLD. All other features are the same—method by which radiation exposure leads to the trapping of electrons and the process by which scintillation photons are emitted following thermal heating (TLD) or laser irradiation (OSLD). Both are used for personnel dosimetry and have replaced photographic film-based dosimeters. The advantage of the OSLD

over the TLD is that laser exposure can be used to release only a fraction of the trapped electrons, thus allowing for multiple dosimetry readouts for OSLDs. *(Pg. 704)*

19. **A**  The primary inorganic scintillator used in optically stimulated luminescent dosimeters (OSLDs) is aluminum oxide carbon activated: $Al_2O_3(C)$. *(Pg. 704)*

20. **D**  The primary distinction between an insulator and a semiconductor is the size of the forbidden energy gap between the valence electron band and the conduction electron band in these two materials. The gap energy is approximately 10 eV in the insulator, while it is only approximately 1 eV in the semiconductor. Energy deposition by incident radiation thus promote an electron from the valence to conduction band more readily in the semiconductor *(Pg. 705)*

21. **B**  Silicon (Si) is a Group IV-B element (see periodic table) and has available four valence electrons, which can pair the valence electrons of four neighboring silicon atoms. To make a p-type Si-based semiconductor, a small fraction of the silicon atoms is replaced with atoms from Group III-B such as boron (B) in which there are only three valence electrons, leaving a "hole" in the location of the fourth electron to be paired with the fourth neighboring silicon atom. This "hole"—literally the absence of an electron—is effectively a location of positive charge (no electron), thus giving us a positive-type (or p-type) silicon semiconductor. The sensitive volume of a semiconductor radiation detector is located near the interface between a p-type and an n-type semiconductor. *(Pg. 704–707)*

22. **D**  Silicon (Si) is a Group IV-B element (see periodic table) and has available four valence electrons, which can pair the valence electrons of four neighboring silicon atoms. To make an n-type Si-based semiconductor, a small fraction of the silicon atoms is replaced with atoms from Group V-B such as phosphorus (P) in which there are five valence electrons, leaving an extra electron available for charge movement under the influence of an applied (or inherent) voltage. The presence of these extra electrons thus gives us a negative-type (or n-type) silicon semiconductor. The sensitive volume of a semiconductor radiation detector is located near the interface between a p-type and an n-type semiconductor. *(Pg. 704–707)*

23. **A**  The sensitive volume of a semiconductor radiation detector coincides with the depletion region located at the interface between a p-type and an n-type semiconductor. This depletion region is formed when the power supply is connected under reverse bias (positive terminal to the n-type semiconductor and negative terminal to the p-type semiconductor) *(Pg. 704–707 and Fig. 17-12)*

24. **B**  The lower-level discriminator (LLD) and upper-level discriminator (ULD) of the single-channel analyzer set the energy window of voltage pulses from photon interaction events, which will be registered as a "count." Energy deposition events below the value of the LLD and those above the value of the ULD will not be considered. The energy window is thus set at 10 keV above and below the Tc-99m gamma-ray energy of 140 keV or 130 to 150 keV. Only 3 of the 10 energy deposition events fall within that energy window. The answer is thus 3 counts. *(Pg. 708–709)*

25. **C**  Pulse heights corresponding to energies between the 32-keV x-rays and the 662-keV gamma-rays from the Ba-137m daughter or Cs-137 may be produced by partial energy deposition of the 662-keV gamma-ray (with the Compton scattered photon leaving the detector), the detection of approximately 200 keV photons created by 180° backscattering of the 662-keV gamma-rays in their Compton collisions with the surrounding Pb shield, or by K-shell Pb x-rays following Compton scattering or photoelectronic absorptions by the 662-keV gamma-rays in the surrounding Pb shield. As the energy of the gamma-ray (662 keV) is below the threshold for pair production in the detector (1.022 MeV), single or double escape peaks of annihilation photons cannot be possible. *(Pg. 711–713, Figs. 17-17 and 17-18)*

26. **B**  For 100 energy deposition events—each of 140 keV (full absorption of the Tc-99m gamma-ray)—a number of detection events must occur before a final voltage pulse is generated. For a scintillation detector of ideal energy resolution, these 100 140-keV energy deposition events would yield 100 voltage pulses of exactly the same pulse height. For this to happen, the following would also have to be exactly the same for each of the 100 events—the number of promoted electrons, the number of scintillation photons emitted during electron de-excitation, the number of scintillation photons internally scattered to the photocathode, and finally the number of photoelectrons ejected into the PMT. For each of these events in the detection signal chain, there are statistical variations and no, they are not all of the same magnitudes. Thus, even though we have 100 140-keV energy deposition events, statistical variations in these intermediate processes lead to a Gaussian shape distribution of pulse height. The mean and most probable pulse height from this distribution should indicate

(if properly energy calibrated) a value of 140-keV energy deposition. Answer B is not true—all gamma-rays emitted from a given radionuclide are unique and fixed in their energy value. Gamma-rays thus are "finger-prints" for specific radionuclides. *(Pg. 714–715)*

27. **C**   A dose calibrator is a well-geometry ion chamber filled with pressurized argon and is used to confirm the total radioactivity of a radiopharmaceutical prior to administration to the patient. *(Pg. 719–720)*

28. **B**   Binary processes may be modeled by the binomial distribution, which functionally includes $N$ as the total number of trials of the measurement, $p$ is the probability of success in a single trial, and $x$ is the number of successes. The Poisson and Gaussian distributions are approximations to the Binomial distribution that are often used when $x$ or $N$ is large. *(Pg. 725)*

29. **C**   The net count rate (r) is the difference between the gross count rate ($g = G/t_G$) and the background count rate ($b = B/tB$). Thus, $r = (1,000/2) - (500/10) = 450$ cpm (counts per minute). *(Pg. 727–730)*

30. **A**   We use the error propagation equation to report the standard error of the net count rate $\sigma_r$.

$$\text{Thus, } \sigma_r = \sqrt{\frac{G}{t_G^2} + \frac{B}{t_B^2}} = \sqrt{\frac{1000}{2^2} + \frac{500}{10^2}} = \sqrt{250 + 5} = 16 \text{ cpm} \quad \text{(Pg. 727–730)}$$

# Section III Key Equations and Symbols

| QUANTITY | EQUATION(S) | EQ NO./PAGE/COMMENTS |
|---|---|---|
| Absolute detection efficiency | $\text{Efficiency} = \dfrac{\text{Number detected}}{\text{Number emitted}}$ | Eq. 17-1/Pg. 690 |
| Absolute detection efficiency | $\text{Efficiency} = \text{Geometric efficiency} \times \text{Intrinsic efficiency}$ | Eq. 17-2/Pg. 690 |
| Intrinsic detection efficiency | $\text{Intrinsic efficiency} = 1 - e^{-\mu x} = 1 - e^{-(\mu/\rho)\rho x}$ | Eq. 17-3/Pg. 691 |
| Energy resolution | $\text{Energy resolution} = \dfrac{\text{FWHM}}{\text{Pulse amplitude at center of peak}} \times 100\%$ | Eq. 17-4/Pg. 715 |
| Mo-99 concentration test | $\text{Concentration} = K \cdot \dfrac{A_{\text{vial in container}} - A_{\text{empty container}}}{A_{\text{vial}}}$ | Eq. 17-5/Pg. 722 |
| Mean value of a set of measurements $x$ | $\bar{x} = \dfrac{x_1 + x_2 + \cdots + x_N}{N}$ | Eq. 17-6/Pg. 724 |
| The variance of a set of measurements $x$ | $\sigma^2 = \dfrac{(x_1 - \bar{x})^2 + (x_2 - \bar{x})^2 + \cdots + (x_N - \bar{x})^2}{N - 1}$ | Eq. 17-7/Pg. 724 |
| Standard deviation is the square root of the variance | $\sigma = \sqrt{\sigma^2}$ | Eq. 17-8/Pg. 724 |
| Fractional standard deviation (coefficient of variation) | $\text{Fractional standard deviation} = \sigma / \bar{x}$ | Eq. 17-9/Pg. 724 |
| Binomial distribution | $P(x) = \dfrac{N!}{x!(N-x)!} p^x (1-p)^{N-x}$ | Eq. 17-10/Pg. 725 |
| Factorial notation | $N! = N \cdot (N-1) \cdot (N-2) \cdots 3 \cdot 2 \cdot 1$ | Eq. 17-11/Pg. 725 |
| Mean and standard deviation of the binomial distribution | $\bar{x} = pN$ and $\sigma = \sqrt{pN(1-p)}$ | Eq. 17-12/Pg. 725 |
| Approximation of the standard deviation of the binomial distribution | $\sigma = \sqrt{pN(1-p)} \approx \sqrt{pN} = \sqrt{\bar{x}}$ | Eq. 17-13/Pg. 726 |
| An approximate estimate of the standard deviation of a single measurement $x$ | $\sigma \approx \sqrt{x}$ | Eq. 17-14/Pg. 727 |
| The fractional error of a single measurement $x$ | $\text{Fractional error} = \dfrac{\sigma}{x} \approx \dfrac{\sqrt{x}}{x} = \dfrac{1}{\sqrt{x}}$ | Eq. 17-15/Pg. 727 |

# Nuclear Imaging—The Gamma Camera

## 18.0 INTRODUCTION

The focus of this chapter is the underlying principles and components of the gamma camera and its use in planar single photon nuclear imaging. Clinical understanding includes that of the photon detector itself; conversion of radioactive decay parent gamma-ray (γ-ray) (or decay daughter x-ray) photon interaction into deposited energy and spatial position; collimation; imaging performance characteristics and their measurement; quality control; and incorporation of digital computers and modes of acquisition.

## 18.1 PLANAR NUCLEAR IMAGING: THE ANGER SCINTILLATION CAMERA

The gamma camera most commonly used for nuclear imaging is the so-called Anger camera, named after its inventor, Hal O. Anger. It is also called a scintillation camera, as it employs a thallium-activated sodium iodide [NaI(Tl)] crystal that converts the energy of an incoming x- or γ-ray into secondary, blue visible to ultra-violet range scintillation photons, from which energy deposited and spatial (x-y) position are obtained.

1. *Anger scintillation camera:* nuclear imager consisting of five major components (Fig. 18-1):
   a. Modern camera: a rectangular crystal, typically 0.95 cm (⅜ inch) or 1.59 cm (⅝ inch) thick, with dimensions/field-of-view (FOV) of approximately 59 cm × 44 cm/54 cm × 40 cm (21 inch × 15.5 inch).
   b. A large number (59 to 91) of 5.1-cm to 7.6-cm (2- to 3-inch) diameter photomultiplier tubes (PMTs) optically coupled to the crystal.
   c. A Lucite light pipe between the crystal's rear glass window and the PMTs, to improve the spatial uniformity of the light response function. (Some camera designs employ a so-called "digital" light pipe, where the PMTs are directly coupled to the glass window and digital circuitry performs the function of a physical light pipe.)
   d. PMT analog output signal preamplifiers.
   e. A collimator, usually made of lead, that only allows x- or γ-rays approaching from certain directions to reach the crystal.

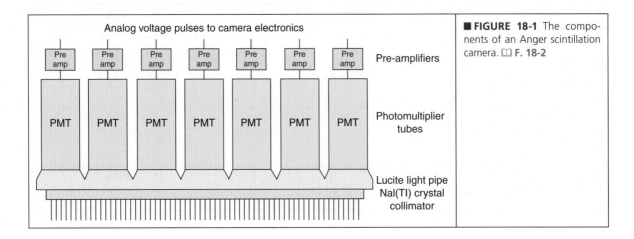

■ **FIGURE 18-1** The components of an Anger scintillation camera. 📖 **F. 18-2**

2. *Anger logic*: algorithm using circuitry that converts PMT preamplifier outputs from an incoming photon interaction to event energy and *x-y* position (Fig. 18-2). Energy is the simple sum of PMT signals, and *x* and *y* are distance-from-center weighted sums of PMT signals.

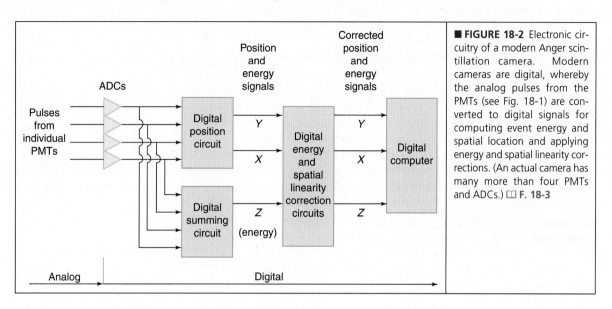

■ **FIGURE 18-2** Electronic circuitry of a modern Anger scintillation camera. Modern cameras are digital, whereby the analog pulses from the PMTs (see Fig. 18-1) are converted to digital signals for computing event energy and spatial location and applying energy and spatial linearity corrections. (An actual camera has many more than four PMTs and ADCs.) ▢ **F. 18-3**

3. *Collimator*: device that allows image formation by restricting photons reaching the detector to only those from certain directions (projection by absorption technique).
   **a.** Most collimators are constructed of lead, with tungsten as the alternative.
   **b.** Spatial resolution and sensitivity are controlled by hole diameter, length, and septal thickness.
   **c.** Septal penetration decreases with decreasing photon energy and increasing septal thickness.
   **d.** Classes of collimators (Fig. 18-3): parallel-hole (general-purpose, magnification *m* = 1); pinhole (thyroid imaging, image inverted, *m* >> 1 decreases and FOV increases with distance *d*); converging (small object imaging, *m* > 1 increases and FOV decreases with *d*); diverging (imaging of objects larger than the detector physical FOV, *m* < 1 decreases and FOV increases with *d*).

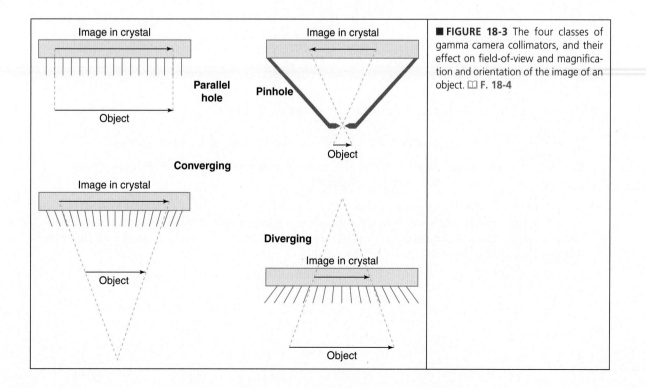

■ **FIGURE 18-3** The four classes of gamma camera collimators, and their effect on field-of-view and magnification and orientation of the image of an object. ▢ **F. 18-4**

4. *Multielement camera:* is an alternative detector design, consisting of a two-dimensional array of independently functioning small crystals (pixels); either NaI(Tl) or CsI(Tl) coupled to either position-sensitive PMTs or a matched array of photodiodes (indirect conversion to position and energy electronic signals) or CZT solid state detectors (direct conversion to position and energy).

5. *Performance:* characteristics of a gamma camera are as follows:
   **a.** Energy resolution (intrinsic detector)
   **b.** Detection efficiency (product of intrinsic photopeak and collimator geometric)
   **c.** Sensitivity (system)
   **d.** Spatial resolution (intrinsic and system including the effect of the collimator)
   **e.** Uniformity (intrinsic, and system including the effect of the collimator)
   **f.** Spatial linearity (intrinsic; Anger camera only)
   **g.** Count rate/dead-time (multielement camera maximum count rate much higher than Anger)
   **h.** Multiple-window spatial registration (for imaging $^{67}$Ga, $^{111}$In; Anger camera only)

6. *Design factors determining performance:* include choice of crystal material (NaI(Tl), CsI(Tl) or CZT) and thickness; number, shape and size of PMTs (Anger camera) or detector pixel size (multielement); collimator material (lead or tungsten), hole area $A$ (*i.e.*, shape and diameter), length ($l$) and septal thickness ($t$); energy, linearity and uniformity corrections; and analog-to-digitial signal processing conversion point (PMT output or downstream)
   **a.** Energy resolution ($^{99m}$Tc 140 keV) is approximately 6% for CZT, approximately 8% for CsI(Tl) and approximately 10% for NaI(Tl); and generally improves with increasing photon energy.
   **b.** Efficiency decreases with decreasing crystal thickness and increasing photon energy (Fig. 18-4).

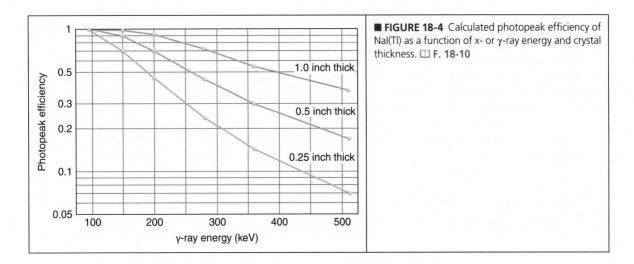

■ **FIGURE 18-4** Calculated photopeak efficiency of NaI(Tl) as a function of x- or γ-ray energy and crystal thickness. 📖 **F. 18-10**

   **c.** Geometric efficiency of a parallel-hole collimator is approximated as:

   $$E_c \approx \frac{A}{4\pi l^2} g$$ ; $A$ = hole area, $l$ = hole length, $g$ = FOV fraction not covered by septa. Increased $E_C$ = decreased spatial resolution (FWHM $\propto A/l$), and vice versa (pinhole $E_C$ decreases, converging $E_C$ increases, and diverging $E_C$ decreases, with distance).

   **d.** System resolution (FWHM) degrades with distance (Fig. 18-5), as $R'_S = \sqrt{R_C^2 + (R_I/m)^2}$. $R_I$ is intrinsic and $R'_C$ is collimator ($\approx d[l_{eff} + b]/(l_{eff}m)$; $d$ = hole diameter, $l_{eff}$ = effective hole length, $b$ = source distance). $m = 1$ (parallel-hole), $f/(f - x)$ (converging), $f/(f + x)$ (diverging), $f/y$ (pinhole); $f$ = crystal-to-focal point, $x$ = crystal-to-object, $y$ = focal point-to-object.

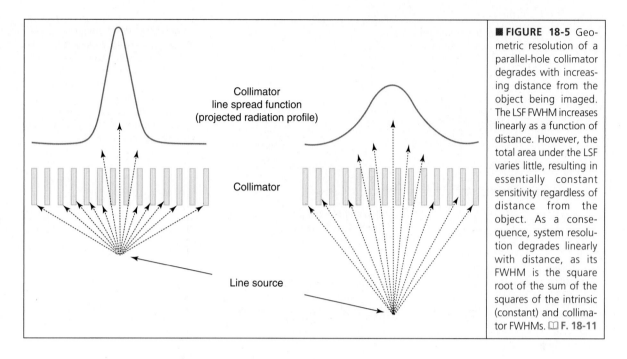

■ **FIGURE 18-5** Geometric resolution of a parallel-hole collimator degrades with increasing distance from the object being imaged. The LSF FWHM increases linearly as a function of distance. However, the total area under the LSF varies little, resulting in essentially constant sensitivity regardless of distance from the object. As a consequence, system resolution degrades linearly with distance, as its FWHM is the square root of the sum of the squares of the intrinsic (constant) and collimator FWHMs. 📖 **F. 18-11**

**e.** Uniformity variation is inherent in all gamma cameras; intrinsic due to variations in total signal output for a given energy deposition, and system due to both variations in crystal efficiency and collimator septa and imperfections. Spatial nonlinearity is inherent in an Anger camera, due to the nonlinear signal response of a PMT versus event distance from its center. Thus, energy, linearity, and uniformity corrections are required. Figure 18-6 shows example images with corrections off (top) and on (bottom). Figure 18-7 shows schematics of nonlinearity and energy corrections.

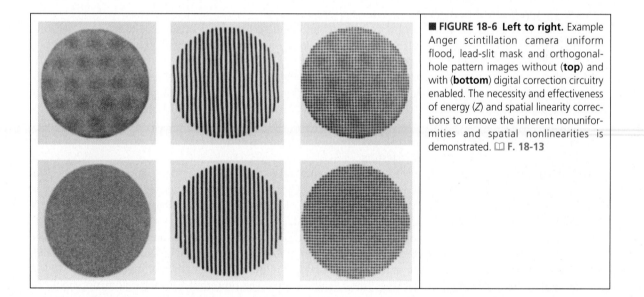

■ **FIGURE 18-6 Left to right.** Example Anger scintillation camera uniform flood, lead-slit mask and orthogonal-hole pattern images without (**top**) and with (**bottom**) digital correction circuitry enabled. The necessity and effectiveness of energy (*Z*) and spatial linearity corrections to remove the inherent nonuniformities and spatial nonlinearities is demonstrated. 📖 **F. 18-13**

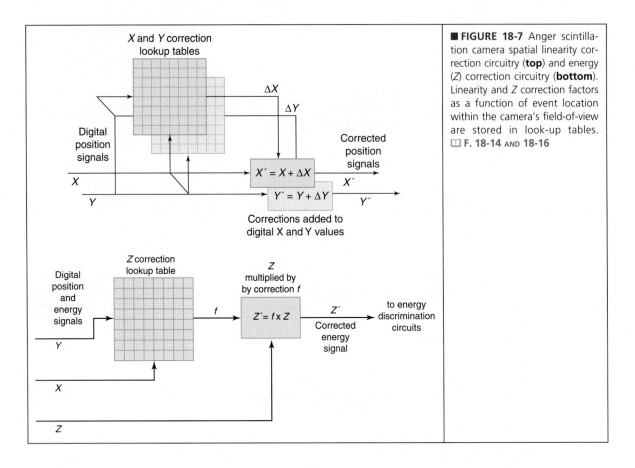

**■ FIGURE 18-7** Anger scintillation camera spatial linearity correction circuitry (**top**) and energy (Z) correction circuitry (**bottom**). Linearity and Z correction factors as a function of event location within the camera's field-of-view are stored in look-up tables. 📖 **F. 18-14** AND **18-16**

7. *Attenuation, scatter and collimator resolution*: cause a nonideal two-dimensional projection gamma camera image of a three-dimensional object.

   **a.** Attenuation reduces the number of photons reaching the detector exponentially as a function of depth in tissue ($e^{-\mu x}$, where $\mu$ = attenuation coefficient [$cm^{-1}$, decreasing with increasing photon energy, *e.g.*, $\mu_{Tl\text{-}201}$ = 0.19 and $\mu_{Tc\text{-}99m}$ = 0.15 for soft tissue] and $x$ = cm depth).

   **b.** Compton scatter photons in the patient may pass through the collimator holes and be detected, resulting in a loss of contrast and an increase in random noise. The energy window must be wide enough to capture the majority of the photopeak, a consequence of which is acceptance of narrow-angle scatter (CZT has better energy resolution than NaI(Tl), which allows a narrower energy window, and, thus, a reduced relative contribution of scatter).

8. *Gamma camera routine quality control*: consists of daily peaking and uniformity; weekly spatial resolution and linearity; and annual performance testing.

   **a.** Peaking: centering energy window(s) on the photopeak(s) of a radionuclide. Daily adjustment or check of the Tc-99m or Co-57 photopeak is performed, using a scatter-free source; other radionuclides are peaked less frequently (*e.g.*, after major calibration). Examples of centered (A, C) and shifted (B) Tc-99m 140 keV photopeaks are illustrated on the left side of Figure 18-8.

   **b.** Uniformity (daily and after repair): assessment of the response of the detector to a uniform flux of photons. A Tc-99m or Co-57 point source (intrinsic uniformity) or Co-57 planar source (system uniformity) is used. Five to fifteen million counts are obtained, and images are evaluated visually and quantitatively (NEMA analysis). The uniformity test will reveal most malfunctions. The uniformity of each collimator should be evaluated periodically. Figure 18-8 upper right shows examples of good (A) and bad (PMT failure) (B) uniformity flood images.

   **c.** Spatial resolution and spatial linearity (weekly): assessment of the ability of the camera to visualize small objects with correct spatial positioning (not applicable to a multielement camera). A four-quadrant bar phantom is typically used, imaged with four 90-degree rotations (alternating 180-degree horizontal and vertical flips) over every 4 weeks, to evaluate all quadrants of the camera equally. Since the bars are manufactured straight, spatial linearity is assessed at the same time. If system resolution is assessed, the same collimation is used every week. A Co-57 sheet source system resolution image of a bar pattern is shown on the lower right of Figure 18-8.

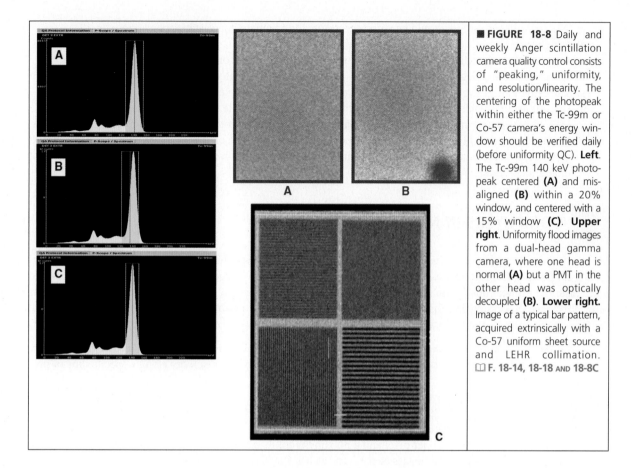

**■ FIGURE  18-8** Daily and weekly Anger scintillation camera quality control consists of "peaking," uniformity, and resolution/linearity. The centering of the photopeak within either the Tc-99m or Co-57 camera's energy window should be verified daily (before uniformity QC). **Left**. The Tc-99m 140 keV photopeak centered **(A)** and misaligned **(B)** within a 20% window, and centered with a 15% window **(C)**. **Upper right**. Uniformity flood images from a dual-head gamma camera, where one head is normal **(A)** but a PMT in the other head was optically decoupled **(B)**. **Lower right.** Image of a typical bar pattern, acquired extrinsically with a Co-57 uniform sheet source and LEHR collimation. ▢ F. 18-14, 18-18 AND 18-8C

d. Efficiency of each camera head should be measured periodically, by calculating the count rate per unit activity from the recorded number of counts and duration of an acquired image of a source of known activity in a consistent geometry.

e. Annual performance evaluation of each camera should be conducted, which includes peaking (all radionuclides imaged); uniformity; efficiency; spatial resolution; multienergy spatial registration (Anger cameras only); energy resolution; and count-rate performance. Relevant tests should also be performed after each repair or adjustment.

f. Acceptance testing of new cameras should be performed by an experienced medical physicist, to ensure the camera's performance meets the purchase specifications prior to first clinical use and establish baseline values for routine quality control testing.

9. *Computers, whole body scanning, and SPECT*:
   a. A digital computer is now used on all gamma cameras to
      (i)   Acquire, process and display digital images
      (ii)  Control camera head movement
   b. Many large FOV gamma cameras can perform whole-body scanning:
      (i)   Some older systems: The camera moves past a stationary patient table (less floor space required).
      (ii)  Modern systems: The table and patient move past a stationary camera.
      (iii) The position of the camera head relative to the patient table is sensed.
      (iv)  Values specifying the camera-relative-to-table position are added to *X-Y* position signals.
      (v)   Older cameras (round or hexagonal crystal): two passes, one over each half of the patient.
      (vi)  Modern rectangular-head: a single pass over entirety of all but extremely obese patients (considerable time savings, superior image statistics).
   c. Many modern gamma cameras are capable of single-photon emission computed tomography:
      (i)   The heads rotate automatically around the patient.
      (ii)  Planar images (projections) are acquired at regular angular increments over 180° or 360°.
      (iii) A computer mathematically manipulates projection images to produce cross-sectional images.

10. *Obtaining high-quality images*:
   a. A sufficient total number of counts must be acquired, so image quantum mottle does not mask lesions.
   b. Imaging times must be as long as possible, consistent with patient throughput and minimizing intra-scan patient motion.

   c. Whole-body scan speed should be sufficiently slow for adequate image statistics.
   d. A higher resolution collimator may improve spatial resolution.
   e. A narrower energy window to reduce scatter may improve image contrast.
   f. Spatial resolution degrades as collimator-to-patient distance increases.
   g. The camera head should always be as close to the patient as possible.
   h. Discourage thick pillow and mattress on table usage for under-table image acquisition.
   i. Patient motion and metal objects worn by patients or in patients' clothing are common sources of artifacts. Metal objects should be identified and removed from the patient or the FOV. The technologist should remain in the room during imaging to minimize patient motion; for safety, a patient should never be left unattended under a moving camera.

## 18.2    COMPUTERS IN NUCLEAR IMAGING

Modern nuclear medicine computer systems consist of commercially available computers with hardware and software added for acquisition, processing, and display of gamma camera images. Two computers may be provided with a gamma camera, one for image acquisition and formation and camera control in the camera itself, and the other for image processing and display; otherwise, a single computer performs both functions. Modern gamma cameras output pairs of digital X- and Y-position signals to the acquisition computer for digital image formation.

1. *Digital image formats in gamma camera imaging*: consist of square or rectangular arrays of numbers, where each element, or pixel, represents the number of counts accumulated from activity along a specific line of projection through the patient.
   a. Gamma cameras have relatively low spatial resolution.
   b. Low-resolution $64^2$ and $128^2$ pixel formats are common, and $256^2$ is occasionally used.
   c. Whole-body images are stored as 256 by 1,024 pixels, reflecting the rectangular scan FOV.
   d. Byte mode: one byte (8 bits) per pixel and a maximum count value of 255; word mode: two bytes (16 bits) and 65,535, respectively. All images in modern nuclear medicine computers are word mode.
2. *Image acquisition*: in nuclear medicine is either frame-mode or list-mode.
   Frame-mode acquisition is illustrated in Figure 18-9. Computer memory is reserved for the image; and it is formed from many pairs of position signals, each increasing a pixel value by one.

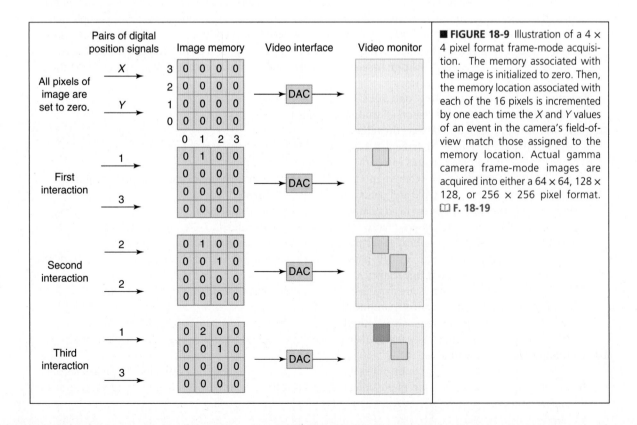

■ **FIGURE 18-9** Illustration of a 4 × 4 pixel format frame-mode acquisition. The memory associated with the image is initialized to zero. Then, the memory location associated with each of the 16 pixels is incremented by one each time the X and Y values of an event in the camera's field-of-view match those assigned to the memory location. Actual gamma camera frame-mode images are acquired into either a 64 × 64, 128 × 128, or 256 × 256 pixel format. 📖 **F. 18-19**

a. **Static:** a single image is acquired for a preset duration or preset number of total counts (*e.g.*, bone spot view, thyroid uptake).

b. **Dynamic:** a sequential acquisition of a series of images for a preset time per image (*e.g.*, kidney flow and excretion, gastric emptying).

c. **Gated:** a repetitive, cyclic acquisition of a set of images, each cycle triggered by an ECG QRS complex pulse (myocardial perfusion or blood pool cardiac mechanical function). Figure 18-10 depicts gated acquisition. Computer memory is reserved for 8 to 24 images. Then,

   **(i)** An average time per cardiac cycle *T* is determined from a sampling of cardiac (R wave-to-R wave) cycles (*e.g.*, 10).

   **(ii)** The time *t* per image is calculated as *T* divided by the number of gated frames.

   **(iii)** When a trigger pulse is received, counts are added to the first image for a time *t*, then the second image for a time *t*, and so on, until the next trigger pulse, when the process restarts at the first image.

   **(iv)** Acquisition continues for a preset duration (*e.g.*, 10 min), which results in a statistically valid depiction of an average cardiac cycle.

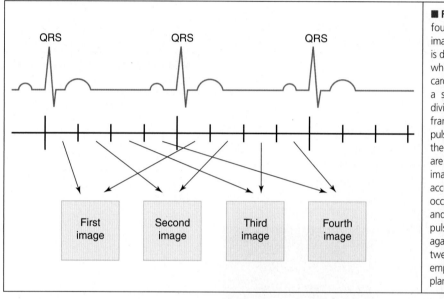

■ **FIGURE 18-10** Illustration of a four-frame gated cardiac planar image acquisition. The cardiac cycle is divided into four equal time bins, where the bin width is an average cardiac (R-to-R) cycle time based on a sampling of cycles (*e.g.*, 10), divided by the number of gated frames. Next, whenever a trigger pulse is generated from detection of the ECG QRS complex, event data are accumulated in the first gated image for a time interval T. Then, accumulation in the second image occurs for the same time interval, and so on. When the next trigger pulse occurs, the cycle starts over again at the first image. Sixteen to twenty-four frames are typically employed for actual gated cardiac planar acquisition. ▭ **F. 18-20**

List-mode acquisition stores position pairs in a list along with periodic timing marks (and trigger marks if gated), as opposed to being immediately added to an image in memory; the data are retrospectively formatted into conventional images for display and processing (Fig. 18-11). List-mode allows flexibility in forming images from the entire set of position pairs. However, large amounts of data are generated, requiring more memory and disk space than frame-mode; the data must be postprocessed to provide images for viewing and processing.

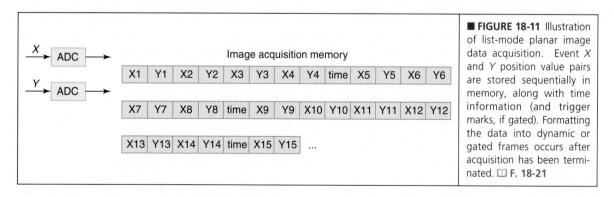

■ **FIGURE 18-11** Illustration of list-mode planar image data acquisition. Event *X* and *Y* position value pairs are stored sequentially in memory, along with time information (and trigger marks, if gated). Formatting the data into dynamic or gated frames occurs after acquisition has been terminated. ▭ **F. 18-21**

3. ***Image processing in nuclear medicine:*** consists of a wide variety of image and region of interest manipulations and analyses. Examples of common image processing are as follows:

   a. **Image subtraction:** Pixel-by-pixel count differences are computed, with negatives set to zero, depicting the change in activity between acquired images (*e.g.*, gated blood pool stroke volume image = end diastolic (ED) image − end systolic (ES) image).

**b.** Region of interest (ROI) and time-activity curve (TAC): An ROI is a closed boundary, drawn manually or automatically, superimposed on an image, within which the sum of pixel counts indicates the activity in a particular region of the patient. A TAC for a dynamic study is created from the total counts in each dynamic image within an ROI drawn on one image of the sequence. The ROI counts versus image number are plotted, indicating the activity in a particular region of the patient as a function of time.

**c.** Spatial filtering: Smoothing (a type of convolution filtering) is applied to reduce quantum mottle present in nuclear medicine images, due to the statistical nature of the acquisition process, at a cost of degraded spatial resolution. The amount of smoothing is a compromise between noise reduction and preservation of clinically significant detail.

**d.** Left ventricular ejection fraction (LVEF): It is a measure of the mechanical performance of the heart, defined as the fraction of end diastolic (ED) volume ($V$) ejected per cardiac cycle ($[V_{ED} - V_{ES}]/V_{ED}$). Nuclear medicine LVEF is commonly derived from a left anterior oblique gated blood pool planar acquisition, based on the assumption that the total number of counts within the LV is directly proportional to LV volume, and is computed from the total number of counts within manually or automatically drawn ED image and ES image ROIs, after subtraction of background computed from average counts in a ROI adjacent to the LV at ES. A volume curve, usually interpolated from ED and ES ROI TACs, depicting LV volume change over the cardiac cycle, is also generated. A typical LVEF display is shown in Figure 18-12.

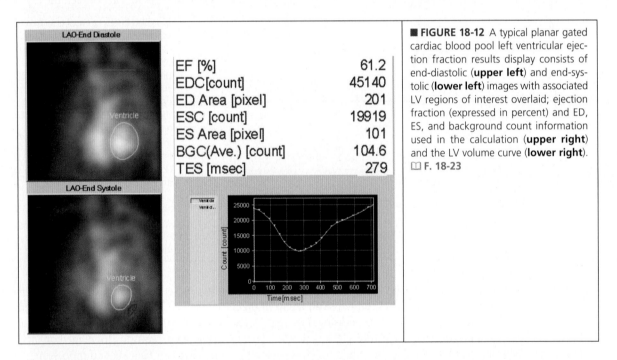

■ **FIGURE 18-12** A typical planar gated cardiac blood pool left ventricular ejection fraction results display consists of end-diastolic (**upper left**) and end-systolic (**lower left**) images with associated LV regions of interest overlaid; ejection fraction (expressed in percent) and ED, ES, and background count information used in the calculation (**upper right**) and the LV volume curve (**lower right**). 📖 F. 18-23

**e.** Other quantitative nuclear medicine imaging studies: Examples are (1) regional lung ventilation (Xe-133, Tc-99m DTPA aerosol or Tc-99m pertechnetate superheated gas)/Tc-99m MAA perfusion (V/Q) mismatch; (2) radioiodine or Tc-99m pertechnetate thyroid uptake; (3) gastric emptying (Tc-99m sulfur colloid solid, Tc-99m or In-111 DTPA liquid); and (4) Tc-99m HIDA with CCK stimulation gall bladder ejection fraction.

# Section II Questions and Answers

1. The location of an interaction in the NaI(Tl) crystal of a scintillation camera is determined by the:
   A. sum of pulses from PMTs
   B. total amount of light emitted in the crystal
   C. relative magnitudes of pulses from PMTs
   D. use of a single channel analyser
   E. use of a multichannel analyzer

2. How does increasing the crystal thickness of a gamma camera affect its performance?
   A. It improves spatial resolution and efficiency.
   B. It degrades spatial resolution and improves efficiency.
   C. It improves spatial resolution and reduces efficiency.
   D. It degrades spatial resolution and reduces efficiency.
   E. It improves efficiency, but has no effect on spatial resolution.

3. For what is the energy (Z) signal produced in a gamma camera primarily used?
   A. Initiation of image acquisition
   B. Specifying position of an interaction in the crystal
   C. Termination of image acquisition
   D. Rejection of interaction energies substantially different from emitted photon energies
   E. Determination of appropriate projection angle during reconstruction

4. A gamma camera reduces the effects of scatter by using:
   A. a collimator to intercept most scattered x- and γ-rays
   B. energy (pulse height) discrimination
   C. an air gap between the patient and camera head
   D. fast electronic circuits
   E. a rotating camera head

5. What electronic devices are used to transform Anger camera PMT event pulses into numeric values for input to position and energy correction circuitry?
   A. Analog-to-digital converters
   B. Amplifiers
   C. Logic circuits
   D. Pre-amplifiers

6. Which component of an Anger camera alters the optical photon response in order to improve spatial linearity and uniformity?
   A. Collimator
   B. PMT cathode coating material
   C. Thallium-doping of the sodium-iodide crystal
   D. Matched index of refraction between the crystal and glass cover
   E. Light pipe and spatially varying light absorbers

7. What is the single most significant factor limiting the quality of gamma camera images?
   A. speed of the camera's electronics
   B. design compromise between intrinsic efficiency and intrinsic spatial resolution
   C. design compromise between collimator efficiency and collimator resolution
   D. number of photomultiplier tubes
   E. crystal thickness

8. The energy resolution at 140 keV is best for which of the following crystals?
   A. bismuth germinate (BGO)
   B. cadmium-zinc-telluride (CZT)
   C. thallium-doped cesium-iodide (CsI(Tl))
   D. thallium-doped sodium-iodide (NaI(Tl))
   E. lutetium orthosilicate (LSO)

9. The collimator type that produces an inverted projection image is a:
   A. pinhole
   B. converging
   C. parallel-hole
   D. diverging
   E. fan-beam

10. When a source is moved away from a parallel-hole collimator:
    A. sensitivity increases and spatial resolution improves
    B. sensitivity decreases and spatial resolution worsens
    C. sensitivity is constant and spatial resolution is constant
    D. sensitivity decreases and spatial resolution is constant
    E. sensitivity is constant and spatial resolution worsens

11. The collimator type that allows imaging of an object that is larger than the field-of-view of the gamma camera is a:
    A. pinhole
    B. converging
    C. parallel-hole
    D. diverging
    E. fan-beam

12. Which of the following statements regarding collimator septal penetration is true?
    A. Septal penetration increases with decreasing photon energy and increasing septal thickness.
    B. Septal penetration decreases with decreasing photon energy and decreasing septal thickness.
    C. Septal penetration increases with increasing photon energy and decreasing septal thickness.
    D. Septal penetration decreases with increasing photon energy and increasing septal thickness.

13. A performance characteristic that is not associated with a multielement gamma camera is:
    A. spatial resolution
    B. C and E
    C. spatial linearity
    D. uniformity
    E. multiple-window spatial registration

14. Which of the following statements regarding parallel-hole collimator geometric efficiency, $E_c$, is false?
    A. $E_c$ is inversely proportional to hole length.
    B. $E_c$ is inversely proportional to hole length squared.
    C. $E_c$ is proportional to hole area.
    D. $E_c$ is proportional to fraction of collimator FOV not covered by septa.
    E. $E_c$ is proportional to septal thickness.

15. The system resolution (FWHM) of a gamma camera with parallel-hole collimation is calculated as the:
    A. sum of the squares of intrinsic and collimator resolutions
    B. sum of intrinsic and collimator resolutions
    C. square-root of the sum of the squares of intrinsic and collimator resolutions
    D. square-root of the sum of the intrinsic and collimator resolutions
    E. square-root of square of intrinsic resolution plus collimator resolution

16. The intrinsic resolution of a multielement gamma camera is best described by which of the following functions in one dimension?
    A. Gaussian
    B. Sine
    C. Sinc
    D. Rectangle
    E. Poisson

17. Which of the following will increase the relative contribution of Compton scatter from a patient in a gamma camera photopeak image?
    A. Decrease in patient thickness
    B. Increase in collimator septal thickness
    C. Shift in the energy window to the low side
    D. Shift in the energy window to the high side
    E. Decrease in energy window width

18. How often should a check of the centering of the photopeak within a gamma camera's energy window for $^{99m}$Tc (or $^{57}$Co as a surrogate) be performed as part of quality control?
    A. Daily
    B. Weekly
    C. Monthly
    D. Quarterly
    E. Annually

19. Gamma camera characteristics typically included in an annual performance evaluation are all of the following except:
    A. energy resolution
    B. spatial resolution
    C. uniformity
    D. system sensitivity
    E. spatial linearity

20. Daily extrinsic uniformity quality control is not useful for detecting:
    A. collimator damage
    B. invalid correction map
    C. PMT gain drift
    D. spatial nonlinearity
    E. PMT failure

21. The collimator that is best suited for weekly bar pattern resolution quality control is:
    A. high-energy (HE)
    B. low-energy high-resolution (LEHR)
    C. converging
    D. medium-energy (ME)
    E. low-energy high-sensitivity (LEHS)

22. What is not required for thorough and consistent weekly evaluation of gamma camera system resolution and linearity with a four-quadrant bar pattern?
    A. Using a pattern with the same bar widths
    B. Acquiring the same number of counts
    C. using the same collimator
    D. Using the same $^{57}$Co sheet source
    E. Week by week alternating horizontal and vertical bar pattern flips

23. Which of the following is not a function performed by a digital computer connected to a modern gamma camera?
    A. Detector energy and linearity corrections
    B. Camera motion control
    C. Image acquisition
    D. Image processing
    E. Image display

24. All of the following are true regarding whole body scanning with a modern dual-detector, large FOV gamma camera except:
    A. the entire patient may be scanned in a single pass
    B. camera-relative-to-table axial location value is added to detector event Y position signals
    C. the camera moves past a stationary table
    D. the position of the camera head relative to the patient table is sensed
    E. sensors are used to minimize detector-to-patient distance, improving resolution

25. The planar gamma camera scanning technique associated with sequential acquisition of a series of images for a preset time per image is:
    A. gated
    B. whole body
    C. dynamic
    D. static
    E. SPECT

26. An important factor in obtaining high-quality gamma camera images is:
    A. increasing whole body scan speed
    B. reducing image acquisition time
    C. widening the photopeak energy window
    D. using high-sensitivity collimation
    E. minimizing detector-to-patient distance

27. Which digital image matrix is never used in gamma camera imaging?
    A. $64^2$
    B. $512^2$
    C. $128^2$
    D. $256^2$
    E. $256 \times 1024$

28. Acquisition that consists of a repetitive, cyclic collection of counts into a fixed number of images is:
    A. list-mode
    B. dynamic
    C. whole body
    D. static
    E. gated

29. Retrospective formatting of acquired gamma camera x-y position pairs into conventional images of different matrix sizes and durations is allowed by:
    A. list-mode acquisition
    B. dynamic acquisition
    C. whole body acquisition
    D. static acquisition
    E. gated acquisition

30. Which of the following is not an example of nuclear medicine image processing?
    A. List-mode reframing
    B. Left ventricular ejection fraction
    C. Image subtraction
    D. Region of interest and time-activity curve generation
    E. Spatial filtering

# Answers

1. **C** The pulses produced by photomultiplier tubes (PMTs) near the interaction in the crystal are larger than those from PMTs further away. The position logic circuit of the scintillation camera determines the centroid (middlemost point) of the light distribution from the relative amplitudes of the pulses from the PMTs. *(Pg. 735)*

2. **B** Increasing the thickness of the crystal of a gamma camera increases the intrinsic efficiency but degrades its spatial resolution (just as increasing the thickness of a radiographic intensifying screen increases its efficiency but degrades spatial resolution). A thicker crystal absorbs more of the incident x- and γ-rays but permits more spreading of the light before it reaches the PMTs. *(Pg. 746)*

3. **D** An interaction in the crystal does not become a count in the image unless the energy discrimination circuits (pulse height analyzers) of a gamma camera accept the interaction. They accept the interaction only when the energy (Z) signal is within the selected energy window or windows. Energy discrimination reduces the fraction of counts in the image due to scattered photons, because scattered photons are of lower energy than unscattered photons. Most coincident events (two or more interactions happening at almost the same time) produce Z signals that are above the energy window and are also rejected. *(Pg. 735)*

4. **B** Energy (pulse height) discrimination. The collimator rejects about the same fractions of primary and scattered photons. A gap between the patient and camera face merely degrades spatial resolution without reducing the scatter fraction. In pulse height discrimination, interactions whose deposited energies are outside an energy window are rejected. Scattered photons have lower energies than primary photons and, thus, pulse height discrimination of the sum of all the PMT outputs can reject much of the scatter. *(Pg. 738)*

5. **A** The electronic pulse from a PMT is an analog signal. Analog-to-digital converters either directly digitally sample and integrate a PMT's pre-amplifier pulse or convert the pulse height after shaping by an amplifier circuit to a digital value, for further processing by digital acquisition hardware and software. *(Pg. 734)*

6. **E** A Lucite light pipe along with spatially varying light absorbers is one means of improving Anger camera spatial linearity and uniformity, by altering the light distribution between PMTs as a function of event position. Modern Anger cameras employ digital correction circuitry to perform this function. *(Pg. 752)*

7. **C** Almost any modification to a collimator to improve its spatial resolution reduces its efficiency, and vice versa. (The efficiency of a collimator is the fraction of emitted photons that pass through the collimator.) *(Pg. 736)*

8. **B** A distinct advantage of the solid-state crystal cadmium-zinc-telluride (CZT) for imaging Tc-99m is its superior (~6%) energy resolution compared to either CsI(Tl) (~8%) or NaI(Tl) (~10%). However, CZT is limited to low-energy x- or γ-ray imaging, due to cost and performance constraints on crystal thickness. The energy resolutions of BGO and LSO are unacceptably poor at 140 keV (due to their relatively low light output compared to NaI(Tl)), which limits their use to 511 keV PET imaging. *(Pg. 740)*

9. **A** A pinhole collimator functions identically to the pinhole of a pinhole photographic camera, where the image of an object is magnified and inverted in both the horizontal and vertical directions. *(Pg. 736)*

10. **E** Gamma camera system sensitivity (total FOV count rate per unit of activity) is essentially constant with respect to source distance from a parallel-hole collimator; whereas, spatial resolution worsens (FWHM increases) with increasing source-to-collimator distance. *(Pg. 746)*

11. **D** The holes of a diverging collimator focus to a point in back of the gamma camera detector, and, thus, diverge outward from the detector, resulting in an object FOV that is larger than the camera's FOV, and minification of an imaged object in both the horizontal and vertical directions, that increases with distance from the collimator. *(Pg. 736)*

12. **C** The transmitted, or penetrating, fraction of x- or γ-rays incident on a material decreases exponentially with depth ($e^{-\mu x}$). A material's attenuation coefficient (μ) decreases, and thus penetration fraction increases, with increasing energy; and the penetration fraction at a given energy increases with decreasing thickness ($x$). *(Pg. 748)*

13. **B** Multielement gamma cameras are pixelated and are, therefore, not susceptible to the effects of nonlinearity and multiple-energy window misregistration associated with the Anger logic event spatial positioning that is employed by conventional PMT-based scintillation cameras. *(Pg. 750)*

14. **E** The geometric efficiency of a parallel-hole collimator is approximated by the equation $E_c \approx \dfrac{A}{4\pi l^2}g$, where $A$ = hole area, $l$ = hole length, and $g$ = FOV fraction not covered by septa, which is inversely proportional to septal thickness, $t$; therefore, $E_C$ is also inversely proportional to $t$. *(Pg. 747)*

15. **C** Both intrinsic and collimator resolution ($R_I$ and $R_C$) of a gamma camera are modeled as Gaussian functions, whose FWHMs add in quadrature. The combined system resolution ($R_S$) is calculated according to the equation $R_S^2 = R_I^2 + R_C^2$. *(Pg. 741)*

16. **D** The intrinsic resolution of a multielement gamma camera is, by definition, its detector element dimensions, as there is no signal sharing between the element in which an incoming photon interacts and other elements. A multielement detector consists of a two-dimensional array of square elements (or pixels); thus, the spatial resolution of each in any direction is equivalent to a rectangle function. *(Pg. 739)*

17. **C** Compton scatter photons from a patient have lower energy than primary photons and, thus, would be detected predominantly below the peak within a centered energy window. A shift in the window to the low side increases Compton scatter photon collection, while decreasing primary photon collection, which is symmetric around the peak, resulting in an increase in the relative contribution of Compton scatter in an image of a patient. *(Pg. 753)*

18. **A** Peaking of $^{99m}$Tc, the primary radionuclide imaged with a gamma camera (or $^{57}$Co as a surrogate) should be performed on each day of use, with a scatter-free source and prior to scanning patients. Peaking of all radionuclides imaged must be performed at acceptance, and afterward at least annually and after any detector major repair or replacement. *(Pg. 753)*

19. **E** Various Anger camera performance characteristics should be tested on an annual basis, including energy (peaking of all radionuclides imaged, and energy resolution); uniformity (intrinsic and system); counting (sensitivity, and maximum count rate or dead time); system spatial resolution; and multiple-window spatial registration (Anger cameras only). The spatial linearity of the bars in an image of a resolution pattern is assessed visually on a weekly basis. *(Pg. 755)*

20. **D** A daily gamma camera image of a uniform flood source can detect a number of different detector problems, including gain drift or failure of a PMT; a correction map that is no longer valid due to a change in a detector's overall response; and damage to a collimator. However, a uniformity quality control image will only be able to detect severe spatial nonlinearity. A weekly bar pattern image will reveal any significant amount of spatial nonlinearity, as the bars are, but would not appear, straight. *(Pg. 755)*

21. **B** Bar patterns consist of bars with widths typically less than 5 mm and are designed primarily for evaluating intrinsic spatial resolution. However, the system resolution at the face of LEHR collimators is sufficient for visualizing one or more sets of such bars with high contrast. LEHS collimators emphasize geometric efficiency and not resolution, and therefore, bar widths less than 5 mm will not be visualized with high contrast. Bar pattern images for both ME and HE collimators will contain aliasing and other artifacts, due to poor geometric resolution, thick septa, and hexagonal holes. Imaging of bar patterns is not applicable to converging collimators, due to geometric distortion. *(Pg. 742)*

22. **D** Optimum and consistent weekly system resolution and linearity quality control using a four-quadrant bar pattern requires that the bar widths, collimator, and a statistically sufficient total number of acquired counts be kept constant; and allowing each quadrant of the detector to image each of the four quadrant's bar widths every 4 weeks. The use of the identical $^{57}$Co sheet source each week is not a pre-requisite, as it only affects the duration of the acquisition, and $^{57}$Co sources must be replaced periodically due to radioactive decay. *(Pg. 742)*

23. **A** On a modern gamma camera, aside from detector corrections such as energy and linearity, that are applied on an event-by-event basis in firmware within the detector itself, all other operations, including image acquisition, processing, display, and motion, are controlled by a connected digital computer. *(Pg. 755)*

24. **C**   All modern dual-detector, large FOV gamma cameras can perform whole body scanning (although systems may be purchased without that feature). The entirety of all but extremely obese patients may be scanned in a single pass; the patient's contour may be tracked to minimize detector-to-patient distance, improving resolution. Sensing the axial position of the heads relative to table and adding the corresponding position value to each event's $Y$ position signal from the detector are required, in order to form the image. The table moves past a stationary camera, which although requiring more floor space, is safer than having an entire gamma camera moving past a stationary table. *(Pg. 756)*

25. **C**   Gamma camera planar image acquisition modes are static (termination by time or total counts); dynamic (sequential acquisition at a preset time per image); gated (ECG-triggered cyclic acquisition of a series of images); and whole body (preset length and scan speed). SPECT is a technique whereby the detectors rotate around the patient at a fixed time per image, in order to reconstruct a stack of three-dimensional image of an assumed static distribution of activity. *(Pg. 758)*

26. **E**   Sufficient resolution and acquired counts are both keys to obtaining high-quality gamma camera images. Image acquisition time reduction or whole body scan speed increase to reduce motion artifacts is limited by the need to collect enough counts for acceptable quantum mottle. Widening the photopeak energy window increases counting efficiency but increases acceptance of scatter that negatively affects contrast. High-sensitivity collimation increases counting efficiency, but at the expense of spatial resolution. Minimizing detector-to-patient distance maximizes spatial resolution with no penalty in counting efficiency. *(Pg. 756)*

27. **B**   Gamma camera image spatial resolution is low, and quantum mottle is high, relative to all other diagnostic imaging modalities. Therefore, formatting acquired counts into a large digital matrix with a very small pixel size, such as $512^2$, is of no benefit. Aside from the special case of $256 \times 1024$ for whole body scan mode, gamma camera images are predominantly $64^2$ or $128^2$, and occasionally $256^2$. *(Pg. 757)*

28. **E**   Gated acquisition mode is employed for evaluating cardiac mechanical function (ejection fraction and wall motion), where each acquisition cycle is triggered by the patient's ECG QRS complex, and counts are added to the first gated frame for a time $t$, then the second for a time $t$, etc., until the next trigger restarts acquisition at the first frame. After a preset total acquisition time, the result is a depiction of an average cardiac cycle. *(Pg. 758)*

29. **A**   Static, dynamic, gated and whole body are frame-mode acquisitions, where counts are placed on-the-fly into fixed digital matrices in reserved computer memory. List-mode stores acquired count data as a list of $x$-$y$ position pairs along with timing marks (and possibly gated trigger marks), which can be retrospectively formatted into conventional images of various durations and matrix sizes, but at the expense of more disk space usage than frame-mode. *(Pg. 759)*

30. **A**   Nuclear medicine image processing tasks utilizing computers, such as subtraction, regions of interest definition, time-activity curve generation, spatial filtering, and quantitative analysis (*e.g.*, LVEF), are performed on conventional digital-matrix images. List-mode reframing is not considered image processing, as it is merely a method of formatting acquired list-mode data into conventional images for possible later processing. *(Pg. 759)*

# Section III Key Equations and Symbols

| QUANTITY | EQUATION | EQ#/ PAGE/COMMENTS |
|---|---|---|
| System spatial resolution FWHM—parallel-hole collimator | $R_{\mathrm{s}} = \sqrt{R_{\mathrm{C}}^2 + R_{\mathrm{I}}^2}$ | Eq. 18-1; Pg. 741. System LSF FWHM (see Fig. 18-7) is computed as the square-root of the sum of the squares of collimator FWHM, $R_c$, and detector intrinsic FWHM, $R_\mathrm{I}$. $R_c$ increases with distance (see Fig. 18-11). |
| System spatial resolution FWHM—non-parallel-hole collimator | $R_{\mathrm{s}}' = \sqrt{R_{\mathrm{C}}'^2 + \left(R_{\mathrm{I}}/m\right)^2}$ | Eq. 18-2; Pg. 741. $R_c'$ is $R_C/m$, where $m$ is a magnification factor specific to the class of collimator. |
| Spatial resolution FWHM estimated from a bar pattern | $R_{\mathrm{s}} \approx 1.7 \times$ (size smallest bars resolved) | Eq. 18-3; Pg. 742. FWHM approximation technique based on visual assessment of a bar pattern. |
| System efficiency | $E_{\mathrm{s}} = E_{\mathrm{c}} \times E_{\mathrm{i}} \times f$ | Eq. 18-4; Pg. 743. Three factors affect overall efficiency: collimator efficiency, $E_c$, intrinsic efficiency, $E_i$, and photopeak fraction, $f$. |
| Intrinsic efficiency | $E_{\mathrm{i}} = 1 - e^{-\mu x}$ | Eq. 18-5; Pg. 744. Intrinsic efficiency depends upon photon energy attenuation coefficient, $\mu$, and crystal thickness, $x$. |
| Photopeak efficiency | $E_{\mathrm{p}} = E_{\mathrm{i}} \times f$ | Eq. 18-6; Pg. 744. Photopeak efficiency depends on both intrinsic efficiency, $E_i$, and the fraction of interactions within the energy window, $f$ (see fig. 18-10). |
| Parallel-hole collimator geometric efficiency | $E_{\mathrm{c}} \approx \dfrac{A}{4\pi l^2} g$ | Eq. 18-7; Pg. 747. Neglecting septal penetration. Collimator geometric efficiency depends upon hole area, $A$, and length, $l$, and fraction not blocked by septa, $g$. |
| Pinhole collimator spatial resolution along its central axis | $R_{\mathrm{c}}' \approx d\dfrac{f + x}{f}$ | Eq. 18-8; Pg. 747. Approximate pinhole FWHM, corrected for collimator magnification, depends upon pinhole diameter, $d$, crystal-to-pinhole distance, $f$, and pinhole-to-object distance, $x$. |
| Pinhole collimator efficiency along its central axis | $E_{\mathrm{c}} = d^2/16x^2$ | Eq. 18-9; Pg. 747. Neglecting penetration around the pinhole, pinhole collimator efficiency depends upon pinhole diameter, $d$, and pinhole-to-object distance, $x$. |
| Example of calculated system resolution at collimator face | $R_{\mathrm{s}} = \sqrt{\left(1.5\,\mathrm{mm}\right)^2 + \left(4.0\,\mathrm{mm}\right)^2} = 4.3\,\mathrm{mm}$ at 0 cm | Eq. 18-10a; Pg. 748. For one manufacturer's LEHR collimator with 1.5 mm FWHM at 0 cm, and 4.0 mm intrinsic FWHM. |

*(Continued)*

*(Continued)*

| QUANTITY | EQUATION | EQ#/ PAGE/COMMENTS |
|---|---|---|
| Example of calculated system resolution at 10 cm from collimator face | $R_s = \sqrt{(6.4\ \text{mm})^2 + (4.0\ \text{mm})^2} = 7.5\ \text{mm at 10 cm}$ | Eq. 18-10b; Pg. 749. For one manufacturer's LEHR collimator with 6.4 mm FWHM at 10 cm, and 4.0 mm intrinsic FWHM. |
| Left ventricular ejection fraction | $\text{LVEF} = (V_{ED} - V_{ES})/V_{ED}$ | Eq. 18-11; Pg. 760. LVEF is defined as the fraction of the end-diastolic volume, $V_{ED}$, ejected per beat, equal to the ratio of $V_{ED}$ – end-systolic volume, $V_{ES}$, to $V_{ED}$. |
| Equilibrium-gated blood pool LVEF ROI crosstalk counts | $\text{Counts crosstalk} = \dfrac{\dfrac{(\text{Counts in crosstalk ROI})}{(\text{Pixels in LV ROI})}}{(\text{Pixels in crosstalk ROI})}$ | Eq. 18-12; Pg. 761. Counts crosstalk in a LV ROI, commonly called background, is computed by scaling total counts in a background ROI by the ratio of pixel areas of the LV and background ROIs. |
| Equilibrium-gated blood pool LVEF calculation | $\text{LVEF} = \dfrac{(\text{Counts ED} - \text{Counts crosstalk ED}) - (\text{Counts ES} - \text{Counts crosstalk ES})}{(\text{Counts ED} - \text{Counts crosstalk ED})}$ | Eq. 18-13; Pg. 762. LVEF is computed as the difference between ED and ES ROI counts divided by ED ROI counts, each corrected for background. |

| SYMBOL | QUANTITY | UNITS |
|---|---|---|
| $R_I$ | Intrinsic resolution full width at half-maximum (FWHM) | mm |
| $R_C$ | Collimator resolution FWHM | mm |
| $R_S$ | System (also called extrinsic) resolution FWHM | mm |
| $E_i$ | Intrinsic efficiency | NA |
| $E_c$ | Collimator efficiency | NA |
| $E_s$ | System efficiency (sensitivity) | NA |
| $\mu$ | Linear attenuation coefficient | $\text{cm}^{-1}$ |
| $f$ | Intrinsic photopeak fraction | NA |
| $A$ | Collimator hole cross-sectional area | $\text{mm}^2$ |
| $l$ | Collimator hole length | mm |
| $g$ | Fraction of collimator area not blocked by septa (total area of holes/total area) | NA |
| $d$ | Diameter of pinhole collimator | mm |
| $f$ | Distance from crystal to pinhole | mm |
| $x$ | Distance from pinhole to object | mm |
| LVEF | Left ventricular ejection fraction | % |
| $V_{ED}$ | End-diastolic volume of the ventricle | ml |

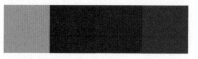

# Nuclear Tomographic Imaging— Single Photon and Positron Emission Tomography (SPECT and PET)

## 19.0 INTRODUCTION

The focus of this chapter is SPECT and PET imaging. Specifically, the chapter covers the principles of operation, image acquisition and reconstruction, data corrections, performance, and quality control for both of these nuclear tomographic imaging modalities. The chapter also covers dual modality imaging (SPECT/CT, PET/CT, and PET/MR) and other recent developments in SPECT and PET imaging. A section on PET image quantification and detrimental factors affecting the quantitative accuracy is also included. Finally, the chapter concludes with a comparison of these two imaging modalities.

## 19.1 FOCAL PLANE TOMOGRAPHY IN NUCLEAR MEDICINE

1. *Focal plane tomography* was the dominant nuclear medicine (NM) tomographic technique prior to the development of SPECT. Many such devices were developed:
    a. Rectilinear scanner with focused collimators.
    b. Anger tomoscanner (two opposed small cameras, converging collimators, raster scanning, multiple coronal whole-body tomographic images).
    c. Anger camera with a seven-pinhole collimator (cardiac short-axis images).
    d. Planar gamma camera imaging is weakly tomographic.
        (i) Spatial resolution degrades with distance (closer structures sharper).
        (ii) Photon attenuation increases with depth (closer structures more visible).

## 19.2 SINGLE-PHOTON EMISSION COMPUTED TOMOGRAPHY

1. *SPECT* is a rotational NM tomographic technique, invented in the early 1960s, but did not become routine until the 1980s. Examples of SPECT scanners are shown in Figure 19-1.
    a. Planar gamma camera images are acquired over 180° (cardiac) or 360° around the patient.
    b. Transverse images are formed by filtered backprojection (FBP) or iterative reconstruction.

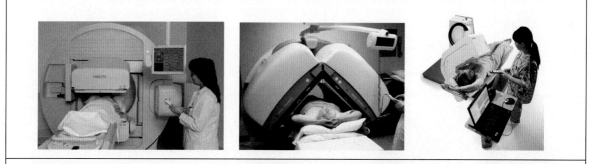

■ **FIGURE 19-1 Left to Right.** Examples of patient positioning for 180° configuration body and 90° configuration cardiac SPECT scans on a large field-of-view dual-head camera and on a dedicated cardiac dual-head camera.

2. *Image acquisition* consists of one or more SPECT camera heads revolving about the patient, and acquiring projections (Fig. 19-2):
   a. Continuous mode: images acquired over angular intervals as the head moves continuously
   b. "Step-and-shoot" mode: images acquired when the head stops at evenly spaced angles
   c. Pixel format usually $64^2$ or $128^2$, but large enough to not degrade resolution due to pixel size
   d. Zoom factor typically approximately 1.5 for $64^2$ cardiac, to reduce pixel size and, thus, improve resolution
   e. Typically, 60–64 ($64^2$) or 120–128 ($128^2$) projections, to reduce reconstruction streak artifacts
   f. Circular orbit: brain imaging (on systems with a small camera head physical edge-to-useful field-of-view edge distance or on systems with a head holder beyond the patient table; resulting in higher resolution compared to body imaging, due to a small radius within the patient's shoulders)
   g. Noncircular ("body contouring") orbit (NCO): body imaging (for a circular orbit, camera heads would be many centimeter from the body surface for anterior and posterior projections, resulting in a loss of spatial resolution). NCO manually specified on some older systems, but automatically determined on modern systems.

Ideally, a 180° arc of projections would be sufficient for reconstruction, as opposed projections would be mirror images. However, due to a large amount of attenuation of photons from activity in the half of the patient opposite the camera head and spatial resolution degradation with distance, projections over a complete revolution (360°) about the patient are required. An exception is cardiac SPECT, where a 180° arc symmetric about the heart, from right anterior oblique to left posterior oblique, is employed. Artifacts can be introduced, but resolution and contrast improve, as projections opposite the heart have poorer resolution and contrast due to greater distance and attenuation than those on the same side as the heart.

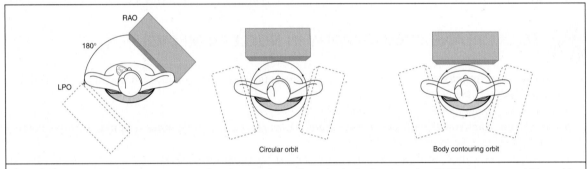

Circular orbit                    Body contouring orbit

■ **FIGURE 19-2 Left to Right.** Illustration of cardiac, circular, and noncircular body-contouring SPECT detector acquisition orbits. 📖 **F. 19-2 AND 19-3**

3. *Transverse image reconstruction*: is performed using either FBP or an iterative algorithm, after uniformity and center-of-rotation correction of projection images.
   Filtered backprojection reconstruction (Fig. 19-3):
   a. Projection images are mathematically filtered.

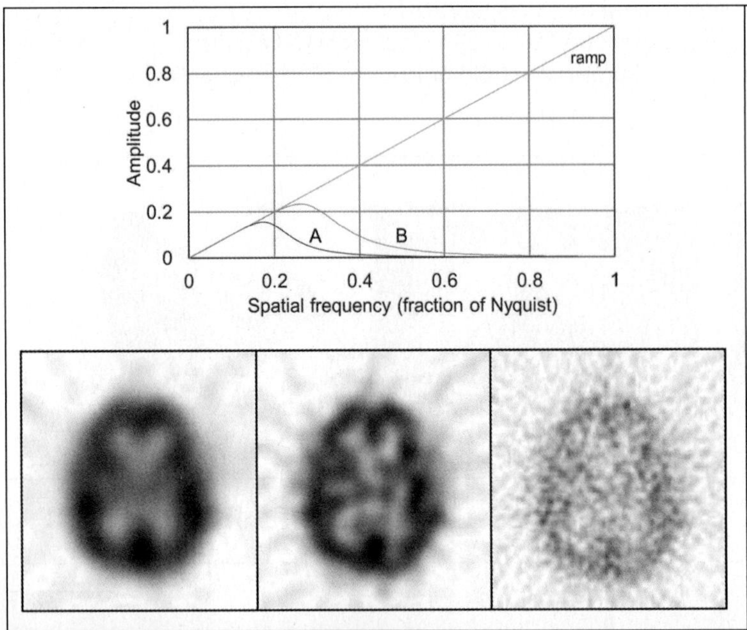

■ **FIGURE 19-3** Illustration of the effect of low-pass filter choice on SPECT filtered backprojection resolution and noise. **Top.** Frequency domain plots of backprojection ideal ramp times low-pass filter kernels. Kernel *A* is a ramp times 0.20 Nyquist critical frequency (amplitude 0.5), fifth-order Butterworth; and *B* is a ramp times 0.30, fifth-order Butterworth. The ideal 1.0 Nyquist cut-off frequency ramp filter with no low-pass filtering is also shown. A lower critical or cut-off frequency results in improved signal-to-noise, but at the expense of resolution. **Bottom.** Tc-99m-HMPAO brain perfusion SPECT slice reconstructed with (*left* to *right*) filter kernels *A*, *B*, and *ramp*. 📖 **F. 19-4 AND 19-5**

**b.** Each transverse slice is formed by backprojection of the corresponding row of projections.

**c.** The theoretical ideal kernel is a ramp filter in the spatial frequency domain.

**d.** Projections contain substantial statistical noise (radioactive decay process, low pixel counts).

**e.** High frequencies in the spatial frequency domain are dominated by statistical noise.

**f.** Gamma camera resolution reduces higher spatial frequency information of imaged structures, increasingly with distance.

**g.** Ideal ramp FBP results in unacceptable noise in transverse slices.

**h.** Projections are smoothed by ramp filter "roll-off" at higher spatial frequencies.

**i.** Filter kernel "roll-off" reduces noise at the expense of spatial resolution.

**j.** Filter kernel selection is a compromise between resolution and noise.

**k.** Different kernels are employed for different SPECT studies, based on the spatial resolution (due to collimator and detector-to-imaged organ distance) and amount of statistical noise (due to amount of activity injected, collimator and acquisition time per projection).

**l.** A filter with a higher spatial frequency cutoff is required for projections of better spatial resolution and less quantum mottle, to avoid unnecessary reconstruction resolution loss.

**m.** A filter with a lower spatial frequency cutoff is required for projections of poorer spatial resolution and greater quantum mottle, to avoid excessive reconstructed quantum mottle.

Iterative reconstruction (Fig. 19-4):

**a.** Filtered backprojection is computationally efficient but assumes perfect projection images of a three-dimensional object, which is not true, due to photon attenuation by the patient, the inclusion of Compton scatter, and collimator resolution degradation with distance.

**b.** The initial activity distribution assumption is uniform or the result of simple backprojection.

**c.** Projection images of the initial distribution are then calculated and compared to the actual (acquired) projection images.

**d.** The activity distribution is adjusted based upon the projection image comparison.

**e.** Distribution projection, projection comparison, and distribution adjustment are repeated until the calculated projection images are approximately equal to the actual projection images.

**f.** Projection calculation can incorporate and thus compensate for
 
  **(i)** Decreasing system resolution point spread function with distance from the camera
  
  **(ii)** Effects of attenuation using a map of attenuation coefficients ($\mu$) in the patient
  
  **(iii)** A model of photon scattering
  
   **a)** Modified PSF
   
   **b)** Secondary energy window images (dual- or triple-energy window), or
   
   **c)** Photopeak transverse images and attenuation and material density maps (effective scatter source estimation)

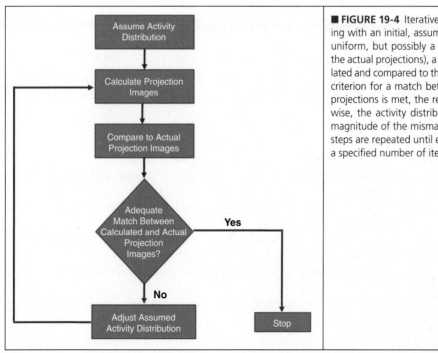

■ **FIGURE 19-4** Iterative reconstruction flowchart. Starting with an initial, assumed activity distribution (typically uniform, but possibly a ramp filtered backprojection of the actual projections), a set of projection images is calculated and compared to the actual projection images. If the criterion for a match between the calculated and actual projections is met, the reconstruction terminates. Otherwise, the activity distribution adjustment based on the magnitude of the mismatch, projection, and comparison steps are repeated until either the criterion is met or until a specified number of iterations is reached. ▢ **F. 19-6**

g. Reconstructed images can be of either higher quality than FBP images or equivalent quality with less administered activity or reduced scan time.

h. Iterative reconstruction is computationally less efficient than FBP, but feasible due to increasing computer speed, the small SPECT matrix sizes, and computationally efficient algorithms such as ordered subset expectation maximization.

i. Three-dimensional spatial filtering is usually applied afterward, due to substantial noise in images reconstructed from projections with relatively poor counting statistics.

4. *Attenuation correction in SPECT*: Radioactivity whose photons traverse long paths through the patient produces fewer projection image counts than activity near the patient surface. This is exhibited as a gradual decrease in activity toward the center of reconstructed images of a uniform cylinder of radioactivity (Fig. 19-5, **left**). Many methods have been developed for attenuation correction (AC):

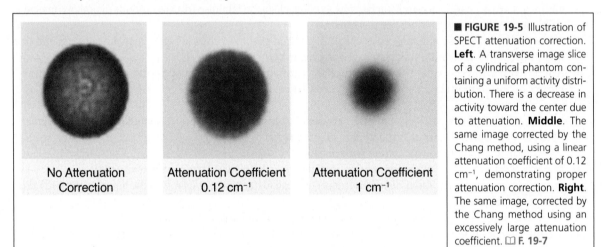

No Attenuation Correction

Attenuation Coefficient 0.12 cm⁻¹

Attenuation Coefficient 1 cm⁻¹

■ **FIGURE 19-5** Illustration of SPECT attenuation correction. **Left**. A transverse image slice of a cylindrical phantom containing a uniform activity distribution. There is a decrease in activity toward the center due to attenuation. **Middle**. The same image corrected by the Chang method, using a linear attenuation coefficient of 0.12 cm⁻¹, demonstrating proper attenuation correction. **Right**. The same image, corrected by the Chang method using an excessively large attenuation coefficient. 📖 **F. 19-7**

a. The Chang approximation method for FBP assumes a constant $\mu$ value; may be used for brain and abdominal studies where $\mu$ is relatively constant; cannot attenuation correct thorax studies, where $\mu$ is highly variable; and should be verified (including $\mu$ value) with a phantom before clinical use (Fig. 19-5, **middle and right**).

b. Sealed radioactive sources (commonly Gd-153, which emits 97- and 103-keV $\gamma$-rays) to measure attenuation were added by several SPECT camera manufacturers in the 1990s:

   **(i)** Transmission projection images were acquired and reconstructed to generate transverse $\mu$ maps similar to x-ray CT images.

   **(ii)** The $\mu$ maps were then used for iterative reconstruction AC.

   **(iii)** Several transmission-sealed source configurations were developed.

      **a)** Scanning collimated line used with parallel-hole collimators

      **b)** Arrays of fixed line used with parallel-hole collimators (cardiac only)

      **c)** A fixed line located at the focal point of a fan-beam collimator

   **(iv)** Transmission data were usually acquired simultaneously with emission data (performing the two separately posed significant transmission-emission data spatial alignment problems and greatly increased total imaging time).

   **(v)** The transmission radionuclide was one with primary $\gamma$-ray emissions significantly lower in energy than those of the radiopharmaceutical.

   **(vi)** Separate transmission and emission photon energy window images were acquired.

   **(vii)** Scattering of higher energy emission photons in the patient and detector produced cross-talk in the lower energy transmission window.

c. Hybrid SPECT/CT scanners, where x-ray CT image data can be used for radionuclide emission data AC, have supplanted radioactive transmission sources.

d. Extensive studies of radioactive source- and x-ray CT-based myocardial perfusion SPECT AC have demonstrated a reduction in attenuation artifacts and improved diagnostic performance.

e. Other studies have shown that emission data and $\mu$ map spatial misalignment can cause AC artifacts in myocardial perfusion SPECT images.

f. A period of transition is needed to retrain even experienced clinicians to interpret attenuation-corrected myocardial perfusion SPECT images.

5. *Generation of coronal, sagittal, and oblique images*:
   a. Coronal and sagittal slices are commonly generated by simple reordering of the pixels from the transverse slices.
   b. Oblique images parallel (vertical and horizontal long-axis images) and perpendicular (short-axis images) to the long axis of the left ventricle are standard for cardiac SPECT.
   c. Due to considerable anatomic variation among patients, the long axis of the heart must be determined before the computer can create the oblique images.
   d. The long axis is commonly defined manually by a technologist, although the software on most systems is now capable of correct automatic reorientation, with operator verification and override.
6. *Collimators for SPECT* are most commonly parallel-hole. Fan-beam collimators (converging and parallel-hole in the x- and y-directions, respectively, Fig. 19-6 **left**), which have better spatial resolution and efficiency, but a smaller transaxial FOV, than parallel-hole, have been designed for brain SPECT (FOV truncation artifacts would occur if used for body SPECT). A variable focal length converging collimator for cardiac imaging has been developed, where the focal length increases from the center outward, ending up parallel-hole at the edge. A heart-centric orbit is employed to achieve an approximately fourfold increase in sensitivity (Fig. 19-6 **right**).

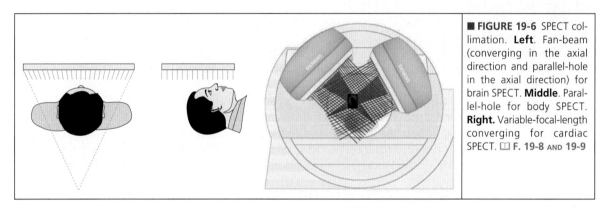

■ **FIGURE 19-6** SPECT collimation. **Left**. Fan-beam (converging in the axial direction and parallel-hole in the axial direction) for brain SPECT. **Middle**. Parallel-hole for body SPECT. **Right**. Variable-focal-length converging for cardiac SPECT. 📖 F. **19-8** AND **19-9**

7. *Multihead SPECT cameras* have been developed to reduce the limitations imposed on SPECT by collimation and limited time per view, and permit the use of higher resolution collimators than a single-head system for a given level of quantum mottle. Severe requirements upon the electrical and mechanical stability of the camera heads are imposed (*X* and *Y* offsets and *X* and *Y* magnification factors of all heads must be precisely matched throughout the rotation about the patient.), but current multihead systems are very stable and provide high-quality tomographic images. Configurations (Fig. 19-1) are
   a. Double-head, 180° opposed heads: head and body SPECT, whole-body (WB) planar
   b. Triple-head, fixed-angle: head and body SPECT, but limited crystal width (no WB planar)
   c. Double-head, variable-angle: head and body SPECT and WB planar (180° opposed), and cardiac SPECT (90° perpendicular)
8. *Multielement detector SPECT cameras* that employ a multitude of small or curved detectors and alternative scanning techniques are now commercially available. For example:
   a. Veriton general purpose (Spectrum Dynamics Medical, Fig. 19-7 **left**)
      (i) Twelve detectors equally spaced over 360° around the patient
      (ii) Detector: 16 (*x*) × 128 (*y*) 6-mm-thick CZT crystals; 2.46 × 2.46 mm elements

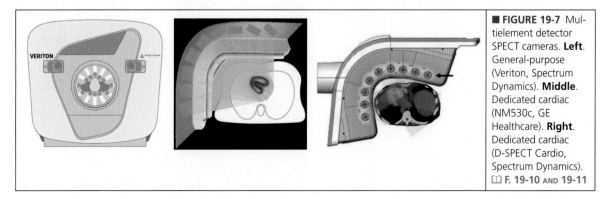

■ **FIGURE 19-7** Multielement detector SPECT cameras. **Left**. General-purpose (Veriton, Spectrum Dynamics). **Middle**. Dedicated cardiac (NM530c, GE Healthcare). **Right**. Dedicated cardiac (D-SPECT Cardio, Spectrum Dynamics). 📖 F. **19-10** AND **19-11**

(iii) Integrated parallel-hole tungsten collimator

(iv) Each (31.5 cm axial) SPECT FOV scan: a combination of detector swivel, rotation, and auto-contouring

(v) Volume sensitivity approximately 3 times that of a dual-head NaI(Tl)/LEHR SPECT camera

(vi) 40 to 220 keV energy range

b. NM530c dedicated cardiac (GE Healthcare, Fig. 19-7 **middle**)

(i) Nine 8 × 8 cm, 5-mm-thick CZT crystals; 2.46 × 2.46 mm elements

(ii) Equally spaced along a stationary L-shaped gantry

(iii) Detector orientations and pinhole collimation allows all views to be acquired simultaneously without detector motion

(iv) Counting efficiency approximately 5 times that of a conventional NaI(Tl)/LEHR SPECT camera

c. D-SPECT Cardio dedicated cardiac (Spectrum Dynamics Medical, Fig. 19-7 **right**)

(i) Nine 4 × 16 cm, 6-mm-thick CZT crystals, 2.46 × 2.46 mm elements

(ii) Parallel-hole tungsten collimation and an L-shaped gantry

(iii) Scanning of the heart achieved by translation and swivel of each detector

(iv) Approximately 8 times the sensitivity of a conventional NaI(Tl)/LEHR SPECT camera

d. CardiArc dedicated cardiac (CardiArc Inc.)

(i) Three adjacent curved NaI(Tl) crystals and an array of photomultiplier tubes

(ii) "Slit-hole" scanning

(iii) One stationary series of lead sheets with horizontal gaps

(iv) A second curved lead sheet with six vertical slits rotates back and forth in electronic synchrony with six corresponding regions of the crystals

(v) Sensitivity gain of approximately 4 compared to a conventional NaI(Tl)/LEHR SPECT camera

9. **SPECT spatial resolution** depends upon a number of factors, including the radionuclide, collimation, radius of rotation, orbit (circular or body-contouring), and reconstruction filter. Brain SPECT resolution is better than that for body SPECT, due to a smaller orbit radius. SPECT resolution can be measured by acquiring and reconstructing a line source, such as a capillary tube, placed along the axis of rotation, for which NEMA has developed a protocol (Fig. 19-8):

a. A 22-cm diameter, cylindrical plastic water-filled phantom.

b. Three Co-57 solid or Tc-99m liquid line inserts (one on the central axis, two offset by 7.5 cm).

c. A 15-cm radius circular orbit, 360° acquisition; and ramp FBP (a "roll-off" reduces resolution).

d. Typical reconstructed FWHMs (LEHR collimator) are 9.5 to 12 mm (central), 7 to 8 mm (tangential), and 9.4 to 12 mm (radial).

NEMA resolution, while a useful index, does not depict clinical resolution. Patient studies may involve larger radii of rotation, shorter acquisition times, and possibly a higher-efficiency, lower-resolution collimation than the NEMA protocol; and a ramp filter "roll-off" to reduce noise, which introduces more blurring (larger FWHM). Furthermore, the NEMA protocol is not applicable to iterative reconstruction with resolution, attenuation, and scatter compensations.

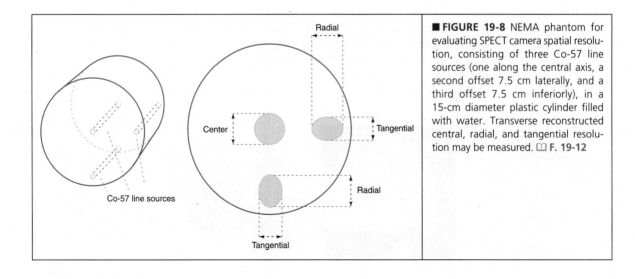

**■ FIGURE 19-8** NEMA phantom for evaluating SPECT camera spatial resolution, consisting of three Co-57 line sources (one along the central axis, a second offset 7.5 cm laterally, and a third offset 7.5 cm inferiorly), in a 15-cm diameter plastic cylinder filled with water. Transverse reconstructed central, radial, and tangential resolution may be measured. 📖 **F. 19-12**

10. ***Comparison of SPECT to conventional planar gamma camera imaging:*** SPECT resolution should be equivalent to that of planar, but FBP clinical resolution is typically slightly worse. The camera may be placed closer to the patient when acquiring a planar image, clinical FBP SPECT requires smoothing for noise reduction and obtaining a sufficient number of SPECT counts may require lower-resolution collimation than for planar. However, iterative reconstruction SPECT with system resolution compensation can result in better resolution than planar. The main advantage of SPECT is the removal of overlapping structures of nonuniform activity, leading to improved contrast and reduced structural noise. Iterative reconstruction can partially compensate for patient scatter, collimator spatial resolution decrease versus distance and septal penetration, and patient photon attenuation using maps from radioactive source or x-ray CT.

11. ***Quality control in SPECT*** is critical to identify malfunctions or maladjustments that can result in a loss of resolution and significant artifacts that may mimic pathology. Following acceptance testing by a medical physicist, a QC program should be established that ensures system SPECT performance remains comparable to that at acceptance.

    a. *X* and *Y* magnification factors (gains) relate distances in the object to numbers of pixels in the acquired image, determined by imaging two point sources a known distance apart, along a line parallel to the camera's *X* and *Y* axes:

    $$X_{mag} (\text{or } Y_{mag}) = \frac{\text{actual distance between centers of points sources}}{\text{number of pixels between centers of point sources}}$$

    and should be equal to one another, as well as between detectors of a multihead system, to prevent projection, coronal, sagittal, and oblique image distortion.

    b. Multienergy spatial registration is important in SPECT for both imaging radionuclides which emit photons of more than one energy (*e.g.*, In-111, Ga-67), and for uniformity and axis-of-rotation (AOR) corrections determined with one radionuclide to be valid for others. Gain and multienergy registration errors are not applicable to multielement cameras, as detector elements are square and the number of element rows and columns is fixed.

    c. Center-of-rotation (COR) calibration aligns projection images to the AOR (an imaginary line about which the SPECT camera revolves).

    **(i)** Misalignment may be mechanical (*e.g.*, camera head not centered in the gantry), electronic, or a digital setting.

    **(ii)** Misalignment may be constant or vary versus camera head angle, and may vary along the AOR.

    **(iii)** Four other possible misalignments are axial tilt, detector-to-detector axial shift, yoke swivel, and axial swivel with respect to the AOR.

    **(iv)** If small, a loss of resolution will result, but if large enough, a reconstructed point or line source will appear as a "doughnut" (Fig. 19-9, **first three images left to right**).

    **(v)** COR alignment is assessed by acquiring SPECT projection images of one or more point sources, or a line source (placed along the AOR) and analyzing them with the SPECT system's computer.

    **(vi)** COR misalignment is corrected by shifting each clinical projection image in the *x*-direction by the proper number of pixels prior to reconstruction.

    **(vii)** When a line source or multiple points are used for calibration, a unique correction can be derived and applied for each transverse slice.

    **(viii)** If misalignment varies with camera head angle, it can only be corrected if angle-by-angle correction is permitted by the system's computer.

    **(ix)** Separate COR corrections are required for different collimators and dual-head configurations (*e.g.*, 180° and 90°) and, on some systems, for different camera zoom factors and image formats (*e.g.*, $64^2$ versus $128^2$).

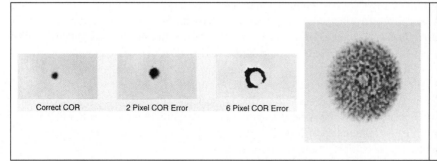

Correct COR    2 Pixel COR Error    6 Pixel COR Error

■ **FIGURE 19-9** Illustration of the effect of SPECT projection acquisition center-of-rotation (COR) misalignment (left) and image nonuniformity (right) on reconstructed image quality. Small COR errors result in a loss of spatial resolution, whereas larger errors result in "tiny doughnut" artifacts. Significant nonuniformities result in ring artifacts. ▭ **F. 19-13** AND **19-14**

**d.** Uniformity of a camera head is important, and more so for SPECT versus planar imaging.

  **(i)**   Slight nonuniformities in projection images are magnified by reconstruction.

  **(ii)**  Nonuniformities appear as rings centered about the AOR (Fig. 19-9, **far right image**).

  **(iii)** Partial rings appear when multihead SPECT projections are not acquired by all heads over a 360° arc.

  **(iv)**  Ring artifacts are most apparent in high count density studies, such as liver scans, but may be most harmful in studies such as myocardial perfusion with poor counting statistics and large variations in count density, where they may be misinterpreted as physiologic variations.

  **(v)**   Modern gamma cameras have digital circuits for energy and linearity correction but not for local nonuniformity due to, for example, collimator dents or manufacturing defects.

  **(vi)**  Minor local nonuniformities are corrected by acquiring a very high count uniform flood image (at least 30 million counts for a $64^2$ pixel format and 120 million for $128^2$) and computing each pixel correction factor as the ratio of the average pixel count in the image to the count in that pixel. Projection images are uniformity-corrected before COR correction and reconstruction.

  **(vii)** Uniformity correction images for each camera head and collimator are typically updated weekly to monthly, and for some cameras, separate intrinsic correction images for each radionuclide are also required.

  **(viii)** Uniformity correction effectiveness can be assessed by inspecting for ring artifacts, the transverse slices of a SPECT scan of a uniform cylinder, or SPECT performance phantom filled with Tc-99m in solution but is limited to the parts of the detector containing the projected image of the phantom.

**e.** Camera head tilt causes a loss of reconstructed spatial resolution and contrast (less toward the center and greatest toward the edge), as out-of-slice activity will be backprojected into each transverse slice (Fig. 19-10), as the camera head is assumed to be aligned with the AOR (exactly parallel for most collimators).

  **(i)**   Head tilt may be tested with a bubble level on a camera head with a flat surface parallel to the collimator face.

  **(ii)**  Some older cameras require manual head tilt adjustment; on others, it is automatic.

  **(iii)** Head tilt accuracy should be periodically tested, with either a bubble level, or (better) by a SPECT acquisition of a point source in the camera FOV, centered in the axial ($y$) direction, but near the edge in the transverse ($x$) direction. The position of the point source will vary in the $y$ direction from image to image, visualized in a cine of the projection images if there is head tilt.

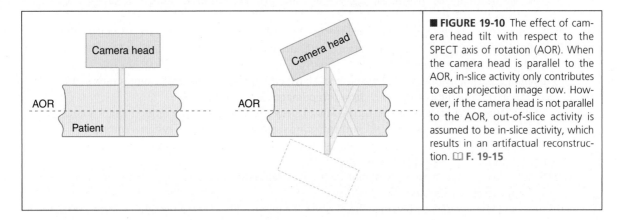

■ **FIGURE 19-10** The effect of camera head tilt with respect to the SPECT axis of rotation (AOR). When the camera head is parallel to the AOR, in-slice activity only contributes to each projection image row. However, if the camera head is not parallel to the AOR, out-of-slice activity is assumed to be in-slice activity, which results in an artifactual reconstruction. 📖 F. 19-15

**12.** *SPECT quality control phantoms* fillable with Tc-99m or other radionuclide solutions are commercially available (*e.g.*, Jaszczak ACR SPECT phantom). Resolution, contrast, and uniformity (although only over a relatively small portion of the SPECT FOV) can be semiquantitatively assessed and are used for system acceptance testing and then periodic (*e.g.*, quarterly) testing.

**13.** *Dual modality imaging—SPECT/X-ray CT systems* incorporate two camera heads capable of planar imaging and SPECT and an x-ray CT system, and a common patient bed; some have an x-ray CT system for attenuation coefficient (mu) map generation and image coregistration only, whereas others can produce diagnostic quality CT images. The advantages and disadvantages are the same as those for PET/CT.

**a.** Advantages:

  **(i)**   Acquisition is much faster than radioactive sealed source CT acquisition.

  **(ii)**  Attenuation information has less statistical noise than that for sealed source CT.

  **(iii)** Nonuniform attenuation in myocardial perfusion imaging, particularly by the diaphragm and, in women, the breasts, can cause apparent perfusion defects. X-ray CT-based AC has been reported to improve diagnostic accuracy by compensating for these artifacts.

**b.** Disadvantages:
   **(i)** γ-Ray energy linear attenuation coefficient must be estimated from CT HU number.
   **(ii)** Artifacts can occur due to incorrect an incorrect mu values or high atomic number material (*e.g.*, metal objects and concentrated contrast material).
   **(iii)** SPECT and x-ray CT information are not acquired simultaneously, and interscan organ motion can result in SPECT-CT misregistration and, therefore, SPECT artifacts.
   **(iv)** SPECT x-ray CT heart misregistration can cause myocardial perfusion artifacts.
SPECT/CT is supplanting SPECT-only imaging, as it has become mainstream and systems have proliferated. SPECT/CT does require the additional QC step of SPECT and CT alignment verification in every clinical examination for optimum visual and quantitative accuracy.

## 19.3 POSITRON EMISSION TOMOGRAPHY

PET generates images depicting the distribution of positron-emitting nuclides in patients. Nearly, all PET systems today are coupled to x-ray CT systems to create what is referred to as a PET/CT scanner (Fig. 19-11).

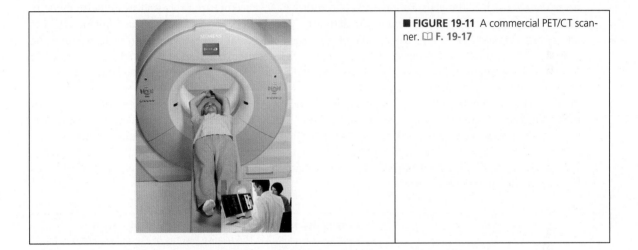

■ **FIGURE 19-11** A commercial PET/CT scanner. □ **F. 19-17**

1. *Design and principles of operation:* In a typical PET system, several rings of detectors surround the patient. PET scanners use annihilation coincidence detection (ACD) instead of collimation to obtain projections of the activity distribution in the subject. The PET system's computer then reconstructs the transverse images from the projection data, as does the computer of an x-ray CT or SPECT system. Modern PET scanners are multislice devices, permitting the simultaneous acquisition of many transverse images over a preset axial distance.
   **a.** *Annihilation Coincidence Detection:* Positron emission results in two 511-keV photons that are emitted in nearly opposite directions (Fig. 19-12). If both photons from an annihilation are detected in the scanner at nearly the same time, a process called ACD, then the line in space connecting the locations of the two interactions, which is known as a line of response (LOR), establishes the trajectories of the detected photons.

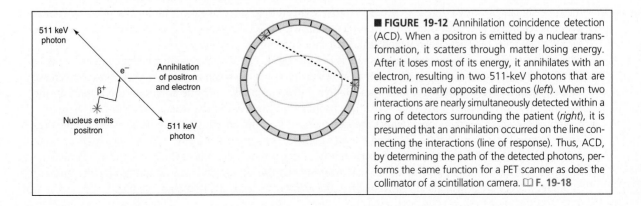

■ **FIGURE 19-12** Annihilation coincidence detection (ACD). When a positron is emitted by a nuclear transformation, it scatters through matter losing energy. After it loses most of its energy, it annihilates with an electron, resulting in two 511-keV photons that are emitted in nearly opposite directions (*left*). When two interactions are nearly simultaneously detected within a ring of detectors surrounding the patient (*right*), it is presumed that an annihilation occurred on the line connecting the interactions (line of response). Thus, ACD, by determining the path of the detected photons, performs the same function for a PET scanner as does the collimator of a scintillation camera. □ **F. 19-18**

**b.** *True, random, and scatter coincidences:* Figure 19-13

   **(i)**   True coincidence is the nearly simultaneous interaction with the detectors of emissions resulting from a single nuclear transformation.

   **(ii)**  A random coincidence (also called an accidental or chance coincidence) occurs when emissions from *different* nuclear transformations interact nearly simultaneously with the detectors.

   **(iii)** A scatter coincidence occurs when one or both of the photons from a single annihilation are scattered, and both are detected.

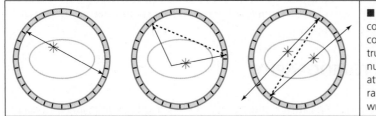

■ **FIGURE 19-13** True coincidence (**left**), scatter coincidence (**center**), and random (accidental) coincidence (**right**). A scatter coincidence is a true coincidence, because it is caused by a single nuclear transformation, but results in a count attributed to the wrong LOR (*dashed line*). The random coincidence is also attributed to the wrong LOR. 📖 **F. 19-19**

**c.** *Detection of interactions:* Scintillation crystals optically coupled to photomultiplier tubes (PMTs) or other light detectors are used. The signals from the PMTs or other light detectors are processed using pulse mode to create signals identifying the position in the detector, deposited energy, and time of each interaction. The energy signal is used for energy discrimination to reduce mispositioned events due to scattering and the time signal is used for coincidence detection. Original PET detector designs had one scintillator coupled to one PMT. However, due to cost and limitations on PMT size, current systems use a block of scintillation crystals coupled to a smaller number of PMTs (Fig. 19-14). The relative magnitudes of the signals from the PMTs coupled to the detector block are then used to identify the location of the crystal within the detector block that had a photon interaction, as in a scintillation camera. The ideal scintillation detector characteristics include prompt light output (short decay constant), high linear attenuation coefficient (stopping power), high conversion efficiency, and high energy resolution to discriminate against scattered events. Originally, BGO used to be the dominant scintillation crystal material in PET scanners. Recently, LSO (LYSO) has become the dominant crystal material.

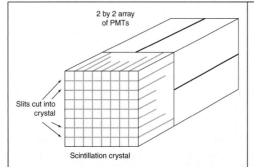

2 by 2 array of PMTs

Slits cut into crystal

Scintillation crystal

■ **FIGURE 19-14** A technique for coupling scintillation crystals to photomultiplier tubes (PMTs). The relative heights of the pulses from the four PMTs are used to determine the position of each interaction in the crystal. The thick (2 to 3 cm) crystal is necessary to provide a reasonable detection efficiency for the 511-keV annihilation photons. The slits cut in the scintillation crystal form light pipes, limiting the spread of light from interactions in the front portion of the crystal, which otherwise would reduce the spatial resolution. This design permits four PMTs to serve 64 detector elements. 📖 **F. 19-20**

**d.** *Timing of interactions and detection of coincidences:* The timing of the interaction of an annihilation photon with the scintillation detector is determined from the leading edge of the electrical signal from the PMTs. When the time signals from two detectors occur within a selected time interval called the time window, a coincidence is recorded. A typical time window for a system with BGO detectors is 12 ns. A typical time window for a system with LSO detectors, which emit light more promptly, is 4.5 ns.

**e.** *True versus random coincidences:* Randoms rate is defined by: $R_{random} = \tau S_1 S_2$, where $\tau$ is the coincidence time window and $S1$ and $S2$ are the actual count rates of the detectors, often called *singles rates*. Randoms decrease linearly with decreasing timing window and increase proportionally with the square of the activity in the patient. This is contrasted with an approximate proportional increase in the true coincident rate.

**f.** *Scatter coincidences:* Scatter coincidences are dependent upon the amount of scattering material and thus occur less in head than in body imaging. Scatter coincidences in PET imaging can be very high (60% to 70% of the acquired coincidence data), particularly in larger cross-sections of the body and when data are acquired in three dimensions. The use of narrower energy discrimination window can reduce the number of scattered events but will also negatively affect the number of recorded true coincidences.

g. *Two-dimensional and three-Dimensional data acquisition:* PET coincidence data can be acquired in two-dimensional (slice) or three-dimensional (volume) mode (Fig. 19-15). In slice mode, coincidences are detected and recorded only within each ring of detector elements or within a few adjacent rings of detector elements. Septa (made from tungsten) prevents coincidences outside an axial slice from reaching the detector ring of that slice hence limiting the acquisition to two-dimensional mode. In volume mode, the absence of the septa allows coincidences to be recorded from the whole detector volume. In volume mode, the total number of recorded events is substantially increased (increase in scanner detection efficiency), but so is the number of recorded scattered and random events. In volume mode, the scanner sensitivity increases linearly from the edges of the scanner to the center of the scanner (Fig. 19-16). This variation in scanner sensitivity requires overlapping of bed positions in situations where patient imaging extends beyond the physical axial length of the scanner. Overlapping of bed position reduces the effect of this variability or the resultant images. Some PET systems are capable of acquiring data in two or three-dimensional mode using retractable septa, but most new PET systems can only acquire data in volume mode.

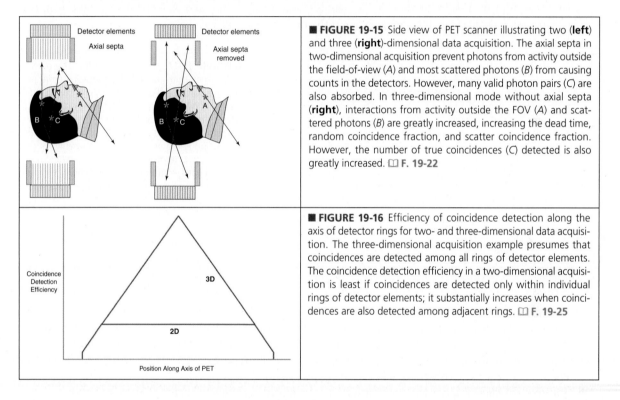

■ **FIGURE 19-15** Side view of PET scanner illustrating two (**left**) and three (**right**)-dimensional data acquisition. The axial septa in two-dimensional acquisition prevent photons from activity outside the field-of-view (*A*) and most scattered photons (*B*) from causing counts in the detectors. However, many valid photon pairs (*C*) are also absorbed. In three-dimensional mode without axial septa (**right**), interactions from activity outside the FOV (*A*) and scattered photons (*B*) are greatly increased, increasing the dead time, random coincidence fraction, and scatter coincidence fraction. However, the number of true coincidences (*C*) detected is also greatly increased. ⌑ **F. 19-22**

■ **FIGURE 19-16** Efficiency of coincidence detection along the axis of detector rings for two- and three-dimensional data acquisition. The three-dimensional acquisition example presumes that coincidences are detected among all rings of detector elements. The coincidence detection efficiency in a two-dimensional acquisition is least if coincidences are detected only within individual rings of detector elements; it substantially increases when coincidences are also detected among adjacent rings. ⌑ **F. 19-25**

h. *Transverse Image reconstruction:* Following the acquisition of the LORs, the data are corrected for several confounding factors and reconstructed using iterative or analytical techniques. Image reconstruction in two-dimensional mode follows similar approaches to SPECT, while three-dimensional mode requires techniques that capture the volumetric data.

2. **Data Correction:** Several data corrections are required to ensure that the resultant PET image truly depicts the radiopharmaceutical biodistribution in the body. These corrections are
   a. *Normalization correction:* conducted to adjust for performance variability among the thousands of detectors in the scanner.
   b. *Randoms correction:* conducted to subtract random events from the recorded total number of events. Two approaches are used: randoms assessment from delays or randoms assessment from singles with the latter resulting in a more accurate correction.
   c. *Scatter correction:* conducted to subtract scatter events from the recorded total number of events. Two approaches are used: scatter is estimated from reconstructed PET and attenuation images while employing computer modeling of photon interactions or scatter is estimated from fitting smoothly varying continuous functions to the tails of the projection profile outside the imaged object. The first approach is mainly used on new hybrid PET/CT systems where the CT scan is used as the attenuation map.
   d. *Deadtime correction:* conducted to account for pulse pileup and deadtime effects whereby various factors are applied to correct any deviation of the scanner count rate performance from a linear response with increasing activity concentrations.

**e.** *Decay correction:* conducted to correct for radioactivity decay during the imaging time (Eq. 19-2).

**f.** *Attenuation correction:* conducted to account for the attenuation of annihilation photons in the patient. Attenuation in PET is more severe than gamma camera or SPECT since both annihilation photons need to escape the patient's body and be detected. Furthermore, attenuation in PET is dependent on the total path length that the annihilation photons travel in the body (Eq. 19-3) and not the depth of the photon in the body (Fig. 19-17) as is the case in gamma camera or SPECT imaging. Three general approaches have been used to correct for attenuation in PET. These are as follows:

**(i)** Approximate methods that assume a uniform attenuation coefficient throughout the object being imaged; historically used in brain imaging.

**(ii)** Radioactive sources that are extended inside the scanner and rotate around the imaged object to measure the transmission profiles of photons from the radioactive sources through the object. These transmission profiles are then used to correct the acquired emission data for attenuation. This approach is still used in dedicated PET scanners.

**(iii)** Use of CT images (in hybrid PET/CT scanners) as a surrogate attenuation map to correct the acquired emission data. This is the approach currently used in hybrid PET/CT systems.

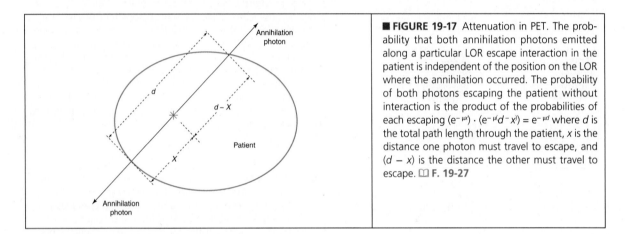

■ **FIGURE 19-17** Attenuation in PET. The probability that both annihilation photons emitted along a particular LOR escape interaction in the patient is independent of the position on the LOR where the annihilation occurred. The probability of both photons escaping the patient without interaction is the product of the probabilities of each escaping $(e^{-\mu x}) \cdot (e^{-\mu(d-x)}) = e^{-\mu d}$ where $d$ is the total path length through the patient, $x$ is the distance one photon must travel to escape, and $(d - x)$ is the distance the other must travel to escape. 📖 **F. 19-27**

**3.** *Quantitation and Detrimental Factors:*

**a.** *Quantitative nature of PET imaging:* Pixel (Voxel) values in PET mages are proportional to the number of counts recorded in that anatomical location in the scanner field of view. The number of counts are in turn proportional to the activity concentration in that location. In that regard, PET images depict the quantitative distribution of activity concentration of a radiopharmaceutical in the body.

**b.** *Scanner calibration:* is the process of transforming the recorded counts following all data correction to activity concentration. The transformation uses a global scale factor that is applied to all image voxel values. The scale factor is obtained by imaging a uniform water cylinder of known activity concentration and determining the ratio of the reconstructed number of counts per pixel to the known activity concentration.

**c.** *Standardized uptake value (SUV):* is a ratio that correlates the activity concentration in a region of interest to the total administered activity. The SUV is primarily used to assist in characterizing tissues that accumulate the administered radiopharmaceutical, particularly in distinguishing benign from malignant lesions or in monitoring tumor therapy. It is defined as follows:

$$SUV = \frac{\text{Activity concentration in a voxel or region}}{\text{Activity administered} / \text{Body mass}}$$

**d.** The SUV has units of density (g/mL) when body mass is described in units of (g). Some modifications of SUV include the use of body lean mass or body surface area in place of body mass. Those, however, are less used since these values are more challenging to obtain on patients.

e. *Factors affecting image quantification:* Several factors affect the magnitude of the measured SUV. These factors are grouped into three categories:

   (i)   Technical factors include all factors that originate from the scanner itself and its support equipment such as dose calibrator errors, residual activity, time synchronization, infiltration, and error in body mass measurement.

   (ii)  Biological factors include all factors that originate from the patient such as patient physiological condition that could affect the radiopharmaceutical biodistribution, scan start time post radiopharmaceutical administration, patient motion during the scan, and patient anxiety/comfort during the radiopharmaceutical biodistribution phase prior to imaging.

   (iii) Physical factors include all factors related to the scanner itself such as scan acquisition parameters, reconstruction parameters, scanner resolution, region of interest size, and scanner quality control performance.

   One approach to mitigate these effects is to harmonize their impact in longitudinal studies leaving any changes in SUV measurements to be truly reflective of radiopharmaceutical uptake in the region of interest. In multicenter clinical trials, such harmonization becomes further complicated by variations in imaging system performance and clinical practices.

4. *Performance:* PET scanner performance can be assessed by evaluating the spatial resolution and sensitivity (efficiency).

   a. *Spatial resolution* usually is on the order of approximately 5 mm in the center of the FOV for current whole-body scanners. Spatial resolution is limited by four factors: (1) detector size ($R_d$)—most dominant factor, (2) positron range before annihilation ($R_r$), (3) the fact that the annihilation photons are not emitted in exactly opposite directions from each other ($R_c$), and (4) the inaccuracy in determining the exact location of the interacting photon in the detector block ($R_l$). The overall system resolution is then equal to the square root of the sum of the squares of all of these factors. Spatial resolution in PET imaging is nonstationary, with the best resolution at the center of the FOV and degrades as one moves out radially from the center. The degradation is primarily due to photons emitted from activity away from the center strike the detectors from oblique angles leading to uncertainty in the depth of interaction and consequently positioning of the LOR (Fig. 19-18).

   b. *Efficiency in annihilation coincidence detection:* Current PET scanner efficiency in two- and three-dimensional mode is 0.1% to 0.3% and 1% to 2%, respectively. Scanner efficiency can be improved by decreasing scanner bore diameter (currently 60 to 80 cm) and increasing scanner axial extent (currently 15 to 30 cm). Both, however, have limitations due to patient size, claustrophobia, and cost.

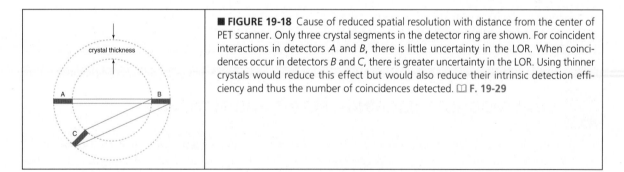

■ **FIGURE 19-18** Cause of reduced spatial resolution with distance from the center of PET scanner. Only three crystal segments in the detector ring are shown. For coincident interactions in detectors *A* and *B*, there is little uncertainty in the LOR. When coincidences occur in detectors *B* and *C*, there is greater uncertainty in the LOR. Using thinner crystals would reduce this effect but would also reduce their intrinsic detection efficiency and thus the number of coincidences detected. 📖 **F. 19-29**

5. *Quality control in PET:* A quality control and assurance program specifically designed for PET imaging is necessary to ensure the proper performance of the scanner. Elements of this program and the frequency of testing are listed in Table 19-1 including tests for the CT component of hybrid scanners. Accreditation and professional bodies such as the ACR and AAPM TG126 have developed similar routine testing schedules for PET. Acceptance testing of PET scanners is performed at the time of scanner installation or following a scanner relocation. These tests follow the NEMA NU2 standard. The results of these tests should be compared to manufacturer specifications.

**TABLE 19-1 ROUTINE TESTS FOR PET**

| TEST | DAILY | WEEKLY | QUARTERLY | SEMIANNUAL | ANNUAL |
|---|---|---|---|---|---|
| CT QC | X | | | | |
| PET QC | X | | | | |
| PET Update Gains and Coincidence Timing | | X | | | |
| PET Normalization | | | X[a] | | |
| PET Calibration | | | X[a] | | |
| Preventive Maintenance and Inspection | | | | X | |
| Source Replacement | | | | | X |
| PET Spatial Resolution | | | | | X |
| PET & CT Registration | | | X[b] | | |
| PET Sensitivity | | | | | X[a] |
| PET Count Rate Performance | | | | | X[c] |
| PET Accuracy of Corrections | | | | | X |
| PET Image Contrast and Scatter/ Attenuation Evaluation | | | X | | |
| PET Image Uniformity Assessment | | | | | X[d] |
| Image Display Monitor Evaluation | | | | | X |
| Emergency Buttons Testing | | | | | X |
| Synchronize System Clocks | | X | | | |
| **Additional Daily Tests[d]** | | | | | |
| Restart Computers | X | | | | |
| Manufacturer-Recommended CT Warm-up Cycle and Calibrations | X | | | | |
| Archive Patient Data | X | | | | |
| Clear Scheduler | X | | | | |
| Clear Local, Network, and Film Queries | X | | | | |

[a]Or if a detector module is replaced.
[b]Or after the gantry is opened.
[c]Or if the electronic boards are replaced.
[d]Philips recommends these tests to be done on a quarterly basis.
📖 T. 19-4

## 19.4 DUAL MODALITY IMAGING—PET/CT AND PET/MRI

Dual modality PET/CT or PET/MRI result in combined images that show anatomy and function superimposed onto one another without the need for image registration (Fig. 19-19). In dual-modality imaging, the patient lies on a bed that passes through the bores of both systems. In PET/CT, the CT images are also used for AC of the PET data. Advantages of using CT images over radioactive sources include faster attenuation scans, increased patient throughput, less statistical noise in the attenuation map, and higher spatial resolution attenuation maps. Nearly, all PET systems sold today are dual-modality (PET/CT or PET/MR) scanners.

1. *Attenuation correction in PET/CT:* CT images represent the average linear attenuation coefficients, averaged over the x-ray energy spectrum, for individual voxels of the patient. To use these values for the AC of PET images requires transforming these values from the average x-ray energy spectrum to 511 keV photon energy used in PET. This is done using a bilinear transformation.

$$\mu_{511\,keV} = \left(9.6 \times 10^{-5}\,cm^{-1}\right) \cdot \left(CT\;number + 1{,}000\right) \quad \left[-1{,}000 < CT\;number < 0\right]$$

$$\mu_{511\,keV} = m \cdot \left(CT\;number\right) + b \quad \left[CT\;number > 0\right]$$

where *m* and *b* are empirically determined constants that differ with the kV used by the x-ray CT system. These values are usually stored in a lookup table and used during the transformation of CT images to PET attenuation maps.

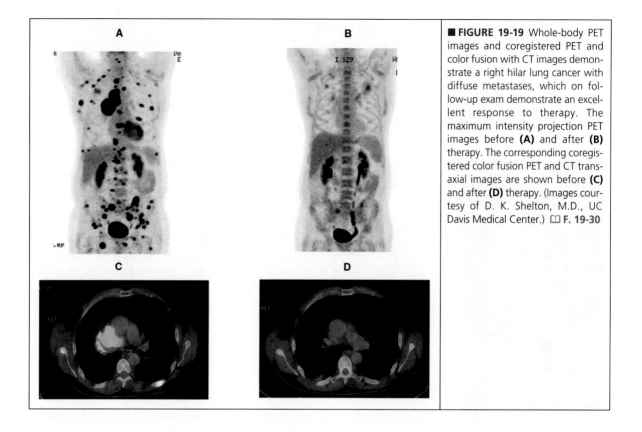

■ **FIGURE 19-19** Whole-body PET images and coregistered PET and color fusion with CT images demonstrate a right hilar lung cancer with diffuse metastases, which on follow-up exam demonstrate an excellent response to therapy. The maximum intensity projection PET images before **(A)** and after **(B)** therapy. The corresponding coregistered color fusion PET and CT transaxial images are shown before **(C)** and after **(D)** therapy. (Images courtesy of D. K. Shelton, M.D., UC Davis Medical Center.) 📖 **F. 19-30**

2. *Artifacts in PET/CT imaging:* Artifacts on CT images that are translated to the PET attenuation map such as metal artifacts or patient motion will lead to artifacts on PET/CT images. Additionally, PET/CT artifacts can arise from the interaction of these two image sets.

    a. *Spatial misregistration artifacts:* Occur since the PET and CT images are not acquired simultaneously. Further, the CT scans are of short duration and acquired over a single breath-hold compared to PET scans that require relatively longer duration and acquired over several breathing cycles. This mismatch results in anatomical misregistration between PET and CT most visible in areas that exhibit large breathing motion such as the dome of the liver (Fig. 19-20). Respiratory gating or matching the CT with the average location of the PET images can help offset this artifact.

    b. *Attenuation correction artifacts:* Occurs when high attenuating material (such as metal or high concentration of CT contrast) artificially increases the CT numbers in the CT image. This artificial increase, in turn, leads

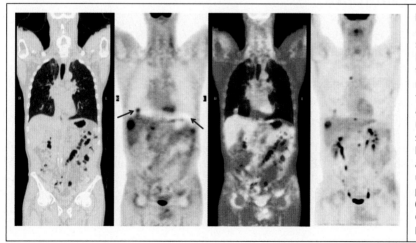

■ **FIGURE 19-20** PET/CT study showing diaphragmatic misregistration with superimposition of a hypermetabolic liver nodule over the right lung base on the fused PET-CT. **Left to right.** coronal CT, attenuation-corrected PET, fused attenuation corrected PET-CT and attenuation-corrected PET maximum intensity projection images. CT shows no nodule in the right lung base, and attenuation-corrected PET and fused PET-CT images show a nodule and a clear band above the diaphragm (*arrows*) due to misregistration. (Images and interpretation courtesy of George M. Segall, M.D., VA Palo Alto Health Care System.) 📖 **F. 19-31**

to an artificial increase in the AC map which ultimately results in an increase in activity concentration in the resultant PET image (Fig. 19-21). The use of nonattenuated corrected PET images which are not affected by this artifact should be used in such cases to confirm the presence of the artifact.

c.  *Truncation artifact:* Occurs due to the difference in the transverse FOV between CT (50 cm) and PET (70 cm). Consequently, objects (patients) that extend beyond the CT FOV (large body girth or patients scanned with arms down) will not be properly attenuated corrected on the resultant PET image. Some PET/CT scanner manufacturers can synthetically increase the CT FOV to match the PET thereby overcoming this limitation.

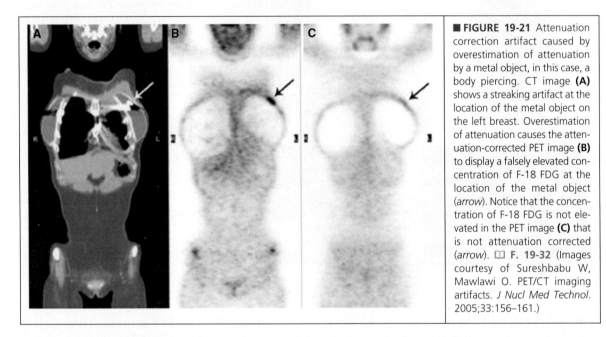

■ **FIGURE 19-21** Attenuation correction artifact caused by overestimation of attenuation by a metal object, in this case, a body piercing. CT image **(A)** shows a streaking artifact at the location of the metal object on the left breast. Overestimation of attenuation causes the attenuation-corrected PET image **(B)** to display a falsely elevated concentration of F-18 FDG at the location of the metal object (*arrow*). Notice that the concentration of F-18 FDG is not elevated in the PET image **(C)** that is not attenuation corrected (*arrow*). 📖 **F. 19-32** (Images courtesy of Sureshbabu W, Mawlawi O. PET/CT imaging artifacts. *J Nucl Med Technol.* 2005;33:156–161.)

3.  **PET/MRI systems:** More recently introduced. Like PET/CT, result in combined images that show anatomy and function superimposed onto one another, and the MRI images are also used for AC. With PET/MRI, both PET and MRI images can be acquired simultaneously and represent a potential advantage over PET/CT. PET/MRI systems require semiconductor detectors since PMTs do not work in the presence of the MRI strong magnetic fields.

4.  **Quality control of dual modality imaging systems** should include QC of PET as well as CT and MRI components. Additionally, testing of the combined system as a whole should include spatial coregistration of the images (PET and CT [MRI]) and accuracy of AC.

## 19.5   ADVANCES IN PET IMAGING

1.  **Time of flight imaging (TOF):** With fast scintillation detectors such as LSO and LYSO, information about the detection (arrival) time of the annihilation photons can be recorded. This knowledge in turn can be used during image reconstruction to inform on where, along a LOR, an annihilation event occurred in the FOV of the scanner, as compared to conventional PET systems that do not have this capability. The knowledge about the arrival times has been shown to improve the resultant signal-to-noise ratio (SNR) of reconstructed PET images. Improving timing resolution (decreasing the value) improves the SNR of resultant images. Current systems have timing resolutions on the order of 250 to 500 ps.

2.  **Digital detectors:** refers to the use of silicon PMT (SiPM) semiconductor detectors to replace the conventional PMTs in PET scanners. Initially developed for PET/MR systems to overcome the effect of the strong magnetic fields of MR scanners on conventional PMT. SiPMs have the advantage of small size (compared to PMTs) potentially improving the PET image resolution, improved light absorption, and conversion as well as event timing. Most PET/CT scanners today use digital detectors.

3. *Continuous bed motion (CBM):* refers to the continuous motion of the scanner bed during the whole-body acquisition of PET data as compared to the conventional step and shoot mode of imaging. CBM has several potential advantages over conventional step and shoot imaging such as improved image uniformity along the axial direction. This advantage diminishes with increasing bed overlap in step and shoot mode. Another advantage is to provide a more flexible imaging workflow which in turn can potentially be used to decrease the x-ray radiation dose in certain imaging situations.

4. *Resolution recovery:* better known as PSF (point spread function) reconstruction, refers to the correction for the degradation in PET image resolution in the transverse FOV due to depth of interaction effects (Fig. 19-18). PET image reconstruction techniques can correct for this resolution degradation. One concern with PSF reconstruction is its tendency to artificially increase the signal intensity (activity concentration) at the edges of objects in the image thereby biasing the quantitative PET measurement.

5. *Motion compensation:* refers to the ability to compensate for (1) mismatch between PET and CT images due to the sequential nature of the imaging and the scan duration differences and (2) motion blur in PET images due to motion during the PET image acquisition. Motion compensation can be achieved using 4D PET/CT or quiescent phase or amplitude PET imaging.

6. *Data-driven gating (DDG):* refers to a novel approach to derive the patient breathing cycle needed to perform motion compensation described above. Conventionally, a patient breathing pattern is recorded using external devices that are not user-friendly. With data-driven techniques, the patient breathing pattern is extracted from the PET data itself with minimal user intervention. Data-driven techniques depend on a high SNR to allow the extraction of the patient breathing pattern from background noise.

7. *Longer axial field of view:* Refers to the new generation of PET scanners with long axial extents. Conventionally PET scanners had axial FOVs of 15 to 20 cm. Newer scanners increase this extent to 30 cm or longer with one manufacturer offering a 194-cm system. Large axial extent scanners have many advantages: (1) higher sensitivity that leads to better image quality, (2) cover a larger axial extent of the patient thereby reducing total scan time which in turn increases scanner throughput and improves patient experience, (3) the improved sensitivity and body coverage can be traded for reduced administered activity (and reduced patient radiation dose) without largely affecting image quality, and (4) allow multiple organ dynamic imaging used for the biodistribution and kinetics studies of novel radiopharmaceuticals.

8. *Improved image reconstruction:* refers to novel image reconstruction techniques that have started to become commercially available. One such technique is regularized reconstruction that constrains the noise in the resultant images. Another is maximum a posteriori (MAP) that preserves edges in the resultant PET image by using priors from CT or MR images or maximum likelihood reconstruction of attenuation and activity (MLAA) that can approximate both the attenuation map and final PET image from the acquired PET data without the need of a separate attenuation map. Finally, artificial intelligence techniques are starting to be used in PET imaging especially with their potential to suppress image noise.

## 19.6 CLINICAL ASPECTS, COMPARISON OF PET AND SPECT, AND DOSE

1. *PET radiopharmaceuticals:* Primarily centered on F-18 labeled radiopharmaceuticals due to its relatively long half-life (110 min) thereby eliminating the need for a nearby or on-site cyclotron. This is in contrast to other positron-emitting radioisotopes of common biochemical elements such as carbon, nitrogen, and oxygen with half-lives of 20, 10, and 2 min, respectively. (F-18) 2-fluoro-2-deoxy-D-glucose (F-18 FDG), one of the most commonly used FDA-approved PET radiopharmaceuticals, is a glucose analog that accumulates in cells at a rate proportional to the local extracellular concentration and glucose uptake and mainly used in oncology to evaluate and assess the efficacy of treatment. Other FDA-approved PET radiopharmaceuticals include fluorine-18 as sodium fluoride for skeletal imaging, gallium-68 Dotatate (NetSpot) for neuroendocrine cancer, fluorine-18 Fluciclovine (Axumin) for prostate cancer, and rubidium-82 chloride for myocardial perfusion imaging.

2. *Radiation doses:* For dual modality, the total patient radiation dose is the sum of the dose from the radiopharmaceutical as well as the x-ray CT dose. For a 370 MBq (10 mCi) administered activity of FDG, the effective dose to an adult is about 7 mSv. The CT dose on the other hand can be in the range of 4 to 16 mSv depending on the technique used.

3. *Comparison of SPECT and PET:* Table 19-2 shows a comparison of these nuclear imaging modalities.

**TABLE 19-2 COMPARISON OF SPECT AND PET**

| | SPECT | PET |
|---|---|---|
| Principle of projection data collection | Collimation | Annihilation coincidence detection (ACD) |
| Transverse image reconstruction | Iterative methods or filtered backprojection | Iterative methods or filtered backprojection |
| Radionuclides | Any emitting x-rays, gamma rays, or annihilation photons. Optimal performance for photon energies of 100–200 keV | Positron emitters only |
| Spatial resolution | Depends upon collimator and camera orbit | Relatively constant across transaxial image, best at center |
| | Within a transaxial image, the resolution in the radial direction is relatively uniform, but the tangential resolution is degraded toward the center | Typically 4.5–5 mm FWHM at center |
| | Typically about 10 mm FWHM at center for a 30-cm diameter orbit and Tc-99m | |
| | Larger camera orbits produce worse resolution | |
| Attenuation | Attenuation less severe. Radioactive attenuation correction sources or x-ray CT can correct for attenuation | Attenuation more severe. Radioactive attenuation correction sources or x-ray CT can correct for attenuation |

📖 T. 19-6

# Section II Questions and Answers

1. The main advantage of SPECT over planar imaging with a scintillation camera is
   A. better spatial resolution
   B. a smaller activity of radiopharmaceutical to be administered to the patient is permitted
   C. shorter imaging time
   D. improved contrast by removing counts from overlapping structures
   E. lower susceptibility to image artifacts

2. Which of the following reduces SPECT reconstruction streak artifacts?
   A. Step-and-shoot acquisition mode
   B. Acquiring a number of projections approximately equal to the pixel format
   C. Acquiring projections over only 180°
   D. Continuous acquisition mode
   E. A smaller pixel format

3. Brain SPECT with higher resolution than body SPECT may be achieved by:
   A. continuous acquisition
   B. acquiring with a noncircular orbit
   C. acquiring with a zoom factor
   D. step-and-shoot acquisition
   E. acquiring with a smaller orbit radius within the patient's shoulders

4. Which of the following is not a reason a 180° arc of projections is insufficient for SPECT reconstruction?
   A. Opposing views are not mirror images of each other
   B. 360° of projections are required for rotational tomography
   C. Spatial resolution degrades with distance from the camera head
   D. Photon attenuation from activity in the half of the patient opposite the camera head is higher than that in the half of the patient on the same side as the camera head
   E. The amount and distribution of scatter in opposing views is different

5. The filter in the spatial frequency domain that is the ideal kernel for filtered backprojection reconstruction is:

A. 1.0 Nyquist cutoff ramp
B. high-frequency "roll-off" ramp
C. low-frequency "roll-off" ramp
D. 0.5 Nyquist frequency cutoff ramp
E. spatial resolution versus noise compromise

6. Which of the following statements regarding SPECT transverse image reconstruction is false?
   A. Projections contain substantial statistical noise.
   B. Filter kernel selection is a compromise between resolution and noise.
   C. Low frequencies in the spatial frequency domain are dominated by statistical noise.
   D. Filter kernel "roll-off" reduces noise at the expense of spatial resolution
   E. Gamma camera resolution reduces higher spatial frequency information

7. Which of these statements is true regarding SPECT transverse image reconstruction?
   A. Noise is increased at the expense of spatial resolution by filter kernel "roll-off."
   B. Filter kernel selection is a compromise between contrast and resolution.
   C. Ideal ramp filtered backprojection results in acceptable noise in transverse slices.
   D. A filter with a higher spatial frequency cutoff is required for projections of better spatial resolution and less quantum mottle.
   E. A filter with a higher spatial frequency cutoff is required for projections of poorer spatial resolution and greater quantum mottle.

8. Iterative reconstruction can model all aspects of, and thus compensate for, the SPECT imaging process, except:
   A. activity calibration
   B. attenuation of photons by the patient
   C. system resolution as a function of distance
   D. scattering of photons by the collimator
   E. scattering of photons by the patient

9. The model of photon scattering by the patient incorporated into SPECT iterative reconstruction, which utilizes the current iteration of the photopeak reconstruction, along with maps of

attenuation coefficient and material density in the patient is:

A. triple-energy window
B. modified point spread function
C. dual-energy window
D. wide-beam attenuation map
E. effective scatter source estimation

10. What is the primary purpose of postiterative reconstruction three-dimensional spatial filtering?

A. Spatial resolution enhancement
B. Signal-to-noise reduction
C. Noise reduction
D. Spatial resolution degradation
E. Compensation for the effect of scatter

11. A computationally efficient iterative reconstruction technique that substantially reduces total reconstruction time is:

A. maximum likelihood
B. least squares
C. maximum a posteriori
D. ordered subset
E. expectation maximization

12. Which attenuation correction method is only applicable to SPECT imaging of objects with a constant attenuation coefficient ($\mu$ value)?

A. Scanning collimated line source
B. Fixed line source
C. Array of fixed line sources
D. Chang approximation
E. X-ray CT-based

13. Which of the following collimators is designed specifically for cardiac SPECT scanning?

A. Fan-beam
B. variable focal length
C. converging
D. pinhole
E. parallel-hole

14. When quantifying SPECT resolution using the NEMA triple-line phantom and protocol:

A. tangential resolution is superior to central and radial resolution
B. central resolution is superior to radial and tangential resolution
C. central and radial resolution are equal and superior to tangential resolution
D. radial resolution is superior to tangential and central resolution
E. central, radial, and tangential resolution are equal

15. What type of correction is required if a SPECT camera's COR misalignment varies as the camera rotates around an object?

A. Image zoom-dependent
B. Image matrix size-dependent
C. Slice-by-slice
D. Angle-by-angle
E. Multienergy

16. All of the following tests are part of SPECT annual performance evaluation except:

A. image contrast
B. center-of-rotation misalignment
C. artifact assessment
D. uniformity
E. high-contrast spatial resolution

17. A "doughnut" artifact in the reconstruction of a line source may occur due to which of the following SPECT acquisition misalignments?

A. Detector-to-detector axial shift
B. X-direction shift
C. Y-direction shift
D. Axial tilt
E. Yoke swivel

18. A ring artifact that appears in the SPECT images produced by a gamma camera due to slight damage to a small area of the collimator can probably be corrected by:

A. determining COR and applying COR correction
B. appropriate modifications to the reconstruction filter
C. acquiring a uniformity image and using it to correct the raw projection images
D. adjusting the energy window
E. increasing the image acquisition time

19. The SPECT acquisition misalignment that results in backprojection of out-of-slice activity into each transverse slice is:

A. axial tilt
B. yoke swivel
C. x-direction shift
D. y-direction shift
E. detector-to-detector axial shift

20. Which of the following performance characteristics is not typically evaluated with a SPECT quality control phantom?

A. Uniformity
B. Attenuation correction
C. Image contrast
D. Spatial resolution
E. Sensitivity

21. In PET, a method of reducing the fraction of detected coincidences due to scatter coincidences is:

A. administering less activity to the patient
B. using a scintillation material with prompter light output
C. using 2-D (slice) image acquisition with axial collimation instead of 3-D acquisition
D. using a shorter coincidence time window
E. using attenuation correction

22. In PET, what is a major advantage of using a scintillation material that emits light very promptly after each interaction?
    A. Improved detection efficiency
    B. Improved rejection of scatter coincidences
    C. Reduced rate of random coincidences
    D. Better spatial resolution
    E. Reduced effects of attenuation of photons in the patient

23. The detectors in most PET scanners are:
    A. argon-filled ionization chambers
    B. xenon-filled ionization chambers
    C. semiconductor detectors
    D. scintillation crystals coupled to photomultiplier tubes
    E. semiconductor detectors coupled to photodiodes

24. If the intrinsic detection efficiencies of the detectors of a PET system are reduced by half, the number of true coincidences detected will:
    A. not change
    B. be reduced to 90%
    C. be reduced to 75%
    D. be reduced to 50%
    E. be reduced to 25%

25. What is an advantage of using x-ray CT to obtain information for attenuation correction in PET/CT scanners, instead of the radioactive sources used in PET systems?
    A. X-ray CT attenuation maps correspond more accurately to the geometry of the PET data.
    B. X-ray CT provides more accurate estimation of attenuation of 511 keV photons.
    C. X-ray CT reduces the likelihood of beam hardening artifacts.
    D. X-ray CT reduces the likelihood of artifacts from implanted metal objects.
    E. X-ray CT reduces the time needed to acquire the attenuation information.

26. In PET imaging, the main advantage of time-of-flight measurements is:
    A. attenuation correction of PET data is not necessary
    B. the location of each annihilation can be accurately determined
    C. improved rejection of scatter coincidences
    D. improved spatial resolution
    E. improved signal to noise ratio

27. What is least likely to cause attenuation artifacts resulting in falsely elevated FDG concentrations in attenuation-corrected $^{18}$F-FDG PET/CT images?
    A. Small metal objects, such as orthopedic devices and pacemakers, in the body
    B. Metal body piercings

C. Concentrated barium contrast following fluoroscopic GI studies
D. Large volume metal objects such as a hip implant
E. Respiratory motion

28. In PET imaging, increasing the activity in the FOV of the scanner by two times (2✕) will lead to a:
    A. two times increase in the number of scatter events
    B. three times increase in the number of true events
    C. four times increase in the number of random events
    D. five times increase in the number of random events
    E. no increase in the number of prompt events

29. In PET imaging, if the diameter of a uniform object being scanned increases by 2 times, the attenuation:
    A. increases by ln 2
    B. decreases by ln 2
    C. increases by 2
    D. decreases by 2
    E. stays the same

30. In PET imaging of a uniform phantom with 20 cm diameter, the attenuation ratio of an annihilation event at the center to that at the edge of the phantom is:
    A. 1/2
    B. 1/4
    C. 2
    D. 4
    E. 1

31. In a uniform water phantom, if the administered activity is increased from 1 to 3 mCi, then the resultant SUV will (assume a water density of 1):
    A. increase by 2
    B. decrease by 2
    C. increase by 50%
    D. decrease by 50%
    E. remain the same

32. The unit of SUV is:
    A. uCi/cc
    B. counts/sec
    C. uCi
    D. unitless
    E. g/cc

33. In PET imaging, if the weight of the patient is doubled, the SUV will:
    A. increase by two times
    B. increase by four times
    C. decrease by two times
    D. decrease by four times
    E. remain the same

34. In PET/CT imaging, the presence of small metal objects in the patient will result in:
    A. artificial increase in activity concentration in that location
    B. artificial decrease in activity concentration in that location
    C. no effect on the activity concentration in that location
    D. artificial decrease in CT attenuation coefficient
    E. no effect on the CT attenuation coefficient

35. In time-of-flight PET imaging, a timing resolution of 200 ps will result in identifying the location of the annihilation event to about:
    A. 2 cm
    B. 4 cm
    C. 6 cm
    D. 8 cm
    E. 10 cm

36. Advantages of continuous bed motion in PET imaging include improvement in:
    A. scanner sensitivity
    B. image resolution
    C. scanner efficiency
    D. image uniformity
    E. scanner count rate

37. Image resolution of PET compared to SPECT (with 30 cm orbit) when measured at the center of the FOV is:
    A. better by about 2 times
    B. better by about 4 times
    C. is the same
    D. worse by about 2 times
    E. worse by about 2 times

38. According to professional societies and accreditation bodies, the PET scanner calibration is recommended to be conducted:
    A. daily
    B. weekly
    C. monthly
    D. quarterly
    E. annually

39. Compared to conventional PET imaging, the signal to noise ratio in time of flight imaging increases with
    A. increasing scanner diameter
    B. decreasing detector length
    C. increasing object diameter
    D. decreasing detector density
    E. increasing scanner axial dimension

40. The factor that has the most impact on current PET scanner image resolution when using a point source of F-18 placed at the center of the FOV is:
    A. positron range
    B. detector size
    C. scanner diameter
    D. detector material
    E. scanner axial extent

41. Which of the following results in the highest improvement in PET scanner sensitivity?
    A. Changing the detector material from BGO to LSO
    B. Changing the timing resolution from 200 to 500 ps
    C. Changing the detector length from 20 to 30 mm
    D. Changing the scanner axial extent from 15 to 30 cm
    E. Changing the scanner diameter from 70 to 80 cm

42. Truncation artifacts in PET/CT imaging:
    A. occur because the CT FOV is larger than PET
    B. occur because the PET is acquired after the CT
    C. occur because the CT FOV is smaller than PET
    D. occur when the CT is acquired after the PET
    E. occur because of high CT attenuation coefficients

# Answers

1. **D**  The main advantage of SPECT over planar imaging with a scintillation camera is that it provides improved contrast by removing counts from overlapping structures. Planar imaging usually provides better spatial resolution because the camera head is closer to the patient and generally requires shorter imaging times. Larger activities of radiopharmaceuticals are often administered to the patient for SPECT to obtain adequate count statistics in the images. *(Pg. 777)*

2. **B**  SPECT reconstruction artifacts are reduced by acquiring a sufficient number of projections. A good "rule of thumb" is to acquire a number of projections that is approximately equal to the pixel format, for example, 120 to 128 projections for $128^2$. *(Pg. 766)*

3. **E**  Acquisition with a smaller-radius orbit makes brain SPECT with higher resolution than body SPECT possible. A small camera head physical edge-to-useful field-of-view edge distance or a head holder beyond the patient table allows an orbit within the patient's shoulders, which is not possible when imaging other parts of the body. *(Pg. 767)*

4. **B**  Ideally, only a 180° arc of projections is required for tomographic reconstruction, as opposing views are mirror images, making those in the second half of a 360° arc redundant. However, spatial resolution loss with distance, higher attenuation of photons from the side of the patient opposite the camera head, and differing amounts and distribution of scatter, all contribute to opposing SPECT projections not being mirrors of each other. Thus, a 360° arc of projections is required, with an exception made for cardiac SPECT. *(Pg. 766)*

5. **A**  According to the theory of reconstruction from projections, the ideal filter to apply, prior to backprojection, is a ramp in the frequency domain, with a cut-off at the Nyquist frequency when implemented digitally, as it is in SPECT. All filters that "roll-off" frequencies below 1.0 Nyquist (including a band-limited ramp) are a trade-off between spatial resolution loss and noise. *(Pg. 767)*

6. **C**  Clinical SPECT projections contain substantial statistical noise, due to low pixel counts as well as the nature of radioactive decay, which is essentially uniform across all spatial frequencies. Information of imaged structures is reduced at higher spatial frequencies, due to the limited spatial resolution of the gamma camera. As a result, high frequencies in the spatial frequency domain are dominated by statistical noise. *(Pg. 767)*

7. **D**  Projections with better spatial resolution and less quantum mottle (statistical noise) require a filter with less smoothing and thus a higher frequency cutoff. Too much smoothing would result in an unnecessary loss of reconstructed resolution with little benefit to reducing quantum mottle. *(Pg. 768)*

8. **A**  SPECT iterative reconstruction can model and thus correct for attenuation and scattering of photons by the patient; the system resolution point spread function with distance from the collimator; and scattering of photons by the collimator. The conversion of reconstructed counts to activity occurs separately, based on a system calibration performed prior to patient scanning. *(Pg. 769)*

9. **E**  Modeling scatter of photons in the patient in SPECT iterative reconstruction with the effective scatter source estimation technique is superior to other scatter approximation methods, such as modified PSF, secondary energy window, and wide-beam attenuation, as patient-specific information (photopeak transverse slices, and attenuation and material density maps) is utilized to estimate the contribution of scatter in the forward projection step. *(Pg. 770)*

10. **C**  SPECT iterative reconstruction from relatively poor counting statistics projections results in reconstructed slices with substantial noise. Postreconstruction three-dimensional smoothing spatial filter is typically employed for signal-to-noise improvement (noise reduction), at the cost of degradation in spatial resolution. *(Pg. 770)*

11. **D**  Ordered subset is an iterative reconstruction technique in which the entire set of projections is divided into a number of unique, equal-sized subsets (*n*), and each iteration consists of n subiterations cycling through the subsets in a given order. The result of one complete ordered subset iteration is essentially equivalent to n conventional iterations with a factor of *n* gain in speed. *(Pg. 770)*

12. **D**  The Chang postreconstruction SPECT attenuation correction approximation technique assumes a constant attenuation coefficient ($\mu$ value) and also requires accurate boundary detection. X-ray or radioactive source-based transmission CT is capable of generating variable $\mu$ value maps for incorporation into SPECT iterative reconstruction of objects consisting of multiple materials with different $\mu$ values. *(Pg. 770)*

13. **B**  A variable focal length collimator has been designed for cardiac SPECT, with greater sensitivity in the region of the heart compared to parallel-hole and without field-of-view truncation artifacts. (Multiple pinhole collimators were used in the distant past for cardiac SPECT.) Fan beam collimators have been developed for improved sensitivity and resolution brain SPECT. (Converging and variable focal length collimators have also been used for brain SPECT.) Parallel-hole collimators are used for SPECT imaging of all organs and the whole body but are not optimized for cardiac or brain SPECT. *(Pg. 772)*

14. **A**  The NEMA protocol for measuring SPECT resolution results in a reconstructed full-width at half maximum in the tangential direction that is smaller than those in the central and radial directions, which are approximately equal. However, NEMA SPECT resolution may not be indicative of clinical resolution, due to the protocol's use of a long acquisition time, small radius-of-rotation, and ideal ramp filtered backprojection. *(Pg. 776)*

15. **D**  A SPECT center-of-rotation misalignment that is not constant as a function of projection image angle can only be corrected by an angel-by-angle correction. *(Pg. 779)*

16. **B**  Electromechanical misalignment with respect to its axis-of-rotation is a characteristic of a SPECT camera that may vary over time and must be corrected. Therefore, it must be tested or calibrated at a higher frequency than once a year, such as monthly. *(Pg. 782)*

17. **B**  An *x*-direction shift in a detector during SPECT acquisition will result in backprojection of all projections for a given slice that are shifted in the radial direction. A small misalignment will result in a loss of resolution, whereas a large misalignment will result in an artifactual "doughnut" reconstruction of a point or line source. *(Pg. 778)*

18. **C**  A nonuniformity in collimator efficiency caused by, for example, physical damage may result in visible ring artifacts in reconstructed phantom or clinical SPECT images. Such artifacts can only be compensated for, by acquiring a new collimator or system uniformity calibration map. *(Pg. 780)*

19. **A**  SPECT reconstruction assumes the detector heads are parallel to the axis of rotation during acquisition. If they are tilted in the axial direction, each row of each projection will be backprojected through a different axial slice from where the projection originated. Axial tilt may be assessed by SPECT acquisition of a point source near the edge of the FOV. An image-to-image variation in the y-direction position of the source indicates axial tilt. *(Pg. 780)*

20. **E**  Commercially available SPECT quality control phantoms consist of a fillable cylindrical tank with a uniform section and sections containing inserts consisting of either "cold" or "hot" rods and spheres of various sizes. These phantoms allow semiquantitative evaluation of uniformity, resolution, contrast, and the effectiveness of attenuation correction (*e.g.*, Chang or x-ray CT-based). SPECT sensitivity is evaluated separately by imaging a source with a known amount of radioactivity. *(Pg. 781)*

21. **C**  2-D (slice) acquisition produces a scatter fraction about half that of 3-D (volume) acquisition. Energy discrimination is also used to reduce the scatter coincidence fraction. Unfortunately, energy discrimination is less successful for scatter reduction in PET than in scintillation camera imaging. The reason for this is that, because of the high energy (511 keV) of the annihilation photons, a substantial fraction of the interactions with the detectors is by Compton scattering instead of by the photoelectric effect. Thus, many of the interactions will not deposit the entire 511 keV in the detector and will not produce counts in the photopeak. Setting an energy window to encompass only the photopeak will therefore reject many valid interactions. *(Pg. 790)*

22. **C**  A major advantage of using a scintillation material that emits light very promptly following each interaction is a reduced rate of random coincidences. This, of course, presumes that the coincidence time window is reduced. Unfortunately, scatter coincidences are true coincidences (both photons causing a scatter coin-

cidence arise from a single positron annihilation) and therefore are not reduced by using a scintillator with faster light emission. Although not listed as a choice in this question, another advantage in PET of using a scintillation material that emits light very promptly is reduced count losses from three or more interactions occurring within the coincidence time window. *(Pg. 788)*

23. **D**  The detectors of all commercially available PET systems are scintillation crystals coupled to photomultiplier tubes. *(Pg. 785)*

24. **E**  If the intrinsic detection efficiencies of the detectors of a PET system are reduced by half, the number of true coincidences detected will be reduced to a fourth of the original number. For a coincidence to be detected, two opposed detectors must each detect an interaction. If the original efficiency is E, the rate of coincidences detected will be proportional to E × E. If the detection efficiency is reduced by half, the detection efficiency of a single detector will be E/2 and the rate of coincidences detected will be proportional to (E/2) × (E/2) = (E × E)/4. This illustrates why detection efficiency is so important in PET. Although some less expensive PET systems use NaI(Tl) crystals, most use crystal scintillators such as BGO, LSO, or GSO, which have linear attenuation coefficients for 511 keV photons over twice that of NaI. *(Pg. 799)*

25. **E**  The advantages to using x-ray CT information for attenuation correction in PET are that the high photon flux of the x-ray CT permits very fast determination of the attenuation maps and provides attenuation maps with very little statistical noise. Dedicated PET systems typically use sealed rod sources of radioactive material for attenuation correction. These sources usually contain a positron-emitting radionuclide, which provides 511 keV photons, or Cs-137, which emits 662 keV photons. There are disadvantages to using the x-ray CT data for PET attenuation correction. The geometry of the x-ray CT attenuation maps does not exactly match the geometry of the PET data, because the CT data are usually acquired during breath-hold, whereas the PET data are acquired with normal breathing. The x-ray CT data describes attenuation at CT x-ray photon energies and so it must be scaled to describe the attenuation of 511 keV photons. (The scaling factors differ with the atomic number of the material. For example, bone requires a different scaling factor than soft tissue.) Beam hardening artifacts are much more likely for the polyenergetic and lower energy x-ray beam used in x-ray CT. Lastly, implanted metal objects often cause artifacts when x-ray CT is used for PET attenuation correction, because of incorrect scaling of attenuation from x-ray CT photon energies to 511 keV. *(Pg. 804)*

26. **E**  In theory, time-of-flight measurements could localize each individual annihilation and make reconstruction unnecessary. However, current detectors cannot determine the time of interaction sufficiently precisely to enable this. Instead, they permit the determination of their location along a line of response within several centimeters. This information can be used in the reconstruction process to substantially improve the signal-to-noise ratio. *(Pg. 808)*

27. **D**  Falsely elevated FDG concentrations in CT attenuation-corrected images are commonly caused by the presence of material, such as metal or concentrated contrast material, that does not fit the assumptions used to estimate the attenuation coefficient for 511 keV photons from the CT number for a particular voxel. This results in an incorrect amplification of the actual radionuclide concentration. However, if there is no positron-emitting radionuclide in a voxel or voxels, there is no concentration to amplify. Zero multiplied by a large number is still zero! Thus, a large volume metal object such as a hip implant may not result in a "hot spot." *(Pg. 807)*

28. **C**  Doubling the amount of activity will increase all the type of events (Trues, Randoms, and Scatter) in a PET scanner. The randoms rate in a PET scanner is given by Equation 19-1 and shows that the rate of random coincidences is approximately proportional to the square of the activity in the patient, so doubling the activity will result in a four times increase in the number of random events. The true coincidence rate, ignoring dead time count losses, is approximately proportional to the activity in the patient. Scatter coincidences are dependent upon the amount of scattering material. *(Pg. 787–788)*

29. **C**  Attenuation in PET is dependent on the total path length in the object being imaged. Attenuation in PET differs from attenuation in SPECT because in PET both annihilation photons must escape the patient to cause a coincident event to be registered. The probability of both photons escaping the patient without interaction is the product of the probabilities of each escaping as shown in Equation 19-3. Doubling the path length will result in doubling the attenuation. *(Pg. 794)*

30. **E**  As mentioned in the previous question, attenuation in PET is dependent on the total path length in the object being imaged and not the depth of the annihilation event. Since the path length in the phantom is the same, the total attenuation will remain the same. *(Pg. 794)*

31. **E**    The SUV Equation (19-4) is directly proportional to the activity concentration in a region of interest and inversely proportional to the ratio of administered activity to the mass of the imaged object. For a uniform phantom and a water density of 1 g/ml, this implies that tripling the administered activity (from 1 to 3 mCi) while everything remains constant will result in tripling the activity concentration in the water phantom, and hence the resultant SUV will remain the same. *(Pg. 796)*

32. **E**    The SUV Equation is given in 19-4. The SUV has units of density, g/cm$^3$. *(Pg. 796)*

33. **C**    For a patient study where the distribution of the radiopharmaceutical in the body is not uniform, doubling the weight of the patient will result in doubling the SUV. *(Pg. 796)*

34. **A**    Material in the patient that does not meet the assumptions inherent in the method to estimate attenuation coefficients for 511-keV photons from x-ray CT data can cause significant errors in attenuation correction. If the attenuation coefficient for 511-keV photons is significantly overestimated, the artifact typically appears as a falsely elevated radionuclide concentration, which can mimic a lesion of clinical relevance. This can occur where there are metallic objects in the body, such as pacemakers, orthopedic devices, or body piercings. *(Pg. 806)*

35. **B**    In time-of-flight imaging, improving (decreasing) the timing resolution improves the ability to pinpoint the location of the annihilation event along the LOR. This can be determined from $\Delta X = (\Delta t/2)c$, where $c$ is the speed of light, $\Delta t$ is the timing resolution of the scanner. *(Pg. 808)*

36. **D**    Several advantages are gained from continuous bed motion (CBM) during PET data acquisition: (1) image uniformity along the axial direction is improved compared to step and shoot given that every imaged section passes through the center of the scanner (which has the highest sensitivity), (2) more flexibility in imaging workflow. With CBM, imaging can be started and stopped at any location along the axial extent of the patient, (3) the flexibility with the imaging workflow has implications on reducing the CT radiation exposure to the patient. *(Pg. 810)*

37. **A**    In SPECT, the spatial resolution and detection efficiency are primarily determined by the collimator. Both are ultimately limited by the compromise between collimator efficiency and collimator spatial resolution that is a consequence of collimated image formation. It is the use of ACD instead of collimation that makes the PET scanner much more efficient than SPECT and also yields its superior spatial resolution. Table 19-2 [Textbook Table 19-6] gives such a comparison. *(Pg. 815–816)*

38. **D** Several professional and accreditation bodies have developed routine testing schedules for PET systems. For scanner calibration, the recommendations suggest that this test be performed quarterly. Table 19-1 [Textbook Table 19-4] lists the routine tests that should be conducted and their frequencies. *(Pg. 801)*

39. **D**    The SNR of time of flight imaging improves over conventional imaging by improving timing resolution as well as the diameter of the imaged object. The equations on page 808 show that larger objects (patients) will benefit more from TOF imaging than smaller objects. *(Pg. 808)*

40. **B**    The spatial resolution of PET scanners is limited by four primary factors: (1) the intrinsic spatial resolution of the detectors ($R_d$), (2) the distances traveled by the positrons before annihilation ($R_r$), (3) the fact that the annihilation photons are not emitted in exactly opposite directions from each other ($R_c$), and (4) the inaccuracy in determining the exact location of the interacting photon in the detector block ($R_l$). The intrinsic resolution of the detectors ($R_d$) which depends on the detector size is the major factor determining the spatial resolution in current scanners. *(Pg. 799)*

41. **D**    An increase in axial extent of the PET scanner has many advantages: it increases scanner throughput by reducing patient scan time, which improves the patient's experience, and it also increases scanner sensitivity, which can be traded for a reduced injected activity and hence a reduced patient radiation dose. All other answers reduce the scanner sensitivity except for answer C where changing the detector length from 20 to 30 mm will increase the detection of more 511 keV photon albeit to a moderate effect given the attenuation coefficient of PET detectors shown in textbook Table 19-2. *(Pg. 813, 786)*

42. **C**    The radial FOVs of the CT and PET systems may differ significantly. Commonly, the PET system has a much larger radial FOV than the CT. If part of a patient, for example, a patient of large girth or a patient imaged with the arms by his or her side, extends outside the FOV of the CT, there will be an error in the attenuation correction of the PET images because attenuation by the portion of the patient outside the CT's FOV is not considered. The acquisition sequence (PET first or CT first) has no impact on truncation artifacts. *(Pg. 807)*

# Section III Key Equations and Symbols

| QUANTITY | EQUATION | EQ NO./PAGE/COMMENTS |
|---|---|---|
| X magnification factor | $X_{mag} = \dfrac{\text{actual distance between centers of points sources}}{\text{number of pixels between centers of point sources}}$ | Pg. 777. $Y$ magnification factor is similarly determined. |
| Rate of random coincidences between any pair of detector pairs | $R_{random} = \tau S_1 S_2$ | Eq. 19-1/Pg. 787/A randoms rate calculated from coincidence time window and detectors' singles rates. |
| Minimum coincidence time window for 70 cm FOV | $\Delta t = 0.7 \text{ m}/(3.0 \times 10^8 \text{ m/s}) = 2.33 \text{ ns}$ | Pg. 788/The minimum allowable coincidence time window is derived from the scanner's FOV. |
| Reduction in number of recorded events for data acquired between time t and t+$\Delta$t | $DF = e^{-(\lambda * t)} * \left[ \dfrac{1 - e^{-(\lambda * \Delta t)}}{\lambda * \Delta t} \right]$ | Eq. 19-2/Pg. 793/The decay factor depends upon the time of acquisition relative to $t = 0$ and the duration of acquisition. |
| Probability of both photons escaping the patient without interaction | $(e^{-\mu x}) \cdot (e^{-\mu(d-x)}) = e^{-\mu d}$ | Eq. 19-3/Pg. 794/Detector-pair coincidence detection probability relative to air depends on the attenuation coefficient and total patient thickness between the detectors. |
| Standardized uptake value | $SUV = \dfrac{\text{activity concentration in a voxel or group of voxels}}{\text{activity administered}/\text{body mass}}$ | Eq. 19-4/Pg. 796/SUV is local activity concentration normalized to the average activity per unit mass of the patient, with units of g/cm³. |
| Overall PET system resolution | $R_{sys}^2 = R_d^2 + R_r^2 + R_c^2 + R_l^2$ | Pg. 799/System resolution depends on detector intrinsic resolution, positron distance traveled before annihilation, noncolinearity of annihilation photons, and uncertainty in determining photon interaction location in detector block. |
| True coincidence rate of a detector pair | $R_T = 2AG\varepsilon^2$ | Eq. 19-5/Pg. 799/True rate is proportional to source positron emission rate, and detector geometric and intrinsic efficiencies. |
| Calculated 511-keV linear attenuation coefficient | $\mu_{511 \text{ keV}} = (9.6 \times 10^{-5} \text{ cm}^{-1}) \cdot (\text{CT number} + 1,000)$ | Pg. 804. CT number-to-511 keV $\mu$ value conversion for tissue densities between air and water. |
| Calculated 511-keV linear attenuation coefficient | $\mu_{511 \text{ keV}} = m \cdot (\text{CT number}) + b$ | Pg. 804. CT number-to-511 keV $\mu$ value conversion for tissue densities above that of water. |
| Time-of-flight signal-to-noise ratio | $SNR_{TOF} \cong \sqrt{\dfrac{D}{\Delta X}} SNR_{Conv} \quad \Delta X = \dfrac{\Delta t}{2}c$ | Pg. 808. SNR increase for TOF relative to non-TOF depends on object diameter and timing resolution. |

*(Continued)*

*(Continued)*

| SYMBOL | QUANTITY | UNITS |
|---|---|---|
| $X_{mag}$ | SPECT X magnification factor | mm/pixel |
| $R_{random}$ | collimator resolution FWHM | counts/sec |
| $\tau$ | coincidence time window | sec |
| $S_1$ | singles rate of one detector of detector pair | counts/sec |
| $S_2$ | singles rate of second detector of detector pair | counts/sec |
| $\lambda$ | Radionuclide decay constant | $sec^{-1}$ |
| $t$ | time | sec |
| $\Delta t$ | time interval | sec |
| DF | decay factor | NA |
| $\mu$ | linear attenuation coefficient | $cm^{-1}$ |
| $d$ | total path length through patient | cm |
| $x$ | distance one photon must travel to escape the patient | cm |
| $\mu/\rho$ | mass attenuation coefficient | $cm^2/g$ |
| SUV | standardized uptake value | $g/cm^3$ |
| $R_d$ | FWHM of detector intrinsic spatial resolution | mm |
| $R_r$ | FWHM of distances traveled by the positrons before annihilation | mm |
| $R_c$ | FWHM due to noncolinearity of annihilation photons | mm |
| $R_l$ | FWHM of determination of photon interaction location in detector block | mm |
| $R_{sys}$ | FWHM of overall PET system resolution | mm |
| $R_T$ | detector pair true coincidence rate | $sec^{-1}$ |
| $A$ | source positron emission rate | $sec^{-1}$ |
| $G$ | detector geometric efficiency | NA |
| $\varepsilon$ | detector intrinsic efficiency | NA |
| $CT_{number}$ | x-ray CT voxel value | HU |
| $m$ | slope | $cm^{-1}$ |
| $b$ | intercept | $cm^{-1}$ |
| $SNR_{TOF}$ | time-of-flight PET signal-to-noise ratio | NA |
| $SNR_{Conv}$ | Conventional PET signal-to-noise ratio | NA |
| $D$ | diameter of the object being imaged | cm |
| $\Delta X$ | time-of-flight distance resolution FWHM | cm |
| $c$ | speed of light | $3 \times 10^8$ m/sec |

# Radiation Biology and Protection

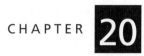

# Radiation Biology

## 20.0 INTRODUCTION

Since the discovery of X-rays and radioactivity over 120 years ago, radiation biology research has amassed more information about the effects of ionizing radiation on living systems than is known about almost any other physical or chemical agent. The biologic response to radiation exposure depends on many factors including variables associated with the radiation source, such as absorbed dose, dose rate, and radiation quality, and biological variables inherent to the cells themselves or to the conditions in the cells at the time of irradiation.

Biologic effects of radiation exposure are classified as follows:

1. **Stochastic effects**: the probability of effect, not severity, increases with dose. Examples include cancer and inherited effects. This leads to the model that risk, for example, of cancer, increases with dose and there is no threshold below which the magnitude of risk goes to zero.
2. **Tissue reactions** (previously called deterministic effects): above a dose threshold, the severity of injury increases with dose, and, in some tissues, the predominant effect is a result of cell killing. Examples of tissue reactions include skin erythema, fibrosis, and hematopoietic damage.

## 20.1 INTERACTION OF RADIATION WITH CELLS AND TISSUES

Observable effects, such as chromosome breakage, cell death, and acute radiation sickness, all have their origin in radiation-induced chemical changes in important biomolecules.

1. Radiation interactions in cells and tissues can produce changes either directly or indirectly.
   a. **Direct action** occurs if a biologic macromolecule such as DNA is ionized or excited by an ionizing particle or photon passing through or near it.
   b. Because cells and tissues are about 70% water, most ionizing radiation interactions will be with water molecules, resulting in production of water-derived free radicals that in turn interact with critical biomolecules like DNA to cause damage, the **indirect action** (Fig. 20-1).
   c. **Free radicals** are atomic or molecular species that have unpaired orbital electrons and are highly reactive.

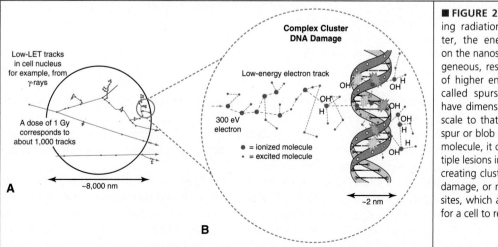

■ **FIGURE 20-1 A.** As ionizing radiation traverses matter, the energy depositions on the nanoscale are inhomogeneous, resulting in regions of higher energy deposition, called spurs or blobs, that have dimensions on a similar scale to that of DNA. **B.** If a spur or blob occurs on a DNA molecule, it can produce multiple lesions in close proximity, creating clustered or complex damage, or multiply damages sites, which are more difficult for a cell to repair accurately.

**d.** The majority of biologically important indirect effects from low-LET radiation are due to reactions of the **hydroxyl radical (·OH)** with DNA.

**e.** The damaging effect of free radicals is enhanced by the presence of oxygen. Oxygen combines with the hydrogen radical to form a highly reactive oxygen species (ROS) such as the hydroperoxyl radical or by reaction with organic radicals, for example, produced on DNA, to form peroxyradicals which are more difficult for a cell to repair.

2. The biological effects of radiation generally increase with increasing LET because the higher specific ionization produces a greater number and more complex clustered DNA damages (Fig. 20-1). The greater effect is quantified using **relative biological effectiveness, RBE**, the ratio of the dose of a reference radiation (usually 250 kV X-rays) to the dose of the high-LET radiation that gives the same level of biological damage.

**a.** RBE tends to increase with LET to a maximum at an LET of about 100 keV/$\mu$m, then decrease at high LET values.

**b.** Although RBE values depend on many factors such as biological system and endpoint, dose, dose rate, and fractionation, they are important for setting radiation weighting factors, $w_R$.

## 20.2 MOLECULAR AND CELLULAR RESPONSE TO RADIATION

1. Ionizing radiation produces a number of types of DNA damages (Fig. 20-2). For mammalian cells, an absorbed dose of 1 Gy from x-rays will produce approximately 40 DSBs, 1,000 SSBs, and 3,000 damaged bases per cell.
2. Regardless of its severity or consequences, the loss or change of a base is considered a type of **mutation**.
3. Chromosome breaks produced by radiation can result in **chromosome aberrations**, which can be observed in cells microscopically during anaphase and metaphase, when the chromosomes are condensed.

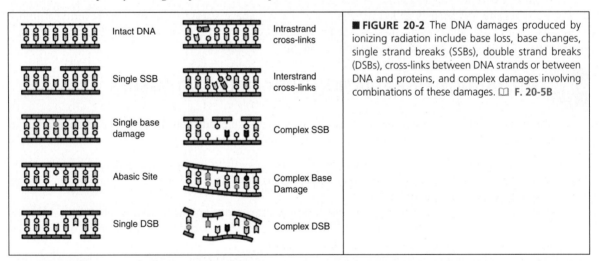

| | |
|---|---|
| Intact DNA | |
| Single SSB | Intrastrand cross-links |
| Single base damage | Interstrand cross-links |
| Abasic Site | Complex SSB |
| Single DSB | Complex Base Damage |
| | Complex DSB |

■ **FIGURE 20-2** The DNA damages produced by ionizing radiation include base loss, base changes, single strand breaks (SSBs), double strand breaks (DSBs), cross-links between DNA strands or between DNA and proteins, and complex damages involving combinations of these damages. 📖 **F. 20-5B**

4. The **DNA damage response (DDR)** in cells may include activation of **cell cycle checkpoints** whereby cell cycle progression is arrested to allow for repair of damaged DNA or incompletely replicated chromosomes or initiation of cell death pathways if the damage is too severe.

**a.** Most of these DNA repair processes occur rapidly (complete within an hour).

**b.** Base excision repair (BER), nucleotide excision repair (NER), mismatch repair (MMR), and homologous recombination repair (HRR) are generally highly accurate, although nonhomologous end joining (NHEJ) is error-prone (Fig. 20-3).

**c.** Defects in the HRR and NHEJ pathways for repair of DSBs can result in increased radiation sensitivity of cells or even in humans who harbor those defective genes.

**d.** Types of **chromosome aberrations** produced by ionizing radiation include fragments, rings, translocations, and dicentrics. Measuring chromosome aberrations in human lymphocytes using fluorescence in situ hybridization (FISH) is a potential way to assess radiation exposure.

For actively proliferating cells, a widely used approach to assess radiation response is the colony formation assay, which assesses the ability of a cell to proliferate indefinitely. **Cell survival curves**, which reflect the relative radiosensitivity of cells, are generally presented as radiation dose plotted on a linear scale on the x-axis and the surviving fraction (SF) from clonogenic assay on a logarithmic scale on the y-axis. Several mathematical models can be used to describe the survival curves, the two most commonly used being the **multitarget (or n-$D_0$) model** (Fig. 20-4) and the **linear-quadratic (LQ) model** (Fig. 20-5).

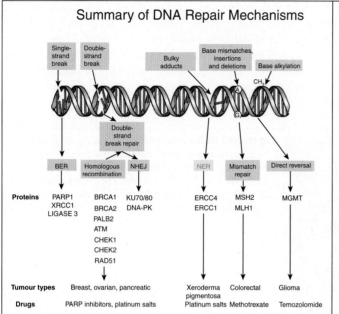

**Summary of DNA Repair Mechanisms**

■ **FIGURE 20-3** Many types of DNA repair exist, including direct repair of a damaged nucleotide, base excision repair (BER), nucleotide excision repair (NER), mismatch repair (MMR), and DSB repair by homologous recombinational repair (HRR) or nonhomologous end-joining (NHEJ), each preferentially working on selected types of damage and each requiring its own set of enzymes. 📖 **F. 20-6A**

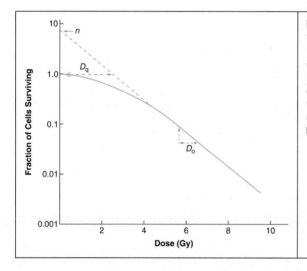

■ **FIGURE 20-4** In the multitarget model, the response to radiation is defined by three parameters: (1) $D_0$, which describes the radiosensitivity of the cell population, is the reciprocal of the slope of the linear portion of the survival curve; (2) the extrapolation number ($n$), which gives a measure of the "shoulder," is found by extrapolating the linear portion of the curve back to its intersection with the $y$-axis; and (3) the quasi-threshold dose ($D_q$), which defines the width of the shoulder region of the survival curve. 📖 **F. 20-10**

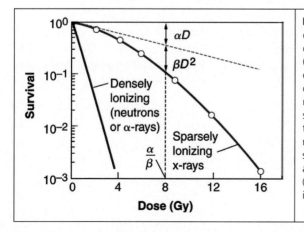

■ **FIGURE 20-5** In the linear-quadratic (LQ) model, now the most often used for survival curves, $SF(D) = e^{-\alpha D + \beta D^2}$ where $D$ is the dose, $\alpha$ is the coefficient of cell killing that is proportional to dose (*i.e.*, the initial linear component on a log-linear plot) and $\beta$ is the coefficient of cell killing that is proportional to the square of the dose (*i.e.*, the quadratic component of the survival curve). The LQ model is useful in radiation therapy because the $\alpha/\beta$ ratio is a measure of the curvature of the cell survival curve and, thus, reflects the sensitivity of different cell types to dose fractionation. Late responding normal tissues, such as spinal cord or lung, that have smaller $\alpha/\beta$ ratios of 3 or 4, are preferentially "spared" by fractionation compared to tumors and early responding normal tissues (gut, skin, bone marrow) where the $\alpha/\beta$ ratio is larger (8 to 12), indicating less repair capacity. 📖 **F. 20-11**

5. Loss of proliferative capacity in irradiated cells can be due to processes such as senescence, quiescence, or terminal differentiation, or because of cell death modes including mitotic catastrophe, apoptosis (Fig. 20-6), autophagy, necroptosis, or necrosis. Most radiation-induced death in proliferating cells results from mitotic death/catastrophe that occurs when cells cannot go through mitosis, generally because of chromosome damage. Nonproliferating cells may be lost through the regulated processes of apoptosis, autophagy or necroptosis, or unregulated necrosis. Each of those processes involves characteristic morphological cell changes and distinct cascades of molecular events.

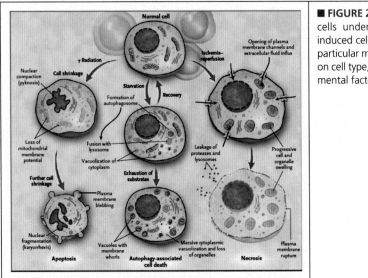

■ **FIGURE 20-6** Comparison of morphological changes in cells undergoing three different modes of radiation-induced cell death: apoptosis, autophagy, and necrosis. A particular mode of cell death may predominate depending on cell type, radiation quality, and dose, and other environmental factors. ▭ **F. 20-12**

   **a.** During **apoptosis,** cells show shrinkage, nuclear condensation, and extensive membrane blebbing, ultimately resulting in cell fragmentation into membrane-bound apoptotic bodies that are eliminated by phagocytosis without causing inflammation. Molecular hallmarks of apoptosis include sequential activation of caspases; interactions of pro- and antiapoptotic members of the Bcl-2 family of proteins, many at the mitochondria; cleavage of multiple proteins; and, ultimately, internucleosomal DNA cleavage. Radiation can induce apoptosis through DNA damage initiating transcription of proapoptotic proteins that activate intrinsic apoptosis or up-regulation of death receptors to initiate extrinsic apoptosis pathways.

   **b. Autophagy** is a process of "self-digestion" of cellular components that can be initiated to obtain energy in cells starved of nutrients or to remove damaged molecules and components, promoting cell survival. It also can be activated by genotoxic stress, such as radiation-induced DNA damage, and if the cell damage is extensive, lead to cell death with characteristic morphology and protein cascades.

6. Radiation response can be influenced by conditional factors such as dose rate, LET, and the presence of oxygen, as well as by inherent biologic factors that are characteristic of the cells themselves, such as mitotic rate, degree of differentiation, and stage of the cell cycle.

   **a.** The rate at which low-LET radiation is delivered affects the degree of biologic damage (Fig. 20-7). In general, high dose rates are more effective at producing biologic damage than low dose rates, presumably because there is more time to repair sublethal damage when the dose is delivered slowly over time.

   **b.** In a similar fashion, if a radiation dose is fractionated into two or more doses with time in between, sublethal damage can be repaired between the fractions, resulting in decreased damage (Fig. 20-8). This concept is fundamental to radiation therapy where, traditionally, dose has been fractionated into multiple daily doses, which "spares" normal tissues, especially late responding normal tissues, relative to tumors.

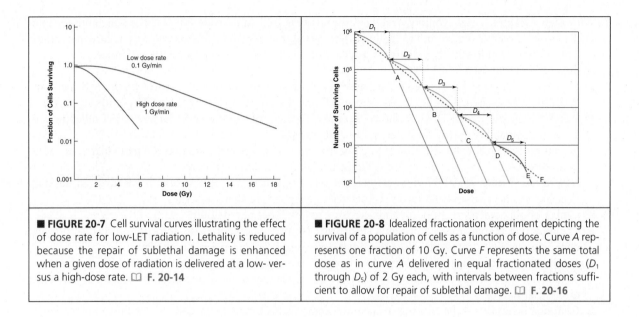

**■ FIGURE 20-7** Cell survival curves illustrating the effect of dose rate for low-LET radiation. Lethality is reduced because the repair of sublethal damage is enhanced when a given dose of radiation is delivered at a low- versus a high-dose rate. 📖 **F. 20-14**

**■ FIGURE 20-8** Idealized fractionation experiment depicting the survival of a population of cells as a function of dose. Curve *A* represents one fraction of 10 Gy. Curve *F* represents the same total dose as in curve *A* delivered in equal fractionated doses ($D_1$ through $D_5$) of 2 Gy each, with intervals between fractions sufficient to allow for repair of sublethal damage. 📖 **F. 20-16**

c. High-LET radiation is considerably more effective in producing cell damage than low-LET radiation (Fig. 20-9) because the dense ionization tracks typically produce more complex, clustered DNA damage that cannot be repaired accurately (Fig. 20-1). Because the complex damage is difficult to repair, there is also a decrease in the dose rate effect as LET increases.

d. Under hypoxic conditions, the level of damage caused by low-LET radiation is decreased, relative to the damage when cells are irradiated in the presence of oxygen (Fig. 20-10). The difference is quantified using the **oxygen enhancement ratio (OER)**, defined as the radiation dose that produces a given biologic response in the absence of oxygen divided by the dose that produces the same biologic response in the presence of oxygen. The OER in well-aerated cells and tissues is 2.5 to 3 with low-LET radiation but decreases to 1.0 (*i.e.*, no oxygen effect) with high-LET radiation. The radiation resistance of hypoxic cells can be important in radiation therapy because some human tumors contain hypoxic regions.

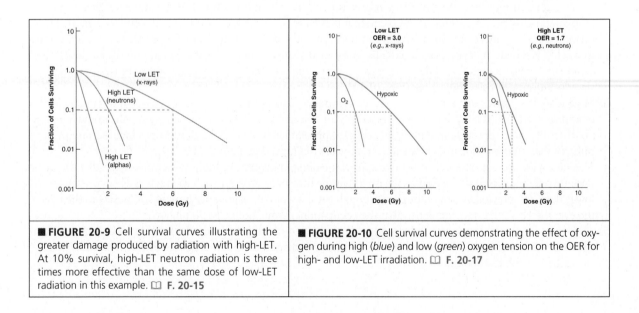

**■ FIGURE 20-9** Cell survival curves illustrating the greater damage produced by radiation with high-LET. At 10% survival, high-LET neutron radiation is three times more effective than the same dose of low-LET radiation in this example. 📖 **F. 20-15**

**■ FIGURE 20-10** Cell survival curves demonstrating the effect of oxygen during high (*blue*) and low (*green*) oxygen tension on the OER for high- and low-LET irradiation. 📖 **F. 20-17**

7. With a few exceptions (*e.g.*, lymphocytes), radiosensitivity is greatest for cells that (1) have a high mitotic rate, (2) have a long mitotic future, and (3) are undifferentiated. For example, bone marrow stem/early progenitor cells are extremely radiosensitive, whereas the fixed postmitotic cells that comprise the central nervous system are relatively radioresistant.

   a. In general, cells exposed to low-LET radiation are most sensitive during mitosis (M phase) and the "gap" between S phase and mitosis ($G_2$), less sensitive during the preparatory period for DNA synthesis ($G_1$), and least sensitive during late DNA synthesis (S phase). The sensitivity differences largely reflect differences in cellular repair ability during the different cell cycle phases.

   b. Radiation also can alter the function of proteins involved in cell cycle checkpoints. Of particular note, radiation can cause cell cycle arrest in proliferating cells in the $G_1$ and $G_2$ phases, with $G_1$ arrest dependent on cells having a wild-type TP53 tumor suppressor gene, producing the p53 protein that is involved not only in cell cycle arrest but in DNA repair and activating apoptosis in some cell types.

8. A number of phenomena might occur after exposure to low doses of radiation.

   a. The **adaptive response** is seen when a small (*e.g.*, 10 mGy) radiation dose, sometimes called a "priming dose," decreases the damaging effect of a larger dose (*e.g.*, 2 Gy) given a few hours later.

   b. The **bystander effect** is the observation of changes, for example, DNA damage or altered gene expression, in cells not traversed by radiation when they are in the vicinity of irradiated cells and receive signals from those irradiated cells.

   c. **Genomic instability** is the occurrence of chromosome changes, mutations, delayed lethality, or other alterations in the progeny of cells that were irradiated but did not appear to show these changes.

## 20.3  TISSUE AND ORGAN SYSTEM RESPONSE TO RADIATION

1. Tissue reactions depend on parenchymal and stem cell killing as well as on complex events including inflammatory, chronic oxidative, and immune reactions, and damage to vasculature and extracellular matrix.

   a. In general, **early reactions**, such as in skin and GI tract, involve killing of the stem/early progenitor cells that supply the mature functional cells in the tissue, as well as inflammatory reactions.

   b. **Late reactions**, for example, in lung, kidney, and brain, involve complex, dynamic interactions among multiple cell types in the tissues and organs and include infiltrating immune cells, production of cytokines, and growth factors, often in persistent, cyclic cascades, and chronic oxidative stress.

2. While radiation-induced skin damage is relatively rare, it is the most commonly encountered tissue reaction following high-dose image-guided interventional procedures. The degree of damage depends on the radiation quantity, quality, and dose rate as well as on the location and size of the irradiated field. Acute effects (days to weeks) can include erythema and edema, moist or dry desquamation or ulceration (after high doses), and changes in pigmentation. Late effects (months to years) include changes in pigmentation, fibrosis, telangiectasia, ulceration, necrosis, and cancer (Fig. 20-11).

3. In general, the gonads are very radiosensitive. Temporary and permanent sterility can occur after acute doses of approximately 500 mGy and 6 Gy, respectively, in the male. In females, the dose that will produce permanent sterility is age-dependent, with higher doses (approximately 10 Gy) required to produce sterility prior to puberty than in premenopausal women over 40 years old (approximately 2 to 3 Gy).

4. The lens of the eye is particularly sensitive to the formation of radiation-induced posterior subcapsular cataracts. Recent epidemiological studies have suggested that the threshold dose for such cataracts is about 0.5 Gy, much lower than had previously been thought. Although the current U.S. regulatory limit is 150 mSv/y to the lens of the eye, the NCRP has recommended that the occupational limit should be 50 mGy/y.

5. Threshold doses and latency periods (time to appearance of damage after irradiation) for normal tissue damage vary substantially with tissue and are dependent on radiation dose and dose rate or fractionation. (Consult Table 20-5 in the textbook.)

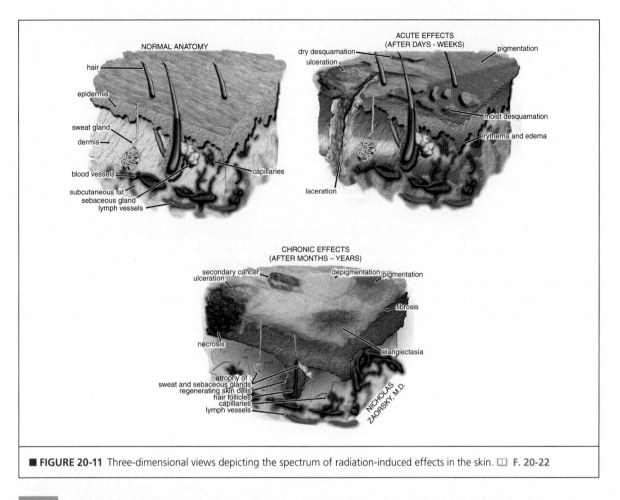

**■ FIGURE 20-11** Three-dimensional views depicting the spectrum of radiation-induced effects in the skin. 📖 **F. 20-22**

## 20.4 WHOLE BODY RESPONSE TO RADIATION: THE ACUTE RADIATION SYNDROME

1. When the whole body (or a large portion of the body) is exposed to a high acute radiation dose, there are a series of characteristic clinical responses known collectively as the **acute radiation syndrome (ARS)**. In order of occurrence with increasing radiation dose, the ARS includes the hematopoietic, gastrointestinal, and neurovascular syndromes. The clinical manifestation of each subsyndrome occurs in a sequence that includes the **prodromal, latent, manifest illness**, and, if the dose is not fatal, recovery stages (Fig. 20-12).

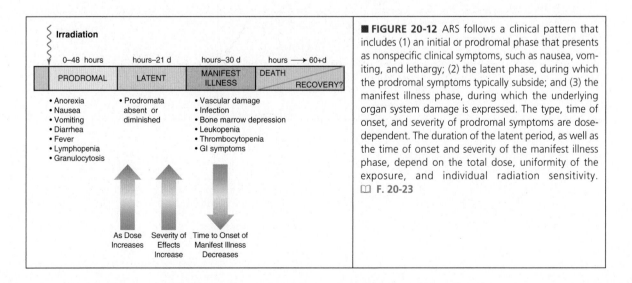

**■ FIGURE 20-12** ARS follows a clinical pattern that includes (1) an initial or prodromal phase that presents as nonspecific clinical symptoms, such as nausea, vomiting, and lethargy; (2) the latent phase, during which the prodromal symptoms typically subside; and (3) the manifest illness phase, during which the underlying organ system damage is expressed. The type, time of onset, and severity of prodromal symptoms are dose-dependent. The duration of the latent period, as well as the time of onset and severity of the manifest illness phase, depend on the total dose, uniformity of the exposure, and individual radiation sensitivity. 📖 **F. 20-23**

a. The **prodromal symptoms** can include anorexia, nausea, lethargy, fever, vomiting, headache, diarrhea, and altered mental status. The time of onset and severity of prodromal symptoms is dose-dependent with a threshold of about 0.5 to 1.0 Gy. The prodromal symptoms subside during the latent period, the length of which is dose-dependent, and then symptoms of the manifest illness occur.

b. Symptoms of the **hematopoietic syndrome** include fever, chills, fatigue, and hemorrhages as a result of loss of circulating blood elements due to radiation sterilization of the mitotically active precursor cells (Fig. 20-13). It occurs after acute radiation doses between 0.5 and 10 Gy. Healthy adults with proper medical care almost always recover from doses lower than 2 Gy, whereas doses greater than 8 Gy are almost always fatal unless advanced therapies such as colony-stimulating factors or bone marrow transplantation are successful.

c. In the absence of medical care, the human **LD$_{50/60}$** (the dose that would be expected to kill 50% of an exposed population within 60 days) is approximately 3.5 to 4.5 Gy total body. The LD$_{50/60}$ may extend to 6 to 7 Gy with supportive care such as transfusions and antibiotics and may be as high as 8 Gy with hematopoietic growth factors in an intensive care setting.

d. At doses greater than 12 Gy, the **gastrointestinal syndrome** becomes prominent and is primarily responsible for lethality. The symptoms of malnutrition, vomiting and diarrhea, anemia, sepsis, dehydration, and acute renal failure from fluid and electrolyte imbalance, reflect the denudation of the mucosal lining of the GI tract due to the loss of reproductive capacity of the intestinal crypt stem cells. These changes in the GI tract are compounded by equally drastic changes in the bone marrow, although those have not reached peak effect in the circulating bloodstream. Death is essentially 100% and occurs within 3 to 10 days after the exposure if no medical care is given or as long as 2 weeks afterward with intensive medical support.

e. Death from the **neurovascular syndrome** (also called cerebrovascular syndrome) occurs within 2 to 3 days after doses in excess of 50 Gy. Death is caused by cardiovascular shock, massive edema, increased intracranial pressure, and cerebral anoxia, in part caused by severe damage to the microvasculature.

f. The clinical features of the manifest illness phase of ARS are summarized in Table 20-1.

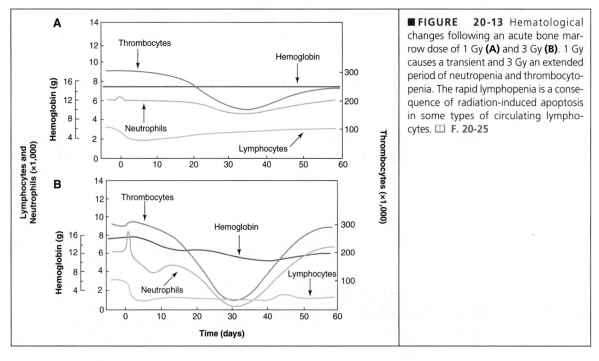

■ **FIGURE 20-13** Hematological changes following an acute bone marrow dose of 1 Gy **(A)** and 3 Gy **(B)**. 1 Gy causes a transient and 3 Gy an extended period of neutropenia and thrombocytopenia. The rapid lymphopenia is a consequence of radiation-induced apoptosis in some types of circulating lymphocytes. 📖 **F. 20-25**

**TABLE 20-1 CLINICAL FEATURES DURING THE MANIFEST ILLNESS PHASE OF ARS** 🕮 T. 20-7

| | | | | | |
|---|---|---|---|---|---|
| | | DEGREE OF ARS AND APPROXIMATE DOSE OF ACUTE WHOLE-BODY EXPOSURE | | | |
| | *MILD (1–2 Gy)* | *MODERATE (2–4 Gy)* | *SEVERE (4–6 Gy)* | *VERY SEVERE (6–8 Gy)* | *LETHAL (>8 Gy)* |
| Onset of signs | >30 d | 18–28 d | 8–18 d | <7 d | <3 d |
| Lymphocytes, G/L[a] | 0.8–1.5 | 0.5–0.8 | 0.3–0.5 | 0.1–0.3 | 0.0–0.1 |
| Platelets, G/L[a] | 60–100 | 30–60 | 25–35 | 15–25 | <20 |
| Percent of patients with cytopenia | 10%–25% | 25%–40% | 40%–80% | 60%–80% | 80%–100%[b] |
| Clinical manifestations | Fatigue, weakness | Fever, infections, bleeding, weakness, epilation | High fever, infections, bleeding, epilation | High fever, diarrhea, vomiting, dizziness and disorientation, hypotension | High fever, diarrhea, unconsciousness |
| Lethality, % | 0–1 | 0–50 | 20–70 | 50–100 | 100 |
| Onset | 6–8 wk | 6–8 wk | 4–8 wk | 1–2 wk | 1–2 wk |
| Medical response | Prophylactic | Special prophylactic treatment from days 14–20; isolation from days 10–20 | Special prophylactic treatment from days 7–10; isolation from the beginning | Special treatment from the first day; isolation from the beginning | 1–2 wk symptomatic only |

[a]G/L, SI units for concentration and refers to $10^9$ per liter.
[b]In very severe cases, with a dose greater than 50 Gy, death precedes cytopenia.
*Source*: Adapted from *Diagnosis and Treatment of Radiation Injuries*. Safety Report Series No. 2. Vienna, Austria: International Atomic Energy Agency; 1998; Koenig KL, Goans RE, Hatchett RJ, et al. Medical treatment of radiological casualties: current concepts. *Ann Emerg Med*. 2005;45:643-652. Copyright © Elsevier.

## 20.5 RADIATION-INDUCED CARCINOGENESIS

1. **Cancer** is the most important delayed somatic effect of radiation exposure. However, radiation is a relatively weak carcinogen at low doses (*e.g.*, occupational and diagnostic exposures), and significantly increased cancer risks cannot be detected at the doses typically encountered in diagnostic imaging.
    a. Baseline cancer rates must be kept in mind when evaluating radiation-induced cancer rates. The baseline annual cancer incidence and mortality age-adjusted rates, for the U.S. population, are approximately 436 and 156 per 100,000, respectively, with males having a higher incidence rate (471 per 100,000) than females (413 per 100,000).
2. Cancer arises from abnormal cell division, with cells in a tumor thought to descend from a common ancestral cell that at some point lost control over normal reproduction.
    a. Two classes of genes, **tumor suppressor genes**, for example, *TP53*, and **oncogenes**, for example, the *RAS* family, which respectively inhibit and encourage cell growth, play major roles in triggering cancer.
    b. In a simplified fashion, cancer formation has been thought of as developing in three stages: (1) **initiation** due to damage in a single cell resulting in a preneoplastic stage followed by (2) **promotion** which permits the cell to successfully proliferate then (3) **progression** during which the transformed cell produces phenotypic clones of which one acquires the advantage of evading the host's defense mechanisms, thus allowing tumor development.
    c. It is now recognized that as cells evolve to a neoplasm, they acquire a succession of capabilities that enable them to become tumorigenic and ultimately malignant. Hanahan and Weinberg originally described six **"Hallmarks of Cancer"**—sustaining proliferative signaling, evading growth suppressors, resisting cell death, enabling replicative immortality, inducing angiogenesis, and activating invasion and metastasis—and more recently have enumerated two enabling characteristics—genome instability and inflammation—and two emerging hallmarks—energy metabolism and evading immune destruction (Fig. 20-14A).
    d. Furthermore, tumors are complex tissues, composed of multiple interacting cell types including stromal cells, such as fibroblasts, and the endothelial cells and pericytes of the vasculature, as well as immune inflammatory cells (Fig. 20-14B). Together, these various cell types create a **tumor microenvironment** that is critical for cancer development and can influence tumor response to treatments, including radiation.

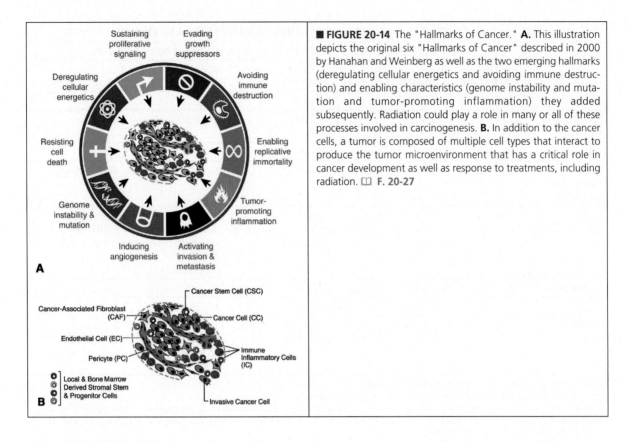

■ **FIGURE 20-14** The "Hallmarks of Cancer." **A.** This illustration depicts the original six "Hallmarks of Cancer" described in 2000 by Hanahan and Weinberg as well as the two emerging hallmarks (deregulating cellular energetics and avoiding immune destruction) and enabling characteristics (genome instability and mutation and tumor-promoting inflammation) they added subsequently. Radiation could play a role in many or all of these processes involved in carcinogenesis. **B.** In addition to the cancer cells, a tumor is composed of multiple cell types that interact to produce the tumor microenvironment that has a critical role in cancer development as well as response to treatments, including radiation. 📖 **F. 20-27**

3. A number of factors such as tobacco, alcohol, diet, sexual behavior, air pollution, and bacterial and viral infections may promote cancer or modify its risk.

4. Risk from radiation (or any other agent) in an exposed population can be expressed in several ways.

    **a.** **Relative risk (RR)** is the ratio of the disease (*e.g.*, cancer) incidence in the exposed population to that in the general (unexposed) population.

    **b.** **Excess relative risk (ERR)** is RR – 1.

    **c.** **Absolute risk (AR)** is the number of excess cancer cases per 100,000 in a population.

    **d.** **Excess absolute risk (EAR)**, also referred to as **excess attributable risk,** is the difference between two absolute risks and is commonly used in radiation epidemiology expressed as the EAR per unit dose.

5. The probability of developing a radiation-induced cancer depends on several physical factors such as radiation quality, dose, and dose rate or fractionation, and biological factors including age, tissue, and sex.

    **a.** RBE values for high-LET radiation (*e.g.*, α-particles) have large uncertainties and range from as high as 20 for liver cancer to 1 for leukemia. Low-energy photons may be more effective than high-energy photons at inducing cancer, presumably because of the higher LET of lower energy secondary electrons, but epidemiological support is lacking.

    **b.** For most types of damage to cells and tissues, the biological effectiveness of the radiation decreases at lower dose rates or with fractionation.

        **(i)** For cancer risk, currently, a **dose and dose-rate effectiveness factor (DDREF)** is used to convert high–dose-rate risk estimates to estimates for exposure at low-dose rates for the purposes of radiation protection.

        **(ii)** At the low doses associated with diagnostic examinations and occupational exposures, dose rate may not affect cancer risk.

    **c.** Latency and the risk of radiation-induced cancers vary with sex, type of cancer, and age at the time of exposure.

        **(i)** For whole-body exposure, females on average have a 40% higher risk of radiogenic cancer than males.

        **(ii)** The organs at greatest risk for radiogenic cancer induction and mortality are breast and lung for women and lung and colon for men.

        **(iii)** The minimal latent period is 2 to 3 years for leukemia, while latent periods for solid tumors range from 5 to 40 years.

    **d.** Mutations in one or more specific genes, while rare, increase susceptibility to developing cancer.

        **(i)** For example, women with inherited mutations in the breast cancer susceptibility genes 1 or 2 (*BRCA1* or *BRCA2*) and a family history of multiple cases of breast cancer carry a lifetime risk of breast cancer that is approximately 5 times higher than for women in the general population.

        **(ii)** Another example is patients with an ataxia-telangiectasia mutated (*ATM*) gene, who are at substantially higher risk of developing cancer than the general population and are also hypersensitive to ionizing radiation because of defective DNA repair mechanisms.

        **(iii)** The extent to which radiation exposure modifies the cancer risk in patients with these inherited mutations is still not clear.

**6.** Although there is general agreement from human epidemiological data that above cumulative doses of 100 to 150 mSv (acute or protracted exposure), exposure to ionizing radiation likely increases the risk of some cancers, insufficient data exist to determine accurately the risks of lower dose radiation exposure to human.

    **a.** The major populations used in epidemiologic investigations of low-dose radiation effects are as follows:

        **(i)** The Life Span Study (LSS) cohort of survivors of the atomic bomb explosions in Hiroshima and Nagasaki

        **(ii)** Patients with medical exposure during treatment of a variety of neoplastic and nonneoplastic diseases

        **(iii)** Persons with occupational exposures

        **(iv)** Populations with high natural background exposures

    **b.** It is very difficult to detect a small increase in the cancer rate due to radiation exposure at low doses (less than ~100 mSv) because radiation is a relatively weak carcinogen, the natural incidence of many types of cancer is high and the latent period for most cancers is long. To rule out statistical fluctuations, a very large irradiated population is required.

    **c.** General points of agreement in many epidemiology studies include the following:

        **(i)** Risk varies according to cancer site.

        **(ii)** Risk is greater when exposures occur at younger ages.

        **(iii)** Risk is greater for females than males.

        **(iv)** Solid cancer risk is consistent with a linear function of dose when all cancers are combined.

        **(v)** Leukemia risk is consistent with a nonlinear function of dose.

        **(vi)** Except for leukemia for which there is a fairly well-defined risk interval following exposure, the risk remains elevated for 50+ years after exposure.

**7.** Scientists have developed dose-response models to predict the risk of cancer in human populations from exposure to low levels of ionizing radiation.

    **a.** The shapes of the radiation dose-response curves for cancer in humans have been characterized as **linear nonthreshold (LNT), linear-quadratic (LQ), threshold, and hormesis** (Fig. 20-15).

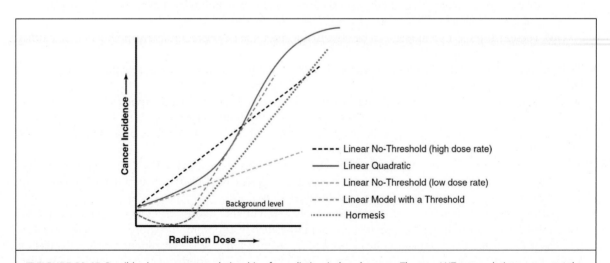

■ **FIGURE 20-15** Possible dose-response relationships for radiation-induced cancer. The two LNT extrapolations represent the high dose and dose rate (*black*) and low dose rate (*orange*) components of the dose-response data. The LQ dose-response curve (*red*) demonstrates reduced effectiveness for radiogenic cancer induction at lower dose and greater effectiveness at higher dose that eventually flattens out due to substantial cell killing. There is also epidemiological evidence for a threshold for some cancers (*blue dashed line*). The hormesis curve (*green*) illustrates a hypothesis that low levels of radiation are beneficial because of the activation of processes such as DNA repair or up-regulation of antioxidant defenses that protect against radiation-induced cancer. ▢ **F. 20-32**

**b.** Although for some types of radiation exposure in specific tissues there appears to be a threshold dose below which no radiogenic cancer risk is evident, the evidence supporting this model is not sufficient to be accepted for general use in assessing cancer risk from radiation exposure. **NCRP, BEIR VII, and ICRP recommend that, based on current epidemiologic data, the LNT model should be used for radiation protection purposes**.

**c.** A DDREF may be used to adjust risk estimates from exposures at high dose and high dose rate to the much lower doses typically encountered in occupational and public settings within a system of radiation protection. The BEIR VII committee applied a DDREF of 1.5 to adjust the response observed in the high-dose range, making it roughly equivalent to the line representing the low-dose response (Fig. 20-16), although UNSCEAR and ICRP use a DDREF of 2.

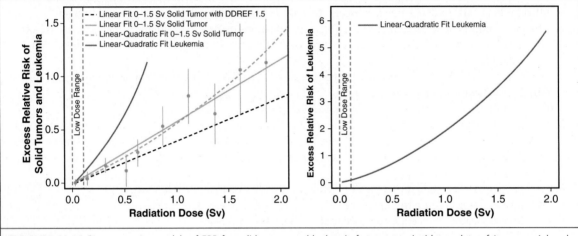

■ **FIGURE 20-16** Dose-response models of ERR for solid cancer and leukemia from cancer incidence data of Japanese A-bomb survivors (averaged over gender and standardized to represent individuals exposed at age 30 who have attained age 60).
📖 F. 20-33

**d.** Estimates of radiation-induced cancer can use multiplicative and/or additive risk models.

   **(i)** The **multiplicative risk-projection model** (also called the relative risk model) is based on the assumption that the excess cancer risk increases in proportion to the baseline cancer rate (Fig. 20-17A).

   **(ii)** The **additive (or absolute) risk model** (expressed in terms of EAR) is based on the assumption that, following the latent period, the excess cancer rate is constant and independent of the spontaneous population and age-specific natural cancer risk (Fig. 20-17B).

   **(iii)** These risk-projection models can be used to transport risk calculated from one population to another dissimilar population.

**8.** Estimates of the total cancer incidence and mortality risk as a function of sex and age at exposure are provided in the BEIR VII report (Fig. 20-18).

   **a.** The increased risk for radiation-induced cancer in children and infants is easily appreciated. Compared to the risk to adults, the risk for a 12-month-old infant is three to four times higher.

   **b.** The increased risk of radiation exposure in females compared to males at all ages is also shown; the magnitude of the difference decreases with age.

   **c.** This overall increase in cancer risk is not the same for all organs nor at all ages. For some organs, there does not appear to be an increase in risk with younger age at exposure (*e.g.*, bladder), and for at least one (lung), there is a decrease in risk with younger exposure age.

**9.** Population-averaged radiation-induced cancer incidence and mortality risk estimates are shown in Table 20-2. To estimate the risk to the general population from low radiation exposure, the approximate values of 11% and 6% per Sv, respectively, for cancer incidence and mortality can be used. As mentioned earlier, the lifetime probabilities of developing or dying from cancer in the United States are approximately 41% and 22%, respectively. According to the linear risk projection model, an acute exposure of 100 people to 100 mSv would add approximately 1 additional cancer case to the 41 normally expected to occur over the lifetime of a group with an age and sex distribution similar to the general population.

**10.** Evaluations of both benefit and risk are important in the use of radiation for medical imaging, and understanding limitations and uncertainties in published epidemiology studies is important for those evaluations.

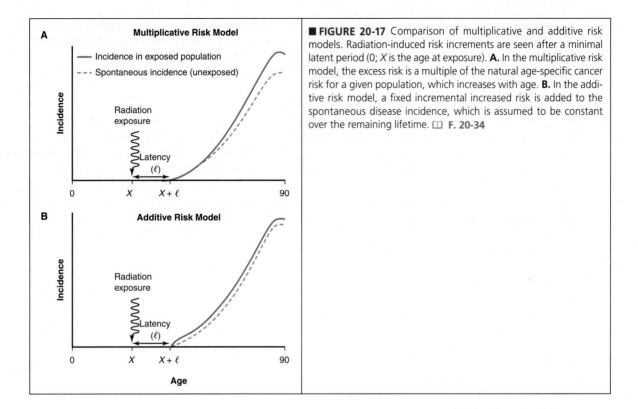

**FIGURE 20-17** Comparison of multiplicative and additive risk models. Radiation-induced risk increments are seen after a minimal latent period (0; *X* is the age at exposure). **A.** In the multiplicative risk model, the excess risk is a multiple of the natural age-specific cancer risk for a given population, which increases with age. **B.** In the additive risk model, a fixed incremental increased risk is added to the spontaneous disease incidence, which is assumed to be constant over the remaining lifetime. 📖 **F. 20-34**

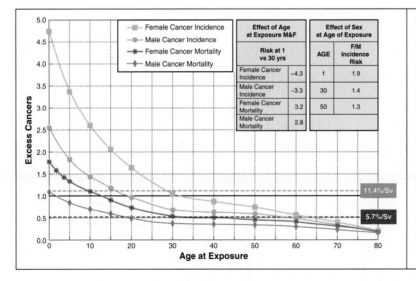

**FIGURE 20-18** Lifetime radiation cancer incidence and mortality as a function of sex and age at exposure. Excess cancer cases per 1,000 following a whole-body dose of 10 mSv (multiply by 10 to convert to percent per Sv). The **table insets** show the relative effect on cancer incidence and mortality for exposures at ages 1 and 30 years old (**left**) and the relative increased radiogenic cancer risk for females compared to males as a function of exposure at 1, 30, and 50 years old (**right**). The population-averaged cancer incidence of 11.4% per Sv (*green line*) and mortality of 5.7% per Sv (*red line*) as calculated from the BEIR VII data are superimposed over the age and sex-specific risk estimates. 📖 **F. 20-36**

**TABLE 20-2 THE U.S. POPULATION AVERAGED RADIATION-INDUCED CANCER INCIDENCE AND MORTALITY RISK ESTIMATES IN PERCENT PER Sv**

| | INCIDENCE | MORTALITY |
|---|---|---|
| Female | 13.7 | 6.6 |
| Male | 9.0 | 4.8 |
| U.S. population average | 11.4 | 5.7 |

*Source:* Calculated from *Health Risks from Exposure to Low Levels of Ionizing Radiation: BEIR VII, Phase 2.* Committee to Assess Health Risks from Exposure to Low Levels of Ionizing Radiation, Board of Radiation Effects, Research Division on Earth and Life Studies, National Research Council of the National Academies. National Academy of Sciences, Washington, DC: National Academies Press; 2006.

a. For example, recent epidemiologic studies of the important question of risks of CT scans during childhood have yielded controversial and contradictory findings. In evaluating the findings, one must realize that study results are subject to significant uncertainties including, but not limited to the following:

   (i) Partial body (or organ) irradiations

   (ii) Lack of historical exposure data

   (iii) Limited organ dosimetry for organs other than the target organ

   (iv) Potential biases because radiologic procedures are often administered for an existing health condition

b. The effective dose concept can be helpful in framing (but not quantifying), the generally small radiation risk associated with CT procedures that are both justified (anticipated benefit greater than the corresponding risk) and optimized (doses utilized are not higher than those required for producing images of diagnostic quality).

c. Communicating with staff, patients, and the public on both benefits and risks of medical imaging procedures is challenging but necessary. To assist in communications, the NCRP has suggested a classification scheme for use of effective dose as a qualitative indicator of radiation detriment for balancing against potential medical benefits, utilizing the following descriptors:

   (i) Negligible (less than 0.1 mSv)

   (ii) Minimal (0.1 to 1 mSv)

   (iii) Minor (greater than 1 to 10 mSv)

   (iv) Low (greater than 10 to 100 mSv)

   (v) Acceptable in the context of the expected benefit (greater than 100 mSv)

d. In this construct, most justified CT examinations could be described as a minimal or minor radiation detriment risk to be balanced with likely individual benefit.

11. Leukemia is one of the most frequently observed radiation-induced cancers.

   a. Excess leukemia cases can be detected as soon as 1 to 2 years after exposure and reach a peak approximately 12 years after the exposure.

   b. The incidence of leukemia is influenced by age at the time of exposure. The incidence of radiation-induced leukemia decreases with age at the time of exposure, but the interval of increased risk is prolonged (Fig. 20-19).

   c. Therefore, it is useful to express risk as a function of time since exposure rather than attained age (Fig. 20-20).

   d. Because the risk estimates for radiation-induced leukemia are based on a LQ function of dose, there was no need to apply a DDREF.

   e. The BEIR VII preferred model for leukemia estimates an excess lifetime risk from an exposure to 0.1 Gy for 100,000 persons with an age distribution similar to that of the U.S. population to be approximately 70 and 100, for females and males, respectively (*i.e.*, approximately 1% per Sv).

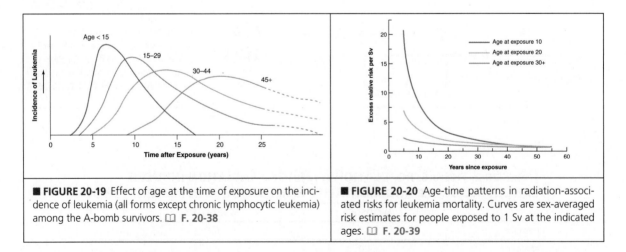

■ **FIGURE 20-19** Effect of age at the time of exposure on the incidence of leukemia (all forms except chronic lymphocytic leukemia) among the A-bomb survivors. 📖 **F. 20-38**

■ **FIGURE 20-20** Age-time patterns in radiation-associated risks for leukemia mortality. Curves are sex-averaged risk estimates for people exposed to 1 Sv at the indicated ages. 📖 **F. 20-39**

12. Estimates of ERR per Sv for a range of site-specific solid cancers are shown in Figure 20-21.

   a. Due to the considerable ability of the thyroid gland to concentrate iodine, the thyroid dose from elemental or ionic radioiodine is typically 1,000 times greater than in other organs in the body. However, the relative

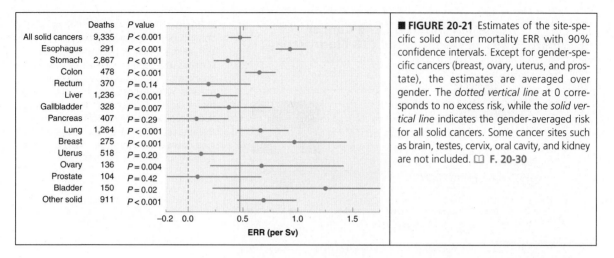

|  | Deaths | P value |
| --- | --- | --- |
| All solid cancers | 9,335 | P < 0.001 |
| Esophagus | 291 | P < 0.001 |
| Stomach | 2,867 | P < 0.001 |
| Colon | 478 | P < 0.001 |
| Rectum | 370 | P = 0.14 |
| Liver | 1,236 | P < 0.001 |
| Gallbladder | 328 | P = 0.007 |
| Pancreas | 407 | P = 0.29 |
| Lung | 1,264 | P < 0.001 |
| Breast | 275 | P < 0.001 |
| Uterus | 518 | P = 0.20 |
| Ovary | 136 | P = 0.004 |
| Prostate | 104 | P = 0.42 |
| Bladder | 150 | P = 0.02 |
| Other solid | 911 | P < 0.001 |

ERR (per Sv)

■ **FIGURE 20-21** Estimates of the site-specific solid cancer mortality ERR with 90% confidence intervals. Except for gender-specific cancers (breast, ovary, uterus, and prostate), the estimates are averaged over gender. The *dotted vertical line* at 0 corresponds to no excess risk, while the *solid vertical line* indicates the gender-averaged risk for all solid cancers. Some cancer sites such as brain, testes, cervix, oral cavity, and kidney are not included. 📖 **F. 20-30**

effectiveness of producing radiogenic thyroid cancer from internally deposited radionuclides has been shown to be approximately 60% to 100% as effective as external x-irradiation. Thus, thyroid cancer is a major concern following exposure to radioiodine, especially in children, as was seen following the Chernobyl nuclear power plant accident.

   **b.** Breast cancer is the most commonly diagnosed cancer among women regardless of race or ethnicity. For women exposed to ionizing radiation during mammography, the potential for an increase in the risk of breast cancer is a concern.

   **(i)** The available epidemiological data on breast cancer fit a linear dose-response model and indicate that fractionation of the dose does not reduce the risk of breast cancer induced by low-LET radiation, although there is some evidence that protracted exposure to radiation in children reduces the risk of radiation-induced breast cancer compared with acute or highly fractionated exposures.

   **(ii)** The latent period ranges from 10 to 40 years, with younger women having longer latencies. In contrast to leukemia, there is no identifiable window of expression; therefore, the risk seems to continue throughout the life of the exposed individual.

   **(iii)** The lifetime attributable risk of developing breast cancer is very age-dependent, being approximately 13 times higher for exposure at age 5 than at age 50.

   **(iv)** Improvements in quality assurance and the introduction of digital mammography, including the use of automatic tube current modulation (TCM) capability, have resulted in a substantial reduction in the dose to the breast. The exposures for mammographic images are substantially below the levels for which significantly increased risks have been detected.

13. The lung is another organ in which there has been considerable debate about the dose-response for cancer and whether there is a sex-specific risk for radiation-induced cancer.

   **a.** An increased risk of lung cancer from radiation has been found in the LSS, which also indicates that the risk is nearly three times greater in women than in men.

   **b.** On the other hand, studies on tuberculosis patients who received frequent chest x-rays to monitor lung collapse therapy and in some occupationally exposed cohorts in the Million Person Study have not shown any increased risk for lung cancer (Fig. 20-22).

   **c.** The reasons for the differences in these dose responses for lung cancer are unclear, although one possibility is the differences in the dose rate.

14. Studies of some radiotherapy patient populations have demonstrated increased risks for diseases other than cancer, particularly cardiovascular disease, mostly at high doses.

   **a.** There is also evidence of an increase in cardiovascular disease at much lower doses among A-bomb survivors; however, there is no statistically significant increase at doses below 0.5 Sv.

   **b.** There is no direct evidence for an increased risk of cardiovascular disease or other noncancer effects at the low doses associated with occupational exposures and diagnostic imaging procedures and, thus far, the data are inadequate to quantify this risk if it exists.

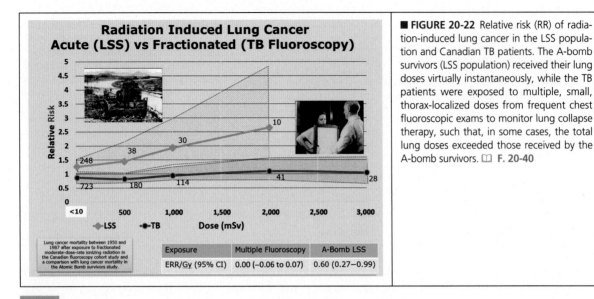

■ **FIGURE 20-22** Relative risk (RR) of radiation-induced lung cancer in the LSS population and Canadian TB patients. The A-bomb survivors (LSS population) received their lung doses virtually instantaneously, while the TB patients were exposed to multiple, small, thorax-localized doses from frequent chest fluoroscopic exams to monitor lung collapse therapy, such that, in some cases, the total lung doses exceeded those received by the A-bomb survivors. ▭ F. 20-40

## 20.6 HEREDITARY EFFECTS OF RADIATION EXPOSURE

1. Although studies in the 1920s and 1950s showed radiation-induced hereditary effects in fruit flies and mice, no human studies have demonstrated significant transgenerational effects from parental irradiation.
   a. Populations that have been studied include children of the survivors of the atomic bombings in Japan, offspring of U.S. radiologic technologists, and children of individuals who had radiotherapy for cancer.
   b. The *doubling dose*, the dose required per generation to double the spontaneous mutation rate, for humans is estimated to be approximately 1 Gy per generation, based on extrapolation from animal data.
   c. The ICRP currently estimates the genetic risks, up to the second generation, to be about 0.2% per Gy, compared to a normal incidence of genetic disorders of about 5%.

## 20.7 RADIATION EFFECTS IN UTERO

1. The effects of radiation exposure in utero depend on the stage of development at the time of exposure (Fig. 20-23) and characteristics of the radiation including dose, dose rate, and quality.
   a. During the preimplantation stage, embryos exhibit an all-or-nothing response such that the exposure is either lethal (with doses of 50 to 100 mGy causing spontaneous abortion in animal studies) or the conceptus shows little evidence of radiation-induced abnormalities.
   b. Particularly in animal studies, embryonic malformations occur more frequently if exposure is during the organogenesis stage.
   c. If exposure is during the fetal growth state, the occurrence of radiation-induced prenatal death and congenital anomalies is negligible; anomalies of the nervous system and sense organs are the primary abnormalities observed.

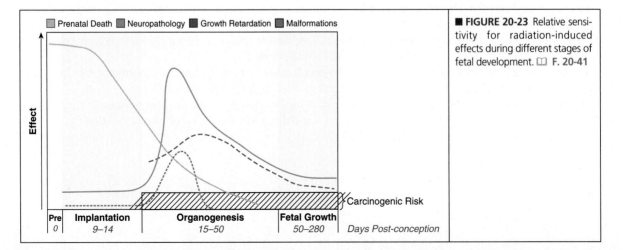

■ **FIGURE 20-23** Relative sensitivity for radiation-induced effects during different stages of fetal development. ▭ F. 20-41

2. In humans, a significant increase in microcephaly and mental retardation has been seen when in utero exposures to the atomic bombs occurred between the 8th and 15th week after conception.
3. Some studies have suggested that the RR for childhood cancer from in utero exposure to radiation is about 1.4, although whether the radiation exposure is causal is controversial.
4. A conceptus dose of 100 mGy does not significantly affect the risks associated with pregnancy; nevertheless, every effort should be made to reduce or avoid fetal exposure.

## 20.8 RADIATION RISK COMMUNICATIONS

1. Radiation risk communication, a key component of good practice in medical imaging, has a major goal of ensuring that patients and their families and/or caregivers receive information about radiation exposures from a procedure in a way that they can understand readily.
2. Because referring medical practitioners outside the radiation fields may have a low level of awareness about radiation doses and associated risks in medical imaging, radiologists play an important role in providing the needed information.
3. There are many challenges in expressing radiation risk to patients and their families. Hence, it is useful to bear in mind clear messages that may convey useful information to a patient, should express risk as absolute risk rather than relative risk, and consider expressing radiation dose and risk in ways that put the information in perspective to enable patients to make a sound judgment about whether or not the radiation risk is acceptable to them.

# Section II Questions and Answers

1. Which of the following is a stochastic effect of ionizing radiation?
   A. Skin erythema
   B. Cancer induction
   C. Denudation of the intestinal epithelium
   D. Loss of circulating lymphocytes
   E. Lung fibrosis

2. Why is it important to understand the difference between direct and indirect action in cells irradiated with low-LET photons?
   A. $H_2O_2$ is a highly damaging species produced by direct action of radiation.
   B. Only direct action produces lethal damage to DNA.
   C. Scavenging ·OH produced by indirect action can decrease radiation damage to cells.
   D. Indirect action is greater with high-LET radiation, thus decreasing cell killing.

3. Which of the following is the primary radiolysis species that is responsible for most biological damage in cells irradiated with low-LET photons?
   A. $H_2O_2$
   B. Hydrogen gas
   C. ·OH
   D. Superoxide anion

4. The term RBE, relative biological effectiveness, describes which of the following?
   A. Ratio of doses to cause a given biological effect for a reference radiation compared to a higher LET radiation
   B. Increased effectiveness of ionizing radiation in hypoxic cells compared to anoxic cells
   C. Enhancement in cell killing seen in the presence of free radicals
   D. Increase in late tissue reactions seen when radiation dose rate is decreased
   E. Change in doses needed to maintain level damage in early versus late responding tissues

5. What is the typical RBE for most diagnostic X-rays?
   A. 0.1          D. 10
   B. 1            E. 30
   C. 3

6. Which of the following is thought to be the most biologically damaging DNA lesion produced by ionizing radiation in mammalian cells?
   A. Clustered lesions
   B. Single-strand breaks
   C. Pyrimidine dimers
   D. DNA-protein crosslinks
   E. DNA-DNA crosslinks

7. Which of the following is a DNA repair process that repairs DNA double-strand breaks?
   A. Base excision repair
   B. Nonhomologous end-joining
   C. Mismatch repair
   D. Nucleotide excision repair

8. Which of the following assays would be most useful for assessing DNA double-strand breaks in irradiated mammalian cells?
   A. Alkali comet
   B. Colony formation
   C. Western blotting
   D. PCR
   E. Foci of γH2AX

9. The base excision repair pathway (BER) is the primary pathway for the repair of which of the following DNA lesions?
   A. Double-strand breaks
   B. Bulky lesions such as pyrimidine dimers
   C. Single-strand breaks
   D. DNA-protein crosslinks
   E. Peptide bond scission

10. Which of the following is NOT a chromosome aberration commonly caused by exposure to ionizing radiation?
    A. Ring
    B. Dicentric
    C. Nonsymmetric translocation
    D. Trisomy

11. In the $n$-$D_0$ mathematical model used to fit clonogenic survival curves for irradiated cells, what is $n$?
    A. Quasithreshold dose
    B. Coefficient representing high radiation dose-response
    C. Slope of the exponential portion of the survival curve
    D. Ratio at which $\alpha$ and $\beta$ are equal
    E. Extrapolation number

12. Which of the following is the coefficient in the LQ model for cell survival curves that provides information on the initial, linear, low dose region of a cell survival curve?
    A. $\alpha$                 C. $d$
    B. $\beta$                 D. $n$

13. What is the cell death mechanism in which cells undergo characteristic morphological changes that include cell shrinkage, nuclear condensation, and extensive membrane blebbing to form membrane-bound bodies that are eliminated by phagocytosis?
    A. Apoptosis
    B. Autophagy
    C. Necroptosis
    D. Senescence
    E. Mitotic catastrophe

14. What is the cell death mechanism in which cells degrade their cytoplasmic components using regulated, catabolic processes?
    A. Apoptosis
    B. Autophagy
    C. Necroptosis
    D. Senescence
    E. Mitotic catastrophe

15. As the radiation dose rate is decreased from about 1 Gy/min to 1 Gy/h, how does the dose-response for cell survival change?
    A. The curve becomes steeper, and the shoulder becomes broader.
    B. The curve becomes steeper, and the shoulder becomes narrower.
    C. The curve becomes less steep and the shoulder broader.
    D. There is no change in the curve.

16. What is the shape of the dose-response curve for induction of chromosome aberrations in cells exposed to high-LET radiation such as alpha particles?
    A. Threshold
    B. Sigmoid
    C. Quadratic
    D. Linear

17. According to Bergonie and Tribondeau, in tissues, radiosensitivity is greatest in cells that have all of the following characteristics EXCEPT:
    A. a high mitotic rate
    B. a long mitotic future
    C. inherent genomic instability
    D. are undifferentiated

18. What is the OER for photons used in the clinic?
    A. 4                 D. 1
    B. 3                 E. 0.5
    C. 2

19. Cells in which phase of the cell cycle are most resistant to radiation?
    A. M                 C. Late S
    B. Late G1                 D. G2

20. Radiation-induced cell cycle arrest during the G1 phase of the cell cycle requires which of the following proteins to be functional?
    A. bcl-2                 D. CD95
    B. p53                 E. RIP
    C. LC3

21. Which of the following terms describes the observation that, under certain conditions, changes can be seen in cells that are not traversed by radiation as a result of radiation energy deposition in other cells?
    A. Bystander effects
    B. Low-dose hypersensitivity
    C. Genomic instability
    D. Adaptive response
    E. Hormesis

22. Based on histological observations of radiation-induced damage, which of the following cell/tissue types is the least radiation sensitive?
    A. Adult bone
    B. Growing bone in a child
    C. Skin
    D. Bone marrow

23. Late tissue reactions after radiation exposure, for example, in the lung, kidneys, and brain, can involve all of the following EXCEPT:
    A. chronic oxidative stress
    B. inflammatory responses
    C. immune reactions
    D. damage to the vasculature
    E. all of the above can occur

24. What is the most common adverse tissue reaction in patients following high-dose image-guided interventional procedures?
    A. Skin cancer
    B. Temporary sterility
    C. Cataracts
    D. Skin damage such as erythema

25. Temporary hair loss (epilation) can occur approximately 3 weeks after exposure to what dose of photon radiation?
    A. Less than 1 Gy
    B. 3 to 6 Gy
    C. 10 to 12 Gy
    D. 15 Gy

26. Which of the following is the most radiosensitive germ cell type?
    A. Spermatozoa
    B. Secondary spermatocytes
    C. Spermatogonia
    D. Spermatids

27. Based on recent epidemiological studies, it is now accepted that the threshold for induction of vision-impairing cataracts is on the order of what dose?
    A. 50 Gy          C. 0.5 Gy
    B. 5 Gy           D. 0.05 Gy

28. The initial phase of the acute radiation syndrome that occurs prior to the latent period and the manifest illness phase is called the:
    A. prodromal syndrome
    B. gastrointestinal syndrome
    C. cerebrovascular syndrome
    D. precarcinogenesis phase
    E. death phase

29. What is the approximate dose for the $LD_{50/60}$ for humans exposed to acute total body irradiation, without medical intervention?
    A. 0.5 to 1.0 Gy
    B. 3.5 to 4.5 Gy
    C. 7 to 10 Gy
    D. 13 to 15 Gy
    E. greater than 20 Gy

30. What is the hematopoietic cell type that shows the most rapid and largest decrease after total body irradiation?
    A. Lymphocytes
    B. Red blood cells
    C. Platelets
    D. Granulocytes
    E. Neutrophils

31. Radiation-induced damage in the GI tract is expressed quickly (less than 2 weeks) because of which of the following?
    A. Low oxygen level in the gut
    B. High radiosensitivity of the GI vasculature
    C. Relatively rapid turnover of the normal epithelial cells
    D. Arrangement of intestinal stem cells in parallel fashion

32. What is the baseline lifetime cancer incidence in the United States?
    A. 10%            D. 60%
    B. 20%            E. 80%
    C. 40%

33. Oncogenes are:
    A. genes that acquire gain of function mutations in cancer
    B. genes that promote mutagenesis
    C. genes that suppress transforming events
    D. genes that code for DNA repair proteins

34. Which of the following is NOT a "Hallmark of Cancer" as described by Hanahan and Weinberg?
    A. Sustaining proliferative signaling
    B. Evading growth suppressors
    C. Resisting cell death
    D. Inhibiting angiogenesis

35. The tumor microenvironment can include all the following EXCEPT:
    A. stromal cells
    B. lymphatics
    C. extracellular matrix
    D. blood vessels
    E. all of the above can be components of a tumor

36. Which of the following describes the gender dependence of risk of radiation-induced cancer?
    A. Females are more sensitive than males.
    B. Males and females are equally sensitive.
    C. Females are less sensitive than males.

37. What is the term for the ratio of the disease (*e.g.*, cancer) incidence in the exposed population to that in the general (unexposed) population called?
    A. Absolute risk
    B. Relative risk
    C. Excess relative risk
    D. Attributable risk

38. Which of the following is a human gene that when mutated is associated with an increased risk of developing cancer?
    A. *BCL-2*         C. *γH2AX*
    B. *ATM*           D. *PDGFA*

39. What is the most widely used source of epidemiologic data for studies of radiation-induced cancer?
    A. SEER database
    B. LSS of atomic bomb survivors in Japan
    C. Medical patients treated for cancer
    D. Phosphorus miners

40. Which of the cancer types listed below have the lowest site-specific solid radiation-induced cancer mortality ERR risk estimates?
    A. Esophagus
    B. Colon
    C. Pancreas
    D. Bladder
    E. Breast

41. What is the shape of the dose-response model for cancer risk that is recommended by most national and international expert committees that have assessed data on radiation-induced cancers to date?
    A. Linear-quadratic
    B. Threshold
    C. Sigmoidal
    D. Linear-no threshold

42. The most commonly used value for DDREF in studies of radiation-induced cancer risk is which of the following?
    A. 0
    B. 0.2 to 0.5
    C. 1.5 to 2
    D. 5 to 7
    E. Greater than 20

43. The multiplicative risk-projection model for radiation-induced cancer is based on which of the following assumptions?
    A. Excess cancer risk increases in proportion to the baseline cancer rate.
    B. Excess cancer rate is constant and independent of the spontaneous population and age-specific natural cancer risk.
    C. Excess cancer risk is independent of age at exposure or attained age.
    D. Excess cancer risk is zero under most conditions.

44. Compared to the risk to adults, the risk of radiation-induced cancer for a 12-month-old infant is how much higher?
    A. The risks are the same
    B. 1 to 2 times higher
    C. 3 to 4 times greater
    D. Approximately 10 times higher

45. In the LSS population, what was the latency period after exposure before the first detection of excess leukemia cases?
    A. 1 to 2 years
    B. 5 to 8 years
    C. 15 to 20 years
    D. Greater than 20 years

46. Studies in which of the following organisms has failed to demonstrate significant levels of radiation-induced genetic effects?
    A. Humans
    B. Fruit flies
    C. Mice
    D. Cultured mammalian cells

47. What is the estimated doubling dose for radiation-induced mutations in humans?
    A. 0.1 Gy per generation
    B. 1 Gy per generation
    C. 10 Gy per generation
    D. 30 Gy per generation

48. What is the most likely detrimental effect seen in humans irradiated in utero during the fetal growth period?
    A. Cancer
    B. Prenatal death
    C. Congenital malformations
    D. Microcephaly

49. A reasonable estimate of the excess risk of childhood cancer from in utero irradiation is approximately which of the following?
    A. Less than 0.01% per Gy
    B. 0.06% to 0.6% per Gy
    C. 0.6% to 6% per Gy
    D. Greater than 10% per Gy

50. Which of the following messages would NOT be considered useful information to convey to a patient?
    A. Low-level background radiation is part of the Earth's natural environment.
    B. The degree of risk associated with exposure to low-level ionizing radiation is thought to be very low.
    C. Scientists agree well about the precise magnitude of this risk.
    D. Any risk from radiation must be balanced against the benefits provided by the activity producing the radiation.

# Answers

1. **B** Stochastic effects of radiation are those whose probability increases with radiation dose, without a threshold, in contrast to tissue reactions whose severity increases with dose. Examples of stochastic effects are cancer and hereditary damage. *(Pg. 822)*

2. **C** It is important to be able to differentiate direct and indirect action of radiation because the indirect action potentially can be modified by scavenging ·OH, thus decreasing radiation damage in cells, but the direct action is not readily modifiable. *(Pg. 825)*

3. **C** The hydroxyl radical, ·OH, is a highly oxidizing species that causes most of the damage from water-derived free radicals that results in biological effects. *(Pg. 825)*

4. **A** RBE is the ratio of the dose of a reference radiation (usually 250 kVp X-rays) to the dose of a high-LET radiation to give the same level of biological damage. *(Pg. 826)*

5. **B** The RBE for most diagnostic X-rays is about 1, meaning the biological effectiveness of the radiation is about the same as the reference radiation, usually taken to be either 250 kVp X-rays or $^{60}$Co gamma rays. *(Pg. 827, Fig. 20-3)*

6. **A** Clustered DNA lesions, composed of several lesions such as strand breaks or base damages within a short distance on the DNA molecule, are the most damaging because they are difficult to repair easily and accurately. *(Pg. 823)*

7. **B** Nonhomologous end joining (NHEJ) and homologous recombination (HRR) repair DNA DSBs, although NHEJ is error-prone while HRR generally is accurate repair. *(Pg. 831)*

8. **E** Use of immunofluorescent labeling of aggregates (foci) of phosphorylated histone H2AX, γH2AX, is a useful assay for the presence of DNA DSBs. *(Pg. 832, Fig. 20-6)*

9. **C** Single-strand breaks and simple base damages are repaired rapidly and accurately by the BER pathway. Bulky lesions and crosslinks are generally repaired by nucleotide excision repair (NER), and DSBs are repaired by homologous recombination (HR) or nonhomologous end-joining (NHEJ). *(Pg. 831, Fig. 20-6)*

10. **D** Trisomy, the presence of three copies of a chromosome, is not caused by radiation exposure. Rings, dicentrics, and translocations can all be produced by exposure of dividing cells to ionizing radiation. *(Pg. 834, Fig. 20-9)*

11. **E** The extrapolation number is *n*, which gives a measure of the "shoulder," or repair capacity, of the cells and is found by extrapolating the linear portion of the cell survival curve back to its intersection with the *y*-axis. $D_0$, which describes the radiosensitivity of the cell population, is the reciprocal of the slope of the linear portion of the survival curve. *(Pg. 835–836, Fig. 20-10)*

12. **A** The linear-quadratic (LQ) model of cell survival curves contains α, which is the coefficient of cell killing that is proportional to dose (*i.e.*, the initial linear component on a log-linear plot), and β, the coefficient of cell killing that is proportional to the square of the dose. *(Pg. 836–837, Fig. 20-11)*

13. **A** Apoptosis is a mode of cell death in which cells undergo characteristic morphological changes that include cell shrinkage, nuclear condensation, and extensive membrane blebbing to form membrane-bound bodies that are eliminated by phagocytosis. On the molecular level, the changes are brought about by cascades of changes in caspases, protein, and, ultimately, DNA degradation. *(Pg. 837–838)*

14. **B** During autophagy, usually brought on by nutrient deprivation or damage to cellular components and molecules, cells initiate a sequence of events to degrade cytoplasmic components by forming autophagosomes containing the damaged components then fusion of the autophagosomes with lysosomes that contain lytic enzymes. *(Pg. 838–839)*

15.  **C**   With decreasing dose rate, there is more time for sublethal damage to be repaired during the radiation exposure and survival increases, resulting in the dose-response curve becoming less steep and the shoulder broadening. *(Pg. 840)*

16.  **D**   With high-LET radiation, there is more clustered DNA damage that is not accurately or readily repaired resulting in a purely linear dose-response curve for chromosome aberrations. *(Pg. 840)*

17.  **C**   The law of Bergonie and Tribondeau states that radiosensitivity is greatest for those cells that (1) have a high mitotic rate, (2) have a long mitotic future, and (3) are undifferentiated. *(Pg. 842)*

18.  **B**   The oxygen enhancement ratio (OER) for low-LET radiation, including clinical energy photons, is about 3. *(Pg. 842)*

19.  **C**   The most radiation-resistant phase of the cell cycle is late S, while M/G2 is the most radiation sensitive. *(Pg. 843)*

20.  **B**   The p53 protein produced by the tumor suppressor gene *TP53* is involved in radiation-induced cell cycle arrest of proliferating cells in the G1 phase of the cell cycle. The protein is also involved in DNA repair and, in some cell types, in the initiation of apoptosis. *(Pg. 844, Fig. 20-19)*

21.  **A**   The radiation-induced bystander effect occurs when cells that are not irradiated show changes, for example, DNA damage or increased expression of certain proteins, as a result of being in the vicinity of cells that are traversed by radiation. *(Pg. 846)*

22.  **A**   Radiation sensitive tissues tend to be those with a significant stem/progenitor cell component that has a high mitotic rate, a long mitotic future, and are undifferentiated. Hence, growing bone, skin, and bone marrow are radiosensitive, but adult bone is radiation resistant. *(Pg. 847–848)*

23.  **E**   Late tissue reactions depend on complex and dynamic interactions among multiple cell types in tissues and organs and include infiltrating immune cells, production of cytokines, and inflammation and chronic oxidative stress, as well as damage to the vasculature and the extracellular matrix (ECM). *(Pg. 847)*

24.  **D**.   Skin damage, which can range from erythema to ulceration at very high doses, is the most common, albeit rare, adverse tissue reaction in patients after high-dose image-guided interventional procedures. *(Pg. 850)*

25.  **B**   Temporary hair loss (epilation) can occur approximately 3 weeks after exposure to 3 to 6 Gy. *(Pg. 851)*

26.  **C**   The testes contain cell populations that range from the most radiosensitive germ cells (*i.e.*, spermatogonia) to the most radioresistant, mature spermatozoa, with the other cell populations with progressively greater differentiation (*i.e.*, primary and secondary spermatocytes and spermatids) of intermediate radiosensitivity. *(Pg. 854)*

27.  **C**   Recent epidemiological studies are consistent with the dose threshold for induction of vision-impairing cataracts being about 0.5 Gy. *(Pg. 856)*

28.  **A**   The prodromal syndrome is the initial stage of acute radiation syndrome (ARS), with symptoms that can include nausea, fatigue, vomiting, headache, and confusion, depending on the dose. *(Pg. 860)*

29.  **B**   The $LD_{50/60}$ (dose that kills 50% of the members of a population within 60 days) for humans after acute total body irradiation, without medical intervention, is about 3.5 to 4.5 Gy. *(Pg. 862)*

30.  **A**   The decline in lymphocyte count in circulating blood can occur within hours and with a dose threshold as low as 0.25 Gy after whole-body irradiation. *(Pg. 863)*

31.  **C**   Radiation-induced damage in the GI tract occurs because of relatively rapid normal turnover of the epithelial cells on the villi that cannot be replaced because of the radiation sterilization of the stem/progenitor cells in the crypts. *(Pg. 864)*

32.  **C**   According to recent statistics on cancer in the United States from the American Cancer Society, the lifetime probability of developing an invasive cancer is 39.4% (40.1% male and 38.7% female) and the probability of dying from cancer is about half that. *(Pg. 865)*

33.  **A**   Oncogenes are genes that have the potential to cause cancer because they are mutated versions of proto-oncogenes (normal genes involved in cell growth and proliferation or inhibition of apoptosis) that have gained, or up-regulated, the function of uncontrolled cell growth. *(Pg. 869–869)*

34.  **D**  The six "Hallmarks of Cancer" originally described by Hanahan and Weinberg are sustaining proliferative signaling, evading growth suppressors, resisting cell death, enabling replicative immortality, inducing angiogenesis, and activating invasion and metastasis. *(Pg. 870, Fig. 20-27A)*

35.  **E**  The tumor microenvironment is composed of multiple interacting cell types such as stromal cells including fibroblasts and the endothelial cells and pericytes of the vasculature, immune inflammatory cells, and lymphatics, as well as the extracellular matrix. *(Pg. 870, Fig. 20-27B)*

36.  **A**  For whole-body exposure, females on average have a 40% higher risk of radiogenic cancer than males. *(Pg. 874)*

37.  **B**  Relative risk (RR) is the ratio of the disease (*e.g.*, cancer) incidence in the exposed population to that in the general (unexposed) population; thus, a RR of 1.2 would indicate a 20% increase over the spontaneous rate that would otherwise have been expected in a population. *(Pg. 871–872)*

38.  **B**  Patients with the ataxia-telangiectasia mutation (ATM) are at substantially higher risk of developing cancer (especially leukemias and lymphomas) than the general population. These patients are also hypersensitive to ionizing radiation exposure because of defective DNA repair mechanisms. *(Pg. 875)*

39.  **B**  The most important source of epidemiological data for assessment of low-dose radiation cancer risk is the LSS (Life Span Study) of the Japanese atomic bomb survivors, who received acute doses of radiation, over a range of doses up to 2 Gy, beyond which errors in dose reconstruction and mortality from complications of the ARS provided limited radioepidemiological information. *(Pg. 876, Fig. 20-29)*

40.  **C**  As shown in Figure 20-30 in the textbook, the pancreas has a lower ERR (per Sv) than the other tissues listed. *(Pg. 881, Fig. 20-30)*

41.  **D**  The NCRP, BEIR VII committee, and ICRP have all concluded that, although there are alternatives to linearity for the shape of the cancer induction dose-response curve, there is no strong evidence supporting the choice of any other form of the dose-response relationship other than the linear-no threshold model. *(Pg. 884)*

42.  **C**  BEIR VII recommended the use of a DDREF (dose and dose-rate effectiveness factor) of 1.5 to adjust risk estimates from exposures at high dose and high dose rate to low doses, although UNSCEAR and ICRP have recommended a value of 2. *(Pg. 886)*

43.  **A**  The multiplicative risk-projection model for radiation-induced cancer is based on the assumption that excess cancer risk increases in proportion to the baseline cancer rate after a latent period. *(Pg. 886–887, Fig. 20-34A)*

44.  **C.**  The risk for radiation-induced cancer of a 12-month-old infant is about 3-4 times higher than that of an adult. *(Pg. 891–892, Fig. 20-36)*

45.  **A**  In the A-bomb survivors, excess leukemia cases were detected as soon as 1 to 2 years after exposure and reached a peak approximately 12 years after the exposure. *(Pg. 897)*

46.  **A**  Epidemiological studies in numerous human populations, including children of the survivors of the atomic bombings in Japan, offspring of U.S. radiologic technologists, and children of individuals who had radiotherapy for cancer, have all failed to show significant levels of transgenerational effects from radiation exposures. *(Pg. 903)*

47.  **B**  The doubling dose for humans is estimated to be approximately 1 Gy per generation; however, this represents an extrapolation from animal data as no significant transgenerational effect has been demonstrated in humans. *(Pg. 904)*

48.  **D**  Individuals exposed in utero at Hiroshima and Nagasaki between the 8th and 15th week after conception showed significant increases in microcephaly and severe mental retardation, in a radiation dose-dependent manner. *(Pg. 907)*

49.  **C**  Although the risk remains controversial, the consensus is that the excess risk of childhood cancer from in utero irradiation is between 0.6% and 6%. *(Pg. 908–909)*

50.  **C.**  It is important to convey that scientists do not agree about the precise magnitude of risks for radiation-induced detriment because these are complex issues. *(Pg. 915)*

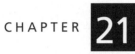 

CHAPTER **21**

# Radiation Protection

## 21.0 INTRODUCTION

It is incumbent upon all individuals who use radiation in medicine to strive for an optimal compromise between its clinical utility and the radiation doses to patients, staff, and the public. Federal and state governments and even some large municipalities have agencies that promulgate regulations regarding the safe use of radiation and radio-active material. Radiation protection programs are designed and implemented to ensure compliance with these regulations. Radiation protection programs include the development of procedures for the safe use of radiation and radioactive material and education of staff about radiation safety principles as well as the risks associated with radiation exposure and contamination.

## 21.1 SOURCES OF EXPOSURE TO IONIZING RADIATION

1. The average annual per capita effective dose from exposure to ionizing radiation in the United States is about 6.2 mSv (about 17 $\mu$Sv per day).
2. Half of the total (3.0 mSv) is from medical exposure of patients, which has increased almost a factor of 6 since the 1080s (Fig. 21-1). The other half (3.1 mSv) is from naturally occurring sources (cosmic rays, cosmogenic radionuclides, and primordial radionuclides and their progeny) (Fig. 21-2).

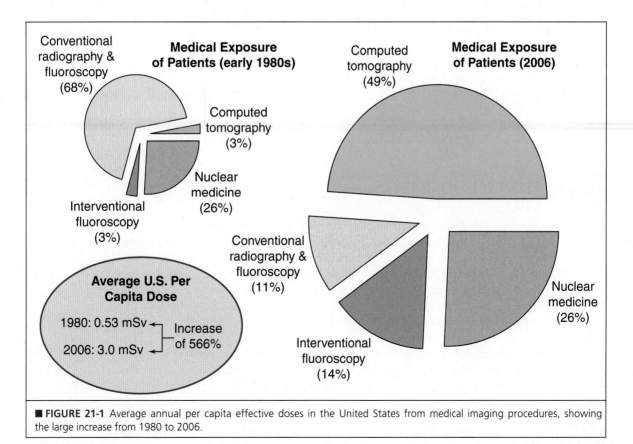

■ **FIGURE 21-1** Average annual per capita effective doses in the United States from medical imaging procedures, showing the large increase from 1980 to 2006.

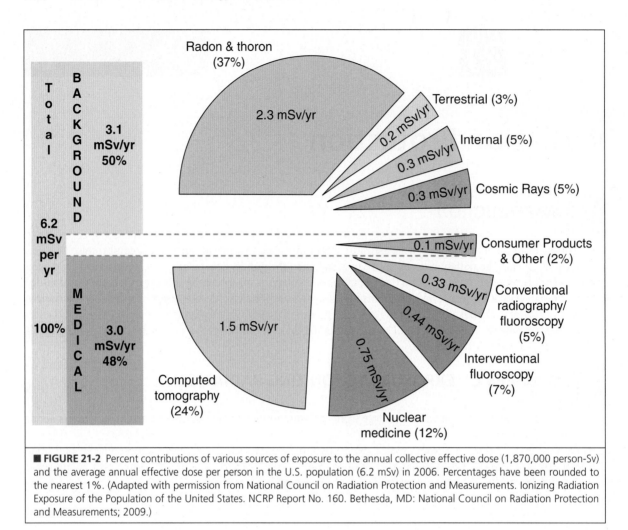

**■ FIGURE 21-2** Percent contributions of various sources of exposure to the annual collective effective dose (1,870,000 person-Sv) and the average annual effective dose per person in the U.S. population (6.2 mSv) in 2006. Percentages have been rounded to the nearest 1%. (Adapted with permission from National Council on Radiation Protection and Measurements. Ionizing Radiation Exposure of the Population of the United States. NCRP Report No. 160. Bethesda, MD: National Council on Radiation Protection and Measurements; 2009.)

3. Consumer products, nuclear power, and fallout from atomic weapons cause only a small fraction of the average population exposure to radiation.
4. Radiation from radon exposure ($^{222}$Rn and progeny) in the United States contributes the greatest effective dose (2.1 mSv) from naturally occurring sources.
5. By 2016 about a 15% to 20% reduction in medical imaging dose had been achieved due to advances in technology, awareness of dose, and optimization of patient doses per procedure.

## 21.2 PERSONNEL DOSIMETRY

1. Personnel radiation exposures are typically monitored by dosimeters using storage phosphors (e.g., TLDs or OSLs) that store energy in trapped electrons. Following the exposure period (typically monthly), the dosimeters are processed ("read") by exposing the phosphors to heat (TLD) or laser energy (OSL). The light emitted from the dosimeter is proportional to the absorbed dose. These phosphor-based dosimeters have largely replaced the older film badge dosimeters for which radiation exposure causes darkening of the film emulsion, which is proportional to the absorbed dose.
   a. TLDs: thermoluminescent dosimeters (Fig. 21-3)
   b. OSLs: optically stimulated luminescent dosimeters
2. Dosimeters are typically provided by a commercial vendor monthly or quarterly with reports listing shallow (skin), eye (lens), and deep (whole-body dose corresponding to penetrating radiations) dose.
3. For radiologists, x-ray technologists, and nuclear medicine technologists, dosimeters are typically worn at waist or shirt-pocket level.
4. For fluoroscopy and interventional procedures, dosimeters are typically placed at collar level in front of the lead apron (and sometimes a second badge is worn under the apron). Effective doses are assessed using algorithms based on the worn badges.

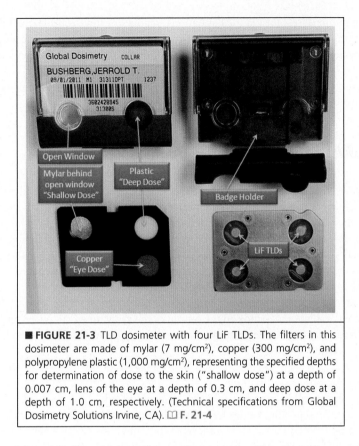

■ **FIGURE 21-3** TLD dosimeter with four LiF TLDs. The filters in this dosimeter are made of mylar (7 mg/cm²), copper (300 mg/cm²), and polypropylene plastic (1,000 mg/cm²), representing the specified depths for determination of dose to the skin ("shallow dose") at a depth of 0.007 cm, lens of the eye at a depth of 0.3 cm, and deep dose at a depth of 1.0 cm, respectively. (Technical specifications from Global Dosimetry Solutions Irvine, CA). 📖 **F. 21-4**

5. A pregnant radiation worker typically wears an additional dosimeter at waist level to assess the fetal dose.
6. Electronic (or self-reading) personal dosimeters with associated alarm functions are supplemental dosimeters that can be used for dose feedback when high doses are expected (*e.g.*, cardiac catheterization or high-dose nuclear medicine therapies).

## 21.3 RADIATION DETECTION EQUIPMENT IN RADIATION SAFETY

1. GM (Geiger-Mueller) survey meters detect the presence and provide an indication of intensities of radiation contamination and fields in units of counts per minute (cpm). GM survey meters can also be properly calibrated for energy and response to provide estimates of exposure rate (mR/h).
2. GM survey meters are useful for locating radioactive material and/or contamination following the use of unsealed radioactive materials (*e.g.*, nuclear medicine or radiopharmacy labs).
3. Ionization chamber survey meters provide accurate measurements of radiation exposure rate (see Chapter 17) and approximate the conditions under which the roentgen is defined (see Chapter 3).
4. Ionization chambers are useful for monitoring dose rates near radiation generating equipment and near patients who have received radioactive material administrations.

## 21.4 FUNDAMENTAL PRINCIPLES AND METHODS OF EXPOSURE CONTROL

1. Three key radiation protection principles: justification, optimization, and limitation of maximum doses.
   a. Justification: benefit of radiation use is higher than the detriment it causes.
   b. Optimization: keeping exposures as low as reasonably achievable (ALARA), implying the lowest dose necessary to produce diagnostic quality. This concept has also been referred to as ALADA, as low as diagnostically acceptable.

c. Limitation of maximum doses: for planned situations, regulatory limits on maximal doses for workers and members of the public. Not applicable to medical exposure of patients and emergency situations.
2. The American College of Radiology (ACR) promulgates appropriate use criteria as evidenced-based guidelines for justification.
3. Methods of exposure control include time (reducing), distance (increasing), shielding (using when appropriate), and controlling contamination.

## 21.5 STRUCTURAL SHIELDING OF IMAGING FACILITIES

1. Shielding design goals, $P$, are stated in terms of $K$ (mGy) at a reference point beyond a protective barrier (*e.g.*, 0.3 m for a wall) delivered over a specified time interval (*e.g.*, weekly, annually). Shielding methods for diagnostic and interventional x-ray rooms are provided in NCRP Report No. 147.
2. A controlled area is an area to which access is controlled for the purposes of radiation protection (procedure rooms, control booths), which under specified exposure conditions is designed not to exceed 0.1 mGy/wk.
3. Uncontrolled areas are other areas (offices, adjacent rooms, hallways, etc.), which under specified exposure conditions are designed not to exceed 0.02 mGy/wk.
4. Exposure sources include primary, scattered, and leakage radiation.
5. The amount of primary radiation depends on the output of the x-ray tube (kV, mGy/min, and mAs) per examination, no. of examinations/week, the fraction of time beam is pointed at a specific barrier ($U$, use factor), and distance to that barrier.
6. Scattered radiation at 1 m from a patient is about 0.1% to 0.15% of the incident exposure to the patient.
7. Lead is the most commonly used material for shielding x-ray facilities (high attenuation and low cost), although gypsum, concrete, glass, and leaded glass are also utilized.
8. Occupancy factor ($T$) represents the average fraction of the time maximally exposed individual is present while x-ray beam is on. Workload ($W$) is the time integral of the x-ray tube current over 1 week (mA-min/wk).
9. In most PET/CT installations, the thick shielding for the annihilation photons is more than sufficient for the lower-energy secondary radiation from the x-ray CT system.
10. Radiologists should obtain the assistance of a qualified medical physicist for the design of shielding.

## 21.6 RADIATION PROTECTION IN DIAGNOSTIC AND INTERVENTIONAL X-RAY IMAGING

1. Protective aprons and collar shields, usually of 0.25- to 0.50-mm lead, protect the torso and thyroid and attenuate greater than 90% of the scattered radiation for fluoroscopy, interventional, and CT-guided procedures.
2. In fluoroscopy, the stray radiation intensity is higher on the side of the patient toward the x-ray source than on the side toward the image receptor (Fig. 21-4).
   a. Keep the x-ray tube under the patient whenever able.
   b. Ceiling mounted, table-mounted, and mobile radiation barriers can reduce operator doses, as can the use of leaded glasses to reduce lens of eye dose.
3. No pregnant or less than 18-year-old individuals should routinely hold patients during examinations.
4. An important goal in diagnostic imaging is to achieve an optimal balance between image quality and dose to the patient.
   a. Patient exposure can often be reduced by using higher kV and lower mAs.
   b. In CT angiography, greater beam filtration and lower kV can improve contrast-to-noise ratio and thus lower dose.
   c. Collimate field size to just necessary volume. Consider shielding other organs (or limbs) when the shadow of the shield does not interfere with anatomy under investigation.
   d. Do not use patient shielding in CT as it interferes with auto-exposure control and introduces artifacts.
5. Fluoroscopy imparts some of the largest imaging tissue doses to individual patients. Patient entrance air kerma is limited to a maximum of 87.3 mGy/min (with auto brightness control) and 44 mGy/min without. The cumulative skin doses in difficult cases or from a series of procedures of a single area of the body can exceed 10 Gy, which can lead to severe radiation-induced skin injuries. Physicians using or directing use should be trained and credentialed.
6. Patient organ doses from CT imaging are typically on the order of 10s of mGy and depend on kV, mA, time per x-ray tube rotation, detector-table motion pitch, and beam filter. Careful protocol settings are necessary (see Chapter 10).

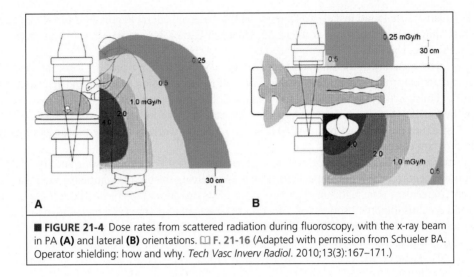

■ **FIGURE 21-4** Dose rates from scattered radiation during fluoroscopy, with the x-ray beam in PA **(A)** and lateral **(B)** orientations. 🕮 **F. 21-16** (Adapted with permission from Schueler BA. Operator shielding: how and why. *Tech Vasc Inverv Radiol*. 2010;13(3):167–171.)

7. Dose optimization, such as automatic exposure control, and right-sizing per patient can result in lower doses and should be considered, especially for thinner patients and pediatrics.
8. National or regional diagnostic reference levels (DRLs, typically 75th percentile) and achievable doses (ADs, typically 50th percentile) can be used to evaluate individual site dose optimization.

## 21.7  RADIATION PROTECTION IN NUCLEAR MEDICINE

1. Minimizing time, maximizing distance, and utilizing shielding when appropriate are important.
2. The use of syringe shields can reduce hand exposure for Tc-99m by as much as 100 fold.
3. Lead aprons utilized in diagnostic radiology are of limited value in the higher-energy photons from radiopharmaceuticals used in nuclear medicine.
4. PET facilities often require shielding (typically lead) of barriers to surrounding areas to attenuate the 511-keV annihilation radiation.
5. Proper contamination control (periodic GM surveys and wipe tests) and lab safety practices (labeling, coats, gloves, goggles, survey hands and clothing, dosimetry, waste disposal, shields where appropriate, no eating/drinking/smoking, etc.) are essential radiation protection methods.
6. Control ordering, receipt, and shipping (per DOT rules) for nuclear medicine.
7. S.W.I.M. for spills—Stop the spill, Warn others, Isolate the area, and Mitigate (cleanup from outside in).
8. Take care with patient identification and double-check prescribed compounds, quantities, and route of administration to prevent medical events.
9. Complete cessation of breastfeeding is suggested for Ga-67 citrate and I-131. Consult available tables and guidance for other radiopharmaceuticals.
10. Consider radiation precautions and instructions per regulations for radionuclide therapy patients.
11. Guidance on the release of patients is found in NCRP Report 155 and ensures doses do not exceed 5 mSv for careers or 1 mSv for members of the public.

## 21.8  REGULATORY AGENCIES AND RADIATION EXPOSURE LIMITS

1. Several regulatory agencies have jurisdiction over various aspects of the use of radiation in medicine. Regulations under their authority carry the force of law.
2. The U.S. Nuclear Regulatory Commission (NRC) regulates special nuclear material (plutonium and uranium enriched in U-233 and U-235), source material (thorium, uranium, and their ores), and by-product material used in nuclear power, research, medicine, and other commercial activities.
3. "Agreement States" have entered into agreements with the NRC to promulgate and enforce regulations similar to those of the NRC. In addition, the agencies of the agreement states typically regulate all sources of ionizing radiation, including diagnostic and interventional x-ray machines and linear accelerators used in radiation oncology.
4. Medical workers must be informed of their rights and responsibilities, including the risks inherent in utilizing radiation sources and their responsibility to follow established safety procedures.

5. NRC regulations are found in Title 10 (Energy) of the Code of Federal Regulations (CFR). Part 20, "Standards for Protection against Radiation" and Part 35, "Medical Use of Byproduct Material" are essential sections of the code for medical staff.

   a. By-product material: In the Atomic Energy Act of 1954, the term by-product material referred primarily to radioactive by-products of nuclear fission in nuclear reactors (fission products and activation products). The Energy Policy Act of 2005 expanded the definition of by-product material to include material made radioactive by use of a particle accelerator. As such, most radiopharmaceuticals are now subject to NRC regulation.

6. Part 20 specifies the maximal permissible doses to radiation workers and the public among other radiation safety program essential elements.

7. Part 35 includes medical use categories, training requirements, precautions, testing and use of dose calibrators, and requirements for the reporting of medical events involving the use of radiopharmaceuticals and radiation.

8. NRC and Agreement State regulatory guidance documents provide acceptable methods for satisfying the regulations and are thus important sources of practical implementation policies and procedures for medical facilities.

9. Other regulatory agencies involved in the use of radiation and radioactive material in medicine include the Food and Drug Agency (FDA), the U.S. Department of Transportation (USDOT), the U.S. Department of Labor (OSHA), the U.S. Office of Human Research Protection (OHRP), and the U.S. Environmental Protection Agency (EPA).

10. Often, x-ray regulations are promulgated at the state level (with additional rules on mammography coming from the FDA) and several states specifically designate definitions of Qualified Medical Physicists.

11. The National Council on Radiation Protection and Measurements (NCRP) and the International Commission on Radiological Protection (ICRP) are recognized professional advisory bodies on radiation, including its use in medicine. The International Atomic Energy Agency (IAEA) provides guidance on the implementation of ICRP recommendations. The United Nations Scientific Committee on the Effects of Atomic Radiation (UNSCEAR) assesses global levels and evaluates the short- and long-term biological effects of ionizing radiation.

12. Other important professional societies develop practical-specific recommendations and guidance in the area of radiation protection of patients and staff that should be consulted by practicing medical physicists, for example, American Association of Physicists in Medicine (AAPM), ACR, Radiological Society of North America (RSNA), Society of Nuclear Medicine and Molecular Imaging (SNMMI), and Health Physics Society (HPS). Ongoing collaborative associations with equipment vendors are also important contributors, for example, Medical Imaging & Technology Alliance (MITA), National Electrical Manufacturer's Association (NEMA), and the International Electrotechnical Commission (IEC).

13. NRC and Agreement State regulations regulate that doses to individuals shall not exceed established limits (Fig. 21-5) and that all exposures shall be kept ALARA, social and economic factors being taken into account.

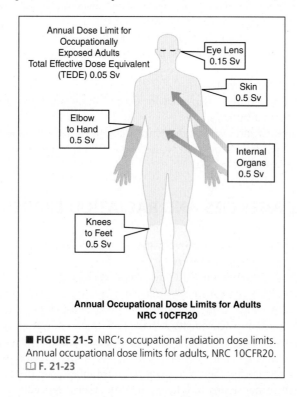

**FIGURE 21-5** NRC's occupational radiation dose limits. Annual occupational dose limits for adults, NRC 10CFR20.
F. 21-23

## 21.9 PREVENTION OF ERRORS

1. A goal of radiation protection programs is to reduce the likelihood and severity of accidents involving radiation and radioactive materials.
    a. Safety culture: represents a set of attributes of an organization, such as a radiology or nuclear medicine department, that are believed to reduce the likelihood of errors; and the behavior and practices resulting from a commitment by leaders and individuals to emphasize safety over competing goals to protect patients, staff, and the public.
2. Policies and procedures may incorporate the following:
    a. The use of a "time out" in which the staff about to perform a clinical procedure jointly verify that the intended procedure is to be properly performed on the intended patient
    b. The use of written or computerized checklists to ensure that essential actions are not omitted
    c. Checks of critical tasks by a second person
    d. Requiring that certain critical communications be in writing
    e. Employing readback in verbal communications, whereby the person hearing information repeats it aloud
    f. Measures to avoid distractions and interruptions during critical tasks, such as prohibiting unnecessary conversations unrelated to a task
3. The incorporation of engineered safety features, such as interlocks that prevent unsafe actions, and automated checks, such as the dose notifications and alerts provided by newer CT scanners, help to avoid accidents due to human errors.
4. When an error or a "near-miss" occurs, an analysis should be performed to determine the root and contributing causes and to devise actions to reduce the likelihood of a recurrence and possibly the severity of a recurrence.
5. The Joint Commission (TJC) is a not-for-profit hospital and other healthcare facility accrediting organization. TJC defines a "sentinel event" as "an unexpected occurrence involving death or serious physical or psychological injury, or the risk thereof." TJC defines as a sentinel event prolonged fluoroscopy with a cumulative dose exceeding 15 Gy to a single field, "a single field" being a location on the skin onto which the x-ray beam is directed.
6. TJC has warned that healthcare organizations must seek new ways to reduce exposure to repeated doses of harmful radiation from diagnostic imaging and fluoroscopy, by raising awareness among staff and patients of the increased risks associated with cumulative doses and by providing the right test and the right dose through effective processes, safe technology, and a culture of safety. TJC emphasizes the use of a diagnostic medical physicist in designing and altering CT scan protocols; centralized quality and safety performance monitoring of all diagnostic imaging equipment; periodic testing of imaging equipment; and implementation of a quality control program.

## 21.10 MANAGEMENT OF RADIATION SAFETY PROGRAMS

1. Radiation safety programs must be designed in such a way as to maintain the safety of staff, patients, and members of the public; compliance with regulations of governmental agencies; and preparedness for emergencies involving radiation and/or radioactive material. Although there are no regulatory limits to the radiation doses that patients may receive as part of their care, the doses to patients should be optimized.
2. Each institution must designate a person, called the RSO, who is responsible for the day-to-day oversight of the radiation safety program and is named on the institution's radioactive material license. The RSO must have appropriate training and qualifications for the role (see 10 CFR 35.50, or equivalent).
3. A radiation safety committee typically meets quarterly and approves policies and procedures, periodically reviews the program, and reviews corrective actions after adverse incidents involving radiation or radioactive material. The radiation safety committee is composed of the RSO, representatives from departments with substantial radiation and radioactive material use (*e.g.*, nuclear medicine, radiology, cardiology, radiation oncology, and nursing), and a member representing hospital management.
4. A radiation safety program should include an audit program to ensure compliance with regulatory requirements, accepted radiation safety practices, and institutional procedures.
5. A diagnostic medical physicist is essential to the radiation safety program of a medical facility performing radiological imaging.

## 21.11 IMAGING OF PREGNANT AND POTENTIALLY PREGNANT PATIENTS

1. The risks of ionizing radiation to the embryo and fetus must be considered when imaging female patients of childbearing age using ionizing radiation and performing therapies using radiopharmaceuticals. See Chapter 20 for additional information on risks.

2. Pregnancy status should be determined for female patients from about 12 to 50 years of age. This is typically based on a documented inquiry to the patient. For some procedures that could impart doses to an embryo or fetus exceeding 100 mSv (*e.g.*, prolonged fluoroscopically guided procedures or multiphase CT examinations of the abdomen or pelvis), a pregnancy test should also be obtained within 72 h prior to the examination.

3. Pregnancy tests should always be obtained prior to radiopharmaceutical therapies.

4. All x-ray imaging examinations, in which the embryo or fetus is not close to the area being imaged, impart doses much less than 100 mSv to the embryo or fetus, and most x-ray examinations of the abdomen and pelvis, including single-phase diagnostic CT examinations, impart doses less than 100 mSv.

## 21.12   MEDICAL EMERGENCIES INVOLVING IONIZING RADIATION

1. Medical institutions should be prepared to respond to emergencies involving radiation and radioactive materials, for example, spills, contamination of personnel, medical events involving errors in the administration of radioactive material, or radiation to patients. Medical emergencies may also include external events, for example, transportation accidents, accidents at nuclear facilities, and radiological or nuclear terrorism.

2. Radiologists and other healthcare professionals, familiar with the properties of radiation, its detection, and biological effects may be called upon to assist in such emergencies and should be prepared to provide guidance and technical assistance to medical staff managing such patients.

3. Each medical facility has or should have a plan for responding to radiation emergencies of varying types and scopes. In particular, the emergency department should be expected to receive and treat injured patients with radioactive contamination.

4. Treatment of severe injuries or life-threatening medical conditions should take priority over decontamination, although very simple and quick measures, such as removal of the patients' clothing and wiping exposed skin with mild soap, tepid water, and a damp cloth, will likely remove most of the contamination.

5. Standard protective clothing commonly worn by the staff is sufficient to protect them from radioactive contamination.

6. Periodic surveys with a GM detector and methods similar to common infection prevention techniques will prevent significant contamination with radioactive material (Fig. 21-6).

7. Decontamination is commonly performed by removing contaminated clothing and washing the contaminated area with soap and water, taking care not to spread contamination to other parts of the body or onto other people, and ensuring that people do not inhale or ingest the radioactive material.

8. Internal contamination may enter the body by inhalation, ingestion, through a wound, by injection, or, for some radioactive material, by absorption through the skin. NCRP Report No. 161 (2008) provides detailed guidance on the treatment of internal contamination.

9. See Chapter 20 for additional information on the acute radiation syndrome.

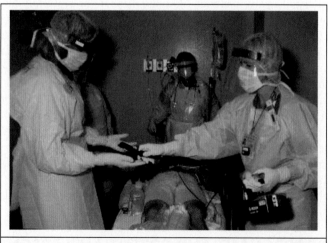

■ **FIGURE 21-6** Standard protective clothing commonly worn by ED staff and periodic surveys with a GM survey meter protect staff from contamination with radioactive material. ▭ **F. 21-24**

# Section II Questions and Answers

1. The exposure rate measured in an office adjacent to a new PET room with an $^{18}$F-FDG patient is 1.28 mR/h with the current wall between the office and the PET room. To reduce this exposure rate to 0.04 mR/h in the office, how much lead shielding is required in this wall? (The half-value layer in lead for 511-keV photons is 4 mm).
   A. 4 mm
   B. 8 mm
   C. 12 mm
   D. 16 mm
   E. 20 mm

2. Which of the following statements is correct?
   A. Radiation mutagenesis is dose rate independent.
   B. The LD50 total-body dose of ionizing radiation for humans is about 20 Gy.
   C. Radiation from medical imaging procedures accounts for about half of the annual per capita estimate of radiation exposure in the United States
   D. Radiation carcinogenesis has a well-defined threshold dose of 100 mSv.
   E. Radon is not a source of exposure for the U.S. population.

3. Which cells/tissues in the below list are considered the most radiosensitive?
   A. Skin cells
   B. Brain cells
   C. Bone marrow stem cells
   D. Spermatids
   E. Lymphoid tissue

4. The effective dose should mainly be used for the which of the following?
   A. Epidemiological studies
   B. Estimating risk of fetal teratogenesis due to irradiation in utero
   C. Prospective dose assessment and comparison for planning and optimization of radiological protection
   D. Calculating radiation dose to the gonads
   E. Activity that will give the same dose to all persons

5. The regulatory effective dose limit for a patient undergoing a cardiac stress test procedure is:
   A. 50 mSv
   B. 20 mSv
   C. 15 mSv
   D. 5 mSv
   E. not limited

6. The current estimated population average natural background radiation exposure in the United States is:
   A. less than 1 mSv
   B. about 1 mSv
   C. about 3 mSv
   D. about 6 mSv
   E. more than 10 mSv

7. When designing the shielding of a diagnostic imaging suite, what is the dose limit in an adjacent unrestricted/uncontrolled area?
   A. 50 mSv in any week
   B. 15 mSv in a year
   C. 0.1 mSv in any hour
   D. 0.02 mSv in any week
   E. unrestricted, no limit

8. How long should nursing mothers be advised to interrupt breastfeeding following administration of iodine-131?
   A. 24 h following administration.
   B. 7 days following administration.
   C. 14 days following administration.
   D. There are no breastfeeding precautions needed.
   E. Permanently for the current baby following administration.

9. According to ICRP Publication 103, what is the tissue weighting factor ($w_T$) for the thyroid?
   A. 0.12
   B. 0.08
   C. 0.05
   D. 0.04
   E. 0.01

10. For quickly estimating effective dose based on the dose-length-product (DLP), which of the following conversion factors ($k$-factor) is most appropriate to use for adult head scans, where $E = DLP(mGy\text{-}cm) * k(mSv/mGy\text{-}cm)$?
    - A. 0.0023
    - B. 0.006
    - C. 0.015
    - D. 0.0021
    - E. 0.05

11. When designing diagnostic imaging suite shielding, what is the most appropriate occupancy factor (T) to be utilized for control booths/rooms?
    - A. 0
    - B. 1
    - C. 1/2
    - D. 1/5
    - E. 1/8

12. When designing a PET/CT suite, which of the following most directly impacts the amount of lead shielding required?
    - A. CT mAs
    - B. DLP
    - C. Activity of PET isotope administered to the patient
    - D. Scatter dose from the CT scanner head
    - E. Humidity

13. According to the NCRP, which of the following recommendations is most applicable for fluoroscopically guided interventional procedures?
    - A. Equipment that is routinely used for pediatric procedures should be appropriately designed, equipped, and configured for this purpose.
    - B. Door interlocks that interrupt x-ray production shall be required at any entrances to FGI procedure rooms.
    - C. Patient dose data are not required to be recorded in the patient's medical record at the conclusion of each procedure.
    - D. Facilities do not have to periodically review radiation doses for patients undergoing FGI procedures.
    - E. All of the above.

14. Medical radiation exposure of patients in the United States was reduced by about 15% to 20% from 2006 to 2016, mainly because which of the following?
    - A. Imaging of fewer individuals than in the past
    - B. Advances in technology, increased awareness, and optimization
    - C. Reductions in CMS coverage of imaging procedures
    - D. Changing the pulses for fluoroscopy cases
    - E. Use of patient shielding

15. Whole-body dosimeters are typically worn on what part of the body?
    - A. Head
    - B. Below the knee
    - C. On the wrist or finger
    - D. Shirt pocket or waist
    - E. Back of the neck

16. When are electronic dosimeters helpful for radiation protection programs?
    - A. As the dose-of-record
    - B. For ongoing dose feedback in cardiac cath or FGI procedures
    - C. For nuclear medicine waiting rooms
    - D. Under a lead apron
    - E. When deployed on walls for area monitoring

17. A common application of GM survey meter in radiation protection is:
    - A. outdoor ground surveys
    - B. when accurate measurements of exposure rate are required
    - C. performing surveys for radioactive contamination
    - D. for calibrating radiotherapy machine output
    - E. in high radiation fields

18. What is the main advantage of ionization chambers for detection?
    - A. Sufficiently accurate for measuring radiation exposure rates in medical imaging.
    - B. Useful when performing contamination surveys after a spill.
    - C. Alpha particles can easily be detected.
    - D. They do not need to be warmed up or stabilized.
    - E. All of the above.

19. What statement best captures the essence of the radiation protection principle of justification with regard to medical imaging?
    - A. The patient's clinical situation does not apply.
    - B. It is only useful for research protocols.
    - C. All medical imaging procedures are justified.
    - D. If insurance providers will pay, then imaging is justified.
    - E. Clinical benefit outweighs the radiation risk.

20. How does optimization best apply to medical imaging?
    - A. Use the newest and best equipment available.
    - B. Use the lowest dose necessary to produce appropriate diagnostic quality or goals of an intervention.
    - C. Reduce the dose until important diagnostic information is lost.
    - D. All of the above.
    - E. None of the above.

21. What is the typical attenuation property of protective aprons and collar shields employed in fluoroscopy settings?
    A. 10%
    B. 25%
    C. 50%
    D. 75%
    E. Greater than 90%

22. Diagnostic Reference Levels are typically set at what percentile of the set of data from a study of dose metrics in medicine?
    A. 10%
    B. 25%
    C. 50%
    D. 75%
    E. Greater than 90%

23. After an emergent spill of radioactive material, what should one keep in mind?
    A. KISS—keep it simple stupid
    B. SING—safety ignores nuclear goofs
    C. SWIM—stop, warn, isolate, and mitigate
    D. RUN—risk under negligence
    E. NADA—nothing as the dose is attenuated

24. Considering the release of patients who have received therapeutic amounts of radioactive material, when are instructions required to be provided?
    A. If the dose to any other individual is likely to exceed 1 mSv
    B. Never
    C. If the dose to a caregiver is likely to exceed 5 mSv
    D. If the patient is thin
    E. If the patient is a child

25. Agreement States typically regulate what areas of radiation control programs?
    A. Only for special nuclear material (plutonium and enriched uranium).
    B. Only for accelerator-produced radioactivity.
    C. Only those areas where they are in agreement.
    D. All sources of ionizing radiation (including medical x-ray use).
    E. There are no agreement states.

26. What sections of the Code of Federal Regulations cover radiation use for hospitals and medical imaging facilities?
    A. Title 10 CFR Part 20 and Title 10 CFR Part 35
    B. Title 11 of the United States Code
    C. Title 49 CFR Part 227
    D. Title 21 CFR Part 25
    E. None of the above

27. What is considered a by-product material in medicine?
    A. Plutonium
    B. Uranium ore
    C. X-rays
    D. Fission, activation, and accelerator-produced products
    E. All of the above

28. The Joint Commission defines a sentinel event as prolonged fluoroscopy with a cumulative dose exceeding what dose to a single field?
    A. 0.15 Gy
    B. 1.5 Gy
    C. 15 Gy
    D. 150 Gy
    E. 15 mGy

29. Which of the following are traits of good safety culture as defined by the NRC?
    A. Trust and respect permeate the organization.
    B. Leaders demonstrate a commitment to safety.
    C. Work activities are planned and conducted safely.
    D. Communications maintain a focus on safety.
    E. All of the above.

30. The radiation safety committee is composed of the radiation safety officer, a member representing hospital management, and representatives of what other departments?
    A. Nuclear medicine, radiology, cardiology, radiation oncology, and nursing
    B. Facilities, social work, billing, and food services
    C. Janitorial services, admitting, psychiatry, and behavioral sciences
    D. Physical therapy, obstetrics, ophthalmology, and orthopedics

31. For what clinical visits should a pregnancy test be performed within 72 h before the examination or procedure?
    A. Procedures that could impart doses exceeding 100 mGy to embryo or fetus
    B. Prolonged fluoroscopically guided procedures of the abdomen
    C. Multiphase diagnostic CT examination of the abdomen or pelvis

32. Decontamination of a nuclear medicine technician after a spill should include removing contaminated clothing and washing the contaminated area with:
    A. dilute solution of DTPA
    B. soap and water
    C. a wire brush
    D. isopropyl alcohol
    E. salt and sand

# Answers

1. **E**  The intensity of x- and gamma-rays decreases exponentially as a function of absorber thickness. With a half-value layer (HVL) in lead for 511-keV photons of 4 mm, the intensity of fluorine-18 radiation decreases by ½ for each 4 mm thickness of lead. Therefore, 20 mm (or five HVLs) of lead decreases the exposure rate from 1.28 mR/h to ½ × ½ × ½ × ½ × ½ × 1.28 = 0.04 mR/h. *(Pg. 57–85)*

2. **C**  The advances in medical imaging over the last several decades have significantly increased the average annual background dose per capita in the United States. The $LD_{50}$ total body dose of ionizing radiation for humans is less than 20 Gy—closer to only 4 to 5 Gy. Like many other radiation effects, mutagenesis exhibits a marked dose-rate effect, meaning the frequency of mutagenesis at a given dose increases as the dose rate increases. Radiation carcinogenesis is considered a stochastic effect and (for the purpose of radiation protection) is assumed not to exhibit a threshold dose. *(Pg. 927–931)*

3. **C**  Radiosensitivity is the relative susceptibility of cells, tissues, organs, and organisms to the injurious action of radiation. In general, it has been found that cell radiosensitivity is directly proportional to the rate of cell division and inversely proportional to the degree of cell differentiation. This means that actively dividing cells or those not fully mature are most at risk from radiation. The most radiosensitive cells are those which have a high division rate, have a high metabolic rate, are of a nonspecific type, and have ample nutrients. As such, bone marrow cells have the highest radiosensitivity on this list. *(Pg. 835; 862)*

4. **C**  Effective dose generally reflects the risk of cancer induction and germ cell damage. According to ICRP Publication No. 103, the main uses of effective dose are the prospective dose assessment for planning and optimization in radiological protection and demonstration of compliance with dose limits for regulatory purposes. Effective dose is not recommended for epidemiological evaluations, nor should it be used for detailed specific retrospective investigations of individual exposure and risk. *(Pg. 66–70)*

5. **E**  In applying the principle of optimization of protection of the patient, the benefits and detriments are received by the same individual, the patient, and the dose to the patient is determined principally by the medical needs. Dose constraints or limits for patients are therefore inappropriate. The limitation of dose to the individual patient is not recommended because it may, by reducing the effectiveness of the patient's diagnosis or treatment, do more harm than good. The emphasis is then on the justification of the medical procedures and the optimization of protection. See ICRP Publication 103 and ICRP Publication 105 for additional discussions of this topic. Of course, in complex fluoroscopic procedures, there is a risk for skin tissue effects (deterministic effects) that should be evaluated according to guidance in NCRP Report No. 168. *(Pg. 940)*

6. **C**  NCRP Report No. 160 is the most recent comprehensive evaluation of population average annual radiation exposure in the United States and is based on information up to about 2006. Medical exposure accounts for about 3.00 mSv including CT (1.47 mSv), nuclear medicine (0.77 mSv), interventional fluoroscopy (0.43 mSv), and conventional radiography (0.33 mSv). Ubiquitous background exposure also accounts for about 3 mSv including internal inhalation (2.28 mSv) (radon and thoron), external space (0.33 mSv), internal ingestion (0.29 mSv), and external terrestrial (0.21 mSv). Other exposures account for about 0.09 mSv. The grand total is about 6.2 mSv per year. *(Pg. 927; 931)*

7. **D**  NCRP Report No. 147 notes that based on ICRP and NCRP recommendations for the annual limit of effective dose to a member of the general public, shielding designs shall limit exposure of all individuals in unrestricted areas to an effective dose that does not exceed 1 mSv/y. NCRP has concluded that a suitable source control for shielding individuals in uncontrolled areas in or near medical radiation facilities is an effective dose of 1 mSv in any year. This recommendation can be achieved with a weekly shielding design goal of 0.02 mSv. Note that 10 CFR Part 20.1301(a)(2) further requires that the "dose" in any unrestricted area from external sources not exceed 2 mrem in any 1 h (0.02 mSv in any hour). *(Pg. 950–954)*

8.  **E**   Guidance on precautions for lactating mothers who receive radioactive material can be found in the U.S. Nuclear Regulatory Commission NUREG-1556, Appendix U and ICRP 128, Table D.1. Although there are no universally recognized guidelines, recommended lengths of time nursing mothers should be advised to interrupt breastfeeding as follows: 24 h for $^{99m}$Tc radiopharmaceuticals; 12 to 24 h for $^{18}$F radiopharmaceuticals or $^{68}$Ga radiopharmaceuticals; 7 days for $^{111}$In-white blood cells or $^{123}$I radiopharmaceuticals; 14 days for $^{201}$Tl-chloride, $^{67}$Ga-citrate, or $^{89}$Zr radiopharmaceuticals; and permanently for $^{131}$I or $^{124}$I radiopharmaceuticals. *(Pg. 984; 1115–1121)*

9.  **A**   Different nominal probabilities exist for the occurrence of stochastic radiation effects in various organs and tissues. This different sensitivity is considered in ICRP Publication 103 by the tissue weighting factor ($w_T$), which is used in calculations of effective dose. In 2007, the ICRP Publication 103 set the $w_T$ of the lung to 0.12. *(Pg. 67; 419–420)*

10.  **D**   In AAPM Report 96, effective dose values calculated from Monte Carlo organ coefficients were compared with DLP values for corresponding clinical examinations to determine a set of coefficients, $k$, where the values of $k$ are dependent only on the region of the body being scanned (head, neck, thorax, abdomen, or pelvis). Using this methodology, effective doses can be estimated from the DLP, which is reported on most CT systems. For the adult, the values of $k$ (mSv/mGy-cm) are 0.0021, 0.0059, 0.014, 0.015, and 0.015 for the adult head, neck, chest, abdomen, and pelvis, respectively. Note that for children, the corresponding coefficients are higher, indicating higher effective doses per unit of DLP for children over adults. *(Pg. 437)*

11.  **B**   NCRP Report 147 gives suggested occupancy factors (T) for use as a guide in planning shielding and provides a value of $T = 1$ for control rooms. Work areas fully occupied by an individual during a typical workday should be assigned a $T = 1$. Note a $T = 1/2$ for adjacent rooms used for patient examinations and treatments. *(Pg. 950)*

12.  **C**   AAPM report number 108 provides information helpful for evaluating the shielding requirements of a PET suite. NCRP Report No. 147 provides information helpful for evaluating shielding requirements for CT suites. The higher energy of the most important photons from PET isotopes (0.511 MeV) generally dominates the lower energy of the typical CT x-ray spectra with peak energies of about 120 to 140 kV. Typical CT-only suites require approximately 1/32nd to 1/16th inch lead equivalent shielding. PET reading suites often require 1/8th to ¼ inch lead equivalent shielding, depending on the size of the room and the activity of the PET isotope given to the patient. *(Pg. 956)*

13.  **E**   NCRP Report No. 168 provides an exceptional summary of recommendations applicable for fluoroscopically guided interventional procedures, including (1) equipment that is routinely used for pediatric procedures should be appropriately designed, equipped, and configured for this purpose. (2) Door interlocks that interrupt x-ray production shall not be permitted at any entrances to FGI procedure rooms. (3) Patient dose data shall be recorded in the patient's medical record at the conclusion of each procedure. (4) Facilities shall have a process to review radiation doses for patients undergoing FGI procedures. *(Pg. 964–967)*

14.  **B**   NCRP Report 184 has detailed information on medical radiation exposure of the patients in the United States *(Pg. 931)*

15.  **D**   Whole body exposure monitoring uses an operational quantity for the torso and central organs. *(Pg. 932–936)*

16.  **B**   Electronic dosimeters, while not the dose-of-record, are especially useful as they display total dose (and/or dose rate) and can assist in the optimization of staff protection. *(Pg. 937)*

17.  **C**   GM survey instruments and their probes react quickly during surveys to detect the presence and provide semiquantitative estimates of the intensities of radiation fields. *(Pg. 939)*

18.  **A**   Ion chambers have linear responses over wide ranges of exposure rates and photon energies, and they indicate exposure rates and photon energies. *(Pg. 939–940)*

19.  **E**   ICRP Publication 103 describes justification as any decision that alters the radiation exposure situation should do more good than harm, that is, yield an individual or societal benefit that is higher than the detriment it causes. ICRP Publication 105 gives additional insight with regard to justification in medicine. *(Pg. 940–941)*

20. **B** Reducing an examination dose to the point where important diagnostic information is lost or that results in the examination needing to be repeated is counterproductive and increases rather than decreases the overall risk to the patient. *(Pg. 940–941)*

21. **E** Greater than 90% of the scattered radiation incident on the apron is attenuated by the 0.25 mm thickness at standard x-ray energies. Aprons of 0.35- and 0.50-mm lead equivalents give greater protection. *(Pg. 957–959)*

22. **D** ICRP 2017 and the ACR have noted that DRLs can be used as an investigational level in a quality assurance program to identify possibly excessive doses to patients and are typically set at the 75th percentile. An achievable dose is typically set at the median value of the dose distribution from the study. *(Pg. 441; 971–974)*

23. **C** SWIM—stop, warn, isolate, and mitigate. *(Pg. 983)*

24. **A** Patient release criteria are promulgated in NRC regulations (Title 10 CFR Part 35.75), and guidance is published in Regulatory Guide 8.39 and NCRP Report 155. *(Pg. 987–988)*

25. **D** The Agreement State program is maintained by the NRC and associated states. The Conference of Radiation Control Program Directors (crcpd.org) has developed general guidance for Agreement States. *(Pg. 684; 982; 989)*

26. **A** Title 10 CFR Part 20—Standards for Protection Against Radiation—establishes standards for protection against ionizing radiation resulting from activities conducted under licenses issued by the NRC. The purpose of the regulations in this part is to control the receipt, possession, use, transfer, and disposal of licensed material by any licensee in such a manner that the total dose to an individual (including doses resulting from licensed and unlicensed radioactive material and radiation sources other than background radiation) does not exceed the standards within. Title 10 CFR Part 35—Medical Use of Byproduct Material—contains the requirements and provisions for the medical use of by-product material and issuance of specific licenses authorizing the medical use of this material. These requirements and provisions provide for the radiation safety of workers, the general public, patients, and human research subjects. *(Pg. 684; 985–990)*

27. **D** Title 10 CFR Part 20, paragraph 20.1003 Definitions, codifies the definition of by-product material that includes fission and activation products as well as radium-226 (for commercial, medical, or research activity) and any material that has been made radioactive by use of a particle accelerator, as well as several other specified materials. *(Pg. 985–990)*

28. **C** The Joint Commission defines sentinel events as follows: *A sentinel event is an unexpected occurrence involving death or serious physical or psychological injury, or the risk thereof. Serious injury specifically includes loss of limb or function. The phrase "or the risk thereof" includes any process variation for which a recurrence would carry a significant chance of a serious adverse outcome. Such events are called "sentinel" because they signal the need for immediate investigation and response.* In 2005, the Joint Commission added the following to its list of events that are reviewable under its Sentinel Event Policy: *prolonged fluoroscopy with cumulative dose greater than 1,500 rads to a single field or any delivery of radiotherapy to the wrong region or greater than 25% above the planned dose.* The Joint Commission also elaborated on radiation risks of diagnostic imaging and fluoroscopy in Sentinel Event Alert 47, revised February 2019. *(Pg. 996; 1008)*

29. **E** The U.S. Nuclear Regulatory Commission issued a final safety culture policy statement in 2011 to set forth its expectation that individuals and organizations performing or overseeing regulated activities establish and maintain a positive safety culture commensurate with the safety and security significance of their activities and the nature and complexity of their organizations and functions. Each of the aspects listed in Answers A to D are included as traits therein. *(Pg. 996; 1009)*

30. **A** 10 CFR Part 35, paragraph 35.24, authority and responsibilities for the radiation protection program, requires that medical licensees establish a radiation safety committee. The Committee must include an authorized user of each type of use permitted by the license, the Radiation Safety Officer, a representative of the nursing service, and a representative of management who is neither an authorized user nor a Radiation Safety Officer. The Committee may include other members the licensee considers appropriate. *(Pg. 684; 998)*

31. **A** For procedures that could impart doses to an embryo or fetus exceeding 100 mSv (*e.g.*, prolonged fluoroscopically guided procedures or multiphase CT examinations of the abdomen or pelvis), a pregnancy test should also be obtained within 72 h prior to the examination. While answers A & B are correct, answer C is the most correct as it is most general case and would include answers A&B. *(Pg. 908–915; 999)*

32. **B** Decontamination is commonly performed by removing contaminated clothing and washing the contaminated area with soap and water, taking care not to spread contamination to other parts of the body. *(Pg. 1003)*

# Section III Key Equations, Symbols, Quantities, and Units

| QUANTITY | EQUATION | EQ NO./PAGE/COMMENTS |
|---|---|---|
| Estimates for effective dose equivalent when using personal protective shielding and a single collar dosimeter | $H_E = 0.18 \ H_N$ | Eq. 21-1/Pg. 936/Calculates the effective dose equivalent from the dose recorded by the collar dosimeter $H_N$. 📖 E. 21-1 |
| Estimates for effective dose equivalent when using personal protective shielding and both a collar and waist or chest dosimeter | $H_E = 1.5 \ H_W + 0.04 \ H_N$ | Eq. 21-2/Pg. 936/Calculates the effective dose equivalent from the dose recorded by collar dosimetry $H_N$ and one worn under the apron at the waist or chest, $H_W$, per NCRP Report No. 122. 📖 E. 21-2 |

| SYMBOL | QUANTITY | UNITS |
|---|---|---|
| $D$ | Absorbed dose, the mean energy imparted by ionizing radiation to matter in a volume element divided by the mass of matter in that volume element | Gy<br><br>(1 J/kg = 1 Gy)<br><br>(1 rad = 0.01 Gy) |
| $A$ | Activity, the number of nuclear transformations occurring in a given quantity of material per unit time | Bq<br><br>(1 Bq = 1/s)<br><br>(1 mCi = 37 MBq) |
| $H_T$ | Equivalent dose, the sum of the mean absorbed dose in a tissue or organ weighted by a radiation weighting factor ($w_R$). Note, $w_R = 1$ for photons (x-rays) and electrons (betas) | Sv<br><br>(1 rem = 0.01 Sv) |
| $E$ | Effective dose, the tissue-weighted sum of equivalent doses in all specified tissues and organs of the body. Note, tissue weighting factors range from 0.12 (red bone marrow, colon, lung, stomach, breast, remainders), to 0.08 (gonads), to 0.04 (bladder, esophagus, liver, thyroid), and to 0.01 (bone surface, brain, salivary glands, skin) | Sv<br><br>(1 rem = 0.01 Sv) |

# Appendices

# SI and Derived Units, Physical Constants, Prefixes, Definitions and Conversion Factors, Geometry, and Roman and Greek Symbols Used in Medical Physics

**TABLE A-1  SI BASE UNITS**   📖 T. B-1

| BASE QUANTITY | | BASE UNIT | |
|---|---|---|---|
| *Name* | *Typical Symbol* | *Name* | *Symbol* |
| time | $t$ | second | s |
| length | $l, x, r$, etc. | meter | m |
| mass | $m$ | kilogram | kg |
| electric current | $I, i$ | ampere | A |
| thermodynamic temperature | $T$ | kelvin | K |
| amount of substance | $n$ | mole | mol |
| luminous intensity | $I_v$ | candela | cd |

Reprinted from Bureau International des Poids et Mesures. *The International System of Units (SI)*. 9th ed. 2019. (CC BY 4.0). https://www.bipm.org/utils/common/pdf/si-brochure/SI-Brochure-9.pdf

**TABLE A-2  THE 21 SI UNITS WITH SPECIAL NAMES AND SYMBOLS**   📖 T. B-2

| DERIVED QUANTITY | SPECIAL NAME OF UNIT | UNIT EXPRESSED IN TERMS OF BASE UNITS[a] | UNIT EXPRESSED IN TERMS OF OTHER SI UNITS |
|---|---|---|---|
| plane angle | radian[b] | $\text{rad} = \text{m/m}$ | |
| solid angle | steradian[c] | $\text{sr} = \text{m}^2/\text{m}^2$ | |
| frequency | hertz[d] | $\text{Hz} = \text{s}^{-1}$ | |
| force | Newton | $\text{N} = \text{kg m s}^{-2}$ | |
| pressure, stress | Pascal | $\text{Pa} = \text{kg m}^{-1}\text{ s}^{-2}$ | |
| energy, work, amount of heat | joule | $\text{J} = \text{kg m}^2\text{ s}^{-2}$ | Nm |
| power, radiant flux | watt | $\text{W} = \text{kg m}^2\text{ s}^{-3}$ | J/s |
| electric charge[a] | coulomb | $\text{C} = \text{A s}$ | |
| electric potential difference[e] | volt | $\text{V} = \text{kg m}^2\text{ s}^{-3}\text{ A}^{-1}$ | W/A |
| capacitance | farad | $\text{F} = \text{kg}^{-1}\text{ m}^{-2}\text{ s}^4\text{ A}^2$ | C/V |
| electric resistance | ohm | $\Omega = \text{kg m}^2\text{ s}^{-3}\text{ A}^{-2}$ | V/A |
| electric conductance | siemens | $\text{S} = \text{kg}^{-1}\text{ m}^2\text{ s}^3\text{ A}^2$ | A/V |
| magnetic flux | weber | $\text{Wb} = \text{kg m}^2\text{ s}^{-2}\text{ A}^{-1}$ | Vs |
| magnetic flux density | tesla | $\text{T} = \text{kg s}^{-2}\text{ A}^{-1}$ | Wb/m$^2$ |

*(Continued)*

**TABLE A-2  THE 21 SI UNITS WITH SPECIAL NAMES AND SYMBOLS** *(Continued)*

| DERIVED QUANTITY | SPECIAL NAME OF UNIT | UNIT EXPRESSED IN TERMS OF BASE UNITS[a] | UNIT EXPRESSED IN TERMS OF OTHER SI UNITS |
|---|---|---|---|
| inductance | henry | $H = kg\ m^2\ s^{-2}\ A^{-2}$ | Wb/A |
| Celsius temperature | degree Celsius[f] | $°C = K$ | |
| luminous flux | lumen | $lm = cd\ sr$[g] | cd sr |
| illuminance | lux | $lx = cd\ sr\ m^{-2}$ | $lm/m^2$ |
| activity referred to a radionuclide[d,h] | becquerel | $Bq = s^{-1}$ | |
| absorbed dose, kerma | gray | $Gy = m^2\ s^{-2}$ | J/kg |
| dose equivalent | sievert[i] | $Sv = m^2\ s^{-2}$ | J/kg |

[a]Under the 2019 redefinition of the SI base units, which took effect on May 20, 2019, the elementary charge (*i.e.*, the charge of the proton or electron and other fundamental particles) was defined as exactly $1.602176634 \times 10^{-19}$ coulombs. Thus the coulomb is the charge of exactly $1/(1.602176634 \times 10^{-19})$ elementary charges, which is approximately $6.2415090744 \times 10^{18}$ elementary charges. The intention was to reflect the underlying physics of the corresponding quantity equations although for some more complex derived units this may not be possible.
[b]The radian is the coherent unit for plane angle. One radian is the angle subtended at the center of a circle by an arc that is equal in length to the radius. It is also the unit for phase angle. For periodic phenomena, the phase angle increases by $2\pi$ rad in one period. The radian was formerly an SI supplementary unit, but this category was abolished in 1995.
[c]The steradian is the coherent unit for solid angle. One steradian is the solid angle subtended at the center of a sphere by an area of the surface that is equal to the squared radius. Like the radian, the steradian was formerly an SI supplementary unit.
[d]The hertz shall only be used for periodic phenomena and the becquerel shall only be used for stochastic processes in activity referred to a radionuclide.
[e]Electric potential difference is also called "voltage" in many countries, as well as "electric tension" or simply "tension" in some countries.
[f]The degree Celsius is used to express Celsius temperatures. The numerical value of a temperature difference or temperature interval is the same when expressed in either degrees Celsius or in kelvin.
[g]In photometry the name steradian and the symbol sr are usually retained in expressions for units.
[h]Activity referred to a radionuclide is sometimes incorrectly called radioactivity.
[i]The special name sievert is also used from the radiation protection quantity effective dose as specified by the International Commission on Radiological Protection (ICRP).
Adapted from Bureau International des Poids et Mesures. *The International System of Units (SI)*. 9th ed. 2019. (CC BY 4.0). https://www.bipm.org/utils/common/pdf/si-brochure/SI-Brochure-9.pdf

**TABLE A-3  SELECTION OF COHERENT DERIVED UNITS IN THE SI EXPRESSED IN TERMS OF BASE UNITS**  📖 T. B-3

| DERIVED QUANTITY | TYPICAL SYMBOL OF QUANTITY | DERIVED UNIT EXPRESSED IN TERMS OF BASE UNITS |
|---|---|---|
| area | $A$ | $m^2$ |
| volume | $V$ | $m^3$ |
| speed, velocity | $v$ | $m\ s^{-1}$ |
| acceleration | $a$ | $m\ s^{-2}$ |
| wavenumber | $\sigma$ | $m^{-1}$ |
| density, mass density | $\rho$ | $kg\ m^{-3}$ |
| surface density | $\rho a$ | $kg\ m^{-2}$ |
| specific volume | $v$ | $m^3\ kg^{-1}$ |
| current density | $j$ | $A\ m^{-2}$ |
| magnetic field strength | $H$ | $A\ m^{-1}$ |
| amount of substance concentration | $c$ | $mol\ m^{-3}$ |
| mass concentration | $\rho, \gamma$ | $kg\ m^{-3}$ |
| luminance | $L_v$ | $cd\ m^{-2}$ |

Reprinted from Bureau International des Poids et Mesures. *The International System of Units (SI)*. 9th ed. 2019. (CC BY 4.0). https://www.bipm.org/utils/common/pdf/si-brochure/SI-Brochure-9.pdf

**TABLE A-4 SI DERIVED UNITS**[a]   📖 T. B-4

| DERIVED QUANTITY | NAME OF COHERENT DERIVED UNIT | SYMBOL | DERIVED UNIT EXPRESSED IN TERMS OF BASE UNITS |
|---|---|---|---|
| moment of force | newton meter | N m | $kg\ m^2\ s^{-2}$ |
| surface tension | newton per meter | N m$^{-1}$ | $kg\ s^{-2}$ |
| angular velocity, angular frequency | radian per second | rad s$^{-1}$ | $s^{-1}$ |
| angular acceleration | radian per second squared | rad s$^{-2}$ | $s^{-2}$ |
| heat flux density, irradiance | watt per square meter | W m$^{-2}$ | $kg\ s^{-3}$ |
| heat capacity, entropy | joule per kelvin | J K$^{-1}$ | $kg\ m^2\ s^{-2}\ K^{-1}$ |
| specific heat capacity, specific entropy | joule per kilogram kelvin | J K$^{-1}$ kg$^{-1}$ | $m^2\ s^{-2}\ K^{-1}$ |
| specific energy | joule per kilogram | J kg$^{-1}$ | $m^2\ s^{-2}$ |
| thermal conductivity | watt per meter kelvin | W m$^{-1}$ K$^{-1}$ | $kg\ m\ s^{-3}\ K^{-1}$ |
| energy density | joule per cubic meter | J m$^{-3}$ | $kg\ m^{-1}\ s^{-2}$ |
| electric field strength | volt per meter | V m$^{-1}$ | $kg\ m\ s^{-3}\ A^{-1}$ |
| electric charge density | coulomb per cubic meter | C m$^{-3}$ | $A\ s\ m^{-3}$ |
| surface charge density | coulomb per square meter | C m$^{-2}$ | $A\ s\ m^{-2}$ |
| electric flux density, electric displacement | coulomb per square meter | C m$^{-2}$ | $A\ s\ m^{-2}$ |
| permittivity | farad per meter | F m$^{-1}$ | $kg^{-1}\ m^{-3}\ s^4\ A^2$ |
| permeability | henry per meter | H m$^{-1}$ | $kg\ m\ s^{-2}\ A^{-2}$ |
| exposure (x- and γ-rays) | coulomb per kilogram | C kg$^{-1}$ | $A\ s\ kg^{-1}$ |
| absorbed dose | gray | Gy | $m^2\ s^{-2}$ |
| radiance | watt per square meter steradian | W sr$^{-1}$ m$^{-2}$ | $kg\ s^{-3}$ |

It is important to emphasize that each physical quantity has only one coherent SI unit, even though this unit can be expressed in different forms by using some of the special names and symbols. The converse, however, is not true, because in general several different quantities may share the same SI unit. For example, specific energy and absorbed dose are derived quantities that are both expressed in SI base units of $m^2\ s^{-2}$. It is therefore important not to use the unit alone to specify the quantity.

[a]Names and symbols include SI coherent derived units with special names and symbols.

Adapted from Bureau International des Poids et Mesures. *The International System of Units (SI)*. 9th ed. 2019. (CC BY 4.0). https://www.bipm.org/utils/common/pdf/si-brochure/SI-Brochure-9.pdf

**TABLE A-5 PHYSICAL CONSTANTS**   📖 T. B-5

| SYMBOL | CONSTANT | VALUE | SI UNITS |
|---|---|---|---|
| $c$ | Velocity of light in vacuum | $2.997925 \times 10^8$ | m s$^{-1}$ |
| $e$ | Elementary charge | $1.602177 \times 10^{-19}$ | C |
| $F$ | Faraday constant | $9.64853 \times 10^4$ | C mol$^{-1}$ |
| $g$ | Standard acceleration of free fall | 9.80665 | m s$^{-2}$ |
| $h$ | Planck constant | $6.626070 \times 10^{-34}$ | J s |
|  |  | $4.1357 \times 10^{-15}$ | eV s |
| $k_B$ | Boltzmann constant | $1.380649 \times 10^{-23}$ | J K$^{-1}$ |
|  |  | $8.617343 \times 10^{-5}$ | eV K$^{-1}$ |
| $m_e$ | Electron rest mass | $9.109383 \times 10^{-31}$ | kg |
| $m_e c^2$ | Electron rest energy | $8.187105 \times 10^{-14}$ | J |
|  |  | $5.10999 \times 10^5$ | eV |
| $m_p$ | Proton rest mass | $1.672622 \times 10^{-27}$ | kg |
| $N_A$ | Avogadro number | $6.022141 \times 10^{23}$ | mol$^{-1}$ |
| $r_e$ | Classical electron radius | $2.817940 \times 10^{-15}$ | m |
| $R$ | Gas constant | 8.31446 | J mol$^{-1}$ K$^{-1}$ |

*(Continued)*

## TABLE A-5  PHYSICAL CONSTANTS *(Continued)*

| SYMBOL | CONSTANT | VALUE | SI UNITS |
|---|---|---|---|
| $u$ | Mass unit ($^{12}$C standard) | $1.660539 \times 10^{-27}$ | kg |
| $uc^2$ | Mass unit (energy units) | $9.31494 \times 10^8$ | eV |
| $\varepsilon_0$ | Electrical permittivity of free space | $8.85419 \times 10^{-12}$ | $C^2\,N^{-1}\,m^{-2}$ |
| $\lambda_C$ | Compton wavelength of electron | $2.42631 \times 10^{-12}$ | m |
| $\mu_B$ | Bohr magneton | $9.274010 \times 10^{-24}$ | $J\,T^{-1}$ |
| $\mu_0$ | Magnetic permeability of space | $4\pi \times 10^{-7} \sim 12.566 \times 10^{-7}$ | $T\,m\,A^{-1}$ |
| $\mu_N$ | Nuclear magneton | $5.050784 \times 10^{-27}$ | $J\,T^{-1}$ |
| $m_n$ | Neutron rest mass | $1.674929310227$ | kg |
| $\gamma$ | Gyromagnetic ratio of proton | $42.5764$ | $MHz\,T^{-1}$ |

## TABLE A-6  PREFIXES  📖 T. B-6

| PREFIXES | |
|---|---|
| yotta (Y) | $10^{24}$ |
| zetta (Z) | $10^{21}$ |
| exa (E) | $10^{18}$ |
| peta (P) | $10^{15}$ |
| tera (T) | $10^{12}$ |
| giga (G) | $10^9$ |
| mega (M) | $10^6$ |
| kilo (k) | $10^3$ |
| hecto (h) | $10^2$ |
| deca (da) | $10^1$ |
| deci (d) | $10^{-1}$ |
| centi (c) | $10^{-2}$ |
| milli (m) | $10^{-3}$ |
| micro ($\mu$) | $10^{-6}$ |
| nano (n) | $10^{-9}$ |
| pico (p) | $10^{-12}$ |
| femto (f) | $10^{-15}$ |
| atto (a) | $10^{-18}$ |
| zepto (z) | $10^{-21}$ |
| yocto (y) | $10^{-24}$ |

## TABLE A-7  DEFINITIONS AND CONVERSION FACTORS    📖 T. B-7

| | |
|---|---|
| **ANGLE** | |
| 1 radian | $360°/2\pi \approx 57.2958°$ |
| **CURRENT** | |
| 1 ampere | 1 C/s |
| 1 ampere | $6.241 \times 10^{18}$ electrons/s |
| **ENERGY** | |
| 1 electron volt (eV) | $1.6022 \times 10^{-19}$ J |
| 1 calorie | 4.187 J |
| **LENGTH** | |
| 1 inch | 25.4 mm |
| 1 inch | 2.54 cm |
| 1 Angstrom | $10^{-10}$ m |
| **MAGNETIC FLUX DENSITY** | |
| 1 Gauss | $10^{-4}$ T |
| **MASS** | |
| 1 pound | 0.45359 kg |
| 1 kg | 2.02046 pound |
| **POWER** | |
| 1 watt (W) | J/s |
| **RADIOLOGIC UNITS** | |
| 1 roentgen (R) | $2.58 \times 10^{-4}$ C/kg |
| 1 roentgen (R) | 8.76 mGy air kerma |
| 1 mGy air kerma | 114.2 mR |
| 1 gray (Gy) | 100 rad |
| 1 sievert (Sv) | 100 rem |
| 1 curie (Ci) | $3.7 \times 10^{10}$ becquerel (Bq) |
| 1 becquerel (Bq) | 1 disintegration $s^{-1}$ (dps) |
| **TEMPERATURE** | |
| °C (Celsius) | $5/9 \times (°F - 32)$ |
| °F (Fahrenheit) | $9/5 \times (°C + 32)$ |
| °K (Kelvin) | °C + 273.16 |
| **VOLUME** | |
| 1 US gallon | 3.7854 L |
| 1 liter (L) | 1,000 cm³ |

## TABLE A-8  GEOMETRY    📖 T. B-8

| | |
|---|---|
| Area of circle | $\pi r^2$ |
| Circumference of circle | $2\pi r$ |
| Surface area of sphere | $4\pi r^2$ |
| Volume of sphere | $(4/3)\pi r^3$ |
| Area of triangle | $(1/2)$ base $\times$ height |

## TABLE A-9 THE GREEK ALPHABET 📖 T. B-10

| GREEK NAME | CAPITAL | LOWERCASE | GREEK NAME | CAPITAL | LOWERCASE |
|---|---|---|---|---|---|
| Alpha | A | α | Nu | N | ν |
| Beta | B | β | Xi | Ξ | ξ |
| Gamma | Γ | γ | Omicron | O | o |
| Delta | Δ | δ | Pi | Π | π |
| Epsilon | E | ε | Rho | P | ρ |
| Zeta | Z | ζ | Sigma | Σ | σ |
| Eta | H | η | Tau | T | τ |
| Theta | Θ | θ | Upsilon | Y | μ |
| Iota | I | ι | Phi | Φ | φ |
| Kappa | K | κ | Chi | X | χ |
| Lambda | Λ | λ | Psi | Ψ | ψ |
| Mu | M | μ | Omega | Ω | ω |

# Effective Doses, Organ Doses, and Fetal Doses from Medical Imaging Procedures

Estimates of effective dose and organ doses for a specific diagnostic procedure extend over a range of values and are dependent on many parameters such as image quality (signal-to-noise and contrast-to-noise ratios), patient size, x-ray acquisition techniques, and the application of dose reduction technologies. Methods to reduce radiation dose include the utilization of higher quantum detection efficiency digital radiographic detectors and application of image processing algorithms to reduce noise. In CT, they include the implementation of automatic tube current modulation as a function of tube angle and patient attenuation and deployment of statistical iterative reconstruction techniques. As technology advances and improves, a trend toward lower radiation dose should occur, which for many procedures will result in lower effective doses than the values listed in these tables. The numbers of days of typical background radiation equal to the average effective dose of the examination are provided to help to place the magnitude of the exposure into perspective.

Tables B-1 and B-2 list typical adult and pediatric effective doses for various diagnostic radiology procedures. Table B-3 provides specific information for adult interventional examinations. Table B-4 provides values of

### TABLE B-1  ADULT EFFECTIVE DOSES FOR VARIOUS DIAGNOSTIC RADIOLOGY PROCEDURES (2016)   📖 T. E-1

| EXAMINATION | AVERAGE EFFECTIVE DOSE (mSv)[a] | DAYS OF EQUIVALENT BACKGROUND RADIATION[b] | NO. OF PROCEDURES |
|---|---|---|---|
| **Radiography** | | | |
| Urography | 3.0 | 352 | 647,000 |
| Lumbar spine | 1.4 | 164 | 11,255,000 |
| Thoracic spine | 1.0 | 117 | 2,509,000 |
| Esophagus | 0.7 | 82 | 2,105,000 |
| Abdomen | 0.6 | 70 | 12,228,000 |
| Pelvis | 0.4 | 47 | 5,411,000 |
| Hip | 0.4 | 47 | 14,995,000 |
| Cervical spine | 0.36 | 42 | 4,884,000 |
| Other head and neck | 0.22 | 26 | 1,121,000 |
| Skull | 0.14 | 16 | 229,000 |
| Chest | 0.10 | 12 | 110,388,000 |
| Shoulder | 0.006 | 0.7 | 11,951,000 |
| Knees | 0.003 | 0.35 | 25,757,000 |
| Hands and feet | <0.001 | <0.12 | 31,194,000 |
| **Diagnostic Fluoroscopy** | | | |
| Upper gastrointestinal | 6.0 | 704 | 938,000 |
| Barium enema | 6.0 | 704 | 192,000 |
| **Mammography** | | | |
| Mammography | 0.36 | 42 | 39,252,000 |

[a]Based on ICRP Publication 103 radiation and tissue weighting factors.
[b]Based upon a background effective dose rate of 3.1 mSv/y.

*Source:* Adapted with permission from National Council on Radiation Protection and Measurements (NCRP). *Report No. 184 Medical Radiation Exposure of Patients in the United States (2019).* http://NCRPonline.org

**TABLE B-2  PEDIATRIC EFFECTIVE DOSES FOR VARIOUS DIAGNOSTIC RADIOLOGY PROCEDURES (2016)**   📖 **T. E-2**

| EXAMINATION | AVERAGE EFFECTIVE DOSE (mSv)[a] | DAYS OF EQUIVALENT BACKGROUND RADIATION[b] | NO. OF PROCEDURES |
|---|---|---|---|
| **Radiography** | | | |
| Spine | 0.60 | 70 | 1,250,000 |
| Abdomen | 0.10 | 12 | 1,250,000 |
| Chest | 0.05 | 6 | 5,000,000 |
| Pelvis | 0.05 | 6 | 1,250,000 |
| Extremity | 0.005 | 1 | 15,000,000 |
| **Diagnostic Fluoroscopy** | | | |
| Contrast enema | 2.0 | 235 | 156,000 |
| Other | 2.0 | 235 | 31,000 |
| Upper gastrointestinal | 1.5 | 176 | 156,000 |
| Cystogram | 0.2 | 23 | 281,000 |

[a]Based on ICRP Publication 103 radiation and tissue weighting factors.
[b]Based upon a background effective dose rate of 3.1 mSv/y.

*Source:* Adapted with permission from National Council on Radiation Protection and Measurements (NCRP). *Report No. 184 Medical Radiation Exposure of Patients in the United States (2019).* http://NCRPonline.org

effective dose for adult CT imaging, along with the numbers of annual CT procedures and CT scans as of the year 2016 (NCRP Report No. 184). Information on pediatric CT exposures is given in Tables B-5 and B-6. The values of effective dose in adult dental radiographic procedures are given in Table B-7.

Table B-8 provides information on *organ doses* based on typical techniques for adult radiography and CT procedures. Table B-9 lists *organ doses* determined from direct measurements of a 6-year-old pediatric anthropomorphic phantom for "routine" abdominal and chest CT examination techniques at seven different sites in Japan, along with the effective dose. Table B-10 lists *effective dose* estimates of various pediatric examinations including the common chest radiograph as well as CT of the head and abdomen as a function of age, from neonate to 15 years old. Table B-11 lists the conceptus dose for various CT, radiography, and fluoroscopy imaging procedures.

**TABLE B-3  ADULT EFFECTIVE DOSES FOR VARIOUS FLUOROSCOPICALLY GUIDED INTERVENTIONAL CARDIAC PROCEDURES (2016)**   📖 **T. E-3**

| EXAMINATION | AVERAGE EFFECTIVE DOSE (mSv)[a] | DAYS OF EQUIVALENT BACKGROUND RADIATION[b] | NO. OF PROCEDURES |
|---|---|---|---|
| Percutaneous intervention | 23 | 2,699 | 850,000 |
| Diagnostic arteriography | 7 | 822 | 2,500,000 |
| Electrophysiology nonpacemaker | 3.2 | 376 | 350,000 |
| Pacemaker | 1 | 117 | 360,000 |

[a]Based on ICRP Publication 103 radiation and tissue weighting factors.
[b]Based upon a background effective dose rate of 3.1 mSv/y.

*Source:* Adapted with permission from National Council on Radiation Protection and Measurements (NCRP). *Report No. 184 Medical Radiation Exposure of Patients in the United States (2019).* http://NCRPonline.org

**TABLE B-4  ADULT EFFECTIVE DOSES FOR VARIOUS COMPUTED TOMOGRAPHY PROCEDURES (2016)   📖 T. E-4**

| EXAMINATION | AVERAGE EFFECTIVE DOSE (mSv)[a] | DAYS OF EQUIVALENT BACKGROUND RADIATION[b] | NO. OF CT PROCEDURES | NO. OF CT SCANS |
|---|---|---|---|---|
| PET/CT | 10.0 | 1,174 | 1,821,610 | 1,821,610 |
| Spine | 8.8 | 1,033 | 6,400,000 | 6,457,522 |
| Cardiac | 8.7 | 1,021 | 281,920 | 281,920 |
| Abdomen and pelvis | 7.7 | 904 | 20,100,000 | 22,137,153 |
| CT colonography | 6.6 | 775 | 200,000 | 200,000 |
| Chest | 6.2 | 728 | 12,700,000 | 13,250,657 |
| CT angiography (noncardiac) | 5.1 | 599 | 6,600,000 | 13,027,708 |
| Interventional | 5.0 | 587 | 863,280 | 863,280 |
| Miscellaneous | 5.0 | 587 | 300,000 | 300,000 |
| Lower extremity | 3.2 | 376 | 1,203,716 | 1,223,064 |
| SPECT/CT | 3.0 | 352 | 314,206 | 314,206 |
| Calcium scoring | 1.7 | 200 | 57,492 | 57,492 |
| Upper extremity | 1.7 | 200 | 471,100 | 479,288 |
| Brain | 1.6 | 188 | 15,300,000 | 15,891,371 |
| Head and neck | 1.2 | 141 | 7,200,000 | 7,700,481 |

[a]Based on ICRP Publication 103 radiation and tissue weighting factors.
[b]Based upon a background effective dose rate of 3.1 mSv/y.

*Source:* Adapted with permission from National Council on Radiation Protection and Measurements (NCRP). *Report No. 184 Medical Radiation Exposure of Patients in the United States (2019).* http://NCRPonline.org

**TABLE B-5  DISTRIBUTION OF EFFECTIVE DOSES AND MEAN ORGAN DOSES FROM COMPUTED TOMOGRAPHY BY ANATOMIC REGION AND PATIENT AGE[a]**

| | HEAD | | | ABDOMEN/PELVIS | | | CHEST | | | SPINE | | |
|---|---|---|---|---|---|---|---|---|---|---|---|---|
| | <5 Y | 5–9 Y | 10–14 Y | <5 Y | 5–9 Y | 10–14 Y | <5 Y | 5–9 Y | 10–14 Y | <5 Y | 5–9 Y | 10–14 Y |
| Patients, No. | 98 | 79 | 102 | 72 | 89 | 115 | 52 | 37 | 58 | 10 | 14 | 18 |
| **Effective dose, percentile** | | | | | | | | | | | | |
| Mean | 3.5 | 1.5 | 1.1 | 10.6 | 11.1 | 14.8 | 5.3 | 7.5 | 6.4 | 5.8 | 7.7 | 8.8 |
| 25th | 1.4 | 0.5 | 0.6 | 3.2 | 3.5 | 6.4 | 2.5 | 2.6 | 3.1 | 0.6 | 1.5 | 2.5 |
| 50th | 2.6 | 1.2 | 1.0 | 4.7 | 8.0 | 11.1 | 3.1 | 3.9 | 5.3 | 2.9 | 4.1 | 5.3 |
| 75th | 4.8 | 2.0 | 1.6 | 14.4 | 14.8 | 20.0 | 4.8 | 10.5 | 8.6 | 6.3 | 10.5 | 10.3 |
| 95th | 11.2 | 3.2 | 2.6 | 30.2 | 32.9 | 35.0 | 20.5 | 26.1 | 18.4 | 26.6 | 26.7 | 42.0 |
| Dose ≥20 mSv, % of patients | 0.0 | 0.0 | 0.0 | 13.9 | 15.7 | 25.2 | 5.8 | 8.1 | 3.4 | 10.0 | 14.3 | 5.6 |
| **Mean organ dose, mGy** | | | | | | | | | | | | |
| Brain | 28.8 | 25.3 | 29.8 | 0.1 | 0.1 | 0.1 | 0.3 | 0.4 | 0.3 | 0.8 | 1.1 | 0.7 |
| Thyroid | 11.8 | 1.2 | 1.0 | 1.0 | 0.6 | 0.6 | 11.4 | 17.5 | 13.6 | 10.8 | 11.4 | 6.4 |
| Esophagus | 3.7 | 0.6 | 0.4 | 5.1 | 5.2 | 6.9 | 8.4 | 12.4 | 10.3 | 8.4 | 7.6 | 8.5 |
| Lungs | 1.9 | 0.4 | 0.3 | 7.6 | 6.2 | 8.1 | 10.2 | 15.0 | 13.2 | 7.7 | 7.1 | 9.7 |
| Breast | 0.9 | 0.1 | 0.1 | 14.8 | 13.0 | 14.0 | 7.8 | 10.6 | 9.9 | 8.3 | 13.0 | 9.7 |
| Stomach wall | 0.7 | 0.1 | 0.0 | 15.9 | 18.1 | 25.3 | 6.1 | 8.7 | 8.0 | 7.5 | 14.5 | 17.9 |
| Liver | 0.8 | 0.1 | 0.0 | 16.3 | 18.0 | 25.3 | 6.9 | 9.9 | 8.9 | 8.6 | 14.9 | 20.3 |
| Colon wall | 0.3 | 0.0 | 0.0 | 16.0 | 18.8 | 26.2 | 2.3 | 2.7 | 2.2 | 3.6 | 5.9 | 4.7 |
| Rectosigmoid wall | 0.1 | 0.0 | 0.0 | 12.1 | 13.8 | 16.7 | 0.7 | 0.6 | 0.2 | 1.0 | 1.2 | 0.7 |
| Bladder wall | 0.1 | 0.0 | 0.0 | 13.0 | 14.6 | 16.6 | 0.7 | 0.4 | 0.1 | 0.7 | 0.7 | 0.4 |
| Prostate | 0.1 | 0.0 | 0.0 | 9.0 | 10.1 | 11.0 | 0.7 | 0.1 | 0.1 | 0.1 | 0.1 | 0.2 |

*(Continued)*

**TABLE B-5  DISTRIBUTION OF EFFECTIVE DOSES AND MEAN ORGAN DOSES FROM COMPUTED TOMOGRAPHY BY ANATOMIC REGION AND PATIENT AGE[a]** *(Continued)*

|  | HEAD | | | ABDOMEN/PELVIS | | | CHEST | | | SPINE | | |
|---|---|---|---|---|---|---|---|---|---|---|---|---|
|  | <5 Y | 5–9 Y | 10–14 Y | <5 Y | 5–9 Y | 10–14 Y | <5 Y | 5–9 Y | 10–14 Y | <5 Y | 5–9 Y | 10–14 Y |
| Uterus | 0.1 | 0.0 | 0.0 | 12.6 | 13.5 | 16.9 | 0.4 | 0.6 | 0.1 | 1.2 | 1.5 | 0.2 |
| Ovaries | 0.1 | 0.0 | 0.0 | 14.6 | 15.4 | 19.6 | 0.5 | 0.7 | 0.1 | 1.8 | 1.8 | 0.2 |
| Red bone marrow | 10.6 | 6.5 | 4.2 | 5.1 | 5.6 | 9.2 | 3.3 | 3.9 | 3.6 | 4.4 | 3.0 | 3.9 |

[a]The doses to the breast, uterus, and ovaries are for girls only; the doses to the prostate are for boys only.

*Source:* Miglioretti DL, Johnson E, Williams A, et al. The use of computed tomography in pediatrics and the associated radiation exposure and estimated cancer risk. *JAMA Pediatr.* 2013;167(8):700–707. doi:10.1001/jamapediatrics.2013.311.

**TABLE B-6  PEDIATRIC EFFECTIVE DOSES FOR VARIOUS COMPUTED TOMOGRAPHY PROCEDURES (2016)** 📖 T. E-6

| EXAMINATION | AVERAGE EFFECTIVE DOSE (mSv)[a] | DAYS OF EQUIVALENT BACKGROUND RADIATION[b] | EFFECTIVE DOSE RANGE (mSv) | NO. OF CT PROCEDURES |
|---|---|---|---|---|
| Abdominopelvis | 7.0 | 822 | 2.9–10.0 | 1,300,000 |
| Spine | 3.5 | 411 | 2.5–5.0 | 520,000 |
| Chest | 3.0 | 352 | 1.3–6.0 | 260,000 |
| Head | 2.0 | 235 | 0.8–3.0 | 2,860,000 |
| Other | 2.0 | 235 | NA | 260,000 |

[a]Based on ICRP Publication 103 radiation and tissue weighting factors.
[b]Based upon a background effective dose rate of 3.1 mSv/y.

*Source:* Adapted with permission from National Council on Radiation Protection and Measurements (NCRP). *Report No. 184 Medical Radiation Exposure of Patients in the United States (2019)*. http://NCRPonline.org

**TABLE B-7  ADULT EFFECTIVE DOSES FOR VARIOUS DENTAL RADIOLOGY PROCEDURES (2016)** 📖 T. E-7

| EXAMINATION | AVERAGE EFFECTIVE DOSE (µSv)[a] | DAYS OF EQUIVALENT BACKGROUND RADIATION[b] | NO. OF PROCEDURES |
|---|---|---|---|
| Intraoral | 43 | 5 | 296,000,000 |
| Panoramic | 26 | 3 | 21,000,000 |
| Cone beam CT | 176.0 | 21 | 5,200,000 |
| Cephalometric | 5–10 | 0.6–1.2 | <1% |

[a]Based on ICRP Publication 103 radiation and tissue weighting factors.
[b]Based upon a background effective dose rate of 3.1 mSv/y.

*Source:* Adapted with permission from National Council on Radiation Protection and Measurements (NCRP). *Report No. 184 Medical Radiation Exposure of Patients in the United States (2019)*. http://NCRPonline.org

**TABLE B-8 TYPICAL ORGAN-SPECIFIC RADIATION DOSES RESULTING FROM VARIOUS RADIOLOGY PROCEDURES    ⊞ T. E-8**

| EXAMINATION | ORGAN | ORGAN-SPECIFIC RADIATION DOSE (mGy) |
|---|---|---|
| PA chest radiography | Lung | 0.01 |
| Mammography | Breast | 3.5 |
| CT chest | Breast | 21.4 |
| CT coronary angiography | Breast | 51.0 |
| Abdominal radiography | Stomach | 0.25 |
| CT abdomen | Stomach | 10.0 |
| | Colon | 4.0 |
| Barium enema | Colon | 15.0 |

*Source:* Reproduced from Davies HE, Wathen CG, Gleeson FV. The risks of radiation exposure related to diagnostic imaging and how to minimise them. *BMJ.* 2011;342:d947. doi:10.1136/bmj.d947. Copyright © 2011, with permissions from British Medical Journal Publishing Group.

**TABLE B-9 ORGAN DOSE AVERAGES FOR A 6-YEAR PEDIATRIC ANTHROPOMORPHIC PHANTOM USING ROUTINE TECHNIQUES AT SEVEN CT SCANNER SITES    ⊞ T. E-9**

| TISSUE OR ORGAN | ORGAN DOSE (mGy) ± σ | |
|---|---|---|
| | *Pediatric Abdomen* | *Pediatric Chest* |
| Thyroid gland | 0.3 ± 0.2 | 10.5 ± 6.6 |
| Lung | 4.2 ± 2.1 | 9.1 ± 4.2 |
| Breast | 2.3 ± 1.8 | 8.4 ± 4.7 |
| Esophagus | 4.2 ± 2.0 | 9.0 ± 4.4 |
| Liver | 8.8 ± 3.5 | 8.0 ± 3.7 |
| Stomach | 9.5 ± 3.9 | 4.7 ± 2.8 |
| Kidneys | 9.0 ± 3.5 | 4.3 ± 2.2 |
| Colon | 9.4 ± 3.5 | 0.6 ± 0.3 |
| Ovary | 9.0 ± 3.1 | 0.1 ± 0.1 |
| Bladder | 9.1 ± 3.3 | 0.1 ± 0.0 |
| Testis | 7.8 ± 3.7 | 0.1 ± 0.0 |
| Bone surface | 8.1 ± 2.8 | 8.5 ± 3.8 |

σ, standard deviation.

*Source*: Republished with permission of British Institute of Radiology from Fujii K, Aoyama T, Koyama S, et al. Comparative evaluation of organ and effective doses for paediatric patients with those for adults in chest and abdominal CT examinations. *Br J Radiol.* 2007;80(956):657–667.

## TABLE B-10 CTDI$_{VOL}$, DLP, AND EFFECTIVE DOSE FROM PEDIATRIC CT IMAGING AS A FUNCTION OF PATIENT AGE ▭ T. E-10

| CT PROTOCOL | CTDI$_{VOL16}$ (mGy) | | DLP$_{16}$ (mGy-cm) | | AVERAGE EFFECTIVE DOSE (mSv)[a] | DAYS OF EQUIVALENT BACKGROUND RADIATION[b] |
|---|---|---|---|---|---|---|
| | Mean | Range | Mean | Range | | |
| **Head/Brain CT** | | | | | | |
| Newborn | 18.8 ± 18.2 | 4.2–67.2 | 225.0 ± 177.9 | 39–665 | 2.1 | 246 |
| ≤1 year | 29.3 ± 17.9 | 8.6–71.6 | 439.0 ± 313.6 | 103–1,163 | 3.3 | 387 |
| 2–5 year | 29.6 ± 15.3 | 13.1–56.0 | 401.0 ± 164.7 | 231–735 | 1.8 | 211 |
| 6–10 year | 38.1 ± 18.0 | 7.01–80.6 | 645.0 ± 318.0 | 190–1,617 | 2.1 | 246 |
| ≤15 year | 44.0 ± 15.0 | 14.9–77.3 | 728.0 ± 270.4 | 209–1,477 | 1.8 | 211 |
| **Chest CT** | | | | | | |
| Newborn | 3.2 ± 2.2 | 1.85–5.84 | 37.0 ± 20.8 | 20–60 | Not Reported | — |
| ≤1 year | 3.6 ± 2.3 | 0.8–7.2 | 720.0 ± 5.7 | 12–166 | 2.8 | 329 |
| 2–5 year | 5.3 ± 2.2 | 1.8–9.4 | 128.0 ± 6.8 | 41–288 | 2.6 | 305 |
| 6–10 year | 7.2 ± 3.9 | 3.1–15.6 | 205.0 ± 9.3 | 26–458 | 2.6 | 305 |
| ≤15 year | 11.4 ± 5.9 | 4.0–21.8 | 375.0 ± 199.5 | 148–800 | 3.1 | 364 |
| **Abdominopelvic CT** | | | | | | |
| Newborn | 5.1 ± 4.5 | 2.9–10.2 | 93.0 ± 74.8 | 46–205 | Not Reported | — |
| ≤1 year | 5.6 ± 2.4 | 4.5–10.4 | 162.0 ± 7.5 | 72–324 | 5.0 | 587 |
| 2–5 year | 6.7 ± 2.9 | 3.3–12.8 | 249.0 ± 137.8 | 88–508 | 5.9 | 692 |
| 6–10 year | 10.1 ± 5.5 | 3.5–28.1 | 412.0 ± 246.5 | 88–972 | 6.3 | 739 |
| ≤15 year | 13.1 ± 7.1 | 4.1–33.9 | 607.0 ± 371.5 | 172–1,714 | 6.0 | 704 |

[a]Values of effective dose are derived from the product of the third quartile values of DLP and the effective dose coefficients from Deak PD, Smal Y, Kalender WA. Multisection CT protocols: sex and age-specific conversion factors used to determine effective dose from dose-length product. *Radiology*. 2010;257:158–166.
[b]Based upon a background effective dose rate of 3.1 mSv/y.

Adapted with permission from Hwang J-Y, Do K-H, Yang D, et al. A survey of pediatric CT protocols and radiation doses in South Korean hospitals to optimize the radiation dose for pediatric CT scanning. *Medicine*. 2015;94(50):e2146.

**TABLE B-11** **ESTIMATED CONCEPTUS DOSES FROM COMMON RADIOGRAPHIC, FLUOROSCOPIC, AND CT EXAMINATIONS**    📖 **T. E-11**

**ESTIMATED CONCEPTUS DOSES FROM SINGLE CT ACQUISITION**

| EXAMINATION | DOSE LEVEL | TYPICAL CONCEPTUS DOSE (mGy) |
|---|---|---|
| **Extra-Abdominal** | | |
| Head CT | Standard | 0 |
| Chest CT | | |
| Routine | Standard | 0.2 |
| Pulmonary embolus | Standard | 0.2 |
| CT angiography of coronary arteries | Standard | 0.1 |
| **Abdominal** | | |
| Abdomen, routine | Standard | 4 |
| Abdomen/pelvis, routine | Standard | 25 |
| CT angiography of aorta (chest through pelvis) | Standard | 34 |
| Abdomen/pelvis, stone protocol[a] | Reduced | 10 |

**ESTIMATED CONCEPTUS DOSES FROM RADIOGRAPHIC AND FLUOROSCOPIC EXAMINATIONS**

| EXAMINATION | TYPICAL CONCEPTUS DOSE (mGy) |
|---|---|
| Cervical spine (AP, lat) | <0.001 |
| Extremities | <0.001 |
| Chest (PA, lat) | 0.002 |
| Thoracic spine (AP, lat) | 0.003 |
| Abdomen (AP) | |
| 21-cm patient thickness | 1 |
| 33-cm patient thickness | 3 |
| Lumbar spine (AP, lat) | 1 |
| Limited IVP[b] | 6 |
| Small-bowel study[c] | 7 |
| Double-contrast barium enema study[d] | 7 |

[a]Anatomic coverage is the same as for routine abdominopelvic CT, but the tube current is decreased and the pitch is increased because standard image quality is not necessary for detection of high-contrast stones.
[b]Limited IVP is assumed to include four abdominopelvic images. A patient thickness of 21 cm is assumed.
[c]A small-bowel study is assumed to include a 6-min fluoroscopic examination with the acquisition of 20 digital spot images.
[d]A double-contrast barium enema study is assumed to include a 4-min fluoroscopic examination with the acquisition of 12 digital spot images.

AP, anteroposterior projection; lat, lateral projection; PA, posteroanterior projection.

Reprinted with permission from McCollough CH, Schueler BA, Atwell TD, et al. Radiation exposure and pregnancy: when should we be concerned? *Radiographics*. 2007;27:909–917. doi:10.1148/rg.274065149. Copyright © Radiological Society of North America.

# Radiopharmaceutical Characteristics and Dosimetry

**TABLE C-1  SUMMARY OF TYPICALLY ADMINISTERED ADULT DOSE; ORGAN RECEIVING THE HIGHEST RADIATION DOSE AND ITS DOSE; GONADAL DOSE; EFFECTIVE DOSE, AND EFFECTIVE DOSE PER ADMINISTERED ACTIVITY FOR FDA-APPROVED RADIOPHARMACEUTICALS  ⊞ T. F-2**

| RADIOPHARMACEUTICAL | TYPICAL ADULT ADMINISTERED ACTIVITY MBq | mCi | ORGAN RECEIVING HIGHEST DOSE | ORGAN DOSE mGy | rad | GONADAL DOSE mGy | | rad | EFFECTIVE DOSE mSv | rem | EFFECTIVE DOSE COEFFICIENT mSv/MBq | rem/mCi | SOURCE |
|---|---|---|---|---|---|---|---|---|---|---|---|---|---|
| C-11 Choline | 555(370–740) | 15(10–20) | Pancreas | 16 | 1.6 | 0.75 (ts) 1.1 (ov) | | 0.075 (ts) 0.11 (ov) | 2.4 | 0.24 | 0.0044 | 0.016 | PI |
| C-11 Urea (PYtest) | 0.037 | 0.001 | BE | 1.22E-03 | 1.22E-04 | 8.88E-04 (ts) 8.88E-04 (ov) | | 8.88E-05 (ts) 8.88E-05 (ov) | 1.15E-03 | 1.15E-04 | 0.031 | 0.115 | ICRP Publication 128 |
| F-18 Florbetaben (Neuraceq) | 300 | 8.1 | UB wall | 21 | 2.1 | 2.7 (ts) 4.8 (ov) | | 0.27 (ts) 0.48 (ov) | 5.7 | 0.57 | 0.019 | 0.070 | PI |
| F-18 Florbetapir (Amyvid) | 370 | 10 | GB wall | 53 | 5.3 | 2.6 (ts) 6.7 (ov) | | 0.26 (ts) 0.67 (ov) | 7.0 | 0.70 | 0.019 | 0.070 | PI |
| F-18 Flortaucipir (TAUVID) | 370 | 10 | Upper large intestine wall | 36 | 3.6 | 2.6 (ts) 7.8 (ov) | | 0.26 (ts) 0.78 (ov) | 8.9 | 0.89 | 0.024 | 0.089 | PI |
| F-18 Fluciclovine (Axumin) | 370 | 10 | Pancreas | 38 | 3.8 | 6.3 (ts) 4.8 (ov) | | 0.63 (ts) 0.48 (ov) | 8.1 | 0.81 | 0.022 | 0.081 | PI |
| F-18 Sodium Fluoride | 375(300–450) | 10(8–12) | UB wall | 56 | 5.6 | 2.3 (ts) 3.1 (ov) | | 0.23 (ts) 0.31 (ov) | 6.4 | 0.64 | 0.017 | 0.063 | ICRP Publication 128 |
| F-18 Fluorodeoxyglucose (FDG) | 280(185–370) | 7.6(5–10) | UB wall | 36 | 3.6 | 3.1 (ts) 3.9 (ov) | | 0.31 (ts) 0.39 (ov) | 5.3 | 0.53 | 0.019 | 0.070 | ICRP Publication 128 |
| F-18 Fluoroestradiol (CERIANNA) | 222(111–222) | 6(3–6) | Liver | 28 | 2.8 | 2.7 (ts) 4.0 (ov) | | 0.27 (ts) 0.40 (ov) | 4.9 | 0.49 | 0.022 | 0.081 | PI |
| F-18 Flutemetamol (Vizamyl) | 185 | 5 | GB wall | 53 | 5.3 | 1.5 (ts) 4.6 (ov) | | 0.15 (ts) 0.46 (ov) | 5.9 | 0.59 | 0.032 | 0.118 | PI |
| Ga-67 Citrate | 130(74–185) | 3.5(2–5) | BE | 82 | 8.2 | 7.3 (ts) 11 (ov) | | 0.73 (ts) 1.1 (ov) | 13 | 1.3 | 0.100 | 0.370 | ICRP Publication 128 |
| Ga-68 Dotatate (NETSPOT) | 150(2 MBq/kg) | 4.1(0.05 mCi/kg) | Spleen | 16 | 1.6 | 1.5 (ts) 2.4 (ov) | | 0.15 (ts) 0.24 (ov) | 3.2 | 0.32 | 0.021 | 0.078 | PI |
| Ga-68 Dotatoc | 148 | 4 | UB wall | 18 | 1.8 | 2.1 (ts) 2.1 (ov) | | 0.21 (ts) 0.21 (ov) | 3.1 | 0.31 | 0.021 | 0.078 | PI |

*(Continued)*

**TABLE C-1  SUMMARY OF TYPICALLY ADMINISTERED ADULT DOSE; ORGAN RECEIVING THE HIGHEST RADIATION DOSE AND ITS DOSE; GONADAL DOSE; EFFECTIVE DOSE, AND EFFECTIVE DOSE PER ADMINISTERED ACTIVITY FOR FDA-APPROVED RADIOPHARMACEUTICALS** *Continued)*

| RADIOPHARMACEUTICAL | TYPICAL ADULT ADMINISTERED ACTIVITY MBq | mCi | ORGAN RECEIVING HIGHEST DOSE | ORGAN DOSE mGy | rad | GONADAL DOSE mGy | rad | EFFECTIVE DOSE mSv | rem | EFF DOSE COEFF mSv/MBq | rem/mCi | SOURCE |
|---|---|---|---|---|---|---|---|---|---|---|---|---|
| In-111 Chloride (Used only for radiolabeling—see text book Appendix F-1) | | | | | | | | | | | | |
| In-111 Oxyquinoline (Labeled Leukocytes) | 13(7.4–18.5) | 0.35(0.2–0.5) | Spleen | 200 | 20 | ts 0.14 / ov 2.0 | ts 0.014 / ov 0.20 | 3.7 | 0.37 | 0.170 | 0.629 | PI |
| In-111 Pentetate (DTPA) | 18.5 | 0.5 | UB wall | 4.6 | 0.46 | ts 0.22 / ov 0.33 | ts 0.022 / ov 0.033 | 0.46 | 0.046 | 0.025 | 0.093 | ICRP Publication 53 |
| In-111 Pentetreotide (Octreoscan) | 222 (SPECT) | 6 (SPECT) | Kidneys | 91 | 9.1 | ts 3.8 / ov 6.0 | ts 0.38 / ov 0.6 | 12 | 1.2 | 0.054 | 0.200 | ICRP Publication 128 |
| I-123 Iobenguane (MIBG) | 370 | 10 | Liver | 25 | 2.5 | ts 2.1 / ov 3.0 | ts 0.21 / ov 0.30 | 4.8 | 0.48 | 0.013 | 0.048 | ICRP Publication 80 |
| I-123 Ioflupane (DaTscan) | 148(111–185) | 4(3–5) | UB wall | 7.9 | 0.79 | ts 1.3 / ov 2.5 | ts 0.13 / ov 0.25 | 3.2 | 0.32 | 0.021 | 0.079 | PI |
| I-123 Sodium Iodine Capsules | 9.3(3.7–14.8) | 0.25(0.1–0.4) | Thyroid | 37 | 3.7 | ts 0.037 / ov 0.065 | ts 0.0037 / ov 0.0065 | 2.0 | 0.20 | 0.220 | 0.814 | ICRP Publication 128 (medium uptake) |
| I-125 Human Serum Albumin (HSA) | | | | Organ dosimetry not provided in PI — Whole-body dose estimated at 0.25 mSv | | | | | | | | |
| I-125 Iothalamate | 0.74(0.37–1.11) | 0.02(0.01–0.03) | UB wall | 0.6 | 0.06 | ts 0.021 / ov 0.0085 | ts 0.0021 / ov 0.00085 | 0.011 | 0.0011 | 0.015 | 0.056 | PI |
| I-131 HSA (Megatope) | 1.85 | 0.05 | Thyroid (blocked) | 13 | 1.3 | ts 1 / ov 4.5 | ts 0.10 / ov 0.45 | 0.5 | 0.05 | 0.270 | 1.00 | PI |
| I-131 Iobenguane (AZEDRA) | 18,500 (therapy) | 500 | Salivary glands | 2.8E+04 | 2.8E+03 | ts 1,129 / ov 2,331 | ts 113 / ov 233 | Not applicable | | | | PI |
| I-131 Sodium Iodide | 3,700 (therapy) | 100 | Thyroid (not blocked) | 1.6E+06 | 1.6E+05 | ts 85 / ov 133 | ts 8.5 / ov 13.3 | Not applicable | | | | ICRP Publication 128 (medium uptake) |
| Lu-177 Dotatate (LUTATHERA) | 4 × 7,400 (therapy) | 4 × 200 | Spleen | 2.5E+04 | 2.5E+03 | ts 800 / ov 900 | ts 80 / ov 90 | Not applicable | | | | PI |

| Radiopharmaceutical | Administered Activity MBq | (mCi) | Critical Organ | Critical Organ Dose mGy | (rad) | Gonadal Dose mGy (ts/ov) | Gonadal Dose rad (ts/ov) | Effective Dose mSv | (rem) | mSv/MBq | rem/mCi | Reference |
|---|---|---|---|---|---|---|---|---|---|---|---|---|
| N-13 Ammonia | 555(370–740) | 15(10–20) | UB wall | 4.5 | 0.45 | ts 1.0 / ov 0.94 | ts 0.10 / ov 0.094 | 1.50 | 0.15 | 0.003 | 0.010 | ICRP Publication 53 |
| Ra-223 Dichloride (Xofigo) | 3.5 | 0.095 | BE | 4,032 | 403 | ts 0.28 / ov 1.72 | ts 0.028 / ov 0.172 | Not applicable | | Not applicable | | PI |
| Rb-82 Chloride | 2,220 | 60 | Kidneys | 21 | 2.1 | ts 0.58 / ov 1.1 | ts 0.058 / ov 0.11 | 2.4 | 0.24 | 0.0011 | 0.0041 | ICRP Publication 128 |
| Sm-153 Lexidronam (Quadramet) | 2,590 | 70 | BE | 1.73E+04 | 1.73E+03 | ts 14 / ov 22 | ts 1.4 / ov 2.2 | Not applicable | | Not applicable | | PI |
| Sr-89 Chloride (Metastron) | 148 | 4 | BE | 2,516 | 252 | ts 115 / ov 115 | ts 11.5 / ov 11.5 | Not applicable | | Not applicable | | ICRP Publication 53 |
| Tc-99m Bicisate (ECD) | 740(370–1,110) | 20(10–30) | UB wall | 37 | 3.7 | ts 2.0 / ov 5.8 | ts 0.20 / ov 0.58 | 5.7 | 0.57 | 0.0077 | 0.0285 | ICRP Publication 128 |
| Tc-99m Exametazime (HMPAO) | 590(260–925) | 16(7–25) | Kidneys | 20 | 2.0 | ts 1.4 / ov 3.9 | ts 0.14 / ov 0.39 | 5.5 | 0.55 | 0.0093 | 0.0344 | ICRP Publication 128 |
| Tc-99m MAA | 93(37–148) | 2.5(1–4) | Lung | 6.1 | 0.61 | ts 0.10 / ov 0.17 | ts 0.01 / ov 0.017 | 1.02 | 0.102 | 0.011 | 0.041 | ICRP Publication 128 |
| Tc-99m Mebrofenin (Choletec) | 130(74–185) | 3.5(2–5) | GB wall | 14 | 1.4 | ts 0.13 / ov 2.3 | ts 0.013 / ov 0.23 | 2.1 | 0.21 | 0.016 | 0.059 | ICRP Publication 128 |
| Tc-99m Medronate (MDP) | 555(370–740) | 15(10–20) | UB wall (normal uptake/excretion) | 26 | 2.6 | ts 1.3 / ov 2.0 | ts 0.13 / ov 0.20 | 2.7 | 0.27 | 0.0049 | 0.0181 | ICRP Publication 128 |
| Tc-99m Mertiatide (MAG3) | 280(185–370) | 7.6(5–10) | UB wall (normal renal function) | 31 | 3.1 | ts 1.0 / ov 1.5 | ts 0.10 / ov 0.15 | 2.0 | 0.20 | 0.007 | 0.026 | ICRP Publication 128 |
| Tc-99m Oxidronate (HDP) | 555(370–740) | 15(10–20) | UB wall (normal uptake/excretion) | 26 | 2.6 | ts 1.3 / ov 2.0 | ts 0.13 / ov 0.20 | 2.7 | 0.27 | 0.0049 | 0.0181 | ICRP Publication 128 |
| Tc-99m Pentetate (DTPA) | 555(370–740) | 15(10–20) | UB wall (normal renal function) | 34 | 3.4 | ts 1.6 / ov 2.3 | ts 0.16 / ov 0.23 | 2.7 | 0.27 | 0.0049 | 0.0181 | ICRP Publication 128 |
| Tc-99m Pyrophosphate (TechneScan) | 370(185–555) | 10(5–15) | UB wall (normal uptake/excretion) | 17 | 1.7 | ts 0.9 / ov 1.3 | ts 0.09 / ov 0.13 | 1.8 | 0.18 | 0.0049 | 0.0181 | ICRP Publication 128 |
| Tc-99m Red Blood Cells (UltraTag) | 555(370–740) | 15(10–20) | Heart wall | 13 | 1.3 | ts 1.3 / ov 2.1 | ts 0.13 / ov 0.21 | 3.9 | 0.39 | 0.007 | 0.026 | ICRP Publication 128 |
| Tc-99m Sestamibi | 740(370–1,110) | 20(10–30) | GB wall (resting subject) | 29 | 2.9 | ts 2.8 / ov 6.7 | ts 0.28 / ov 0.67 | 6.7 | 0.67 | 0.009 | 0.033 | ICRP Publication 128 |

*(Continued)*

**TABLE C-1  SUMMARY OF TYPICALLY ADMINISTERED ADULT DOSE; ORGAN RECEIVING THE HIGHEST RADIATION DOSE AND ITS DOSE; GONADAL DOSE; EFFECTIVE DOSE, AND EFFECTIVE DOSE PER ADMINISTERED ACTIVITY FOR FDA-APPROVED RADIOPHARMACEUTICALS** *(Continued)*

| RADIOPHARMACEUTICAL | TYPICAL ADULT ADMINISTERED ACTIVITY MBq | mCi | ORGAN RECEIVING HIGHEST DOSE | ORGAN DOSE mGy | rad | GONADAL DOSE mGy | | rad | EFFECTIVE DOSE mSv | rem | EFFECTIVE DOSE COEFFICIENT mSv/MBq | rem/mCi | SOURCE |
|---|---|---|---|---|---|---|---|---|---|---|---|---|---|
| Tc-99m Sodium Pertechnetate | 740(18.5–1,110) | 20(0.5–30) | Upper large intestine wall (IV admin/no blocking agent) | 41 | 4.1 | ts 2.1 | ov 7.3 | 0.21 0.73 | 9.6 | 0.96 | 0.013 | 0.048 | ICRP Publication 128 |
| Tc-99m Succimer (DMSA) | 148(72–222) | 4(2–6) | Kidneys | 27 | 2.7 | ts 0.27 | ov 0.52 | 0.027 0.052 | 1.3 | 0.13 | 0.0088 | 0.0326 | ICRP Publication 128 |
| Tc-99m Sulfur Colloid | 240(37–444) | 6.5(1–12) | Spleen (normal liver function) | 18 | 1.8 | ts 0.13 | ov 0.53 | 0.013 0.053 | 2.2 | 0.22 | 0.0091 | 0.034 | ICRP Publication 128 |
| Tc-99m Tetrofosmin (Myoview) | 740(185–1,221) | 20(5–33) | GB wall (resting subject) | 27 | 2.7 | ts 2.3 | ov 6.5 | 0.23 0.65 | 5.9 | 0.59 | 0.008 | 0.030 | ICRP Publication 128 |
| Tc-99m Tilmanocept (Lymphoseek) | 18.5 | 0.5 | Breast (injection site) (breast cancer) | 1.7 | 0.17 | ts 0.05 | ov 0.19 | 0.005 0.019 | 0.33 | 0.033 | 0.018 | 0.067 | PI |
| Tl-201 Chloride | 56(37–74) | 1.5(1–2) | Kidneys | 27 | 2.7 | ts 10 | ov 6.7 | 1.0 0.67 | 7.8 | 0.78 | 0.140 | 0.518 | ICRP Publication 128 |
| Xe-133 Gas | 740(370–1,110) | 20(10–30) | Lungs (single inhalation) | 0.61 | 0.061 | ts 0.070 | ov 0.074 | 0.007 0.007 | 0.13 | 0.013 | 0.00018 | 0.00067 | ICRP Publication 128 |
| Y-90 Chloride (used only for radiolabeling) | | | | | | | | | | | | | |
| Y-90 Ibritumomab Tiuxetan | 1,184 | 32 | Spleen | 11,130 | 1,113 | ts 1,776 | ov 474 | 178 47 | Not applicable | | | | PI |

Note: PI = Package Insert.

ICRP 128 = ICRP, 2015. Radiation Dose to Patients from Radiopharmaceuticals: A Compendium of Current Information Related to Frequently Used Substances. ICRP Publication 128. Ann. ICRP 44(2S).

ICRP 80 = ICRP, 1998. Radiation Dose to Patients from Radiopharmaceuticals (Addendum to ICRP Publication 53). ICRP Publication 80. Ann. ICRP 28 (3).

ICRP 53 = ICRP, 1988. Radiation Dose to Patients from Radiopharmaceuticals. ICRP Publication 53. Ann. ICRP 18 (1-4).

## TABLE C-2A EFFECTIVE DOSE PER UNIT ACTIVITY ADMINISTERED TO PEDIATRIC PATIENTS (1, 5, 10, AND 15 YEARS) FOR FDA-APPROVED RADIOPHARMACEUTICALS ▢ T. F-3A

| RADIOPHARMACEUTICAL | EFFECTIVE DOSE COEFFICIENT | | | | | | | | SOURCE |
| --- | --- | --- | --- | --- | --- | --- | --- | --- | --- |
| | 15-YEAR-OLD | | 10-YEAR-OLD | | 5-YEAR-OLD | | 1-YEAR-OLD | | |
| | mSv/MBq | rem/mCi | mSv/MBq | rem/mCi | mSv/MBq | rem/mCi | mSv/MBq | rem/mCi | |
| F-18 Fluorodeoxyglucose (FDG) | 0.024 | 0.089 | 0.037 | 0.137 | 0.056 | 0.207 | 0.095 | 0.352 | ICRP Publication 128 |
| Ga-67 Citrate | 0.130 | 0.481 | 0.200 | 0.740 | 0.330 | 1.221 | 0.640 | 2.368 | ICRP Publication 128 |
| In-111 Pentetate (DTPA) | 0.031 | 0.115 | 0.045 | 0.167 | 0.067 | 0.248 | 0.120 | 0.444 | ICRP Publication 53 |
| In-111 Pentetreotide (Octreoscan) | 0.071 | 0.263 | 0.100 | 0.370 | 0.160 | 0.592 | 0.280 | 1.036 | ICRP Publication 128 |
| I-123 Iobenguane (MIBG) | 0.017 | 0.063 | 0.026 | 0.096 | 0.037 | 0.137 | 0.068 | 0.252 | ICRP Publication 80 |
| I-123 Sodium Iodine Capsules | 0.350 | 1.295 | 0.520 | 1.924 | 1.100 | 4.070 | 2.100 | 7.770 | ICRP Publication 128 |
| I-131 Sodium Iodide | 35 | 130 | 53 | 196 | 110 | 407 | 180 | 666 | ICRP Publication 128 |
| Tc-99m Bicisate (ECD) | 0.010 | 0.037 | 0.015 | 0.056 | 0.022 | 0.081 | 0.040 | 0.148 | ICRP Publication 128 |
| Tc-99m Exametazime (HMPAO) | 0.011 | 0.041 | 0.017 | 0.063 | 0.027 | 0.100 | 0.049 | 0.181 | ICRP Publication 128 |
| Tc-99m MAA | 0.016 | 0.059 | 0.023 | 0.085 | 0.034 | 0.126 | 0.063 | 0.233 | ICRP Publication 128 |
| Tc-99m Mebrofenin (Choletec) | 0.020 | 0.074 | 0.027 | 0.100 | 0.043 | 0.159 | 0.100 | 0.370 | ICRP Publication 128 |
| Tc-99m Medronate (MDP) | 0.0057 | 0.021 | 0.0086 | 0.032 | 0.012 | 0.044 | 0.018 | 0.067 | ICRP Publication 128 |
| Tc-99m Mertiatide (MAG3) | 0.009 | 0.033 | 0.012 | 0.044 | 0.012 | 0.044 | 0.022 | 0.081 | ICRP Publication 128 |
| Tc-99m Pentetate (DTPA) | 0.0063 | 0.023 | 0.0094 | 0.035 | 0.012 | 0.044 | 0.016 | 0.059 | ICRP Publication 128 |
| Tc-99m Red Blood Cells (UltraTag) | 0.009 | 0.033 | 0.014 | 0.052 | 0.021 | 0.078 | 0.039 | 0.144 | ICRP Publication 128 |
| Tc-99m Sestamibi | 0.012 | 0.044 | 0.018 | 0.067 | 0.028 | 0.104 | 0.053 | 0.196 | ICRP Publication 128 |
| Tc-99m Sodium Pertechnetate | 0.017 | 0.0629 | 0.026 | 0.0962 | 0.042 | 0.1554 | 0.079 | 0.2923 | ICRP Publication 128 |
| Tc-99m Succimer (DMSA) | 0.011 | 0.041 | 0.015 | 0.056 | 0.021 | 0.078 | 0.037 | 0.137 | ICRP Publication 128 |
| Tc-99m Sulfur Colloid | 0.012 | 0.0444 | 0.018 | 0.0666 | 0.027 | 0.0999 | 0.049 | 0.1813 | ICRP Publication 128 |
| Tl-201 Chloride | 0.200 | 0.740 | 0.560 | 2.072 | 0.790 | 2.923 | 1.300 | 4.810 | ICRP Publication 128 |
| Xe-133 Gas | 0.00026 | 0.00096 | 0.00040 | 0.00148 | 0.00065 | 0.00241 | 0.00130 | 0.00481 | ICRP Publication 128 |

ICRP 128 = ICRP, 2015. Radiation Dose to Patients from Radiopharmaceuticals: A Compendium of Current Information Related to Frequently Used Substances. ICRP Publication 128. Ann. ICRP 44(2S).

ICRP 80 = ICRP, 1998. Radiation Dose to Patients from Radiopharmaceuticals (Addendum to ICRP Publication 53). ICRP Publication 80. Ann. ICRP 28 (3).

ICRP 53 = ICRP, 1988. Radiation Dose to Patients from Radiopharmaceuticals. ICRP Publication 53. Ann. ICRP 18 (1-4).

## TABLE C-2B NORTH AMERICAN CONSENSUS GUIDELINES FOR PEDIATRIC ADMINISTERED RADIOPHARMACEUTICAL ACTIVITIES—2016 UPDATE ▢ T. F-3B

| RADIOPHARMACEUTICAL | IMAGING TASK | NOTES | ADMINISTERED ACTIVITY (MBq/kg) | (mCi/kg) | MINIMUM (MBq) | (mCi) | MAXIMUM (MBq) | (mCi) |
|---|---|---|---|---|---|---|---|---|
| I-123 MIBG | Cancer detection | A | 5.2 | 0.14 | 37 | 1.0 | 370 | 10.0 |
| Tc-99m MDP | Bone imaging | A | 9.3 | | 37 | 1.0 | | |
| F-18 FDG | Body imaging | A, B | 3.7–5.2 | 0.10–0.14 | 26 | 0.7 | | |
| | Brain imaging | A, B | 3.7 | 0.10 | 14 | 0.37 | | |
| Tc-99m DMSA | Kidney function | A | 1.85 | 0.05 | 18.5 | 0.5 | 100 | 2.7 |
| Tc-99m MAG3 | Without flow study | A, C | 3.7 | 0.10 | 37 | 1.0 | 148 | 4.0 |
| | With flow study | A | 5.55 | 0.15 | | | | |
| Tc-99m IDA | Hepatobiliary Imaging | A, D | 1.85 | 0.05 | 18.5 | 0.5 | | |
| Tc-99 MAA | Ventilation study | A | 2.59 | 0.07 | | | | |
| | No ventilation study | A | 1.11 | 0.03 | 14.8 | 0.4 | | |
| Tc-99m Pertechnetate | Meckel diverticulum imaging | A | 1.85 | 0.05 | 9.25 | 0.25 | | |
| F-18 Sodium Fluoride | Bone imaging | A | 2.22 | 0.06 | 14 | 0.38 | | |
| Tc-99m Pertechnetate | Cystography | E | No weight-based dose | | 37 | 1.0 | 37 | 1.0 |
| Tc-99m Sulfur Colloid | Oral liquid gastric emptying | F | No weight-based dose | | 9.25 | 0.25 | 37 | 1.0 |
| Tc-99m Sulfur Colloid | Solid gastric emptying | F | No weight-based dose | | 9.25 | 0.25 | 18.5 | 0.5 |
| Tc-99m HMPAO (Ceretec) | Brain perfusion | | 11.1 | 0.3 | 185 | 5 | 740 | 20 |
| Tc-99m ECD (Neurolite) | Brain perfusion | | 11.1 | 0.3 | 185 | 5 | 740 | 20 |
| Tc-99m Sestamibi (Cardiolite) | Myocardial perfusion (single/first of two) | | 5.55 | 0.15 | 74 | 2 | 370 | 10 |
| Tc-99m Tetrofosmin (Myoview) | Myocardial perfusion (single/first of two) | | 5.55 | 0.15 | 74 | 2 | 370 | 10 |
| Tc-99m Sestamibi (Cardiolite) | Myocardial perfusion (second of two) | | 16.7 | 0.45 | 222 | 6 | 1,110 | 30 |
| Tc-99m Tetrofosmin (Myoview) | Myocardial perfusion (second of two) | | 16.7 | 0.45 | 222 | 6 | 1,110 | 30 |
| I-123 NaI | Thyroid imaging | | 0.28 | 0.0075 | 1 | 0.027 | 11 | 0.3 |
| Tc-99m Pertechnetate | Thyroid imaging | | 1.1 | 0.03 | 7 | 0.19 | 93 | 2.5 |
| Tc-99m RBC | Blood pool imaging | | 11.8 | 0.32 | 74 | 2 | 740 | 20 |

| | | | | | | | | |
|---|---|---|---|---|---|---|---|---|
| Tc-99m WBC | Infection imaging | | 7.4 | 0.2 | 74 | 2 | 555 | 15 |
| Ga-68 DOTATOC | Neuroendocrine tumor imaging | G | 2.7 | 0.074 | 14 | 0.38 | 185 | 5 |
| Ga-68 DOTATATE | Neuroendocrine tumor imaging | G | 2.7 | 0.074 | 14 | 0.38 | 185 | 5 |

*Notes:* This information is intended as a guideline only. Local practice may vary depending on patient population, choice of collimator, and specific requirements of clinical protocols. Administered activity may be adjusted when appropriate by order of the nuclear medicine practitioner. For patients who weigh 0.70 kg, it is recommended that the maximum administered activity not exceed the product of the patient's weight (kg) and the recommended weight-based administered activity. Some practitioners may choose to set a fixed maximum administered activity equal to 70 times the recommended weight-based administered activity, expressed as MBq/kg or mCi/kg (*e.g.*, less than 10 mCi [370 MBq] for 18F-FDG body imaging). The administered activities assume use of a low-energy high-resolution collimator for 99mTc radiopharmaceuticals and a medium-energy collimator for 123I-MIBG. Individual practitioners may use lower administered activities if their equipment or software permits them to do so. Higher administered activities may be required in selected patients. No recommended administered activity is given for intravenous 67Ga-citrate; intravenous 67Ga-citrate should be used very infrequently and only in low doses.

[A] The EANM Dosage Card 2014 version 2 administered activity may also be used.

[B] The low end of the dose range should be considered for smaller patients. Administered activity may take into account patient mass and time available on the PET scanner. The EANM Dosage Card 2014 version 2 administered activity may also be used.

[C] Administered activities assume that image data are reframed at 1 min/image. Administered activity may be reduced if image data are reframed at a longer time per image.

[D] A higher administered activity of 1 mCi may be considered for neonatal jaundice.

[E] 99mTc-sulfur colloid, 99mTc-pertechnetate, 99mTc-DTPA, or possibly other 99mTc radiopharmaceuticals may be used. There is a wide variety of acceptable administration and imaging techniques for 99mTc cystography, many of which will work well with lower administered activities. An example of appropriate lower administered activities is found in the 2014 revision of the EANM Paediatric Dose Card 2.

[F] The administered activity may be based on patient weight or on the age of the child.

[G] The administered activity is based on the EANM Dosage Card 2014 version 2 dosage for a 60-kg patient, using the minimum and maximum doses from the EANM Dosage Card. There was little experience with this radiopharmaceutical in children in North America at the time of preparation of this dosage table.

Note: Page numbers followed by f indicate figures; page numbers followed by t indicate tables